Textbook of
Critical Care Nutrition

Textbook of
Critical Care Nutrition

INDIAN SOCIETY FOR PARENTERAL & ENTERAL NUTRITION — ispen

Editors

Subhal Bhalchandra Dixit
MD (Medicine) FCCM FICCM FICP
Director
Department of Critical Care ICU
Sanjeevan and MJM Hospital
Pune, Maharashtra, India

Kapil Gangadhar Zirpe
MBBS MD (Chest) FICCM FCCM FSNCC
Head
Department of Neuro-Trauma Intensive Care Unit
Grant Medical Foundation
Ruby Hall Clinic
Pune, Maharashtra, India

Atul Prabhakar Kulkarni
MD (Anesthesiology) FISCCM PGDHHM FICCM
Professor and Head
Division of Critical Care Medicine
Department of Anesthesiology, Critical Care and Pain
Tata Memorial Hospital
Homi Bhabha National Institute
Mumbai, Maharashtra, India

Associate Editors

B Ravinder Reddy
MBBS MS FRCS (Edinburgh) FRCS (Glasgow)
Consultant Surgeon
Division of Surgical Gastroenterology
and General Surgery
CARE Hospital Hyderabad, Telangana, India
President, Indian Society for Parenteral and
Enteral Nutrition (ISPEN)

Khalid Ismail Khatib
MD (Medicine) FICCM FICP
Professor
Department of Medicine
Smt Kashibai Navale Medical College
Pune, Maharashtra, India

Forewords
Jean-Louis Vincent
Varsha T

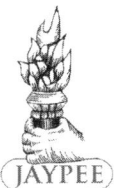

JAYPEE BROTHERS MEDICAL PUBLISHERS
The Health Sciences Publisher
New Delhi | London

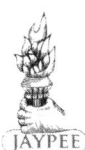

Jaypee Brothers Medical Publishers (P) Ltd

Headquarters

EMCA House
23/23-B, Ansari Road, Daryaganj
New Delhi 110 002, India
Landline: +91-11-23272143, +91-11-23272703
+91-11-23282021, +91-11-23245672
E-mail: jaypee@jaypeebrothers.com

Overseas Office

JP Medical Ltd.
83, Victoria Street, London
SW1H 0HW (UK)
Phone: +44-20 3170 8910
E-mail: info@jpmedpub.com

Corporate Office

Jaypee Brothers Medical Publishers (P) Ltd.
4838/24, Ansari Road, Daryaganj
New Delhi 110 002, India
Phone: +91-11-43574357
Fax: +91-11-43574314
E-mail: jaypee@jaypeebrothers.com

EU GPSR Authorised Representative
Logos Europe, 9 rue Nicolas Poussin 17000,
La Rochelle, France
Phone: +33 (0) 6 67 93 73 78
E-mail: Contact@logoseurope.eu

Website: www.jaypeebrothers.com
Website: www.jaypeedigital.com

© 2024, Jaypee Brothers Medical Publishers

The views and opinions expressed in this book are solely those of the original contributor(s)/author(s) and do not necessarily represent those of editor(s) or publisher of the book.

All rights reserved. No part of this publication may be reproduced, stored or transmitted in any form or by any means, electronic, mechanical, photocopying, recording or otherwise, without the prior permission in writing of the publishers.

All brand names and product names used in this book are trade names, service marks, trademarks or registered trademarks of their respective owners. The publisher is not associated with any product or vendor mentioned in this book.

Medical knowledge and practice change constantly. This book is designed to provide accurate, authoritative information about the subject matter in question. However, readers are advised to check the most current information available on procedures included and check information from the manufacturer of each product to be administered, to verify the recommended dose, formula, method and duration of administration, adverse effects and contraindications. It is the responsibility of the practitioner to take all appropriate safety precautions. Neither the publisher nor the author(s)/editor(s) assume any liability for any injury and/or damage to persons or property arising from or related to use of material in this book.

This book is sold on the understanding that the publisher is not engaged in providing professional medical services. If such advice or services are required, the services of a competent medical professional should be sought.

Every effort has been made where necessary to contact holders of copyright to obtain permission to reproduce copyright material. If any have been inadvertently overlooked, the publisher will be pleased to make the necessary arrangements at the first opportunity.

Inquiries for bulk sales may be solicited at: jaypee@jaypeebrothers.com

Textbook of Critical Care Nutrition

First Edition: 2024, Reprint: **2025**

ISBN: 978-93-5696-315-3

Printed in India

Dedication

*Managing critically ill patients present a formidable encounter.
Each and every patient presents with a unique set of pathological issues, degrees of immune responses and various grades of organ dysfunctions, and necessitating distinctly specific interventions. However, nutritional interventions form the common denominator in each and every patient with critical illness, which plays a pivotal role in achieving a positive clinical outcome. Hence, this book is dedicated to all the critically ill patients who have enabled the evolution of safe nutritional interventions in the critically ill.*

About the Associate Editors

B Ravinder Reddy MBBS MS FRCS (Edinburgh) FRCS (Glasgow) is a Consultant Surgeon, Division of Surgical Gastroenterology and General Surgery, CARE Hospital, Hyderabad, Telangana, India, with special interest in surgery in the critically ill patients, nutrition support in gastrointestinal failure, wound healing and the evolving role of gut microbiota in health and disease. He is the President of Indian Society for Parenteral and Enteral Nutrition (ISPEN). He is the Panel Member of World Health Organizations (WHO) guidelines for "Nutrition Support in Hospitalized Patients in South-East Asia Region (SEAR)". He has authored of multiple book chapters and publications in peer-reviewed national and international journals. He is invited faculty to multiple academic societies in India, Asia, Europe, USA and South America.

Khalid Ismail Khatib MD (Medicine) FICCM FICP is currently working as Professor in the Department of Medicine, Smt Kashibai Navale Medical College, Pune, Maharashtra, India. He has shown keen interest in research and has published more than 40 original articles in national and international journals. He has participated as a speaker in many national and international conferences and won awards in conferences.

Contributors

Adarsh Chaudhary MS FRCS
Chairperson and Head
Department of GI Surgery, GI Oncology
and Minimal Access Surgery
Medanta—The Medicity
Gurugram, Haryana, India

Amit Goyal MBBS DNB PDCC EDIC
Principal Consultant
Department of Critical Care
Max Super Speciality Hospital
New Delhi, India

Anjali Mishra DNB FNB
Consultant
Department of Critical Care Medicine
Holy Family Hospital
New Delhi, India

Anshu Joshi MBBS DCH
Consultant Pediatrician
Department of Pediatrics
Joshi Children Clinic
Chittorgarh, Rajasthan, India

Anuja Phalle MSc (Clinical Nutrition and Dietetics)
Junior Research Fellow and PhD Scholar
Department of Nutrition and Dietetics
Symbiosis Institute of Health Sciences
Symbiosis International University
Pune, Maharashtra, India

Anna Ferreira MD
FELANPE- Federación Latinoamericana
de Terapia Nutricional, Nutrición Clínica y
Metabolismo A.C.
Asunción, Paraguay

Arijit Sardar MD DM
Consultant
Department of Critical Care Medicine
BLK-Max Superspeciality Hospital
New Delhi, India

Arti Bhalerao MSc (Food Science and Nutrition)
Registered Dietician
Certified Nutrigenomics Counselor
Head Dietician
Symbiosis University Hospital and
Research Centre
Symbiosis International University
Pune IDA—Life Member
Symbiosis University Hospital and Research Centre
Symbiosis International (Deemed) University
Pune, Maharashtra, India

Arun Kumar MBBS MD (DrNB)
Registrar (Academic)
Department of Critical Care Medicine
Virinchi Hospital
Hyderabad, Telangana, India

Atul Prabhakar Kulkarni
MD (Anesthesiology) FISCCM PGDHHM FICCM
Professor and Head
Division of Critical Care Medicine
Department of Anesthesiology, Critical Care
and Pain
Tata Memorial Hospital
Homi Bhabha National Institute
Mumbai, Maharashtra, India

B Ravinder Reddy
MBBS MS FRCS (Edinburgh) FRCS (Glasgow)
Consultant Surgeon
Division of Surgical Gastroenterology and
General Surgery
CARE Hospital
Hyderabad, Telangana, India

Balguri Mukesh Kumar
MBBS MD (Anesthesia) FNB (Critical Care) EDIC
Consultant
Department of Critical Care Medicine
CARE Hospital
Hyderabad, Telangana, India

Bamini Arthi G Murugesh MSc RD
Vice President
Nutrition Support Service
Sundaram Medical Foundation
Dr Rangarajan Memorial Hospital
Chennai, Tamil Nadu, India

Barkha Bindu
MBBS MD DNB DM
Consultant
Department of Neuroanesthesiology and
Neurocritical Care
Paras Hospital
Gurugram, Haryana, India

Bharat Jagiasi MD IDCCM FICCM
Director
Department of Critical Care
Kokilaben Dhirubhai Ambani Hospital
Navi Mumbai, Maharashtra, India

Chen Liu MBChB
PhD Candidate
Department of Surgery
Faculty of Medical and Health Sciences
University of Auckland
Grafton, Auckland, New Zealand

Chitra Mahesh MSc RD CNSD
Consultant Dietitian
Department of Clinical Nutrition
Meenakshi Multispeciality Hospital
Chennai, Tamil Nadu, India

Chitra Mehta MD
Director
Department of Cardiac Anesthesia and
Critical Care
Medanta Institute of Critical Care and
Anesthesiology
Medanta—The Medicity
Gurugram, Haryana, India

Daphnee Lovesley PhD RD
Chief Clinical Dietitian
Department of Dietetics
Apollo Main Hospital
Chennai, Tamil Nadu, India

Dedeepiya Devaprasad
MD DNB EDIC FICCM
Lead Consultant
Department of Critical Care
Apollo Speciality Hospital/Apollo Cancer Institute
Chennai, Tamil Nadu, India

Deeksha Kapoor
MBBS DNB (General Surgery)
DNB (Surgical Gastroenterology)
Consultant
Departments of GI Surgery, GI Oncology
and Minimal Access Surgery
Medanta—The Medicity
Gurugram, Haryana, India

Deven Juneja DNB FNB EDIC FICCM
Director
Institute of Critical Care Medicine
Max Super Specialty Hospital, New Delhi
ICU, Max Super Specialty Hospital
New Delhi, India

Dhruva Chaudhry
MD (Medicine) DNB (Medicine) DM (PCCM) FAMS FICCM
Senior Professor and Head
Department of Pulmonary and
Critical Care Medicine
Pt BD Sharma Post Graduate Institute of
Medical Sciences
Rohtak, Haryana, India

Durval Ribas Filho MD
ABRAN - Associação Brasileira de Nutrologia/
Brazilian Association of Nutrology
Catanduva, Sao Paulo, Brazil

Emma Ludlow Master of Nursing
Clinical Nurse Specialist
Department of Surgery
University of Auckland
Auckland, New Zealand

Ganshyam Jagathkar MD FNB FICCM
Director
Department of Critical Care
Medicover Hospital
Hyderabad, Telangana, India

Gil Hardy PhD FRSC FASPEN
Director
Department of Research, Ipanema Trust
Auckland, New Zealand

Gunadhar Padhi
MBBS MD IDCCM FCCCM FIMSA Diploma in ECMO
Senior Consultant
Department of Critical Care Medicine
Apollo Hospital
Navi Mumbai, Maharashtra, India

Hemanshu Prabhakar MD PhD FSNCC (Hon)
Professor
Department of Neuroanesthesiology
and Critical Care
All India Institute of Medical Sciences
New Delhi, India

Ian Bissett MBChB FRACS MD
Professor
Department of Surgery
University of Auckland
Auckland, New Zealand

Idiberto José MD
ABRAN - Associação Brasileira de Nutrologia/
Brazilian Association of Nutrology
Catanduva, Sao Paulo, Brazil

Indu Kapoor MD (Anesthesia)
Additional Professor
Department of Neuroanesthesiology
and Critical Care
All India Institute of Medical Sciences
New Delhi, India

Jagadeesh KN MBBS MD
Associate Consultant, Liver transplant
and GI Critical Care
Department of Critical Care
Medanta—The Medicity
Gurugram, Haryana, India

Kapil Gangadhar Zirpe
MBBS MD (Chest) FICCM FCCM FSNCC
Head
Department of Neuro-Trauma Intensive Care Unit
Grant Medical Foundation, Ruby Hall Clinic
Pune, Maharashtra, India

Keerti Brar MBBS DA IDCCM IFCCM
Attending Consultant
Department of Critical Care
Medanta—The Medicity
Gurugram, Haryana, India

Khalid Ismail Khatib
MD (Medicine) FICCM FICP
Professor
Department of Medicine
Smt Kashibai Navale Medical College
Pune, Maharashtra, India

Khusrav Bajan MD EDIC
Consultant Physician and Intensivist
Department of Medicine and Critical Care
PD Hinduja Hospital
Mumbai, Maharashtra, India

Kirandeep Kaur
MBBS MD (Pharmacology)
Professor
Department of Pharmacology
Dayanand Medical College and Hospital
Ludhiana, Punjab, India

Krishnan Sriram MBBS FRCS(C) FCCM FACS
Intensivist
US Department of Veterans Affairs
Tele-Critical Care West
Chicago, USA

Mahesh Kota
MBBS MD (General Medicine) IDCCM DrNB (Nephrology)
Consultant Nephrologist
Department of Nephrology and Critical Care
Yashoda Hospitals
Hyderabad, Telangana, India

Mahesha P MD FNB EDIC
Consultant Intensivist
Department of Critical Care Medicine
Manipal Hospital
Bengaluru, Karnataka, India

Malissa Warren RD CNSD
Chief Dietician
Department of Surgery
Oregon Health and Science University
Portland, Oregon, USA

Masood Ahmed Chandsha
MBBS MD DrNB (Critical Care Medicine)
Consultant
Department of Critical Care Medicine
HCG-KLE Suchirayu Hospital
Hubballi, Karnataka, India

Nagarajan Ramakrishnan
Diplomate American Board (Internal Medicine and Critical Care) FACP FCCP FCCM FAASM FICCM
Senior Consultant
Department of Critical Care
Director, Critical Care Services
Apollo Hospitals
Chennai, Tamil Nadu, India

Nishanth Aasuri MBBS
Medical Student
Georgia, Ljubljana

PC Gupta MS
Clinical Director and Head
Department of Vascular and Endovascular Surgery
CARE Hospital
Hyderabad, Telangana, India

Penmetsa Vijay Varma
MBBS MD (General Medicine) IDCCM DrNB (Nephrology)
Consultant Nephrologist
Department of Nephrology and Critical Care
Yashoda Hospitals
Hyderabad, Telangana, India

Pooja Tyagi MBBS MD (Anesthesia) FNB
Associate Consultant
Department of Critical Care Medicine
Medanta Institute of Critical Care and Anesthesiology
Medanta—The Medicity
Gurugram, Haryana, India

Priya Mistry MRPharmS
Consultant
Lead Pharmacist
Department of Nutrition Support and Intestinal Failure
University Hospital Southampton NHS Foundation Trust
Southampton, SO16 6YD

Priya Sonavdekar MBBS MHA
ICU Registrar
Kokilaben Dhirubhai Ambani Hospital
Navi Mumbai, Maharashtra, India

Radha Reddy Chada PhD RD
Chief Clinical Dietitian and Head
Department of Clinical Nutrition and Dietetics
AIG Hospitals
Hyderabad, Telangana, India

Rahul Harne MBBS MD
Consultant, Liver Transplant and GI Critical Care
Department of Critical Care
Medanta—The Medicity
Gurugram, Haryana, India

Rajasekara Chakravarthi
MBBS MD (General Medicine) DrNB (Nephrology)
Director and Head
Department of Nephrology
Yashoda Hospital
Hyderabad, Telangana, India

Rajesh Pande MD PDCC FICCM FCCM
Principal Director and Head
Department of Critical care
BLK-Max Centre of Excellence for Critical Care
BLK-Max Superspeciality Hospital
New Delhi, India

Ranil Jayawardena MBBS MSc PhD RNutr
Professor in Nutrition
Department of Physiology, Faculty of Medicine
University of Colombo
Colombo, Sri Lanka

Ritu Sudhakar BSc MSc (Foods & Nutrition) RD CDE
Chief Dietician
Department of Dietetics
Dayanand Medical College and Hospital
Ludhiana, Punjab, India

Robert Martindale MD PhD FASPEN
Professor
Division of Gastrointestinal and General Surgery
Department of Surgery
Medical Director, Hospital Nutrition Services
Oregon Health and Science University
Portland, OR, USA

Sadanand Kulkarni MBBS MD (Clinical Microbiology)
Vice President
Department of Medical Affairs
and Clinical Research
Fresenius Kabi India Pvt Ltd
Pune, Maharashtra, India

Sanjith Saseedharan
DA (Univ) DA (CPS) IDCCM EDIC FNNCC FIMSA
Teacher and Head
Department of Critical Care
SL Raheja Hospital—A Fortis Associate
Mumbai, Maharashtra, India

Sarah Warren MD
Research Assistant
Department of Surgery
Oregon Health and Science University
Portland, Oregon, USA

Shradha K Bajan MBBS
Resident
Department of Pulmonary Medicine
DY Patil University
Navi Mumbai, Maharashtra, India

Shweta Ram Chandankhede
MBBS MD IDCCM IFCCM HCM-ISB
Senior Consultant
Department of Critical Care Medicine
CARE Hospital
Hyderabad, Telangana, India

Shweta Suri Kandpal MBBS MD (Anesthesia)
Fellowship in Indian Association in Cardiac Anesthesiologist
Consultant
Department of Cardiac Anesthesia
Medanta Institute of Critical Care and Anesthesiology
Medanta—The Medicity Gurugram, Haryana, India

Sónia Maria Cabral RD
Dietitian
Department of Clinical Nutrition—Oncology,
Surgery and ICU
Nutritional Sciences of the University of Porto,
Porto, Nutritionist
Instituto Português de Oncologia do Porto,
Francisco Gentil, EPE
Porto, Portugal

Srinivas Samavedam
MD DNB FRCP FNB EDIC FICCM DMLE MBA
Head and Medical Director
Department of Critical Care
Virinchi Hospital
Hyderabad, Telangana, India

Subhal Bhalchandra Dixit
MD (Medicine) FCCM FICCM FICP
Director
Department of Critical Care ICU
Sanjeevan and MJM Hospital
Pune, Maharashtra, India

Subhankar Paul DNB Fellow
Associate Consultant
Department of Critical Care
BLK-Max Centre for Critical Care
BLK-Max Superspeciality Hospital
New Delhi, India

Sunil Honkalas
MBBS MD (Pharmacology)
Manager, Medical Affairs
and Clinical Research
Fresenius Kabi India Pvt Ltd
Pune, Maharashtra, India

Sunil Karanth
MD (Internal Medicine) FNB EDIC FCICM
Chairman, Head and Consultant
Department of Critical Care Medicine
Manipal Hospitals
Bengaluru, Karnataka, India

Sunil T Pandya
MD PDCC (Neuro-Anesthesia) (SCTIMST, Trivandrum)
Post-Doctoral Fellowship-Obstetric
Chief
Department of Anesthesia
Perioperative Medicine and Critical Care
AIG Hospitals, Hyderabad
Consultant
Department of Anesthesia and
Obstetric Critical Care
Fernandez Hospitals, Hyderabad
Director
PACCS Health Care Pvt Ltd
Hyderabad, Telangana, India

Sweta J Patel MBBS DA IDCCM
Senior Consultant
Department of Critical Care Medicine
Medanta Institute of Critical Care and
Anesthesiology
Medanta—The Medicity
Gurugram, Haryana, India

T Mohan S Maharaj
MBBS MD PDCC IDCCM MBA
Director and Head
Department of Critical Care
Medicover Hospital
Visakhapatnam, Andhra Pradesh, India

Urvi Shukla
MD DNB (Anesthesia) MRCA EDIC FICCM
Head
Department of Intensive Care Unit
Symbiosis University Hospital and
Research Centre
Symbiosis International University
Pune, Maharashtra, India

Vanessa Fuchs-Tarlovsky MD PhD RD
Head and Founder
Clinical Nutrition Service and Researcher
Department of Clinical Nutrition in Oncology
Hospital General de México
Parque de los Pirineos #16
Colonia: Parques de la Herradura
CP: 52786
Huixquilucan, Estado de México, Mexico

Varalakshmi Diwakarla
MBBS DA DNB IDCCM EDIC DM
Consultant
Department of Critical Care
Pinnacle Hospital
Visakhapatnam, Andhra Pradesh, India

Varsha M Asrani PhD
Intensivist
Department of Surgery
Surgical and Translational Research (STaR) Centre
School of Medicine, Faculty of Medical and
Health Sciences
University of Auckland
Auckland, New Zealand

Vineela Surapaneni DM
Fellow
Department of Pulmonary and Critical Care Medicine
Pt BD Sharma Post Graduate Institute of Medical
Sciences
Rohtak, Haryana, India

Viswanath Atreyapurapu DrNB (Vascular Surgery)
Consultant
Department of Vascular and Endovascular Surgery
CARE Hospital
Hyderabad, Telangana, India

William Manzanares MD PhD
Full Professor of Intensive Care
Department of Critical Care
Faculty of Medicine
Universidad de la República (UdelaR)
Montevideo, Uruguay

Yatin Mehta MD FRCA MNAMS
Chairman
Department of Cardiac Anesthesia and Critical Care
Institute of Critical Care and Anesthesia
Medanta—The Medicity
Gurugram, Haryana, India

Zotarelli Filho MD
ABRAN - Associação Brasileira de Nutrologia/
Brazilian Association of Nutrology
Catanduva, Sao Paulo, Brazil

Foreword

Of the many forms of organ support used in intensive care, nutrition has frequently been overlooked or considered less urgent. Yet optimal nutrition is essential to ensure the best possible outcome for critically ill patients. Indeed, the crucial role of nutrition in the pathophysiology and management of critical illness has been increasingly highlighted in recent years. A quick search of PubMed indicates an exponential increase in the number of publications on "critical illness" and "nutrition" over the past 3 decades, from just 8 in 1990 to 381 in 2022. These studies have tried to answer questions related to how much, which route, when to start, which components, among others, and have emphasized the need to individualize nutrition. This is a complex area of critical care medicine and it is important to keep up to date with the latest knowledge and expert opinion in the field. This Textbook is therefore highly topical and relevant. Divided into seven clear sections, it provides a comprehensive overview of this multifaceted topic. The first section reviews the role of nutrition and metabolism in the pathophysiology of critical illness and the different techniques to assess nutritional status. Sections 2 to 4 cover the nutritional requirements in critically ill patients and the place of enteral and parenteral nutrition. In sections 5 and 6, optimal nutrition in specific groups of critically ill patients, including those with burns, pancreatitis or renal failure, the obese, and pregnant women is considered, as well as problems associated with overfeeding, and the impact of nutrition on the gut microbiome. The final section includes chapters on nutritional support teams and the cost-effectiveness of intensive care nutrition. Endorsed by ISPEN (Indian Society for Parenteral and Enteral Nutrition) and written by an international faculty, but targeted at the Indian subcontinent, this textbook will provide a solid ground in nutrition knowledge for those involved in the daily management of critically ill patients. I commend the Editors, Dr Subhal Bhalchandra Dixit, Dr Kapil Gangadhar Zirpe, and Dr Atul Prabhakar Kulkarni, and Associate Editors, Dr B Ravinder Reddy and Dr Khalid Ismail Khatib, for their effort drawing together this impressive volume.

Jean-Louis Vincent MD PhD
Professor
Department of Intensive Care Medicine
Université Libre de Bruxelles, Brussels, Belgium
Consultant, Department of Intensive Care
Erasme University Hospital, Brussels, Belgium

Foreword

Indian Society for Parenteral and Enteral Nutrition (ISPEN), a very unique society consisting of Clinical Nutritionists/Dietitians, Doctors, Nurses, Pharmacists, and nutraceutical industry formed with the express intent to promote Clinical Nutrition in Hospitals has been striving for a score and 10 years, since its inception in 1994, to encourage research, education and the exchange of information in the field of Clinical Nutrition, specifically enteral and parenteral nutritional support to improve the quality of patient care.

In keeping with its object to encourage exchange of information and research, besides hosting 17 Annual conferences, ISPEN collaborated for the Joint Annual Conference with Indian Society of Critical Care Medicine—ISCCM in 1996, hosted PENSA (Parenteral and Enteral Nutrition Society of Asia) International conferences in Goa, 2003 and Hyderabad, 2022 and NUTRIFE[A]ST 2008 with Nutrition Society of India and Indian Dietetic Association.

ISPEN spearheaded "The Technical Consultation on Hospital Nutrition Practices in South-East Asia", New Delhi, India, 2010 that addressed the present status of hospital nutrition support services in the Region and the bottlenecks preventing improvements. The panel also discussed the development of a roadmap towards improved protocols and appropriate interventions and World Health Organization Report—2012 presented the deliberations and recommendation of the consultation.

ISPEN is now once more charting a historic collaboration with ISCCM *"Textbook of Critical Care Nutrition."* Critical Care Nutrition is the provision of safe and optimal nutrition to patients who have life-threatening injuries and illnesses and admitted to the intensive care unit (ICU), using evidence-based practice wherein early nutrition therapy is documented to decrease disease severity, decrease complications, reduce length of stay in the ICU and decrease mortality. *This exhaustive compilation of seven sections ranging from basic concepts; planning and nutritional interventions; enteral and parenteral nutrition in critical illness; nutrition in specific situations and special issues in critical illness; as well as organization of Nutritional Support Teams by eighty-one contributors, is a laudable attempt that truly captures the expertise and experience of clinical nutritionist/dietitians as well as critical care physicians as adapted to Indian Practice Scenario.*

Being associated and actively involved with ISPEN right from its inception, throughout its 29 years of existence and having both nurtured and served the organization in various capacities as Project Coordinator, Joint Secretary, Secretary, President (2005–2021) and presently its Immediate Past President, I am convinced under the tutelage of Dr Ravinder Reddy, Present President, it will not be a flash in the pan, but a sustained collaboration that shall grow from strength to strength and will have several new updated versions in the years to come.

Congratulations to both ISPEN and ISCCM for this stupendous effort. Best wishes to the future leadership of ISPEN that will continue formulating and publishing India specific practice guidelines not only for Critical Care but both preventive and effective management of Malnutrition in hospitals and in Day Care Patient Populace.

Varsha T MSc PhD RD CCN CNIS
Founder Chair and Managing Trustee
Indian Institute of Nutritional Sciences (IINS)
Professor and Course Co-ordinator
BSc (Clinical Nutrition)
Institute of Diabetology
Madras Medical College
Chennai, Tamil Nadu, India
President
International Affiliate of the Academy of
Nutrition and Dietetics (IAAND), USA
Adjunct Professor
Nutritional Sciences Division of
the Institute of Human Nutrition and Food
College of Human Ecology
University of the Philippines in
Los Baños (IHNF-CHE, UPLB)
Laguna, Philippines
Past President, ISPEN

Preface

Working on this *Textbook of Critical Care Nutrition* was a great experience and was more Rewarding than I could have ever imagined.

I must start by appreciating my awesome, supportive Editor colleagues Dr Atul Prabhakar Kulkarni, Dr Kapil Gangadhar Zirpe, and Associate Editors Dr B Ravinder Reddy and Dr Khalid Ismail Khatib for guiding and giving me proper advice and support at every stage of the planning of this book. Thank you, Friends.

A special "Thank you" to Dr B Ravinder Reddy for his timely suggestions and endorsing this book as the President of the Indian Society for Parenteral and Enteral Nutrition (ISPEN).

On behalf of the Editorial Board, I sincerely appreciate the contribution of each and every author, both national and international levels for timely completion their chapters and writing them with immense precision. Everyone's contribution has added more credibility to this *Textbook of Critical Care Nutrition* which we all are sure will be helpful to all students and consultants.

I thank for your continued trust on us and look forward for your support to work on future endeavors.

I appreciate the contribution of M/s Jaypee Brothers Medical Publishers (P) Ltd, New Delhi, India, for tireless follow-up and finishing the book within the timeline.

Subhal Bhalchandra Dixit

Acknowledgments

Thanks to all the authors who have contributed immensely and spent hours to pen down the latest, evidence-based literature in the field of nutritional interventions in critical illnesses.

We are indebted to all the Editors, Dr Kapil Gangadhar Zirpe and Dr Atul Prabhakar Kulkarni, and Associate Editors Dr B Ravinder Reddy and Dr Khalid Ismail Khatib, for reading the manuscripts, and for the valuable suggestions.

Special thanks to Dr B Ravinder Reddy, President of Indian Society for Parenteral and Enteral Nutrition (ISPEN), for endorsing this substantially comprehensive *Textbook of Critical Care Nutrition*.

And finally, our gratitude to Shri Jitendar P Vij (Group Chairman), Mr Ankit Vij (Managing Director), Ms Chetna Malhotra (Senior Director—Professional Publishing, Marketing and Business Development), Ms Manpreet Kaur (Development Editor) and all the other team members of M/s Jaypee Brothers Medical Publishers (P) Ltd, New Delhi, India, for trusting and supporting us in the publication of this book.

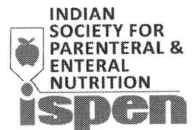

ISPEN Endorsement Letter

Nutrient intake plays a key role, beginning from the time of conception, subsequent progress, growth, development and in the maintenance of optimal health. Furthermore, nutritional status of an individual is a crucial factor in determining the consequence of various disease-states. This is even more important in all of the critically ill patients, who are potentially at a risk of developing nutrient-related deficiencies, which undoubtedly have an impact on recovery and clinical outcomes.

Indian Society for Parenteral and Enteral Nutrition—ISPEN (https://ispen.org.in) is involved in academic, education and training of healthcare professionals in the *"art and science"* of artificial nutrition, since its inception in 1994. It provides evidence-based direction, guidelines, consensus recommendations and state-of-art bedside guidance and safe clinical practice points for various enteral and parenteral nutritional interventions. ISPEN, in academic partnership with the Indian Society of Critical Care Medicine—ISCCM, has been closely associated with the origination of various chapters and their content, as well as author selection of this comprehensive textbook, devoted to various aspects of nutritional support in various acute conditions and critical illnesses.

On behalf of the Members and Executive Committee of ISPEN, it indeed is a pleasure to endorse this *Textbook of Critical Care Nutrition*, being published by M/s Jaypee Brothers Publishers (P) Ltd, New Delhi, India.

B Ravinder Reddy
President—ISPEN

Contents

SECTION 1: Basic Concepts

1. **Pathophysiology of Critical Illness** 3
   Gunadhar Padhi, Masood Ahmed Chandsha
2. **Nutrient Metabolism in Critical Illness** 14
   Dedeepiya Devaprasad, Krishnan Sriram, Nagarajan Ramakrishnan
3. **Immune Responses and Immunometabolism: An Overview** 21
   B Ravinder Reddy
4. **Malnutrition and Body Composition Assessment in Critical Illness** 32
   Radha Reddy Chada
5. **Nutritional Assessment in Critical Illness** 41
   Daphnee Lovesley
6. **Nutrition in Inflammatory Bowel Disease** 58
   Ritu Sudhakar, Kirandeep Kaur

SECTION 2: Planning and Nutritional Interventions

7. **Indirect Calorimetry in Critical Illness** 91
   Sanjith Saseedharan
8. **Macronutrients in Critical Illness: Nutrition Backbones for Survival and Recovery!** 98
   Varsha M Asrani
9. **Micronutrient Physiology and Requirements in Critical Illness** 112
   Ranil Jayawardena
10. **Probiotics, Prebiotics, Synbiotics, and Postbiotics** 118
    B Ravinder Reddy
11. **Mechanical and Metabolic Complications of Parenteral Nutrition** 124
    Subhankar Paul, Rajesh Pande

SECTION 3: Enteral Nutrition in Critical Illness

12. **Enteral Nutrition in Critical Illness: Physiological Benefits and Beyond** 137
    Krishnan Sriram, Chitra Mahesh
13. **Gastrointestinal Disturbances in Critically Ill Patients** 146
    Ganshyam Jagathkar, Radha Reddy Chada
14. **Enteral Access: Device and Selection** 155
    Srinivas Samavedam, Arun Kumar

15. **Initiation, Maintenance, and Progression of Enteral Feeds** 161
    Urvi Shukla, Arti Bhalerao, Anuja Phalle
16. **Monitoring and Management of Complications of Enteral Nutrition** 171
    Deven Juneja, Anjali Mishra

SECTION 4: Parenteral Nutrition in Critical Illness

17. **Parenteral Nutrition: Indications and Formulations** 187
    Arijit Sardar, Rajesh Pande
18. **Intravenous Access for Parenteral Nutrition** 191
    Viswanath Atreyapurapu, PC Gupta
19. **Safe Practices in Parenteral Nutrition Therapy** 198
    Priya Mistry, Gil Hardy
20. **Nutrient–Drug: Interactions and Compatibility** 210
    T Mohan S Maharaj, Varalakshmi Diwakarla
21. **Fluid and Electrolytes in Critical Illness** 227
    Bharat Jagiasi, Priya Sonavdekar

SECTION 5: Nutrition in Specific Situations

22. **Nutrition in Medical ICU Patients** 245
    Chitra Mehta, Yatin Mehta
23. **Nutrition in Pediatric ICUs** 252
    Anshu Joshi
24. **Nutritional Therapy in the Perioperative Period** 258
    Robert Martindale, Sarah Warren, Malissa Warren
25. **Nutrition in Cardiac and Cardiothoracic Intensive Care** 268
    Shweta Suri Kandpal
26. **Clinical Nutrition in Oncology** 281
    Vanessa Fuchs-Tarlovsky
27. **Nutrition in Severe Acute Pancreatitis** 301
    Deeksha Kapoor, Adarsh Chaudhary
28. **Nutrition in Short Bowel Syndrome and Enterocutaneous Fistulas** 313
    Gil Hardy, Chen Liu, Emma Ludlow, Ian Bissett
29. **Nutrition in Critically Ill Patients with Renal Failure** 322
    Penmetsa Vijay Varma, Rajasekara Chakravarthi, Mahesh Kota
30. **Nutrition in Critically Ill Patients with Respiratory Failure** 327
    Dhruva Chaudhry, Vineela Surapaneni
31. **Nutrition in the Critical Patient with Obesity** 334
    Anna Ferreira, Idiberto José, Zotarelli Filho, Durval Ribas Filho

32. Nutrition in Critically Ill Patients with Liver Dysfunction and Failure 342
    Keerti Brar, Rahul Harne, Sweta J Patel
33. Nutrition in Major Trauma and Burns 348
    Khusrav Bajan, Shradha K Bajan
34. Nutrition in Neurology and Neurosurgical Patients 360
    Barkha Bindu, Amit Goyal, Indu Kapoor, Hemanshu Prabhakar
35. Nutrition in Solid Organ Transplantation and Immunocompromised Patients 376
    Pooja Tyagi, Sweta J Patel, Jagadeesh KN
36. Nutritional Support in a Critically Ill Parturient 390
    Sunil T Pandya, Nishanth Aasuri

SECTION 6: Special Issues in Critical Illness

37. Immunonutrition in the Critically Ill 401
    William Manzanares, Gil Hardy
38. Dysglycemia in Critical Illness 413
    Shweta Ram Chandankhede, Balguri Mukesh Kumar
39. Refeeding Syndrome in Critically Ill Adults: Preemptive Strategies 425
    Krishnan Sriram, Chitra Mahesh
40. Nutrition in Severe Hemodynamic Failure and in Noninvasive Ventilation 436
    Khalid Ismail Khatib, Subhal Bhalchandra Dixit
41. Gut Microbiome in Critical Illness 440
    B Ravinder Reddy
42. Evaluation of Sarcopenia in Critical Illness 447
    Deeksha Kapoor
43. Feeding Options in Patients with Intra-abdominal Hypertension 456
    Sunil Karanth, Mahesha P
44. Nutrition and Wound Healing 459
    Sónia Maria Cabral

SECTION 7: Organization of Nutritional Support Teams

45. Nutrition Support Team 471
    Bamini Arthi G Murugesh
46. Is it Cost-effective to Feed Critically Ill Patients? 477
    Sadanand Kulkarni, Sunil Honkalas

Index *485*

SECTION 1: Basic Concepts

1. **Pathophysiology of Critical Illness**
   Gunadhar Padhi, Masood Ahmed Chandsha

2. **Nutrient Metabolism in Critical Illness**
   Dedeepiya Devaprasad, Krishnan Sriram, Nagarajan Ramakrishnan

3. **Immune Responses and Immunometabolism: An Overview**
   B Ravinder Reddy

4. **Malnutrition and Body Composition Assessment in Critical Illness**
   Radha Reddy Chada

5. **Nutritional Assessment in Critical Illness**
   Daphnee Lovesley

6. **Nutrition in Inflammatory Bowel Disease**
   Ritu Sudhakar, Kirandeep Kaur

CHAPTER 1

Pathophysiology of Critical Illness

Gunadhar Padhi, Masood Ahmed Chandsha

GENERAL CONCEPTS IN CRITICAL ILLNESS

Patients admitted in intensive care unit (ICU) with conditions such as sepsis, acute respiratory distress syndrome (ARDS), multiple organ dysfunction syndrome (MODS), and shock. They have severe physiologic derangement resulting in organ failure and/or systemic inflammation.

The pathophysiology of critical illness is complex and multifactorial, and typically involves a combination of several interconnected processes, such as inflammation, hypoxia mitochondrial dysfunction, oxidative stress, coagulopathy, and immune dysfunction.

These pathophysiological processes are linked and can lead to a vicious cycle of organ failure, further exacerbating the critical illness state. Successful critical illness treatment often requires addressing each of these underlying processes, either through supportive care or focused interventions.

Nutrition plays an important role in management of critically ill. Adequate nutrition is important to maintain cellular integrity, support immune function, and promote tissue repair. However, severe disease can disrupt the normal metabolic pathways involved in nutrient absorption, utilization, and storage.

The pathophysiology of nutrition in critical illness can be outlined as altered nutrient metabolism, malabsorption, hypermetabolism, oxidative stress, inflammation, and enteral feeding intolerance secondary to gastrointestinal dysfunction.

These processes can contribute to malnutrition in critically ill patients and lead to additional complications such as impaired wound healing, impaired immune function, and prolonged hospitalization. Critical illness is a hypercatabolic state. And nutritional management may optimize the host response and thereby minimize nutritionally related complications while improving overall outcome. It requires a multidisciplinary approach, including early enteral nutrition, optimization of nutrient tolerance, addition of supplemental parenteral nutrition, and monitoring of nutritional status.

Critical Illness-associated Weakness: A Syndromal Term

Critical illness-associated weakness (CIAW) is a syndromal term used to describe loss of muscle mass and muscle weakness that occurs in critically ill patients. It is a common complication of critical illness and is associated with prolonged mechanical ventilation, increased ICU stays, and is attributed with increased mortality and morbidity.

Critical illness-associated weakness can present as global muscle weakness, challenges in liberation from mechanical ventilation, and limited functional capacity. It is thought that a number of factors contribute to this such as immobility, inflammation, oxidative stress, and metabolic abnormalities.[1]

Critical illness-associated weakness might be triggered by either critical illness polyneuropathy (CIP), critical illness myopathy (CIM), or both. CIAW is a common major illness syndrome that is linked to a significant mortality and morbidity rate for acute major illnesses.[2]

The most frequent causes of neuromuscular weakness in the intensive care setting are CIM, CIP, overlapping, and critical illness polyneuromyopathy (CIPNM). These are frequently under blame for the loss of disassociation from ventilation.[3]

Early mobilization, physical therapy, and rehabilitation can help to prevent and treat CIAW. Adequate nutrition support, particularly sugar control and protein supplementation, can also help to prevent muscle wasting and promote recovery. Other interventions, such as electrical muscle stimulation and pharmacologic agents, are being studied as potential treatments for CIAW.[4]

As a whole, CIAW is a grave complication of critical illness that can have a major impact on patients' long-term outcomes, quality of life, and healthcare utilization.

PATHOPHYSIOLOGICAL STRESSES OR INJURY RESULTING IN CRITICAL ILLNESS

A variety of pathophysiological stresses or injuries to the body results in critical illness. These stresses or injuries are usually from.

- *Infections:* Severe sepsis and septic shock are one of the pressing issues in acute care medicine. The pathophysiology of sepsis as seen as host response to infection in form overly exuberant inflammatory response leading to overstimulation of the immune system, coagulation abnormalities, leading to organ dysfunction and failure.[5]
- *Trauma:* Traumatic injuries can result in critical illness. The severity of the injury and the extent of tissue damage determines the extent of critical illness. Trauma causes activation of nearly all components of the immune system. It activates the neuroendocrine system and local tissue destruction and accumulation of toxic byproducts of metabolic respiration leads to release of mediators. SIRS can lead to tissue destruction in organs not originally affected by the initial trauma with subsequent development of multiorgan dysfunction (MOD).[6]
- *Surgery:* Stress responses to surgery, serious illness, injury, and burns include disruption of metabolic and physiological processes that trigger inflammation, acute phase, hormonal, and genomic responses. The result is hypermetabolism and catabolism leading to muscle weakness, impaired immune function, wound healing, organ failure, and death.[7]
- *Chronic diseases:* Chronic diseases such as diabetes, heart disease, and chronic obstructive pulmonary disease (COPD) can damage organs over time and make them vulnerable to stress or injury, leading to serious illness.
- *Environmental factors:* Exposure to toxins, extreme temperatures, or radiation can damage cells and tissues throughout the body, causing serious illness.

Regardless of the underlying cause, critical illness often results in a complex cascade of physiological changes that can lead to MODS.

The objective of interventional therapy is to minimize the disruption of normal physiological parameters during the initial stage of the stressor. And repair metabolism and avoid organ damage, this encompasses the idea of the "golden hour".[8]

Injury at the Tissue Level

Systemic inflammatory response syndrome (SIRS) is an exaggerated defense response of the body to a noxious stressor (infection, trauma, surgery, acute inflammation, ischemia or reperfusion, or malignancy, to name a few) to localize and then eliminate the endogenous or exogenous source of the insult. It involves the delivery of acute phase reactants that are direct mediators of a wide range of autonomic, endocrine, hematological, and immunological changes in the patient. Although the goal is defense, an unregulated cytokine storm can trigger a massive inflammatory cascade that can lead to reversible or irreversible end-organ dysfunction and even death.

The compensatory anti-inflammatory response syndrome (CARS) limits the severe consequences of SIRS, also happens concurrently with it. In addition, a gradual immune response failure (affecting lymphocytes) with just an elevated risk of immunoparalysis and related infection consequences occurs. Cellular as well as humoral effectors both contribute to the emergence of SIRS and CARS. The most significant body's immune agents include complements, leukotrienes, PAF, proinflammatory (IL-1, IL-6, IL-8, and IL-12), and anti-inflammatory (IL-4 and IL-10) cytokines and chemokines. Neutrophils, monocytes, macrophages, lymphocytes, and endothelial cells are examples of effector cells.[9] The endothelial plays a crucial role in the development of distant organ failure because it has a strong chemoattractive effect on inflammatory cells, permits leukocyte transport within organs and tissues, and encourages more activation through the cytokines that it releases. Besides that, the deterioration of vasoregulatory capabilities and the rise in leakage are associated with muscle edema and depression. The widespread deposits of experiments, which are carried upon by the distributed stimulation of the clotting cascade, may lead to an imbalance in capillaries' blood circulation and, therefore, to hypoxic tissue injury. The major organ failure disorder is brought on by this process, along with a rise in vascular permeability and dilatation (MODS).[10]

Failure of Metabolism

Injuries and severe disease trigger a hypermetabolic reaction that results in higher oxygen and substrate utilization. A gene-driven immunologic decline characterized by various innate immunity deficiencies, as well as a slow mobilization of amino acids from muscle and other sources of protein. The body's attempt to cope with severe trauma is accompanied by significant changes in carbohydrate and protein metabolism. These variations help to support host defenses against infectious disease, anorexia, immobilization, and impairment of hemodynamic resiliency. This metabolic reaction is caused by elevated hormone levels that regulate child behavior. If such a reaction is unchecked and continues, it will eventually result in death. The patient gradually heals from damage, recovers an appreciation for life, and gradually increases activity when the body is able to handle the requirements and properly treat the injuries.[11]

Physicians can adopt an intelligent approach to the nutritional therapy of their critically ill and critically injured patients by studying the chemotactic reaction to harm and its effects after subsequent utilization. The body reacts to severe trauma or serious sickness by initiating a regulated series of measures meant to regain and preserve cardiovascular homeostasis and minimize the extent of the damage. The size of this response is influenced by the wound's or inflammation's severity. Whereas minor operations, such as elective surgery, cause a very moderate metabolic response, serious multiple sclerosis promotes hypermetabolism via neurologic and hormonal stimuli. The brain is alerted to multiple injuries by this neuroendocrine reaction, which also helps the body to maintain proper control and resolution of some wounds while recovering.[12]

Three different stages of biotransformation exist **(Flowchart 1)**. The first stage only lasts a few hours and is mainly focused on increasing blood volume and addressing any irregularities in the circulation of peripheral tissues. When all organs are adequately transfused, the second phase is brought about by a broad breakdown of the lean tissue when amino acids are released from the peripheral tissue into the central circulation. This condition is related to elevated urea production, a negative nitrogen balance, an increase in energy use at rest, and high serum sugar levels are all signs of muscle tissue mobilization after using peripheral. The body gradually recovers the function in the final phase once the patient has begun to recuperate, the injuries are healing, and infections have been contained or eliminated.[12]

Shock

Shock is a sudden and widespread reduction in effective tissue perfusion that results in an imbalance between oxygen demand and supply, anaerobic metabolism, lactic acidosis, cell and organ dysfunction, metabolic disturbances, and, if prolonged, irreversible injury and death.

The pathophysiology of different types of shock is diverse and complex, with hemodynamic and oxygenation changes, changes in fluid compartment composition, and different mediators **(Flowchart 2)**. Shock results from changes in one or a combination of intravascular volume, myocardial function, systemic vascular resistance, or blood flow distribution.

Clinical types of shock include hypovolemic, cardiogenic, distributive (septic), and

Flowchart 1: Stages of biotransformation.

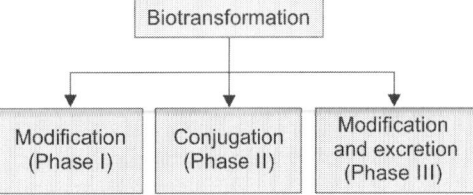

Flowchart 2: Pathophysiology of shock.

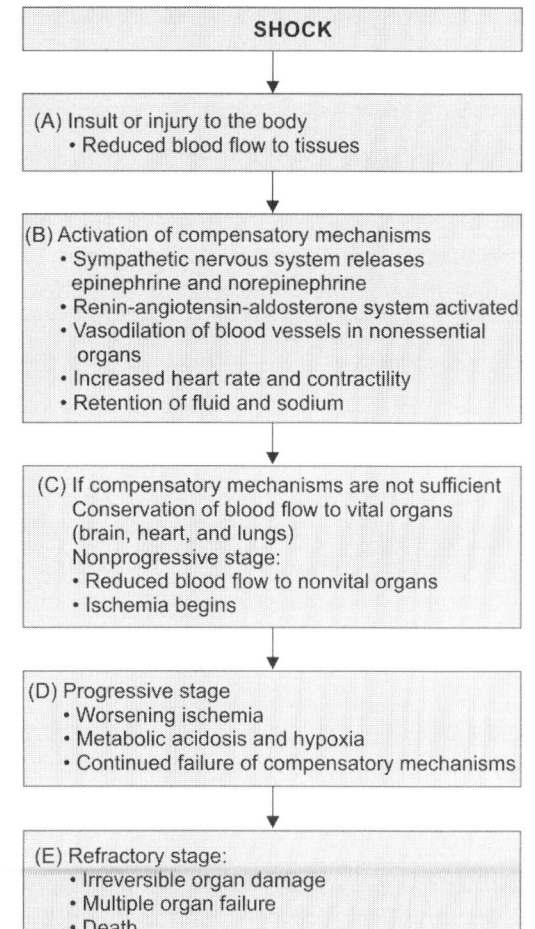

obstructive. A better understanding of the pathophysiological changes, rapid diagnosis, adequate monitoring, and appropriate treatment can reduce the high morbidity and mortality in shock.

In summary, the pathophysiology of shock involves a complex series of physiological responses aimed at restoring adequate blood flow to the body's vital organs. If these compensatory mechanisms fail, the body enters a cycle of worsening ischemia, metabolic acidosis, and hypoxia, which can ultimately lead to irreversible organ damage and death.

PATHOPHYSIOLOGY OF CRITICAL ILLNESS MYOPATHY, CRITICAL ILLNESS POLYNEUROPATHY, AND CRITICAL ILLNESS POLYNEUROMYOPATHY

While having comparable clinical signs within a single patient group, CIM, CIP, and CIPNM have quite various underlying pathologies. Surprisingly, electrophysiological alterations discovered through screening might happen just hours after being admitted to the ICU. A condensed version of the pathophysiology behind CIM, CIP, and CIPNM is shown in **Flowcharts 3 and 4**. Microvascular, molecular, and chemical abnormalities may take place throughout the major illness and affect nerves and muscle tissue as well.[13]

Critical Illness Myopathy

Several pathologic subgroups of CIM exist; conventional CIM exhibits protein loss, severe clinical acute/chronic granulomatous myopathy, and hypercalcemia myopathy. Creatine kinase and data sources are frequently markedly elevated in severe tuberculous myopathy. The main clinical disease resembles use atrophy in appearance, and the test findings agree with type 2 fiber loss. Despite the reality each category has the same clinical course, there are probably various underlying pathogenetic

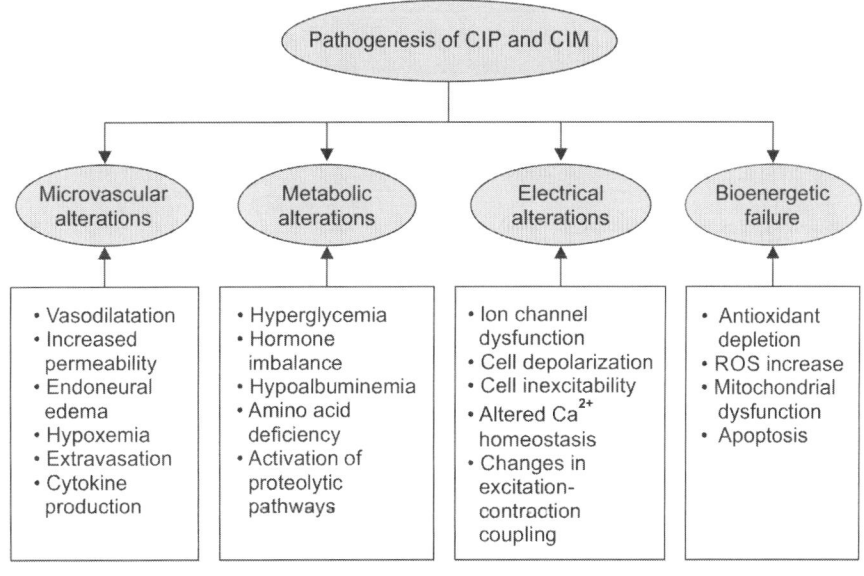

Flowchart 3: Pathophysiology of critical illness myopathy (CIM) and critical illness polyneuropathy (CIP).

(ROS: reactive oxygen species)

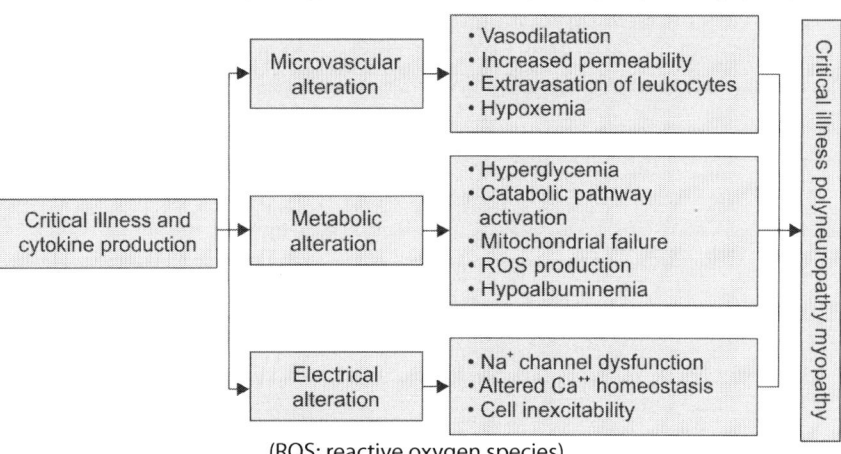

Flowchart 4: Pathophysiology of critical illness polyneuropathy and myopathy.

(ROS: reactive oxygen species)

processes that have not yet been completely understood.[13]

Lack of myosin and further disintegration of the muscle fibers characterize the much more common CIM. Creatinine kinase levels for such a CIM may normally range from regular to slightly raised. Research has shown that nerve muscles subjected to large doses of corticosteroids would selectively lose thick filaments, and that corticosteroid receptor numbers rise after denervation. The exact mechanism by which drugs generate these modifications is unknown. Other chemicals or physiological pressures, such as higher metabolic needs that lead to widespread muscular atrophy, could also be to blame for the decrease in elastin.[14]

Muscle fiber membrane disruption has also been shown to occur in CIM. In the tibialis anterior muscle, Allen et al. used needle electrodes to study-based building nerve impulse and found that while overall nerve conduction velocities were normal, there was a slowing of the conduction within only one muscle, suggesting that muscle fiber glands cannot convert messages. It is unclear if the aberrant calcium resistance is what leads to the myosin loss or what caused it. Animal models have shown that the deactivation of sodium ions could contribute to all this.[15]

The pathophysiology of CIM is intricate and involves changes to the bioenergetic, inflammatory, and metabolic systems. Muscle atrophy and catabolism of proteins are seen in CIM. The proinflammatory cytokines along with enhanced apoptosis cause an upregulation of the ubiquitin-proteasome and calpain proteolytic pathways. Calpain is a calcium-activated protease, hence inflammation and endotoxemia may have an impact on cellular calcium homeostasis. Acute activation of the proteasome-ubiquitin complex and the transforming growth factor-beta/mitogen-activated protein kinase (TGF-β/MAPK) pathway has additionally been proposed as a possible explanation for the loss of muscle. These patients' muscle biopsies show a decline in the concentration of all amino acids, but most notably, glutamine.[13]

Protein synthesis and degradation are both known to be stimulated and inhibited by glutamine. In relation to the rising demands of critically ill patients, there seems to be a relative glutamine deficit. In CIM, myofilament apoptosis and loss may be caused by reduced anabolic hormone levels and elevated catabolic hormone levels. Another pathophysiological mechanism that has been proposed is channelopathy. Frequently, electrodiagnostic investigations reveal the inexcitability of the muscular membrane.[14] This might be connected to a change in the voltage dependency of channel inactivation and sodium-channel inactivation at the resting potential. In sepsis, the interactions of lipopolysaccharide with voltage-gated sodium channels may be a factor in the inexcitability of muscle membranes. Additionally, because nitric oxide plays a role in maintaining the resting potential of muscle fibers, it has been hypothesized that altered gene expression of nitric oxide synthetases may have an impact on the excitability of muscle membranes in CIM. As blood serum from CIM patients was shown to affect both the excitability of muscle fiber membranes and the discharge of calcium from the sarcoplasmic reticulum (SR), it is possible that CIM also involves changes in the excitation-contraction coupling.[15]

It is unclear what causes axon damage in CIP. Endothelial alterations linked to the inflammatory process are one of the possible mechanisms of harm. Anaerobic oxidation is changed as a result of increased cytokine, nitrous oxide, and other forms of reactive oxygen production, which alters remote brain injury and damage.[16]

Pathophysiology of Chronic Illness Polyneuropathy

Without a significant demyelinating element, such as that seen in a few other acute neuropathic disorders (such as the classic Guillain–Barré syndrome/acute inflammatory demyelinating polyneuropathy or mononeuritis multiplex), CIP results from peripheral nerve axonal malfunction and death. A modification to the microvasculature of the axons of peripheral nerves is one suggested mechanism underlying CIP.[17] Bolton et al. proposed that CIP might result from increased access to the vasa nervorum in some early research. The greatly elevated expression of the activation of membrane marker E-selectin observed in human patients with CIP may be the cause of this enhanced permeability. An inflammatory reaction is the resulting transmigration of immune cells into nerve tissue through the release of inflammatory mediators including TNF-α and IL-1.[18] The ensuing edema may cause hypoxia, which would hamper energy production and cause a rise in reactive oxygen species (ROS). Degeneration of axons can follow from energy deficiencies, and elevated ROS can add to bioenergetic failure by structurally harming mitochondria. SIRS has been named for this inflammatory response that occurs in the absence of infection.[19]

As seen in diabetic polyneuropathy, hyperglycemia—a characteristic of persons with critical illnesses—has been hypothesized to exert direct harmful effects on the axons and has been found to impair mitochondrial activity. Two theories may help to explain why hyperglycemia may be more damaging in ICU patients than in diabetics who are not critically ill, despite the fact that the underlying process is yet unknown. The primary assumption is that critical disease causes cellular glucose excess, which has a direct harmful effect. In response to increasing hypoxia, angiotensin II, cytokines, vascular endothelial growth factor (VEGF), endothelin-1, and TGF-β stimulation, glucose transporters are upregulated on a variety of tissue types, including neurons.[13]

The second idea, which may be a continuation of the first, postulates that elevated glucose levels cause an increase in ROS production, specifically superoxide created by the processes of glycolysis and oxidative phosphorylation. Additionally, critically ill patients have a weakness in the scavenging of ROS.[20] The natural ROS defense mechanisms of the cell are severely outmatched by the substantial increase in superoxide molecule production, and unneutralized ROS can subsequently interact with nitric oxide to produce peroxynitrite. Theoretically, peroxynitrites can inhibit the mitochondrial electron transport chain, triggering a cascade of events that ultimately results in cell apoptosis.[14]

Another theory about the pathophysiology of CIP, supported by comparatively little evidence, is that depolarization of the membrane brought on by endoneurial hypoxia or systemic hyperkalemia may have an impact on nerve signal conductance. Increased endoneurial potassium levels cause depolarization of the membrane in renal failure by changing the membrane's subexcitability potential, which eventually causes the axonal membrane to become depolarized.[21] The same changed membrane potential, which has been linked to acute local ischemia at the vasa nervorum level, was also observed in human patients with CIP who did not have renal failure. As a result, it is theorized that the state of membrane depolarization results directly from a drop in oxygen levels and may be a factor in the death of peripheral neurons.[22]

Another theory regarding the cause of neuronal damage in CIP is higher microcirculation, which leads to a rise in leukocytes in the nervous tissue region as well as the development of edema. Similar to the central nervous system, edema can worsen due to hypoalbuminemia and glucose. Moreover, the etiology of nerve failure has been linked to potassium-channel inactivation, which causes fast peripheral nerve hyperexcitability. There is sodium-channel inactivation and a shift in the resting membrane potential, as stated in both CIP and CIM. Its importance of possible nerve injury in the pathophysiology of CIM is highlighted by the ability of concurrent CIP to enhance the effects of CIM. This lends credence to the idea that CIM and CIP are various disease symptoms related to a single basic illness activity.[23]

Pathophysiology of Critical Illness Polyneuromyopathy (Fig. 1)

The pathophysiology of CIPNM has been explained by a number of processes, most of which are complicated and unproven. According to one idea, CIPNM is merely another organ failure that occurs in critically unwell patients. It is well known that individuals with SIRS and sepsis have several alterations in the microvasculature that

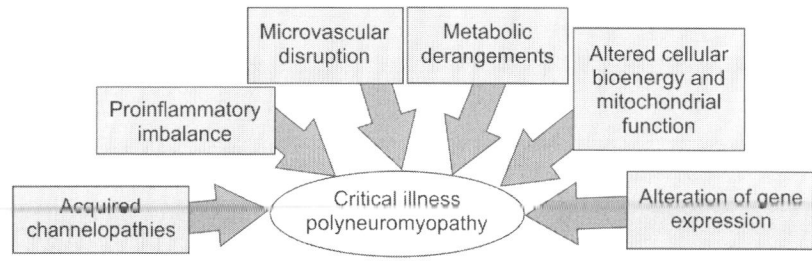

Fig. 1: Multiple pathophysiological mechanisms of critical illness polyneuromyopathy.

TABLE 1: Risk factors associated with ICU-acquired weakness.

Modifiable risk factors	Nonmodifiable risk factors
Prolonged critical illness	Female gender
Neuromuscular junction blockers	Low baseline muscle mass
High-dose corticosteroids	Premorbid malnutrition
High-dose vasopressors	Severe sepsis
Immobility, prolonged bed rest	Multiorgan system failure
Hyperglycemia	Higher severity of illness (high acute physiology and chronic health evaluation and high sequential organ failure assessment scores in the first week)
Use of aminoglycosides	

affect the perfusion of the peripheral nerves and organs. Axonal degeneration may result from sepsis-related variables such as the release of tumor-necrosis factor, macrophages, cytokines, and other free radicals, according to a theory put forth by Bolton et al.[24]

Increased expression of E-selectin in the vascular endothelium may be a mediator in the pathophysiology of CIPNM. Through its part in the buildup of leukocytes at the site of damage, E-selectin, a cell adhesion protein produced on endothelial cells stimulated by proinflammatory cytokines, plays a crucial function in the inflammatory process.[20] This leukocyte recruitment may cause tissue damage, which would increase the production of cytokines. These cytokines, which can affect vasoregulation and raise capillary permeability, are additionally found in sepsis and are similar to histamine in their biological features. Enhanced endothelial edema and enhanced microvascular permeability both contribute to the passage of neurotoxic substances, which can eventually result in hypoxia and loss of energy. Primary axonal degeneration results from these energy supply shortages.[25]

Patients with sepsis and other serious illnesses frequently exhibit hyperglycemia and passive glucose uptake, which has been reported to disrupt the microcirculation of peripheral nerves. ROS are produced more frequently and are less efficiently scavenged by the body, which causes mitochondria to malfunction. Hyperglycemia has also been linked to energy depletion **(Table 1)**. In addition to causing damage to tissues, hypoalbuminemia, and hyperkalemia can encourage endothelial edema and hypoxia.[26]

■ CONCLUSION

The chapter introduces all the essentials facets of critical illness and CIAW, shedding light on the intricate landscape of these conditions within the context of medical care. Critical illness, characterized by severe disruptions in organ function necessitating intensive medical intervention, demands heightened attention, particularly for patients enduring prolonged stays. CIAW is a puzzling phenomenon, denoting muscle discomfort emerging during hospitalization with no apparent extraneous cause apart from the primary infection and its treatment. Neuromuscular weaknesses arising in intensive care settings predominantly manifest as CIM, CIP, and their convergence into CIPNM. The temporal onset of CIAW remains often elusive, adding complexity to its understanding. This abstract delves into the intricate intricacies of these conditions, acknowledging their substantial impact on patients and the healthcare landscape. The intricate interplay of stress response in critical illness has remained a topic of relatively limited exploration, despite its vital role. Pathophysiological stressors, such as SIRS and MODS, usher in critical illness, precipitating a cascade of physiological disturbances. Electrodiagnostic investigations play a pivotal role in the diagnostic journey of CIM, CIP, and CIPNM. While numerous treatment options exist for associated respiratory failures and fatigue, thorough assessment remains paramount. Differentiating neuromuscular from non-neuromuscular origins is imperative in this endeavor, demanding clinical acumen. Electrodiagnostic findings like decreased compound muscle action potential amplitudes in CIM or length-dependent axonal polyneuropathy patterns in CIP offer diagnostic insights. Accurate diagnosis entails a combination of clinical assessment, electrodiagnostic findings, and exclusion of non-neuromuscular causes. Essential diagnostic criteria guide the identification of CIP and myopathy, elucidating distinct attributes and patterns. Effective management strategies entail multidisciplinary approaches, concentrating on the underlying causes of the critical illness. Measures such as glucose control, avoidance of corticosteroids and neuromuscular blocking agents, and appropriate physical therapy are integral to treatment protocols. The varying management strategies for CIM, CIP, and CIPNM recognize the nuanced aspects of each condition.

The prognosis for these conditions varies with severity and extent of damage. Recovery is possible in milder cases, but in severe instances, it may be partial or prolonged, correlating with a higher risk of mortality. While therapeutic options offer hope, the complexity of critical illness and its associated weaknesses reinforces the importance of early intervention, meticulous assessment, and tailored treatment approaches. This chapter provides a comprehensive glimpse into the deep insights of critical illness and its associated weaknesses, offering an overview that underscores the importance of timely diagnosis, appropriate management, and a holistic approach to patient care in critical care settings.

REFERENCES

1. Puthucheary ZA, Rawal J, McPhail M, Connolly B, Ratnayake G, Chan P, et al. Acute skeletal muscle wasting in critical illness. JAMA. 2013;310(15):1591-600.
2. Hermans G, Van den Berghe G. Clinical review: Intensive Care Unit acquired weakness. Crit Care. 2015;19(1):274.
3. Bolton CF, Gilbert JJ, Hahn AF, Sibbald WJ. Polyneuropathy in critically ill patients. J Neurol Neurosurg Psychiatry. 1984;47:1223-31.
4. Hermans G, De Jonghe B, Bruyninckx F, Van den Berghe G. Interventions for preventing critical illness polyneuropathy and critical illness myopathy. Cochrane Database Syst Rev. 2014;2014(1):CD006832.
5. Angus DC, van der PT. Severe sepsis and septic shock. N Engl J Med. 2013;369(9):840-51.
6. Lenz A, Franklin GA, Cheadle WG. Systemic inflammation after trauma. Injury. 2007;38(12):1336-45.
7. Finnerty CC, Mabvuure NT, Ali A, Kozar RA, Herndon DN. The surgically induced stress response. JPEN J Parenter Enteral Nutr. 2013;37(5 Suppl):21S-9S.
8. Bistrian BR, Blackburn GL, Hallowell E, Heddle R. Protein status of general surgical patients. JAMA. 1974;230(6):858-60.
9. American College of Chest Physicians/Society of Critical Care Medicine Consensus Conference. Definitions for sepsis and organ failure and guidelines for the use of innovative therapies in sepsis. Crit Care Med. 1992;20:864-74.

10. Lord JM, Midwinter MJ, Chen Y, Belli A, Brohi K, Kovacs EJ, et al. The systemic immune response to trauma: an overview of pathophysiology and treatment. Lancet. 2014;384:1455-65.
11. Buckley S, Kudsk KA. Metabolic response to critical illness and injury. AACN Clin Issues Crit Care Nurs. 1994;5(4):443-9.
12. Preiser JC, Ichai C, Orban JC, Groeneveld AB. Metabolic response to the stress of critical illness. Br J Anaesth. 2014;113:945-54.
13. Shepherd S, Batra A, Lerner DP. Review of critical illness myopathy and neuropathy. Neurohospitalist. 2017;7(1):41-8.
14. Bercker S, Weber-Carsten SD. Critical illness polyneuropathy and myopathy in patients with acute respiratory distress syndrome. Crit Care Med. 2005;33(4):711-5.
15. Beknarik J, Vondracek P, Dusek L, Moravcova E, Cundrle I. Risk factors for critical illness polyneuromyopathy. J Neurol. 2005;252(3):343-51.
16. Mohr M, Englisch L, Roth A, Burchardi H, Zielmann S. Effects of early treatment with immunoglobulin on critical illness polyneuropathy following multiple organ failure and gram-negative sepsis. Intensive Care Med. 1997;23(11):1144-9.
17. Thiele RI, Jakob H, Hund E, Genzwuerker H, Herold U, Schweiger P, et al. Critical Illness Polyneuropathy: a new iatrogenically induced syndrome after cardiac surgery? Eur J Cardiothorac Surg. 1997;12(6):826-35.
18. Fink MP, Evans TW. Mechanisms of organ dysfunction in critical illness: report from a Round Table Conference held in Brussels. Intensive Care Med. 2002;28(3):369-75.
19. Hermans G, De Jonghe B, Bruyninckx F, Van den Berghe G. Clinical review: Critical Illness Polyneuropathy and myopathy. Crit Care. 2008;12(6):238-44.
20. Zhou C, Wu L, Fenghimg Ni, Ji W, Wu J, Zhang H. Critical Illness Polyneuropathy and myopathy: a systematic review. Neural Regen Res. 2014;9(1):101-10.
21. Tennilä A, Salmi T, Pettila V, Roine RO, Varpula T, Takkunen O. Early signs of critical illness polyneuropathy in ICU patients with systemic inflammatory response syndrome or sepsis. Intensive Care Med. 2000;26(9):1360-3.
22. de Letter MA, Schmitz PI, Visser LH, Verheul FA, Schellens RL, Op de Coul DA, et al. Risk factors for the development of polyneuropathy and myopathy in critically ill patients. Crit Care Med. 2001;29(12):2281-6.
23. Zink W, Kollmar R, Schwab S. Critical illness polyneuropathy and myopathy in the intensive care unit. Nat Rev Neurol. 2009;5(5):372-9.
24. Hermans G, Vanhorebeek I, Derde S, Van den Berghe G. Metabolic aspects of critical illness polyneuromyopathy. Crit Care Med. 2009;37(10):391-7.
25. Latronico N, Guarneri B. Critical illness myopathy and neuropathy. Minerva Anestesiol. 2008;74:319-23.
26. Dhand UK. Clinical approach to the weak patient in the Intensive Care Unit. Respir Care. 2006;51:1024-40.

CHAPTER 2

Nutrient Metabolism in Critical Illness

Dedeepiya Devaprasad, Krishnan Sriram, Nagarajan Ramakrishnan

INTRODUCTION

Nutrients are defined as chemical substances contained in food that are required for growth and maintenance of living organisms. Metabolism refers to all chemical processes that are ongoing in a living cell making it possible for that cell to continue living.

Critical illness is defined as a life-threatening condition that requires pharmacological or mechanical support of the impaired organ in the absence of which death is likely to ensue. A more recent and better definition of critical illness is "a state of ill-health with dysfunction of vital organs and risk of imminent death if immediate care is not provided." Critical care is defined as "the identification, monitoring, and treatment of patients with critical illness with sustained support of organ functions".[1]

In this chapter, we will review the chemical processes (i.e., metabolism) of chemical substances in food or artificial nutrition (i.e., nutrients) that occurs in critical illness.

Carbohydrates (CHO), fats, and proteins, when oxidized outside the body will release energy in the form of heat. However, within the body the oxidization of these nutrients is not wasted by release of heat but "coupled" with specific cellular enzyme systems and electron transport system to help to perform physiological functions.[2]

CARBOHYDRATE METABOLISM

Carbohydrates are the primary source of energy in the resting fed state. They are finally digested into glucose, galactose, and fructose, which are absorbed in the proximal small intestine. Most of the absorbed fructose and almost all the absorbed galactose that reach the liver cells are converted into glucose. Glucose is thus the ultimate CHO source that is transported into the circulation. Glucose is absorbed in the intestine because of glucose sodium cotransporters. The active transport of sodium provides energy for the absorption of glucose against its concentration gradient. This mechanism of glucose transport that exists in the intestinal lumen also exists in the renal cortex and wherever glucose must be transported against a concentration gradient. The passage of glucose from the circulation into the cell is facilitated by the action of insulin on the glucose transporters (GLUT) present on the surface of cells. The glucose that enters the cell undergoes glycolysis to form pyruvate.

Fate and Importance of Pyruvate

There are four potential pathways for further metabolism of pyruvate. It undergoes oxidative decarboxylation to form acetyl coenzyme (acetyl-CoA), can be reduced to lactate, or undergo carboxylation to form oxaloacetate and by further transamination be converted to alanine.[3]

Under normal circumstances, the pyruvate undergoes oxidative decarboxylation to form acetyl-CoA and enters the Krebs cycle to generate adenosine triphosphate (ATP). 686,000 calories are expected to be released during the complete oxidation of each gram of glucose. However, in the cells, for each molecule of glucose degraded to form carbon dioxide and water, a maximum of 38 ATP molecules are released. This translates to 456,000 calories of energy stored in ATP and thus about 66% of maximum efficiency of energy transfer. The remaining 34% of energy is liberated as heat and cannot be utilized by the cells.

However, in ischemic or hypoxic states where cellular oxygen supply is low, the pyruvate undergoes reduction to lactate. Anaerobic glycolysis is an extremely wasteful reaction in terms of energy efficiency because for each molecule of glucose utilized, only 24,000 calories of energy are used to form ATP. This represents only about 3% of the energy stored in glucose.

Lactic acid readily diffuses from the cell into extracellular fluid and intracellular fluids. An elevated serum lactate level may, therefore, serve as a marker of "septic shock" although normal levels do not rule out sepsis. The heart muscle can convert lactate to pyruvate which it can subsequently utilize for energy. However, the greatest interconversion of lactate into pyruvate occurs in the liver whenever cellular oxygen uptake is restored.

Oxaloacetate is not only an intermediary of citric acid cycle but also plays a key role in gluconeogenesis, uric acid cycle, amino acid synthesis, and fatty acid (FA) synthesis. The enzyme serum glutamate oxaloacetic aminotransferase (SGOT), now designated as aspartate amino transaminase (AST), forms aspartate from oxaloacetate by the process of transamination. Likewise, serum glutamic pyruvic transaminase (SGPT), now called alanine aminotransferase (ALT) forms alanine from pyruvate by process of transamination from glutamate. Aspartate plays an important role in the synthesis of asparagine, methionine, lysine, isoleucine, and threonine while pyruvate molecules are involved in the synthesis of alanine, valine, leucine, and isoleucine.

The pyruvate molecule serves to produce ATP by entering the Krebs cycle or by forming lactate. It is also a key molecule in the interconversion of glucose, amino acids, and FA, thus helping in the integration of nutrient metabolism.

Storage of CHO

Excess glucose, not immediately used for metabolic processes, is stored as glycogen in the liver or muscle. While muscle glycogen is available only for muscle tissue, hepatic glycogen is available for the entire body.

FAT METABOLISM
Fat Absorption and Digestion

Fatty acids ingested through our diet forms the main lipid source of energy. However, FA is also synthesized from glucose and amino acids under appropriate conditions. This is facilitated by insulin and inhibited by adrenaline, glucagon, and glucose. The human body is not equipped with the necessary enzymes to produce the long chain of polyunsaturated fatty acids (PUFA), ω-6 linoleic acid and ω-3 α-linolenic acid. Since PUFA cannot be produced endogenously, they are termed essential and have to be obtained from the diet. Sunflower oil, corn oil, and cotton oil are some natural sources of ω-6 acids while fish oil, nut oil, and rapeseed oil are natural sources of ω-3 acids. Soyabean oil acts as a natural source of both ω-6 and ω-3 oils.[4]

Emulsification is the first process in FA digestion. The physical movements (propulsion and retropulsion) of the stomach and the enzymatic action of lingual lipase and gastric lipase help in emulsification. The emulsification is further continued in the duodenum and beyond through the action of bile (bile salts and phospholipids) that are secreted in the liver and released from the gallbladder.[5] Fats and proteins stimulate the release of cholecystokinin (CCK) which stimulates both bile secretion and release.

Short-chain fatty acids (SCFA—a class of saturated FA) are obtained directly from butter or indirectly by bacterial fermentation on the ingested soluble fibers in the colon to acetoacetic, butyric, and propionic acids. The SCFA though absorbed in the intestinal lumen largely serves as a nutrient metabolite for the colonocytes and thus hardly reaches the circulation.

Medium chain fatty acids (MCFA) which are a type of saturated FA are obtained from coconut oil and palm oil. Their digestion begins in the stomach under the action of the lingual and gastric lipases. They are absorbed by the enterocytes and transported predominantly in the unbound form and to a lesser extent after being bound to albumin. They are then transported through the bloodstream to reach the liver.

The long-chain fatty acids (LCFA—also a type of saturated FA) are mainly derived from animal fat. Cocoa is a plant source of LCFA. The digestion of LCFA is predominantly accomplished by the action of pancreatic lipase, phospholipase A2, and cholesterol esterase. Postdigestion absorption is through the brush border of the enterocyte through the lymphatic system. The absorbed products are used for the resynthesis of triglycerides (TG). The resynthesized TGs are incorporated into cholesterol, phospholipids, and lipoproteins and transported as lipoprotein through the lymphatic system (in contrast to MCFA that are transported through the bloodstream and portal venous system) to reach the circulation.

Fat Transport and Distribution

The lipoproteins in the bloodstream are of varying densities. Chylomicrons, very low-density lipoproteins (VLDL), low-density lipoproteins (LDL), and high-density lipoproteins (HDL) represent lipoprotein arrangement in increasing density.

Chylomicrons are transported from the intestinal lumen to the peripheral tissues. The action of lipoprotein lipase presents on the capillary endothelium releases the TGs and free FA from the chylomicrons. The released FA is thus able to act as an energy source of the peripheral tissues.

Very low-density lipoproteins is formed in the liver and transported to the adipocytes where it acts as an energy source. The excess is then used up for storage. LDL is also formed in the liver by the action of hepatic lipase on the VLDL. This serves to remove the TGs from the VLDL and converts it into cholesterol dense LDL. LDL distributes cholesterol to the other peripheral tissues. The distributed cholesterol serves several important functions. It is incorporated into cellular membranes, stored as cholesterol esters, and used for steroid hormone synthesis. HDL transports the excess cholesterol from the peripheral tissues to the liver where it is metabolized and eliminated as biliary salts and acids.

Role of Fat Absorption in Energy Production and Other Functions

Fatty acids are the lipid source of energy. SCFA are used as energy source for enterocytes and colonocytes while MCFA and LCFA that reach the circulation through the bloodstream and lymphatics respectively, serve as energy sources for the rest of the body cells. The MCFA enter the cell, pass into the cytosol, and then into the mitochondria where they undergo β-oxidation to provide energy (only 10–20% of MCFA needs carnitine). LCFA are also absorbed from the circulation into cellular cytosol but need the presence of carnitine on the mitochondrial matrix to be transported inside it before undergoing β-oxidation.

In addition to directly supplying cells with energy the FA serves two additional important purposes that aid in cellular function. FAs are used in the synthesis of phospholipids which are incorporated in cellular membranes and membrane of organelles and thus play an important role in structure and function of cells. FAs are also involved in the formation of eicosanoids through the cyclooxygenase and lipoxygenase pathways and these serve as secondary messengers for cellular function and as inflammatory mediators.[6]

Storage of Fat

Excess CHO, proteins, and triglycerides in the diet are converted into FA in the liver and stored as triglycerides in the adipose tissue. This "White adipose" that is distributed in the subcutaneous tissues is about 15% of the bodyweight of a normal adult and can serve as an energy source for up to 2 months. Whenever there is a need for energy, the triglycerides are broken down into FA in the adipose tissue through the process of lipolysis. The lipolytic function occurs through the action of either lipoprotein lipase or hormone sensitive lipase. The lipolytic hormones (glucagon, cortisol, adrenaline, noradrenaline, adrenocorticotropic hormone, growth hormone, and leptin) bind to certain β-adrenergic receptors on the cell membrane of adipocytes and through complex intracellular signaling activates the intracellular hormone sensitive lipase. The activated hormone sensitive lipase breaks down the triglycerides into its constituent FA and glycerol and the released FA become a source of energy. Intravenously administered lipid emulsions are metabolized by the lipoprotein lipase in capillary endothelium and not by hepatocytes. Although lipolysis may increase in critical illness, as manifested by increase in triglyceride levels, FA gets re-esterified to a great extent, thus precluding fat stores as an efficient mechanism of providing endogenous energy in critical illness.

PROTEIN METABOLISM

Ingested proteins are almost completed digested and absorbed as amino acids (AA). Very rarely whole protein molecules and polypeptides are also absorbed into the bloodstream. The excess AA in the blood are rapidly absorbed by the cells throughout the body, especially the liver cells. The entry of AA into cells is by facilitated diffusion or by participation of carrier molecules. Once inside the cells, under the instruction of the cell's messenger RNA and ribosomal system, AA form cellular proteins and this becomes the main storage form. The concentration of intracellular free AA is thus low. Though the plasma concentration of free AA is low, whenever the concentration falls below the established normal range, the appropriate cellular proteins are degraded to facilitate the release of AA. This helps to maintain the plasma concentration of AA. Thus, the plasma AA and labile proteins in the cells are in a constant interchangeable equilibrium.

The low levels of circulating free AA in the blood are filtered through the glomerulus and actively reabsorbed into the proximal tubule up to a maximum upper limit of transport.

The unabsorbed free AA are then excreted in the urine. Ammonia in the urine, urinary creatinine, urinary uric acid, urea, peptides, and urinary AA are the various nitrogenous compounds excreted in the urine. The urea nitrogen excreted in the urine over 24 hours may help to estimate the nitrogen balance in patients, although this has limited clinical application.

During prolonged starvation, inevitably there is more proteolysis to maintain adequate plasma glucose and free AA. Growth hormone and insulin increase the formation of tissue proteins while adrenocorticotropic hormone (ACTH) increases the concentration of plasma AAs.

In the resting fed state, CHO and fats can be referred to as protein sparers. They are so-called because they are metabolized to produce energy for cellular needs, thereby preventing protein from being used for energy primarily. However, about 20–30 g of protein is metabolized and lost every day in the absence of intake, and this is referred to as "obligatory protein loss". It is therefore recommended that we provide at least 1.2 g/kg/day of protein in critical illness. This translates to 70–80 g protein/day and provides a higher safety limit for the obligatory protein loss. In addition to this obligatory loss, in prolonged starvation or inadequate provision of calories and protein to critically ill patients, there will be additional protein loss as the proteins will be utilized to provide energy. This is amplified by the effect of "hormonal" and "inflammatory" mediators' protein catabolism. The protein in the cells of the liver, kidney, intestinal mucosa, and muscle are the major source of this proteolytic phenomenon.[7] Approximately 3.5 g of glucose is derived from 6.25 g of protein. The minimum amount of glucose needed for obligatory metabolic processes is 150 g, which is derived from 270 g of protein (dry weight) or 675 g of protein per day.

All body proteins except the proteins in the chromosome, collagen, and structural proteins of muscle undergo proteolysis. This leads to loss of body cell mass (BCM)/lean body mass and is responsible for the muscle wasting, sarcopenia and frailty associated with critical illness. The loss of BCM can also impair host defense and increase the mortality and morbidity associated with critical illness.[8] The urinary excretion of nitrogen has been estimated to be around 8/day in trauma, failure which is the equivalent of 60 g of protein.[9] As compared to normal individuals the negative nitrogen balance is about six times higher in those with severe injury and eight times higher in the severely burnt patient. Increasing nitrogen intake does not reduce the nitrogen loss but improves the nitrogen balance. Kinetic studies have indicated that beyond a protein intake of 1.5 g/kg/day nitrogen balance may not be improved but would merely increase the rate of protein synthesis and protein break down. The optimal protein and calorie intake in critical illness is still unclear.[10]

INTEGRATED METABOLISM AND INTERCONVERSION

Glucose is the predominant energy source of the body. In the fasting state or any state where there is a low supply of glucose, the first response is to provide the needed glucose by glycogenolysis of the stored glycogen in the liver. After 24 hours when the glycogen storage exhausted, proteins stored in the muscles and other protein stores are broken down to release glucogenic amino acids. Alanine, glutamine, and other such AA that get released are transported into the liver where they are used to form glucose through the gluconeogenesis pathway. The nervous tissues and erythrocytes continue to require glucose as an energy source at least partially while other tissues become adapted to start utilizing FA and lactate for energy beyond 24 hours of fasting or glucose restricted state.

The oxidation of FA provides energy and results in the excess generation of acetyl CoA. Acetyl CoA is subsequently converted into ketone bodies (KB) through the ketogenic pathway. The FA and KB then become the principal source of energy for the peripheral tissues (chiefly muscular tissues).[11] In the continued fasting state, the initial adaptation to use body proteins to generate glucose reduces over a period of time until KB are used as an alternative fuel. This adaptation to use KB occurs even in the central nervous system. Muscles, renal cortex, and small intestine are other tissues where this adaptation occurs.

CLINICAL CORRELATES

Importance of Early Feeding

Most patients without comorbidities are usually nutritionally well supported and are in an adequate resting fed state. When they become acutely critically ill, they are subjected to starvation (due to delay in feeding) and catabolic responses (because of the critical illness). The stored glucose reservoirs are quickly depleted and under the influence of the catabolic hormones, the protein reservoir in the muscle is used to produce glucose. Some cells adapt to utilize FA but the near complete adaptation and switch from glucose to FA and ketone bodies as fuel may take up to 2 months. Hence, it is essential to initiate early feeding in the intensive care unit (ICU) and provides adequate glucose and thus reduces the lipolytic and proteolytic process. Studies have focused on early enteral feeding and have indeed shown a reduction in mortality if feeding was initiated in the ICU within 48–72 hours of admission.[12,13]

Understanding the Catabolic Response

Patients admitted to the ICU are heterogenous in terms of the disease type and organs involved.[14] The stress response of the burnt victim is higher than that of a polytrauma patient which in-turn is more than a septic ventilated patient. Consequently, the caloric and protein needs are not uniform and vary according to the stress response. However, it is clinically not possible at this point of time to measure the catabolic response of each individual patient to decide their caloric needs using affordable and accessible tools. Hence, the recommended calorie-protein intake for each subset of patients' needs to be initiated as per standard guidelines and then tailored to each patient. The assessment of a dynamic hand-grip strength at the bed side of a conscious patient is at present, a useful tool to ascertain the adequacy of protein supplementation.

Insulin Resistance

Perioperative critically ill patients face the problem of insulin-resistant state. When insulin was infused in sufficient amounts to normalize glucose levels, the rest of metabolism was also shown to normalize.[15] This may also be the possible clinical explanation for the demonstration of safety and efficacy of tight glucose control in the critically ill surgical patient. The benefit of a preoperative drink of 200–400 mL of a 12% maltodextrin containing CHO preparation in colorectal surgery patients has also been shown to break the overnight fasted and catabolic state before the onset of operation and enhances insulin sensitivity.[16] This phenomenon of insulin resistance has also been demonstrated in the other subsets of critically ill patients. However, the benefit of tight glucose control has not been demonstrated in the medical critically ill patients.

CONCLUSION

The resting state in health is changed into a starvation and hypercatabolic state in critical illness. The primary response of the body is to produce glucose and alternate energy fuel to cells. The lipolytic and proteolytic response is critical illness continues to a variable extent and duration depending on type of critical illness. Insulin resistance and the usefulness of treating it has been demonstrated in the surgically ill patients. Understanding nutrient metabolism helps us to recognize the importance of early adequate nutrition, equips us with the knowledge to choose wisely among the different product composition available in the medical nutrition industry. It will also help clinicians to pose the appropriate research questions that would hopefully help to clarify the many unanswered clinical nutrition problems we face in our daily critical care practice.

REFERENCES

1. Kayambankadzanja RK, Schell CO, Gerdin Wärnberg M, Tamras T, Mollazadegan H, Holmberg M, et al. Towards definitions of critical illness and critical care using concept analysis. BMJ Open. 2022;12(9): e060972–e060972.
2. Hall JE. Metabolism of Carbohydrates, and Formation of Adenosine Triphosphate. In: Hall JE, Gyton AC (Eds). Guyton and Hall Textbook of Medical Physiology, 12th edition. Philadelphia: Elsevier; 2010. pp. 809-17.
3. Marian M, Roberts S. Carbohydrate Metabolism: A Comparison of Stress and Nonstress States. In: Cresci GA (ed). Nutrition Support for the Critically Ill Patient, 2nd edition. Boca Raton: CRC Press; 2015. pp. 15-31.
4. Linus Pauling Institute | Oregon State University. Essential Fatty Acids. [online] Available from: https://lpi.oregonstate.edu/mic/other-nutrients/essential-fatty-acids. [Last accessed June, 2023].
5. Liao TH, Hamosh P, Hamosh M. Fat Digestion by Lingual Lipase: Mechanism of Lipolysis in the Stomach and Upper Small Intestine. Pediatr Res. 1984;18(5):402-9.
6. Alexander JW. Immunonutrition: the role of ω-3 fatty acids. Nutrition. 1998;14(7–8):627-33.
7. Hall JE. Protein metabolism. In: Hall JE, Gyton AC (Eds). Guyton and Hall Textbook of Medical Physiology, 12th edition. Philadelphia: Elsevier; 2011. pp. 831-5.
8. Cruz-Jentoft AJ, Gonzalez MC, Prado CM. Sarcopenia ≠ low muscle mass. Eur Geriatr Med. 2023;14(2):225-8.
9. Frankenfield DC, Smith JS, Cooney RN. Accelerated nitrogen loss after traumatic injury is not attenuated by achievement of energy balance. JPEN J Parenter Enter Nutr. 1997;21(6):324-9.
10. Hill A, Heyland DK, Ortiz Reyes LA, Laaf E, Wendt S, Elke G, et al. Combination of enteral and parenteral nutrition in the acute phase of critical illness: An updated systematic review and meta-analysis. JPEN J Parenter Enter Nutr. 2022;46(2):395-410.
11. DelMedico NV, Lov J. Ketone bodies as an energy source: regular-grade, premium, or super-fuel to power the mitochondrial engine? J Physiol. 2021;599(3):735-6.
12. Shankar B, Daphnee DK, Ramakrishnan N, Venkataraman R. Feasibility, safety, and outcome of very early enteral nutrition in critically ill patients: Results of an observational study. J Crit Care. 2015;30(3):473-5.
13. Pardo E, Lescot T, Preiser JC, Massanet P, Pons A, Jaber S, et al. Association between early nutrition support and 28-day mortality in critically ill patients: the FRANS prospective nutrition cohort study. Crit Care. 2023;27(1):7.
14. Chan J, Lu YC, Yao MMS, Kosik RO. Correlation between hand grip strength and regional muscle mass in older Asian adults: an observational study. BMC Geriatr. 2022;;22(1):206.
15. Brandi LS, Frediani M, Oleggini M, Mosca F, Cerri M, Boni C, et al. Insulin Resistance after Surgery: Normalization by Insulin Treatment. Clin Sci. 1990;79(5):443-50.
16. Svanfeldt M, Thorell A, Hausel J, Soop M, Nygren J, Ljungqvist O. Effect of "preoperative" oral carbohydrate treatment on insulin action—a randomised cross-over unblinded study in healthy subjects. Clin Nutr. 2005;24(5):815-21.

CHAPTER 3

Immune Responses and Immunometabolism: An Overview

B Ravinder Reddy

The greatest discoveries often lie not in finding new things, but in seeing familiar things in new ways.
— Alexander Fleming

INTRODUCTION

On an average, humans contain about 37 trillion cells and about 39 trillion bacteria, which marginally outnumber human cells at an estimated ratio of about 1.3:1.[1] The intrinsic human cells also include the different types of immune cells involved in innate defenses and acquired immunity. Configuration of their structural form and the control of the different functions of all these numerous cells occur at molecular level, involving various biochemical reactions. These complex physiological mechanisms enable extraction of energy in the form of a small molecule—adenosine triphosphate (ATP) and other provisions from the nutrients. In addition, these metabolic reactions also enable the biosynthesis and assembly of newer molecules, which in turn act as substrates for production of newer reactants and products for further biochemical pathways. Hence, these dynamic intra- and inter-cellular responses are crucial for various metabolic interactions, supporting the various immune cells and facilitating their responses. Therefore, the interactions between metabolism and immunity, termed as *immunometabolism*, can be described as numerous interactions between the various metabolic pathways that sustain and regulate the diverse immune responses.[2] Immunometabolism, which was first described in 2011, is a rapidly evolving field, linking various disciplines and is presently a leading research topic in the field of metabolism. Immunometabolism forms a major mechanism in preserving homeostasis, in facilitating metabolic signaling, and is involved in the pathogenesis of obesity, diabetes, and various other metabolic disorders, inflammation, autoimmune diseases, cancers, infections, and sepsis.[3]

OVERVIEW OF BASIC METABOLIC PATHWAYS

There are seven interconnected metabolic paths, which are essential for growth, sustenance, and survival:

1. Glycolytic pathway
2. Tricarboxylic acid (TCA) cycle
3. Oxidative phosphorylation (OXPHOS)
4. Pentose phosphate pathway (PPP)
5. Fatty acid oxidation (FAO)
6. Fatty acid synthesis (FAS)
7. Amino acid pathways

1. *Glycolytic pathway:* This occurs within the cytoplasm of all the cells, in aerobic as well as anaerobic conditions. A single molecule of glucose produces seven ATPs (aerobic glycolysis) and two ATPs (anaerobic glycolysis, the only pathway that

produces ATP in the absence of oxygen). Though this seems like an inefficient pathway, it actually generates essential biosynthetic precursors for cellular proliferation, such as ribose for synthesis of nucleotides, amino acids, fatty acids (FAs), and enzymes, which act as cofactors (known as the Warburg effect). Glycolysis plays a leading role in all the rapidly dividing cells, including activated white blood cells and neoplastic cells.[4]

2. *Tricarboxylic acid cycle:* This occurs in the mitochondrial matrix and is also known as Krebs cycle or citric acid cycle. The "cycle" commences by accepting acetyl CoA (which is produced by all the three macronutrients—glucose, fatty acids, and amino acids). It has both catabolic (each cycle generates 10 ATPs by breakdown of macronutrients) and anabolic (synthesis of new molecules by providing raw materials), hence termed as amphibolic pathway. An important aspect of TCA cycle is the generation of reducing equivalents, flavin adenine dinucleotide ($FADH_2$), nicotinamide adenine dinucleotide (NADH), and protons (H^+). These energy-rich molecules take part in the electron transport chain (ETC), by moving electrons and enabling oxidative phosphorylation. TCA cycle is an efficient process of ATP generation.[5]

3. *Oxidative phosphorylation:* This occurs in the presence of oxygen, at the inner mitochondrial membrane, and is made up of two components—electron transport chain and chemiosmosis. ETC is made of four extremely complex structures, embedded within the inner mitochondrial membrane (complex I, II, III, and IV). The high-energy electrons, NADH and $FADH_2$ present in the mitochondrial matrix, are transferred serially from one membrane-bound complex to the other (enabled by coenzyme Q10 and cytochrome c), in a series of redox reactions, releasing protons (H^+), and produce energy at each step. This energy is used to pump these protons (which are at a higher concentration in the matrix of the mitochondria) against the concentration gradient into the intermembrane space. Subsequently, by the process of chemiosmosis, these protons within the intermembrane space of mitochondria flow down the concentration gradient through a complex molecule called ATP synthase, producing ATP. Finally, the high-energy protons interact with oxygen and form water. An important by-product of the serial transfer of electrons (e^-) is the generation of reactive oxygen species (ROS), which aid in cell signaling to maintain homeostasis and also contributes to the oxidative stress. On an average, one molecule of glucose generates 30–36 ATPs, thus oxidative phosphorylation is an extremely efficient metabolic process in the generation of energy.[6]

4. *Pentose phosphate pathway:* Like glycolysis, PPP too occurs within the cell cytoplasm and is also called phosphogluconate pathway or hexose monophosphate shunt. A key function is enabling the synthesis of various molecules, by using substrates from glycolytic pathway, to generate nucleic acids, nucleotides, amino acid precursors, FAs, cholesterol, and glutathione. It also plays a major role in the cell defenses by production of the small antioxidant molecules and antioxidant enzymes. PPP has several functions, the most important of which are cell proliferation (anabolic)

and detoxification and neutralization of intracellular ROS (survival), especially in the immune cells.[7]

5. *Fatty acid oxidation:* This process occurs within the mitochondria and utilizes numerous enzymes to generate ATPs and energy-rich NADH and $FADH_2$. It begins within the cytoplasm where the inert FAs are converted into an energy-dense derivative called acyl-coenzyme A ("activation"). It is then transported to mitochondrial matrix by conjugating with carnitine. The medium- and long-chain FAs need carnitine (carnitine shuttle) to be transported into the mitochondria, whereas the short-chain FAs (having less than six carbon atoms) diffuse easily into the mitochondrial matrix. Subsequently, each of the activated FA acyl-coenzyme A undergoes a complex and a repeated process called beta-oxidation, resulting in production of enormous amounts of ATP. For example, palmitic acid, a common form of saturated FA, yields 106 ATPs. FAs are calorie-dense nutrients and have the potential to generate significant amounts of energy when metabolic demands are high.[8]

6. *Fatty acid synthesis:* This occurs in the cell cytoplasm using substrates and metabolic products from other pathways, such as glycolysis, TCA, and PPP, by a complex mechanism. The major source of FAS is by glycolysis, which provides carbon atoms. Glycogen, the stored form of carbohydrates, is limited to about 500 g in the muscles (range from 300 to 700 g) and about 80 g in the liver (range from 0 to 160 g). Therefore, excess glucose undergoes glycolysis, providing the acetyl coenzyme A and NADH + H^+, which are utilized as substrate and generate FAs in a complex biosynthetic pathway. In addition, mechanistic target of rapamycin (mTOR), a molecule that controls growth and metabolism, also controls synthesis of FAs. FAS enables production of lipids, which are essential for growth and proliferation.[9]

7. *Amino acid pathways:* Amino acids are critical for cell and tissue growth, proliferation, and homeostasis. They are essential for locomotion, organ functions, interorgan cross talk, and provide substrates for gluconeogenesis and in inflammatory and immune responses. They are crucial for intra- and extracellular cell signaling and also for the mTOR pathways, which sense the availability of essential amino acids, which in turn control protein synthesis.[10] Additionally, amino acids act as reservoirs and reactants for many diverse molecular, metabolic, and biochemical reactions. Though all of the 20 amino acids are needed for various homeostatic processes, certain amino acids such as glutamine, arginine, and tryptophan play a significant role in immune cell activation and immune responses and serve as immunometabolites and immunotransmitters. Glutamine has multiple roles, noteworthy of which are— it acts as substrates for synthesis of purines and pyrimidines, fuel for immune and other proliferating cells, substrate for neoglucogenesis, expression of heat-shock proteins, ATP production, and FAS. Arginine acts as a substrate for production of nitric acid, nitric oxide, polyamines, and has an essential role in wound healing, releasing of hormones and T cell, and other immune functions. Tryptophan has a positive role in cell proliferation and anabolism and is utilized in different biochemical reactions.

Therefore, amino acids are mandatory for several intracellular and intercellular functions, which enable immune cell activation, differentiation, proliferation, and a robust immune response.[11]

OVERVIEW OF IMMUNE CELLS AND RESPONSES

The following is a brief overview of immune cells and immune responses.

The immune system comprises diverse group of extremely intricate cells, each having a specific nutrient and energy requirements, obtained either from a highly efficient process of OXPHOS or from a process of glycolysis, which has a low efficiency of extraction of energy, but is a major source of substrates for biosynthesis of cellular components and various other molecules. They also have distinct types of proteins, which aid in the many dynamic and complex responses. These processes are extremely efficient in the protection and defense against various microbes and their toxins, from developing malignant tumors, other cancerous conditions, and from foreign substances. They also play a pivotal role in immune tolerance, repair of tissues, and in homeostasis. However, disturbances and dysregulations of immune cells have the potential to induce and provoke abnormalities and various complications ranging from allergies, hypersensitivity, anaphylaxis, autoimmunity, severe and excessive inflammations, infections, and overwhelming sepsis.

Immune cells form an important component of the immune system and originate from the bone marrow hematopoietic precursor cells. Under the influence of specific cytokines, they differentiate either into myeloid series (erythrocytes, monocytes, neutrophils, eosinophils, basophils, and platelets) or lymphoid series [dendritic cells (DCs), natural killer (NK) cells, and T and B lymphocytes], and depending on the types, their lifespan ranges from a few hours or days to several months.[12] The other essential components of immune system comprise a host of distinct proteins that make up the cytokines (small soluble proteins), the complement system (soluble and membrane-bound proteins), antibodies (polypeptide chains), and the innumerable assortment of receptors (intricate proteins), some of which are present on their surfaces in a very precise manner, and some of which are known as cluster of differentiation (CD). Therefore, the myriad types of immune responses depend on the type and the individual characteristics of immune cells, tissues, and organs and include physical barriers such as skin and mucus membranes. A characteristic feature of immune system is the rapid shift of the immune cells from inactive to highly activated state and depend on the availability of energy and the metabolic pathways that occur in these complex arrays of immune cells.[13] Some of the prominent features of the important immune cells, such as neutrophils, macrophages, DCs, NK cells, and lymphocytes, are as follows:

- *Neutrophils:* These short-lived lymphocytes constitute about 50–60% of white blood cells and have multilobed nuclei with abundant cytoplasmic granules. Quiescent neutrophils are activated by interleukin (IL)-1, which prolongs their lifespan from 24 hours to about 5 days and enable their rapid migration to the sites of injury and infections; they play a pivotal role in host defenses by initiating inflammation and phagocytosis. Microbial killing occurs by degranulating their lytic enzymes, generation of hydrogen peroxide, and ROS. They also release extracellular net-like traps, called neutrophil extracellular traps (NETs), made up of their mitochondrial DNA, due to lysis of mitochondria, secondary to increased ROS within them. These NETs trap and bind the microbes to expose them to a high concentration of microbicidal factors. NETs have the potential to cause tissue damage in the vicinity of their formation, which can lead to untended inflammatory cell recruitment and responses.[14]

- *Macrophages:* These immune cells are large and distributed in all body tissues and are derived from monocytes. They are tissue specific, which include alveolar macrophages (lungs), Kupffer cells (liver), microglial cells (central nervous system), and splenic macrophages, Langerhans cells (skin and mucosa), lamina propria macrophages (intestines), histiocytes (connective tissues), osteoclasts (bones), synovial A cells (joints) and peritoneal macrophages (proinflammatory), or by alternate pathways, involving anti-inflammatory cytokines, IL-4 and 13, called M2 macrophages. M1 macrophages secrete proinflammatory cytokines and are involved in recognition, phagocytosis, and destruction of microbes and tumor cells. In overactivated states, they have the potential to cause tissue damage. M2 macrophages induce anti-inflammatory effects and are essential for wound healing and repair.[15]
- *DCs:* These are highly specialized leukocytes present in all the tissues, which constantly sample their immediate environments for antigens and other molecular patterns by diverse group of structures on their surface, called pattern recognition receptors (PRRs). In the presence of foreign antigens and microbial products, DCs mature rapidly and coordinate innate and adaptive responses (which are further described below in the section of activation of T lymphocytes), in addition to recognizing the self-antigens and promoting immune tolerance.[16]
- *NK cells:* These cells, which are a part of the innate immune system, are granular lymphocytes, and respond very rapidly to a wide variety of immune challenges. They are also called group I innate lymphoid cells (ILCs) and belong to the same family as T and B lymphocytes and mount a direct toxicity, as well as by antibody-dependent cytotoxicity. They have a crucial role in the immune defense, immune-surveillance, and by targeting tumor cells and especially those infected with viruses.[17]
- *T and B lymphocytes:* These lymphocytes form a crucial component of acquired immune system. Though morphologically similar, they have distinct functions, with T cells being involved in cell-mediated B cells, which produce antibodies and form plasma cells that are involved in humoral immunity. Based on the CD found on their surfaces, T cells are further subclassified into $CD4^+$, $CD8^+$, gamma delta ($\Upsilon\delta$) T cells, and regulatory T cells (T_{regs}). Both T and B cells exist in inactive (or naïve) state and get activated on exposure to various antigens, which can be present either on the surface of infected cells (T cells), or by the antigens present on the surface of bacteria and viruses (B cells). Upon activation, they form the highly efficient effector cells and memory cells.[18]
- *Immune responses:* Immune defenses commence as soon as the physical barriers are breached, either by pathogens or tissue damage by injuries or trauma, and result in specific molecular patterns— pathogenic-associated molecular

patterns (PAMPs) or damage-associated molecular patterns (DAMPs), both of which are recognized by receptors called PRRs, which are present on the surface of the immune cells. In addition, PRRs are present within the cell cytoplasm, cell vesicles, as well as in the soluble forms within the body fluids and blood. Depending on the nature of molecular patterns (PAMPs/DAMPs), phagocytic responses, cytotoxic activation, or biochemical cascades are initiated.[19] Those which occur immediately are the innate immune responses, whereas those that develop a few days after the initial invasion or infection are the acquired or adaptive immune responses, which is an adapted response and more specific to the particular pathogen or a situation.

Innate immunities are quite efficient in eliminating pathogens and initiating the process of repair and regeneration. They include the phagocytes (neutrophils, macrophages, and DCs), NK cells, mast cells, eosinophils, and basophils. On the other hand, when innate responses are insufficient and inadequate, acquired immune responses are induced and activated to provide an effective protection, in the form of cell-mediated responses by T lymphocytes and humoral immune responses by B lymphocytes. The primary or central lymphoid organs, bone marrow and thymus, are involved in the production and processing of lymphocytes. Both T and B lymphocytes have highly specific receptors and other complex molecules on their surfaces, which allow them to recognize a wide spectrum of antigens and result in activation of dormant or quiescent lymphocytes.

- *Activation of T lymphocytes:* The proteins from the pathogenic microbes (and their toxins) are taken up and processed to smaller peptides by specialized cells called antigen-presenting cells (APCs). Important APCs are DCs, macrophages, and B cells. DCs form extremely efficient APCs. On the surface of these APCs are tiny, intricate complexes which are part of major histocompatibility complex (MHC). There are two types of MHCs, class I and II. DCs, which are the prominent form of APCs, have class II MHC molecules. Once the foreign proteins are processed by DCs, they are displayed on its surface, in conjunction class II MHC and are recognized by T cells. It is important to note that T-cell receptors (TCRs) recognize a specific antigen on the APCs, only if presented by class II MHC molecules, and are activated, generally within the draining lymph nodes. In bloodstream infections, the splenic APCs process and present the antigens. Lymph nodes, spleen, and lymphoid tissues associated with gut and other mucosal membranes [gut-associated lymphoid tissue (GALT) and mucosa-associated lymphoid tissue (MALT)], which constitute the peripheral and secondary lymphoid organs also enable antigen processing and presentations. Once activated, the T cells undergo a swift polarization into specific subsets of T helper (Th) cells—Th1, Th2, and Th17. Th1 cells form the core component of cell-mediated immunity and activate neutrophils, macrophages, CD8$^+$ cells, which initiate the process of identification and destruction of intracellular microbes (bacteria and viruses) by inducing cytolysis. They are also essential for the generation of memory T cells. Th2 cells are involved in the eradication of extracellular microbes and parasites, production of anti-inflammatory cytokines, and in the activation of B cells. Th17 cells form the main core of defending the mucosal barriers and surfaces and are also implicated in the pathogenesis of autoimmune diseases. $CD8^+$ are the effective T cells against tumor cells and intracellular microbes (viruses and bacteria). ϒδ T cells (so called because their receptors are made of ϒ and δ chains) form a smaller subset of T cells, which are present within the epithelial cells of intestines and lungs, and initiate protective effects by producing proinflammatory mediators upon activation. T_{regs} play a crucial role in homeostasis by moderating and regulating the excessive immune responses.[20,21]

- *Activation of B lymphocytes:* B cells, which constitute an essential part of acquired immune responses, produce antibodies upon activation. Antibodies, in addition, also form part of the B-cell receptors (BCRs). Different types of biochemically distinct antigens are recognized by BCRs. The antigens include a variety of proteins, lipids, carbohydrates, and other molecules, which are present in soluble forms, as well as cell-associated antigens. This process too occurs in the draining lymph nodes and also within the other components of peripheral lymphoid organs and tissues. B cell can be activated directly when antigens bind to BCRs. Complement proteins with their bound antigens accelerate the process. In addition, they can also be activated by a cell-to-cell interaction with an activated T cell. Therefore, B cells can be activated directly by antigens and also by T-cell-dependent activation. Large quantities of antibodies are secreted by activated B cells (plasma cells).[22]

Though T and B cells have about billions of receptors for numerous antigens, each of them has a highly specific receptor for a specific antigen. Soon after activation, they undergo clonal expansion, which is an energy-intense process, and each cell division takes about 8–12 hours. Hence, it takes a few days after the initial or "first" exposure for initiation of acquired immune responses takes. In addition to the effector responses by the activated lymphocytes, some of these activated T and B cells convert to memory T and B cells, which provide long-term immunity.

Therefore, the immune system has a wide reservoir of specialized cells, which interact with various pathogens, antigens, and other abnormal conditions and mount an effective protection and defense. Metabolism forms the core of these complex responses.

Metabolic Pathways in Immune Cells during Various Immune Responses

Glycolytic pathways in immune cells: Glucose is a vital energy source and glycolysis forms a crucial pathway for the activated immune cells, which have a voracious appetite for readily available glucose. The rapid availability of ATP enables phagocytosis, dendritic functions, production of cytokine, interferon gamma (IFN-γ), and other acute-phase proteins, especially by activated neutrophils, M1 macrophages, NK cells, effector T cells, and B cells, especially during clonal expansion of specific subtypes. B cells especially use glycolysis in all phases of maturation, activation, and differentiation. Additionally, glycolysis, by providing biosynthetic molecules, acts as precursors for PPP, and synthesis of nucleotides, amino acids, and fats (by providing acetyl coenzyme A) and also in the activation of mTOR pathways. Conversely, a block or reduced glycolytic pathway and uptake of glucose has the potential to result in reduced neutrophil functions, hypoinflammation, and the likelihood of immune supression.[23]

Pentose phosphate pathways in immune cells: Forms an essential biochemical route in the immune cells (including M1 macrophages, etc.) during acute inflammatory conditions and sepsis, as there is an increased demand for ROS, followed by facilitation of an effective antioxidant environment. PPP generates adequate amounts of reduced nicotinamide adenine dinucleotide phosphate (NADPH), which results in an effective production of ROS as well as glutathione, a naturally occurring antioxidant, which counteracts the free radicals.[24]

TCA and OXPHOS in immune cells: TCA and OXPHOS are the main pathways in the naïve and quiescent immune cells, including M2 macrophages. In addition, citrate, an important molecule of TCA cycle, enables production of bactericidal compounds (itaconic acid) in M1 macrophages. Succinate, another molecule from the TCA cycle, is involved in the production of hypoxia-inducible factor-1 (HIF-1) and IL-1β. In hypoxic conditions, HIF-1 regulates and activates various responses to maintain homeostasis, switching on genes to adapt to hypoxia, and also in increasing oxygen delivery. Both, TCA and OXPHOS, are the major metabolic pathways in M2 macrophages.[25]

FAO in immune cells: FAO is a common catabolic pathway and provides energy and substrates for TCA cycle and genesis of other molecules. FAO occurs in immune cells, which have a longer lifespan, such as M2 macrophages, T_{regs}, and cells involved in immune memory and immunological tolerance. Reduced FAO leads to abnormal accumulation of FAs, especially within the cardiac myocytes, leading to septic shock. Their accumulation in the macrophages (foam cells) plays a role in the development of atherosclerosis and also induces potent inflammatory responses by expressing IL-1β.[26]

FAS in immune cells: FAS has opposing actions (to FAO) within the immune cells involved in various responses. They provide subunits for synthesis of phospholipids, triglycerides, and some hormones. In the presence of inflammation and sepsis, FAS pathways are enhanced in the macrophages, DCs, and T and B cells, to support their activation, differentiation, and effector functions. A reduction in FAS has been shown to be associated with increase in immature neutrophils (band forms). Thus, FAS is a common pathway in the effector cells of the immune system to support their increased growth and metabolic needs.[27]

Amino acid pathways in immune cells: Proliferating immune cells have an increased demand for protein synthesis and opt for ways that enhance the production of ATPs, especially during activation and differentiation. Additionally, metabolites from the amino acid pathways are involved in activation of mTOR, which has a pivotal function in regulating metabolic functions, by modulating elements of glycolysis and OXPHOS. They are also essential for the generation of cytokines, enzymes, and various cofactors, and especially in providing substrates necessary for meeting the increased demand for all the rapidly proliferating immune cells. Metabolism and metabolites of amino acids are central to the various immune responses, prominent of which are glutamine, branched-chain amino acids, arginine, tryptophan, amongst others. Glutamine (along with glucose) is especially essential for phagocytosis, cytotoxic functions, induction of cytokines (IL-1, etc.), generation of nitric oxide (by enabling arginine synthesis), enhances succinate production (by promoting TCA cycle), and also promote functions of M2 macrophages. Deficiencies of essential amino acids, glutamine, and arginine are associated with decreased levels of immunoglobulins, immunosuppression, and immunoparesis, leading to overwhelming infections. Immune cell metabolism of amino acids plays a central role in immune responses.[28,29]

IMMUNOMETABOLISM IN SEPSIS

The immune system has a primary role in preventing, defending, and limiting serious infections. However, abnormal immune responses lead to sepsis as a result of disturbed and disrupted metabolism in the immune cells. Sepsis-3 defines sepsis as a life-threatening organ dysfunction caused by a severely dysregulated host response to infection.[30,31] The disorder begins with failure of the innate immune responses to clear the pathogenic organisms, which results in a massive release of inflammatory mediators by overactivity of the acquired immune responses, resulting in a serious condition called "cytokine storm." This is thought to be due to severe disruption of the interactions between metabolism and all the prominent types of immune cells. Neutrophils and M1 macrophages show an enormous shift from OXPHOS to glycolysis, with an increase in the expression of glucose transporters (GLUT 1 and 3), and an increase in PPP pathways. There is a massive expansion in the production of immature innate immune cells, the myeloid-derived suppressor cells (MDSCs). Glycolysis, glutaminolysis, and metabolism of amino acids are increased, and FAO is inhibited within the MDSCs, resulting in an increase in anti-inflammatory molecules and immunosuppression. Elevated levels of pro- and anti-inflammatory mediators lead to significant dysregulation of metabolism in the various subsets of T cells, leading to increase in apoptosis (CD4$^+$, CD8$^+$, and ϒδ T cells), B cells, and DCs. There is an increase in resistance to apoptosis in T_{regs}. Along with the increase in MDSCs, the persistence of T_{regs} contributes significantly to immune suppression. Being an energy-intense process, the amplification of these immunometabolic dysregulations lead to paucity of energy supply and defective supply of building blocks, causing ineffective effector immune responses and imperfect memory cell functions. As a consequence, there is a breakdown in the processes of pathogen eradication, with a rapid progression of the disease, reduced tissue perfusion, organ dysfunctions, and overwhelming sepsis and septic shock.[32]

CONCLUSION

The most remarkable aspect of each and every biologic function depends on cell metabolism. A highly regulated metabolism in the immune cells is a mandatory process for their normal production, differentiation, proliferation, activation, and effective function. An abnormally aberrant metabolism is the basis of dysregulated immune responses, resulting in the pathogenesis of various diseases, including sepsis. Immunometabolism, an interaction between immunology and metabolism, is a developing field of investigation evaluating the metabolism within immune cells and immune responses. Understanding the interplay of immunometabolic pathways offers a tremendous potential to strategize therapeutic interventions in various diseases, including critical illness and sepsis.

A detailed and a comprehensive description on the basic metabolic pathways, immunity in health and diseases, immunometabolic pathways, and potential therapies to target immunometabolic factors are beyond the scope of this chapter and can be appraised from the list of references and dedicated textbooks.[33]

REFERENCES

1. Sender R, Fuchs S, Milo R. Revised estimates for the number of human and bacterial cells in the body. PLoS Biology. 2016;14(8): e1002533.
2. Jung J, Zeng H, Horng T. Metabolism as a guiding force for immunity. Nat Cell Biol. 2019;21:85-93.
3. Chi H. Immunometabolism at the intersection of metabolic signalling, cell fate, and systems immunology. Cell Mol Immunol. 2022;19:299-302.
4. Brooks GA. What does glycolysis make and why is it important? J Appl Physiol. 2010;108:1450-1.
5. Martinez-Reyes I, Chandel NS. Mitochondrial TCA cycle metabolites control physiology and disease. Nat Commun. 2020;11:102.
6. Nolfi-Donegan D, Braganza A, Shiva S. Mitochondrial electron transport chain: Oxidative phosphorylation, oxidant production, and methods of measurement. Redox Biol. 2020;37:101674.
7. Britt EC, Lika J, Giese MA, Schoen TJ, Seim GL, Huang Z, et al. Switching to the cyclic pentose phosphate pathway powers the oxidative burst in activated neutrophils. Nat Metab. 2022;4:389-403.
8. Houten SM, Violante S, Ventura FV, Wanders RJA. The biochemistry and physiology of mitochondrial fatty acid β-oxidation and its genetic disorders. Annu Rev Physiol. 2016;78:23-44.
9. Beld J, Lee DJ, Burkart MD. Fatty acid biosynthesis revisited: structure elucidation and metabolic engineering. Molecular Omics. 2015;11(1):38-59.
10. Liy GY, Sabatini DM. mTOR at the nexus of nutrition, growth, ageing, and disease. Nat Rev Mol Cell Biol. 2020;21(4):183-203.
11. Miyajima M. Amino acids: Key sources for immunometabolites and immunotransmitters. Int Immunol. 2020;26(7):435-46.
12. Orkin SH, Zon LI. Hematopoiesis: An evolving paradigm for stem cell biology. Cell. 2008;132(4):631-44.
13. Carroll RG, Timmons GA, Cervantes-Silva MP, Kennedy OD, Curtis AM. Immunometabolism around the Clock. Trends Mol Med. 2019;25(7):612-25.
14. Kolaczkowska E, Kubes P. Neutrophil recruitment in health and inflammation. Nat Rev Immunol. 2013;13(3):159-75.
15. Bai J, Liu F. The Yin-Yang functions of macrophages in metabolic disorders. Life Med. 2022;1(3):319-32.
16. Patente TA, Pinho MP, Oliveira AA, Evangelista GCM, Bergami-Santos PC, Barbuto JAM. Human dendritic cells: their heterogeneity and clinical application potential in cancer immunotherapy. Front Immunol. 2019;9:3176.
17. Abel AM, Yang C, Thakar MS, Malarkannan S. Natural killer cells: development, maturation, and clinical utilization. Front Immunol. 2018;9:1869.
18. Petersone L, Ednet NM, Ovcinnikovs V, Heuts F, Ross EM, Ntavli E, et al. T-cell/B-cell collaboration and autoimmunity: an intimate relationship. Front Immunol. 2018;9:1941.
19. Zindel J, Kubes P. DAMPs, PAMPs, and LAMPs in immunity and sterile inflammation. Annu Rev Pathol. 2020;24(15):493-518.
20. La Gruta NL, Gras S, Daley SR, Thomas PG, Rossjohn J. Understanding the drivers of MHC restriction of T-cell receptors. Nat Rev Immunol. 2018;18(7):467-78.
21. Heimall J. The adaptive cellular immune response: T cells and cytokines. [online] Available from: https://www.uptodate.com/

contents/the-adaptive-cellular-immune-response-t-cells-and-cytokines [Last accessed August, 2023].
22. Ma C, Liu H, Yang S, Li H, Liao X, Kang Y. The emerging roles and therapeutic potential of B cells in sepsis. Front Pharmacol. 2022;13:1034667.
23. Makowski L, Chaib M, Rathmell JC. Immunometabolism: From basic mechanism to translation. Immunol Rev. 2020;295(1):5-14.
24. Ganeshan K, Chawla A. Metabolic regulation of immune responses. Annu Rev Immunol. 2014;32:609-34.
25. Weidemann A, Johnson RS. Biology of HIF-1alpha. Cell Death Differ. 2008;5:621-7.
26. Lusis AJ. Atherosclerosis. Nature. 2000;407:233-41.
27. O'Neill LA, Kishton RJ, Rathmell J. A guide to immunometabolism for immunologists. Nat Rev Immunol. 2016;16(9):533-65.
28. Su Y, Li Y, Zhang Y, Han S. Efficacy of alanyl glutamine in nutritional support therapy for patients with sepsis. Medicine (Baltimore). 2021;100(11):e24861.
29. Hou YC, Pai MH, Wu JM, Yang PJ, Lee PC, Chen KY, et al. Protective effects of glutamine and leucine supplementation on sepsis-induced skeletal muscle injuries. Int J Mol Sci. 2021;22(23):13003.
30. Singer M, Deutschman CS, Seymour CW, Shankar-Hari M, Annane D, Bauer M, et al. The Third International Consensus Definition for Sepsis and Septic Shock. JAMA. 2016;315(8):801-10.
31. Ghnewa YG, Fish M, Jennings A, Carter MJ, Shankar-Hari M. Goodbye SIRS? Innate, trained, and adaptive immunity and pathogenesis of organ dysfunction. Med Klin Intensivmed Notfmed. 2020;Supplement 1:S10-4.
32. Brady J, Horie S, Laffey JG. Role of adaptive immune response in sepsis. Intensive Care Med Exp. 2020;8(1):20.
33. Niels Camara OS, Alves-Filho JC, de Moraes-Vieira PMM, Andrade-Olivera V (Eds). Essential Aspects of Immunometabolism in Health and Disease, 1st edition. Switzerland AG: Springer Nature; 2022.

CHAPTER 4

Malnutrition and Body Composition Assessment in Critical Illness

Radha Reddy Chada

INTRODUCTION

According to estimates, malnutrition affects 40–50% of patients who are critically ill[1,2] and is linked to decreased immune function, longer ventilator reliance, an increase in infectious complications, and an overall increase in morbidity and mortality.[2] Additionally, during and after their initial intensive care unit (ICU) hospitalization, survivors of critical illness are more likely to develop substantial sarcopenia, or loss of muscular mass and strength. Muscle wasting, physical disability, and quality of life deficits brought on by sarcopenia can last for years.[3-6] The best post-ICU recovery and preventing of related consequences depend on identifying patients who are at risk for sarcopenia and malnutrition.

Nutritional risk is an increased likelihood of developing problems as a result of malnutrition or undernutrition. Tools have been developed and validated to identify nutrition risk in critically ill patients. Tools such as the Nutrition Risk Score-2002,[7] and the modified Nutrition Risk in Critically Ill (mNUTRIC) scoring system[8] which have been specifically developed for the ICU population have been validated in a diverse population. Most nutrition screening tools presently focus their decisions on criteria like bodyweight, body mass index (BMI), or weight change prior to hospitalization. The difficulty of BMI to discriminate between different obesity phenotypes, such as sarcopenic obesity, is one of its limitations. The clinically relevant changes in body composition, such as an increase in fluid or fat mass (FM) and/or the loss of lean body mass (LBM) in a patient who is weight-stable, may not be effectively captured by these variables especially in the elderly and obese.[9] Additionally, obtaining an accurate weight history from a critically ill patient may be difficult. The acute-phase response and changes in intravascular volume might influence laboratory data, such as albumin and other blood proteins, rendering them unreliable indicators of nutrition status in critically ill patients.[10,11] Body composition may provide a more accurate assessment of sarcopenia. In the recent years, the Global Leadership Initiative on Malnutrition (GLIM) consisting of three phenotypic and two etiologic criteria for diagnosis and grading of malnutrition has been proposed and evaluated.[12] The GLIM criteria recommend for evaluation of muscle mass by different body composition techniques which may provide a more accurate assessment of sarcopenia among different populations.

There are numerous methods to evaluate body composition, including computed tomography (CT), ultrasound, bioimpedance, dual-energy X-ray absorptiometry (DXA), and magnetic resonance imaging (MRI). Lean and adipose tissue reserves have been measured using these modalities in clinical studies, but hospitalized patients have not always had access to them because of equipment shortages and logistical challenges.[13] Accelerated loss of lean tissue reserves, including skeletal muscle (SM) mass, occurs in the context of malnutrition, sarcopenia, cachexia, elevated inflammatory response, hypermetabolic state, or any combination of these. Therefore, understanding body composition is essential to delivering the right nutritional intervention. In the ICU, nutrition evaluation based on body composition of the patient can assist to identify at-risk patients and provide optimal nutrition therapy. To assess body composition in critically ill patients, the current chapter aims to present a narrative review of the currently available and emerging technologies.

FACTORS THAT INFLUENCE BODY COMPOSITION

Fat Mass in Health

Infants are about 10-15% fat at birth. By 6 months of age, it grows to over 30%, and during early childhood, it starts to steadily diminish. The amount of total body fat rises throughout adolescence. Percent body fat increases in girls between 9 and 20 years but decreases in boys after 13 years as fat-free mass (FFM) rapidly increases. Throughout adulthood, total body fat mass (FM) steadily increases with age. The reference percentage of fat for adults varies by age, race, and sex on the assumption that the body is divided into two compartments: fat and FFM (body weight = fat + fat-free mass).[14-51]

Females accumulate greater body fat than men at birth, indicating sex distinctions in body composition. Over the course of sexual development and the adolescent growth spurt, these disparities become increasingly obvious. Males and females differ in that SM mass, total bone mineral content (especially of the limb skeleton), and FFM typically higher in men, while females have a greater body fat percentage. The gender distinctions formed throughout adolescence continue into adulthood, and as individuals age, certain aspects of their physical body composition vary substantially depending on the sex.

The amount of FFM increases throughout development, remains largely steady during adulthood, and decreases during aging. Total body bone mass is an element of FFM that rises with age as an individual grows and develops to maturity, peaks between the ages of 20 and 30 years, and then declines with age after reaching a peak. In women and men older than 50 years, there is a hormonally associated rapid decrease of bone mineral density. One such element of FFM is SM mass. Growth and development are generally phases of rapidly SM accretion, with pronounced sexual dimorphism emerging throughout adolescence. Up to the age of 30-40 years, the SM mass of an adult is mostly steady, after which the mass starts to decline. The organs of the body constitute a third part of FFM. At birth, the liver and brain each accounted for around 4.5% of total bodyweight, making them the two largest organs in the body. These percentages drop as people age until they are about 20 years old and then remain steady for the majority of a person's lifespan. The next biggest organs are the kidneys and the heart, which together make up roughly 0.45% and 0.54% of an adult's bodyweight. The evidence currently available indicates that these organs' relative sizes gradually decline with age, starting in middle life and continuing until senescence.

Skeletal Muscle Mass

In healthy young people, SM mass makes up around 40% of body weight. At older ages, SM mass drops to around 30% of values for a young adult. About 60% of the body's cell mass is made up of SM. Body cell mass and fat-free mass (FFM = body weight – fat mass) are typically regarded as two components that best describe the entire body's metabolically active tissue. One of the most challenging components to quantify is SM.

Common measurement methods to derive appendicular skeletal muscle (ASM) include DXA, CT, ultrasound, bioimpedance, and MRI. In disease and critically ill states, a measure of SM mass is frequently desired for nutritional intervention purposes.

BODY COMPOSITION AND CLINICAL OUTCOMES IN CRITICAL ILLNESS

Body composition is the compartmentalization and measurement of different parts, such as bone mass or skeleton, LBM, and FM. Generally speaking, LBM is the sum of the body's total protein, carbohydrates, non-fat lipids, soft-tissue minerals, and water.[14] Both the bone mineral portion and LBM are included in FFM. Adipose tissue, which consists of adipocytes, collagen and elastic fibers, fibroblasts, and capillaries, is included in FM. BMI and waist circumference (WC), although widely utilized and easily accessible, do not quantify LBM and SM mass, which have been found to be important determinants of outcomes in critically ill patients.[15-17] Sarcopenia, defined as both low muscle function and low muscle mass, can occur due to poor nutrition and chronic disease. Sarcopenia can be difficult to identify in individuals with obesity when simply considering BMI or bodyweight. Many of the presumptions on which the usual techniques of calculating body composition are based fall apart in the case of extreme obesity. As a result, there is a dearth of knowledge on "normative" body composition in very obese individuals, which has implications for developing effective dietary treatments.[50]

In fact, according to Moisey et al. findings, 47% of elderly patients with traumatic injuries were classified as overweight or obese according to the BMI scale, whereas only 9% of sarcopenic patients were underweight.[15] This study has huge ramifications since critically ill sarcopenic patients typically have longer ICU and hospital stays, greater mortality, and more ventilator days than patients with normal muscle mass.[15,16] Sarcopenia can develop in critically ill patients as a result of both impaired protein synthesis and muscle breakdown.[3] According to some studies, critically ill patients may lose 17–30% of their muscle mass in the first 10 days after being admitted to an ICU.[18] Compared to patients with single organ failure, patients who have multiple organ failure lose greater muscle mass.[5] Up to 5 years following an ICU stay, the combination of inherited and acquired sarcopenia might dramatically worsen physical mobility and cause long-term disability.[4] It is obvious that conventional anthropometric measurements, such as bodyweight or BMI, are insufficiently sensitive to detect sarcopenia in critically ill patients, particularly when obesity is present.[19]

CHOICE OF MODALITIES FOR BODY COMPOSITION ASSESSMENT: BIOELECTRIC IMPEDANCE ANALYSIS TECHNIQUE

Bioelectric impedance analysis (BIA) is an easy, inexpensive, and noninvasive approach to determine body composition.

BIA is based on the body's natural ability to conduct electricity. Measures of bioelectrical conductivity are inversely correlated with total body water (TBW) and high water-concentration body parts such SM and FFM. According to BIA, the body is divided into two compartments: FM and FFM (body weight = FM + FFM).[20,21] BIA is most well-known as a method for calculating body fat percentage. The present review will concentrate on important BIA concepts and clinical results in critically ill patients because other outstanding publications[20-22] have already provided a thorough description of the methods and underlying assumptions of BIA. Resistance, which is an obstacle to the passage of current, and reactance, which is the delay in conduction brought on by cell membranes, tissue surfaces, and nonionic substances are the two frequency-dependent factors which constitute up impedance.[20] In critically ill patients, resistance can be associated with the degree of edema, and reactance to the degree of severity of illness.[33]

Three different technologies of bioimpedance are currently available: single-frequency, multiple frequency, and bioimpedance spectroscopy analysis (BIS). The electrodes are commonly positioned at the wrist and ankles in SF-BIA, which uses a single frequency (50 kHz) to estimate whole-body composition. When estimating TBW in children and adults, the SF-BIA model approach results in larger errors than MF-BIA models. Conflicting findings of the estimate of extracellular water (ECW) and TBW in various age groups in the ICU have been reported for a number of chosen single-frequency BIA equations for predicting FFM.[32,33] No single equation has been validated in all groups. In critically ill patients, electrolyte shifts and alterations in the distribution of fluid between intracellular and extracellular compartments might cause the single frequency BIA's predictions to be inaccurate typically.[20,24,25] Similarly, FFM might be overstated in conditions where ECW enlargement has taken place (heart failure, renal failure, or critical illness).[26] A more precise indication of membrane integrity and water distribution between intracellular and extracellular regions is phase angle, a derived metric developed from direct measurement of resistance and reactance.[27] Studies showing a significant correlation between phase angle and survival in patients with HIV, cancer, hemodialysis, and critical illness have established phase angle as a prognostic indicator.[28-30]

The ability to quantify ECW and TBW at lower and higher frequencies makes the use of MF-BIA advantageous for improved fluid determination within body compartments.[21] Numerous MF-BIA devices are also multisegmented, which divides the body into five distinct cylinders (two upper extremities, two lower extremities, and the trunk) and, in theory, produces estimates that are more accurate while attempting to address the drawbacks of single frequency whole-body BIA.[31] The BIS method advances this by measuring impedance at a minimum of 50 frequencies from around 5 kHz to as high as 1,200 kHz. This offers a theoretical advantage over SF-BIA and MF-BIA in that BIS employs nonlinear least squares curve fitting techniques with all of the impedance data to get whole-body volume and masses instead of relying on prediction formulae. Furthermore, a more thorough measurement of TBW is possible with the use of very high frequencies. Clinical outcomes, particularly death, have been predicted using raw BIA data.[23,30,34-36] Bioimpedance has several important advantages over CT or DXA in that it enables repeated measurements to be carried out at the bedside, despite the individual-level variability. Bioimpedance measures in critically ill patients continue to show promise based on the information that is currently available. Capacitance and phase angle are two unprocessed SF-BIA measures that have been connected to disease severity. However, the variety of illnesses and fluid overload condition present in the majority of critically ill patients continue to provide challenges for bioimpedance technology. To further construct equations that will produce more precise measurements in critically ill patients and enable therapeutic therapy based on such findings, additional research is still required.

COMPUTED TOMOGRAPHY OR MAGNETIC RESONANCE IMAGING

The use of CT or MRI as a reference tool for assessing and tracking alterations in whole-body and regional body composition over time has a lot of support. This methodology does not appear to be a useful measuring tool for use in clinical screening due to the cost involved. However, it must be noted that it is feasible to assess the mass of various organs, total adipose tissue (TAT), and SM in individuals while they are alive. Whole-body multi-slice CT or MRI can be used to assess SM and TAT, including total subcutaneous adipose tissue (TSAT), visceral adipose tissue (VAT), and intermuscular adipose tissue (IMAT).[37]

In order to predict whole-body fat and FFM over a wide range of ages and ethnicities, several teams have validated the use of a single-slice regional analysis [usually mid-third lumbar (mid-L3) vertebral slice].[37-39] Additionally, sarcopenia has been detected using a single-slice CT estimation of the total psoas muscle cross-sectional area (CSA).[14] Because each tissue has a unique range of radiodensity, which describes the quantity of X-ray radiation absorbed by each element in tissue, this distinction of tissues can be achieved.[40,41] This radiodensity is then given a numerical value called the Hounsfield unit (HU) with each tissue having the following typical ranges: −29 to 150 for SM (includes psoas, erector spinae, quadrates lumborum, transverse abdominus, external and internal obliques, and rectus abdominus) and −150 to −50 for visceral, subcutaneous, and intramuscular adipose tissue.[42,43] Conceptually, the slices can detect aberrant muscle or muscle with a large amount of triglycerides. Using software to add the tissue pixels and multiply by the body surface area, the CSA (cm^2) of the detected tissue is then determined. In earlier studies, there was a strong correlation between whole-body DXA measurements and L3 total CSA, FFM, and SM.[37] In 240 ICU patients on mechanical ventilation who were admitted for at least 4 days, a retrospective study of the L3 CT imaging found that 63% of patients had low muscle area, and hospital mortality was significantly higher in sarcopenic patients than in those with normal muscle area in both females and males (47.5% vs 20.0%, and 32.3% vs 7.5%) respectively. Muscle mass, gender, and APACHE II scores all independently predicted hospital mortality in regression analysis.[44] CT scan of L3 intervertebral image of 301 patients who were admitted to the ICU over a 12-month period and noted that 35 of them had at least two CT scans that included L3 imaging[12] which were at least 10 days apart, revealed that there was an average SM decline of 0.49% per day over this time. For SM and adipose tissue CSAs, Moisey et al. examined L3 CT scan pictures of 153, 65 years and older injured elderly patients, who were hospitalized to a Level 1 trauma center.[15] They reported that 38% of the sarcopenic group were overweight, and 9% were obese, and that 71% of patients were sarcopenic at the time of ICU admission determined on CT imaging. Overall mortality was 27% with sarcopenic patients dying twofold as often as nonsarcopenic patients (32 vs 14%). Patients with sarcopenia also had a smaller duration of ventilator-free days, fewer days without being in the ICU, and a lower likelihood of being discharged home early.[15]

Few restrictions apply to CT scans. A mechanically ventilated, sedated patient who needs many support devices might pose a logistical issue while undergoing a CT scan since it demands a high radiation dosage and requires patient transport outside of the ICU. Contrarily, it is usual for critically ill patients to have had abdominal CT imaging performed at least once, if not more than once, allowing for image interpretation in hindsight.

ULTRASOUND

Based on the high-frequency sound waves' reflected amplitude and the velocity at which they traverse the body, ultrasound creates a picture. There is considerable interest in the use of ultrasound to examine SM to detect the existence of sarcopenia and/or malnutrition since it has important benefits over CT scanning, including minimal radiation exposure and the ability to be done at the bedside.[45] Although SM ultrasonography moderately correlates with other body composition measurement techniques, it has been used effectively to capture the loss of muscle mass with prolonged critical illness. It is important to note that external factors, the angle at which the probe is applied to the tissue surface and the orientation of the scanned image (longitudinal or transverse), can also significantly change the echogenicity measures.[46] Gruther et al. captured quadriceps muscle thickness among patients admitted to ICU noted a logarithmic loss of muscle mass that was quite rapid in the first 2-3 weeks and much higher than bedrest experiments conducted in healthy subjects.[47] These findings are in agreement with other studies who have also confirmed rapid decline in muscle thickness in critically ill patients.[3,18,48,49]

Ultrasound measures have been useful in identifying muscle mass loss in critically ill patients, giving healthcare professionals the chance to take action to stop ICU-acquired weakness. However, there is not yet agreement on the best way to utilize ultrasound to forecast FFM or whole-body muscle mass. Researchers have developed a variety of methods that vary in the muscle group they employ, how much underlying tissue is compressed by the ultrasound transducer, and how much muscle thickness or CSA they use. Prior to widespread usage, more sizable clinical trials will be required to create protocols that standardize the ultrasound procedures, such as muscle compression and transducer probe angle.

CONCLUSION

Since the 1990s, a variety of screening techniques have been created and put into use to help to detect patients who are malnourished because to the harmful health consequences of both sarcopenia and malnutrition. Our capacity to identify and treat patients who are at substantial nutritional risk has undergone a paradigm change as a result of the accessible availability of instruments to analyze body composition at the bedside. Among some methodological issues are the following: (1) SM mass atrophy due to bed rest coupled with fluid retention, both of which may be concealed by little change in body weight. (2) Hydration of fat-free body mass changes with disease progression or with medical/pharmacological intervention or treatment. (3) The density of fat-free body mass changes with age, disease progression, or with medical/pharmacological intervention or treatment. The absolute accuracy of approaches for assessing fatness or FFM using the two-compartment model approach in diseased or critically ill states is affected by these between-group discrepancies. Although these methods have been around for a while, there is still need for improvement in their use and validation in critically ill patients. This population also needs more study to fully understand certain unusual changes in body composition, such increases in TBW and in the very obese patients. To further develop standardized methods and prediction equations that allow for elimination of measurement errors and improved body composition measurement, bigger multicenter studies are also required. These research that result in agreement and the creation of standardized methodologies will enable better clinical outcomes correlation and broader application of body composition approaches.

REFERENCES

1. Sriram K, Mizock BA. Critical care nutrition: Are the skeletons still in the closet? Crit Care Med. 2010;38(2):690-1.
2. Heyland D, Dhaliwal R, Drover J, Gramlich L, Dodek P. Canadian clinical practice guidelines for nutrition support in mechanically ventilated, critically ill adult patients. J Parenter Enter Nutr. 2003;27(5):355-73.
3. Puthucheary ZA, Rawal J, McPhail M, Connolly B, Ratnayake G, Chan P, et al. Acute skeletal muscle wasting in critical illness. JAMA. 2013;310(15):1591-600.
4. Herridge MS, Tansey CM, Matté A, Tomlinson G, Diaz-Granados N, Cooper A, et al. Functional disability 5 years after acute respiratory distress syndrome. N Engl J Med. 2011;364(14):1293-304.
5. Paris M, Mourtzakis M. Assessment of skeletal muscle mass in critically ill patients: Considerations for the utility of computed tomography imaging and ultrasonography. Curr Opin Clin Nutr Metab Care. 2016;19(2):125-30.
6. Casaer MP. Muscle weakness and nutrition therapy in ICU. Curr Opin Clin Nutr Metab Care. 2015;18(2):162-8.
7. Kondrup J, Allison SP, Elia M, Vellas B, Plauth M. ESPEN guidelines for nutrition screening 2002. Clin Nutr. 2003;22(4):415-21.
8. Rahman A, Hasan RM, Agarwala R, Martin C, Day AG, Heyland DK. Identifying critically-ill patients who will benefit most from nutritional therapy: Further validation of the "modified NUTRIC" nutritional risk assessment tool. Clin Nutr. 2016;35(1):158-62.
9. Prado CM, Siervo M, Mire E, Heymsfield SB, Stephan BC, Broyles S, et al. A population-based approach to define body-composition phenotypes. Am J Clin Nutr. 2014;99(6):1369-77.
10. Kuzuya M, Izawa S, Enoki H, Okada K, Iguchi A. Is serum albumin a good marker for malnutrition in the physically impaired elderly? Clin Nutr. 2007;26(1):84-90.
11. Gabay C, Kushner I. Acute-phase proteins and other systemic responses to inflammation. N Engl J Med. 1999;340(6):448-54.
12. Braunschweig CA, Sheean PM, Peterson SJ, Gomez Perez S, Freels S, Troy KL, et al. Exploitation of diagnostic computed tomography scans to assess the impact of nutritional support on body composition changes in respiratory failure patients. JPEN J Parenter Enteral Nutr. 2014;38(7):880-5.
13. Cederholm T, Jensen GL, Correia MITD, Gonzalez MC, Fukushima R, Higashiguchi T, et al. GLIM criteria for the diagnosis of malnutrition - a consensus report from the global clinical nutrition community. J Cachexia Sarcopenia Muscle. 2019;10(1):207-17.

14. Prado CMM, Heymsfield SB. Lean tissue imaging. JPEN J Parenter Enteral Nutr. 2014;38(8):940-53.
15. Moisey LL, Mourtzakis M, Cotton BA, Premji T, Heyland DK, Wade CE, et al. Skeletal muscle predicts ventilator-free days, ICU-free days, and mortality in elderly ICU patients. Crit Care. 2013;17(5):R206.
16. Paris MT, Mourtzakis M, Day A, Leung R, Watharkar S, Kozar R, et al. Validation of bedside ultrasound of muscle layer thickness of the quadriceps in the critically ill patient (VALIDUM Study): A prospective multicenter study. J Parenter Enter Nutr. 2017;41(2):171-80.
17. Antoun S, Baracos VE, Birdsell L, Escudier B, Sawyer MB. Low body mass index and sarcopenia associated with dose-limiting toxicity of sorafenib in patients with renal cell carcinoma. Ann Oncol. 2010;21(8):1594-8.
18. Parry SM, El-Ansary D, Cartwright MS, Sarwal A, Berney S, Koopman R, et al. Ultrasonography in the intensive care setting can be used to detect changes in the quality and quantity of muscle and is related to muscle strength and function. J Crit Care. 2015;30(5):1151.e9-1151.e14.
19. Mundi MS, Patel JJ, Martindale R. Body Composition Technology: Implications for the ICU. Nutr Clin Pract. 2019;34(1):48-58.
20. Mulasi U, Kuchnia AJ, Cole AJ, Earthman CP. Bioimpedance at the bedside: Current applications, limitations, and opportunities. Nutr Clin Pract. 2015;30(2):180-93.
21. Kyle UG, Bosaeus I, De Lorenzo AD, Deurenberg P, Elia M, Gómez JM, et al. Bioelectrical impedance analysis—part I: Review of principles and methods. Clin Nutr. 2004;23(5):1226-43.
22. Lukaski HC. Biological indexes considered in the derivation of the bioelectrical impedance analysis. Am J Clin Nutr. 1996; 64(3):397S-404S.
23. Azevedo ZM, Moore DC, de Matos FA, Fonseca VM, Peixoto MV, Gaspar-Elsas MI, et al. Bioelectrical impedance parameters in critically ill children: Importance of reactance and resistance. Clin Nutr. 2013;32(5):824-9.
24. Ellis KJ, Bell SJ, Chertow GM, Chumlea WC, Knox TA, Kotler DP, et al. Bioelectrical impedance methods in clinical research: A follow-up to the NIH technology assessment conference. Nutrition. 1999;15(11):874-80.
25. Earthman CP, Matthie JR, Reid PM, Harper IT, Ravussin E, Howell WH. A comparison of bioimpedance methods for detection of body cell mass change in HIV infection. J Appl Physiol. 2000;88(3):944-56.
26. Savalle M, Gillaizeau F, Maruani G, Puymirat E, Bellenfant F, Houillier P, et al. Assessment of body cell mass at bedside in critically ill patients. Am J Physiol—Endocrinol Metab. 2012;303(3):E389-96.
27. Barbosa-Silva MCG, Barros AJ, Wang J, Heymsfield SB, Pierson RN. Bioelectrical impedance analysis: Population reference values for phase angle by age and sex. Am J Clin Nutr. 2005;82(1):49-52.
28. Schwenk A, Beisenherz A, Römer K, Kremer G, Salzberger B, Elia M. Phase angle from bioelectrical impedance analysis remains an independent predictive marker in HIV-infected patients in the era of highly active antiretroviral treatment. Am J Clin Nutr. 2000;72(2):496-501.
29. Toso S, Piccoli A, Gusella M, Menon D, Bononi A, Crepaldi G, et al. Altered tissue electric properties in lung cancer patients as detected by bioelectric impedance vector analysis. Nutr Burbank Los Angel Cty Calif. 2000;16(2):120-4.
30. Máttar JA. Application of total body bioimpedance to the critically ill patient. Brazilian group for bioimpedance study. New Horiz Baltim Md. 1996;4(4):493-503.
31. Shafer KJ, Siders WA, Johnson LK, Lukaski HC. Validity of segmental multiple-frequency bioelectrical impedance analysis to estimate body composition of adults across a range of body mass indexes. Nutrition. 2009;25(1):25-32.
32. Foley K, Keegan M, Campbell I, Murby B, Hancox D, Pollard B. Use of single-frequency bioimpedance at 50 kHz to estimate total body water in patients with multiple organ failure and fluid overload. Crit Care Med. 1999;27(8):1472-7.

33. Bracco D, Revelly JP, Berger MM, Chiolero RL. Bedside determination of fluid accumulation after cardiac surgery using segmental bioelectrical impedance. Crit Care Med. 1998;26(6):1065-70.
34. Moissl UM, Wabel P, Chamney PW, Bosaeus I, Levin NW, Bosy-Westphal A, et al. Body fluid volume determination via body composition spectroscopy in health and disease. Physiol Meas. 2006;27(9):921-33.
35. Shime N, Ashida H, Chihara E, Kageyama K, Katoh Y, Yamagishi M, et al. Bioelectrical impedance analysis for assessment of severity of illness in pediatric patients after heart surgery. Crit Care Med. 2002; 30(3):518-20.
36. Dabrowski W, Kotlinska-Hasiec E, Schneditz D, Zaluska W, Rzecki Z, De Keulenaer B, et al. Continuous veno-venous hemofiltration to adjust fluid volume excess in septic shock patients reduces intra-abdominal pressure. Clin Nephrol. 2014;82:41-50.
37. Mourtzakis M, Prado CMM, Lieffers JR, Reiman T, McCargar LJ, Baracos VE. A practical and precise approach to quantification of body composition in cancer patients using computed tomography images acquired during routine care. Appl Physiol Nutr Metab Physiol Appl Nutr Metab. 2008;33(5):997-1006.
38. Shen W, Punyanitya M, Wang Z, Gallagher D, St-Onge MP, Albu J, et al. Visceral adipose tissue: Relations between single-slice areas and total volume. Am J Clin Nutr. 2004;80(2):271-8.
39. Shen W, Punyanitya M, Wang Z, Gallagher D, St-Onge MP, Albu J, et al. Total body skeletal muscle and adipose tissue volumes: Estimation from a single abdominal cross-sectional image. J Appl Physiol. 2004;97(6):2333-8.
40. Hounsfield GN. Computed medical imaging. Med Phys. 1980;7(4):283-90.
41. Patel J, Baruah D, Shahir K. A novel computed tomography method to detect normal from abnormal psoas muscle: A pilot feasibility study. JCSM Clin Rep. 2017;2(1):e00014-e00020.
42. Aubrey J, Esfandiari N, Baracos VE, Buteau FA, Frenette J, Putman CT, et al. Measurement of skeletal muscle radiation attenuation and basis of its biological variation. Acta Physiol Oxf Engl. 2014;210(3):489-97.
43. Goodpaster BH, Thaete FL, Kelley DE. Composition of skeletal muscle evaluated with computed tomography. Ann NY Acad Sci. 2000;904(1):18-24.
44. Weijs PJ, Looijaard WG, Dekker IM, Stapel SN, Girbes AR, Oudemans-van Straaten HM, et al. Low skeletal muscle area is a risk factor for mortality in mechanically ventilated critically ill patients. Crit Care. 2014;18(1):R12.
45. Teigen LM, Kuchnia AJ, Mourtzakis M, Earthman CP. The use of technology for estimating body composition: strengths and weaknesses of common modalities in a clinical setting. Nutr Clin Pract. 2017;32(1):20-9.
46. Harris-Love MO, Seamon BA, Teixeira C, Ismail C. Ultrasound estimates of muscle quality in older adults: reliability and comparison of Photoshop and ImageJ for the grayscale analysis of muscle echogenicity. PeerJ. 2016;4:e1721.
47. Gruther W, Benesch T, Zorn C, Paternostro-Sluga T, Quittan M, Fialka-Moser V, et al. Muscle wasting in intensive care patients: Ultrasound observation of the M. quadriceps femoris muscle layer. J Rehabil Med. 2008; 40(3):185-9.
48. Saseedharan S, Chada RR, Rambhad S, Bhurke A, Mathew E, Paradkar K, et al. Muscle Mass Loss in Mechanically Ventilated Critically Ill Patients in Intensive Care Unit. Muscles, Ligaments Tendons J. 2023;13(2):290-6.
49. Reid CL, Campbell IT, Little RA. Muscle wasting and energy balance in critical illness. Clin Nutr. 2004;23(2):273-80.
50. Gallagher D, DeLegge M. Body composition (sarcopenia) in obese patients: implications for care in the intensive care unit. JPEN J Parenter Enteral Nutr. 2011;35 (5 Suppl):21S-8S.
51. Heymsfield SB, Lohman TG, Wang Z, Going SB. Human Body Composition. Champaign, US: Human Kinetics; 2005.

CHAPTER 5

Nutritional Assessment in Critical Illness

Daphnee Lovesley

▮ INTRODUCTION

The prevalence of malnutrition in critically ill patients ranges between 38 and 78%.[1] Malnutrition is independently associated with the patients' increased morbidity, mortality, and hospital-related cost.[1] The increased dependency on mechanical ventilation, length of hospital stay, intensive care unit (ICU) readmission, rate of infection, and risk of hospital mortality associated with undernutrition make it a predicament in the care of ICU patients.[2,3] In addition to poor clinical outcomes, patients experience worsened physical function and long-term disability up to 5 years post-ICU stay.[4,5] Yet, studies associating malnutrition with poor clinical outcomes in the ICU often have contrary results due in part to the inappropriate diagnosis of malnutrition. Despite the prevalence of malnutrition in acute-care hospitals and long-term care centers, a national and global consensus on nutrition screening and malnutrition diagnosis is still lacking.

Early identification and relevant nutritional intervention in malnourished patients have frequently been shown to decrease hospital stay, infectious complications, and overall healthcare costs.[6] While assessing nutrition status is crucial in identifying malnutrition, the recommended indicators for stratifying malnutrition have not been in regular use in routine clinical practice across healthcare settings. There is no gold standard tool for nutritional assessment in critically ill patients to date. Although numerous nutrition screening, nutrition assessment, and diagnosis tools are available, this chapter will target the most common inpatient nutrition screening and malnutrition diagnosis tools for adults that have been validated through widely accepted research.

▮ NUTRITION SCREENING

Nutrition screening is the process of identifying patients who may have a nutrition diagnosis and benefit from nutrition assessment and intervention by a registered dietitian nutritionist (RDN).[7]

Nutritional Risk Screening 2002

Kondrup et al., as part of an ESPEN working group, developed the nutrition risk screening 2002 (NRS-2002) to formulate a screening tool using retrospective analysis of controlled trials that featured nutrition characteristics of participants and outcomes of nutrition interventions.[8] Kondrup et al. reviewed 128 studies and developed a system that used the severity of disease and nutrition status to predict those who would benefit from nutrition support.

The NRS-2002 is used to identify ICU patients at high nutrition risk and includes age, food intake, weight loss, body mass

TABLE 1: Nutritional Risk Screening 2002.

Questions	Points
Does the patient have an impaired nutrition status?	
Weight loss >5% in 3 months or food intake below 50–75% of normal requirements in the preceding week	1
Weight loss >5% in 2 weeks or BMI of 18.5–20.5 with an impaired general condition or food intake 25–50% of normal requirements in the preceding week	2
Weight loss >5% in 1 month (>15% in 3 months) or BMI <18.5 with impaired general condition or food intake 0–25% of normal requirements in the preceding week	3
Rate the severity of the disease, to account for increased needs and stress metabolism	
Normal nutrition requirements	0
Hip fracture, chronic illness, or acute complications such as cirrhosis, COPD, chronic hemodialysis, diabetes, or cancer	1
Major abdominal surgery, stroke, severe pneumonia, or hematologic malignancy	2
Head injury, bone marrow transplant, and intensive care patients	3

Note: To calculate the total score, find the score (0–3) for impaired nutrition status by choosing the variable with the highest score and finding the score for the severity of disease. Add the two scores together. Add 1 to the total score if the patient is ≥70 years of age. If the age-corrected score is ≥3, it is recommended to start nutrition support. (BMI: body mass index; COPD: chronic obstructive pulmonary disease)

index (BMI), and disease severity[9] **(Table 1)**. It has been validated mainly in hospitalized patients.[10] In addition, a score of >5 on admission has predicted ICU mortality.[9]

The European Society for Parenteral and Enteral Nutrition (ESPEN) had recommended NRS-2002 for all hospitalized patients and ASPEN for all critically ill patients.[11,12] This tool identifies patients who could benefit from nutrition support and does not identify the risk of malnutrition.

Malnutrition Screening Tool

Ferguson et al. 1999 originally developed the malnutrition screening tool (MST) for use in medical and surgical patients. Ferguson and the team reviewed 21 questions and chose the combination of questions that produced the highest specificity and sensitivity for the screening tool. The selected questions included are tabulated in **Table 2**.[13]

TABLE 2: Malnutrition screening tool.

Questions	Points
Have you recently lost weight without trying?	
No	0
Unsure	2
If yes, how much weight have you lost?	
2–13 lb (0.9–5.9 kg)	1
14–23 lb (6.4–10.4 kg)	2
24–33 lb (10.9–15 kg)	3
Have you been eating poorly because of a decreased appetite?	
No	0
Yes	1

Note: Add score for weight loss and appetite for final malnutrition screen tool (MST) score. MST score of 0–1: not at malnutrition risk; if the length of stay exceeds 7 days, rescreen and repeat as needed. MST score of 2 or more: at malnutrition risk; rapidly implementing nutrition interventions. Perform nutrition consult within 24–72 hours, depending on risk.

The MST is the recommended screening tool for all care settings by the academy of nutrition and dietetics (AND).[14] The MST was originally validated against the Subjective Global Assessment (SGA) and had a high agreement between interprofessional ratings (RDs and other non-nutrition professionals) that used the tool. Patients who were identified to be at risk for malnutrition with the MST had a significantly longer length of hospital stay. The AND rates the MST as having moderate overall validity with good generalizability, moderate agreement and moderate reliability, and strong quality of evidence.[14] The subjective quality of the questions asked in MST is a weakness, making it ineffective in noncommunicative patients. This is a common issue with the most screening tools in an inpatient setting.

Mininutrition Assessment

In 1996, the mininutrition assessment (MNA) was developed as part of the standard geriatric evaluation to assess nutrition status by the coordinated endeavor of the Centre for Internal Medicine and Clinical Gerontology of Toulouse, the Clinical Nutrition Program at the University of New Mexico, and the Nestlé Research Institute in Switzerland. The 18 components of MNA with subjective and objective measures are separated into four groups: anthropometrics, general assessment, nutrition assessment, and self-assessment take <15 minutes to complete with a maximum score of 30. Hence, the MNA—short form (SF) was also developed for low-risk patients and is faster to complete, containing only six sections with a high score of 14 **(Table 3)**.[15] The ESPEN recommends MNA be used for older adults (aged >65 years). Although the MNA was originally designed as a nutrition assessment tool, it is frequently used as a screening tool,

TABLE 3: Mininutritional assessment—short form.

Questions	Points
A. *Has food intake declined over the past 3 months because of a loss of appetite, digestive problems, or chewing or swallowing difficulties?*	
Severe decrease in food intake	0
Moderate decrease in food intake	1
No decrease in food intake	2
B. *Weight loss during the past 3 months*	
Weight loss of >3 kg (5.5 lb)	0
Does not know the amount of weight loss	1
Weight loss between 1 and 3 kg (2.2–6.6 lb)	2
No weight loss	3
C. *Mobility*	
Chair- or bedbound	0
Able to get out of bed/chair but does not go out	1
Goes out	2
D. *Has the patient experienced psychological stress or acute disease in the past 3 months?*	
Yes	0
No	1
E. *Neuropsychological problems*	
Severe dementia or depression	0
Mild dementia	1
No psychological problems	2
F1. *BMI,[a] kg/m^2*	
<19	0
19 to <21	1
21 to <23	2
≥23	3
F2. *CC*	
<31 cm	0
≥31 cm	3

Note: Maximum score is 14 points. Normal nutrition status, 12–14 points. At risk for malnutrition, 8–11 points. Malnourished, 0–7 points.
(BMI: body mass index; CC: calf circumference)
[a]If BMI is not available, replace question F1 with question F2. Do not answer F2, if F1 is completed.

specifically the MNA-SF. The MNA-SF has also been validated separately against the MNA.[15]

NUTRITION ASSESSMENT

Subjective Global Assessment

Detsky et al. first discussed SGA as a nutrition assessment tool in the 1980s to evaluate the nutritional status at the bedside by analyzing dietary and medical history, weight changes and anthropometrics, and laboratory values.[16,17] The SGA was designed to evaluate the nutrition risk of surgical patients with infectious complications, but it is now widely utilized in all healthcare settings including critically ill patients.[18-20] The SGA depends heavily on clinical skills and the knowledge of the practitioner utilizing it since the tool does not use body composition analysis.

Subjective global assessment comprises an evaluation of the following which is depicted in **Figure 1**.

Researchers in Turkey evaluated the SGA in >100 patients admitted for gastrointestinal surgeries and found it to be efficient and effective in the diagnosis of protein-calorie malnutrition (PCM).[18]

Nutrition Risk in the Critically Ill

Heyland et al. developed the nutrition risk in the critically ill (NUTRIC) score to determine which critically ill patients would benefit most from aggressive nutrition support, and it is not considered a traditional screening tool. The conceptual model originally used to develop the NUTRIC score was by linking starvation, inflammation, nutrition status, and clinical outcomes. A secondary analysis

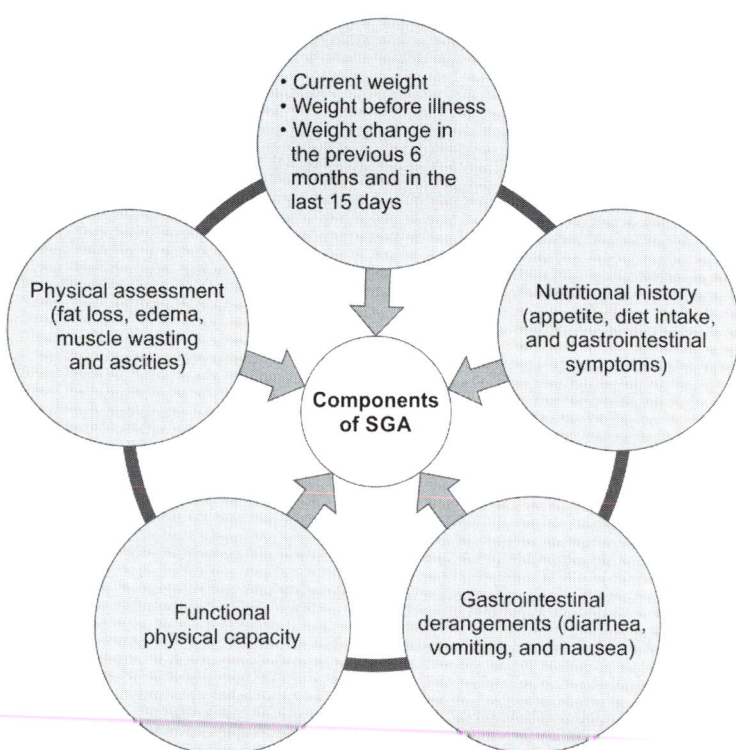

Fig. 1: Components of subjective global assessment (SGA).

of a prospective, observational study in three medical/surgical ICUs was completed by this group. The study evaluated the significance of a multitude of subjective and objective criteria on mortality and ventilator-free days. The combination of age, Acute Physiology, and Chronic Health Evaluation II (APACHE II) score, Sequential Organ Failure Assessment (SOFA) score, number of comorbidities, days from hospital to ICU admission, and interleukin-6 (IL-6) were found to be the best predictors of clinical outcomes. If IL-6 is not available, a modified NUTRIC can also be used. High malnutrition risk is associated with a NUTRIC score ≥6 leading to worse clinical outcomes and ratifying aggressive nutrition support. A score <6 indicates low malnutrition risk. A modified NUTRIC score ≥5 is associated with the same worsened clinical outcomes.[21] The American Society for Parenteral and Enteral Nutrition (ASPEN) recommends the NUTRIC score to screen critically ill patients.[12]

In Heyland and team's original publication, a high NUTRIC score was positively correlated with 28-day mortality and those who achieved their caloric targets showed attenuation in mortality risk. There was no benefit in those with lower NUTRIC scores.[21] Several studies have validated the NUTRIC score in other countries also and the results corroborated the association with 28-day mortality.[22,23]

The NUTRIC score is designed to quantify the risk of critically ill patients developing adverse events that may be modified by aggressive nutrition therapy. The score of 1–10 is based on six variables that are explained below. The scoring system is shown in **Tables 4 to 6**.

Global Leadership Initiative in Malnutrition

Despite numerous published diagnostic criteria, malnutrition diagnosis is still difficult. To address this problem, a varied group of clinicians with a strong experience in nutrition developed the Global Leadership Initiative in Malnutrition (GLIM) in 2016.

TABLE 4: NUTRIC score variables.

Variable	Range	Points
Age	<50	0
	50–<75	1
	≥75	2
APACHE-II	<15	0
	15–<20	1
	20–28	2
	≥28	3
SOFA	<6	0
	6–<10	1
	≥10	2
Number of comorbidities	0–1	0
	≥2	1
Days from hospital to ICU admission	0–<1	0
	≥1	1
IL-6	0–<400	0
	≥400	1

(APACHE II: Acute Physiology, and Chronic Health Evaluation II; ICU: intensive care unit; IL-6: interleukin-6; NUTRIC: nutrition risk in the critically ill; SOFA: Sequential Organ Failure Assessment)

TABLE 5: NUTRIC score scoring system: if IL-6 available.

Sum of points	Category	Explanation
6–10	High score	• Associated with worse clinical outcomes (mortality and ventilation) • These patients are the most likely to benefit from aggressive nutrition therapy
0–5	Low score	These patients have a low malnutrition risk

(IL-6: interleukin-6; NUTRIC: nutrition risk in the critically ill)

TABLE 6: NUTRIC score scoring system: If no IL-6 available.*		
Sum of points	**Category**	**Explanation**
5–9	High score	• Associated with worse clinical outcomes (mortality and ventilation) • These patients are the most likely to benefit from aggressive nutrition therapy
0–4	Low score	These patients have a low malnutrition risk

(IL-6: interleukin-6; NUTRIC: nutrition risk in the critically ill)
*It is acceptable to not include IL-6 data when it is not routinely available; it was shown to contribute very little to the overall prediction of the NUTRIC score.

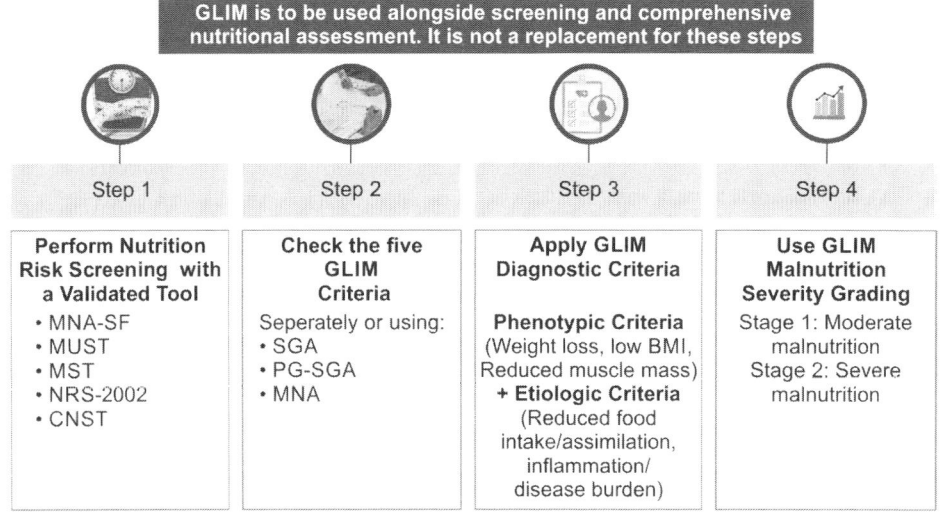

Fig. 2: Steps for diagnosing malnutrition the Global Leadership Initiative on Malnutrition (GLIM) framework is to be used alongside nutritional screening and assessment; it is not a replacement for these steps.
(BMI: body mass index; CNST: Canadian nutrition screening tool; MNA-SF: mininutrition assessment-short form; MST: malnutrition screening tool; MUST: malnutrition universal screening; NRS: nutrition risk screening; PG-SGA: patent generated-subjective global assessment)
Source: Adapted from Prado et al.[27]

The GLIM published a set of evidence-based, clinically relevant criteria to be used in conjunction with a comprehensive nutritional assessment or validated assessment tools, like the SGA, to diagnose adult malnutrition in any healthcare setting **(Fig. 2)**.[24,25]

The GLIM tool analyzes weight loss, muscle mass, BMI, food intake, and inflammation or disease burden, and classifies the data into two groups: phenotypical and etiological markers **(Table 7)**.[26]

Weight loss, reduced muscle mass, and a low BMI are phenotypic characteristics that are classified as moderate, or severe. The etiologic criteria which contribute to the diagnosis include reduced oral intake and inflammatory processes but are more focused on directing the intervention needed and helping to predict clinical outcomes.[26] To adequately diagnose PCM using GLIM, clinicians need at least one criterion to be met in both phenotypic and etiologic categories.

TABLE 7: Global Leadership Initiative in Malnutrition (GLIM) criteria.	
Criteria	
Phenotypic criteria	
Unintended weight loss	
Moderate malnutrition	5–10% in <6 months or 10–20% in >6 months
Severe malnutrition	>10% in <6 months or >20% in >6 months
Low BMI	
Moderate malnutrition	<20 if <70 years of age or <18.5 if <70 years of age
Severe malnutrition	<22 if >70 years of age or <20 in >70 years of age
Reduced muscle mass[a]	
Moderate malnutrition	Reduced by objective measures and/or physical examination
Severe malnutrition	Severe deficit (per validated assessment methods)
Etiologic criteria	
Reduced nutrition intake	<50% of requirements in >1 week; any reduction in >2 weeks; chronic GI disorders with adverse nutrition impact
Inflammation	Chronic disease; acute disease; injury with severe systemic inflammation; and socioeconomic/environmental starvation

Note: Malnutrition diagnosis requires at least one phenotypic criterion and one etiologic criterion. The severity of malnutrition is based on phenotypic criteria only and requires one phenotypic criterion that meets the threshold of moderate or severe malnutrition.
(BMI: body mass index; GI: gastrointestinal)
[a]Validated assessment methods of muscle mass include dual-energy X-ray absorptiometry, bioelectrical impedance analysis, ultrasound, computed tomography or magnetic resonance imaging, calf or arm circumference measurement, and physical examination findings with calibrated handgrip strength.

The GLIM criteria are frequently used in surgical settings. The use of phenotypic criterion in GLIM, i.e., body composition—reduced muscle mass may lead to a greater number of patients identified as having malnutrition, which may otherwise be undetected if screened by other diagnostic tools. Skeletal muscle loss is a defining criterion of malnutrition and frailty. Novel direct and indirect approaches to assess muscle mass in clinical settings may facilitate the identification of patients with or at risk for malnutrition.

Clinical Approaches for Assessing Muscle Mass and Muscle Strength

The nutrition care process in critical care should include measuring muscle mass as a crucial step. When body composition measures are not accessible, doctors in most clinical settings rely on physical examination and anthropometry (e.g., mid-upper arm circumference and calf circumference) to determine muscle loss. These stand-in methods can aid doctors in the early detection of high-risk individuals and prompt intervention to lessen or stop muscle loss. Handgrip strength and physical performance tests (such as the sit-to-stand test and gait speed), which are widely used to evaluate muscular function in the diagnosis of sarcopenia and frailty, should not be utilized as substitutes for measurements of muscle mass (i.e., quantity).[28-31]

Calf Circumference

The direct and indirect measures of skeletal muscle mass are highly correlated with anthropometric measures like calf circumference and thus it is useful in assessing the muscle mass component of the malnutrition and sarcopenia diagnosis.[30-34] In 2019, Asian Working Group[29] and GLIM Body Composition Working Group[30,31] endorsed calf circumference as a screening tool for case finding in different populations when body composition techniques are not available. Additionally, the ability to detect age-related loss of muscle mass appears to be more sensitive in the calf circumference than upper arm circumferences.[33,34] In both inpatient and outpatient settings, measuring calf circumference is a useful tool, but several confounding variables might alter measurement and interpretation, including age, BMI, ethnicity, and edema.

In adults, calf circumference can be used by applying a simple adjustment factor before correlating it to sex-specific cut-off values.[35] Notably, persons with a BMI <18.5 kg/m² who have lost weight or muscle should not be adjusted for BMI, especially in aging and clinical populations. This is because adjustment factors for individuals with low BMI (i.e., BMI <18.5 kg/m²) were generated from "healthy" adults (population-based study), who accounted for only 2% of the overall sample analyzed. The adjustment factor (rounded value: þ 4.0 cm) for this BMI category was thus developed to impede underestimation of calf muscle in healthy adults when using raw measurements, allowing a direct comparison with suggested cut-off values.[35] For older adults and clinical populations presenting with a BMI <18.5 kg/m² who are suspected to have weight or muscle losses, no adjustment value should be applied, as low muscle mass could be concealed if the adjustment factor is applied. Notably, for lower extremity edema also adjustment factors are available.[36] However, as compared to other body composition tests,

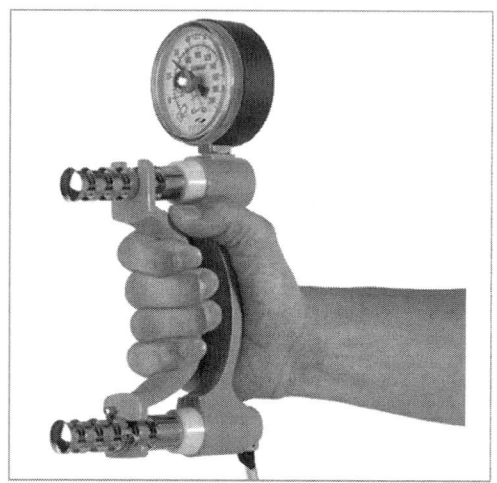

Fig. 3: Handgrip dynamometer.

calf circumference may not be able to detect slight changes in muscle mass, precluding its application in short-term follow-up.

Handgrip Strength

Handgrip strength (HGS) is a simple, bedside, and noninvasive tool to assess muscle strength of the upper extremities and thus, muscle function in clinical practice.[37] Muscle function can be altered by muscle depletion (or wasting) from immobility or sarcopenia secondary to chronic inflammation or aging.

A handgrip dynamometer **(Fig. 3)** is used to measure HGS and provides a surrogate measure of overall muscle strength.[38,39] Patients sat in a chair or bed with the arm by their side of the body and the forearm bent at the elbow to an angle of 90° and unsupported.[40]

Several studies have reported associations between HGS at admission or during hospitalization and postoperative complications, prolonged length of stay, mortality, or impaired health-related quality of life.[41-47]

Allard et al. recruited >1,000 patients from 18 acute care hospitals in Canada and demonstrated that HGS was an independent predictor of outcomes for malnutrition[48] and was associated with 30-day readmission to hospital and SGA.[49] Lower HGS at discharge was associated with 30-day readmission. Identifying patients who have lower HGS for their age and gender and individualizing discharge nutrition care plan may improve the patient's nutritional status and strength as well as reduce the risk of readmission within 30 days.[49]

McNicholl et al., in 2019, demonstrated that HGS is a more practical functional measure for use in a clinical nutrition assessment at the bedside than the 5 m in acute care medical patients. HGS was substantially associated with food intake and barriers to food intake and could be completed on almost all patients and suggesting its potential use for enhancing the clinical nutrition assessment.[50] Handgrip strength may be able to predict the decline in nutrition status before other signs of clinical compromise are apparent.[51]

Sultan et al.[52] found that impaired HGS (<85%) of normal predicted values was associated with possible postoperative complications such as the increased length of hospital stay, higher readmission, and mortality rates.

Advances in Muscle Mass Assessment: Technical Approaches

In clinical and research applications, measuring body composition is crucial to identify patients with low muscle mass or muscle loss and to evaluate the effectiveness of anabolic interventions. The BMI, which is a frequent measure used in clinical settings, is not a good surrogate for determining body composition since it fails to reflect muscle health.[53] Many body composition procedures can be used to assess or estimate muscle mass.[30,31] Each method has unique benefits, drawbacks, and factors to be taken into account. The validity, safety (e.g., radiation exposure), feasibility, and practicality are a few of these factors.[27,54] In inpatient and outpatient settings between research and clinical applications, there may be differences in the overall performance of commonly used techniques. For instance, magnetic resonance imaging (MRI) precisely assesses muscle mass throughout the body, and magnetic resonance-based methods (such as spectroscopy) can be utilized to assess intra- and extracellular lipid content as indicators of muscle composition.[55,56] Although these methods are helpful for research, they are not presently accessible in clinical settings. However, improvements in data collection and analysis may soon make those methods applicable in clinical settings in the future. In research settings, computed tomography scans of selected sites are often used based on clinically obtained images (i.e., from patient's medical records); however, due to high radiation exposure, collecting these images solely for muscle mass assessment is not indicated prospectively. Finally, anthropometry can be considered useful in clinical settings as a marker of muscle mass; it does not measure body composition. Although accessibility and affordability of anthropometric measurements are significant factors, the technique performs poorly as a research tool.

Bioelectrical Impedance Analysis and Phase Angle

Using population-, equation-, and device-specific prediction equations, bioelectrical impedance analysis (BIA) estimates muscle mass; however, when applied to specific patients, these equations may be a potential source of errors.[57,58] Phase angle (PhA), a BIA value obtained from resistance and reactance measurements, is an alternate approach that is emerging as a marker of aberrant body composition. Phase angle has also been linked to indicators of oxidative stress and inflammation.[59]

Measurements from BIA can differ depending on sex, age, and body composition. Along with other physical state changes after ICU admission, changes in body hydration can affect cellular resistance and consequently PhA.[60] In a mixed cohort of medical and surgical, acute, and elective ICU patients, BIA-derived PhA served as an independent predictor of 1-year mortality following ICU admission.[61]

According to research, PhA is related to muscle area and composition and is linked to a higher risk of dysmobility syndrome, which is determined by a score made up of six factors, including osteoporosis, low lean mass, a history of falls, a slow gait speed, low handgrip strength, and a high-fat mass.[57,62]

Furthermore, a systematic review found the prevalence of sarcopenia was higher in patients with low PhA.[63] As the cut-off values of low PhA are population and device-specific, they cannot be used interchangeably. In addition, factors affecting the fluid balance (extracellular and intracellular water) can also impact the PhA measures,[64,65] including obesity, edema, physical activity, and other factors linked to disease. As low PhA may be because of alterations in cell mass and hydration, or impaired cellular function related to disease (e.g., patients with a BMI >40 kg/m^2 showing lower PhA).[66]

Ultrasound

The bedside ultrasound (US) has recently emerged as a tool to evaluate muscle loss in hospitalized and ICU patients as it is widely available, simple to learn and perform,[67] affordable, and minimally invasive.

Due to these benefits, it may be used by bedside clinicians such as RDNs to assess muscle mass. The US can be used to measure the thickness of the muscle mass layer at various body locations, such as the mid-upper arm, forearm, and quadriceps.[5,68-72] The quadriceps muscle is the most often measured site because it represents total LBM[17,73] and it can be easily accessed in majority of the ICU patients, and it corresponds well with ICU LOS.[71]

During the first week of hospitalization in the ICU, serial ultrasound measurements of the quadriceps muscle's cross-sectional area indicated early and rapid muscle loss, which is quantitatively more significant in extremely ill patients.[74] Serial measurements help to identify changes that may occur in response to treatments as well as the amount of muscle loss from baseline. Some studies have mentioned RDNs as the principal clinicians using the US to assess LBM in critically ill patients.[5,68,69,71,72,75] It is rational to train RDNs to conduct bedside US measures for determining muscle mass since dietitians constantly evaluate and monitor ICU patients' nutritional status and can directly include US study measurements into the patient's nutrition evaluation and consequent treatment plan as needed.

The B-mode ultrasonography technique can be used to noninvasively identify myofiber necrosis and fascial inflammation in critically ill patients. In the subacute phase of fasciitis, macrophages predominate and typically follow muscle necrosis. Further research is needed on the pathophysiology underpinning fascial and muscular inflammation and necrosis and as well as the impact of these qualitative changes in skeletal muscle on early mobilization, rehabilitation, and subsequent functional debility.[76]

Due to recent advancements in ultrasound technology, it is now possible to obtain measurements of muscle thickness and architecture that are equal to those obtained with conventional US devices in a pocket-sized package.[77] However, its extensive application in clinical practice remains limited by the absence of standardized methods and cut-off values to identify low muscle mass. Measuring muscle parameters in people who are obese or edematous is difficult since such conditions have been proven to affect muscle echo intensity.[78]

Computed Tomography Imaging

The value of body composition in clinical settings, including patients undergoing surgery, has evolved as a result of the use of computed tomography (CT) imaging for measuring muscle mass. This has tremendously increased our understanding of the association between muscle mass and tolerance to anticancer therapy, side effects, and survival, especially in oncology. However, traditionally, in a CT scan, manual segmentation of the adipose and muscle tissues which is laborious and time-intensive, and unpredictable—was used to separate adipose and muscle tissues in a CT scan. Data demonstrating good agreement between automated and manual analysis are currently available in many software programs for automated CT segmentation.[79] Similar associations with cancer-related mortality have been reported, besides being faster than manual segmentation.[80]

Muscle radiodensity, a predictive indicator of muscle composition, is also an important CT measure.[81] Low preoperative muscle radiodensities were linked to prolonged postoperative hospital stays, higher complication rates, and mortality rates in patients with colorectal cancer.[82,83]

According to a systematic review and meta-analysis of 40 research studies in cancer patients, 75% higher mortality risk in patients with myosteatosis than those without it.[84] Low muscle mass has been correlated with adverse outcomes, including poor survival, stays longer in the hospital, increased requirements for rehabilitation, and surgical complications.[82,85] It has also been observed that "Myosteatosis" is associated with a higher risk of prediabetes and type 2 diabetes mellitus, a higher rate of Homeostasis Model Assessments for Insulin Resistance (HOMa-IR), as well as circulating glucose, insulin, CRP, and interleukin-6 levels.[86] In addition, the risk for poorer outcomes may be greater in patients with myosteatosis and low muscle mass, compared to other conditions alone.[87,88]

The use of CT imaging for body composition analysis is particularly important in surgical oncology, as these images are readily available in the medical records of most patients obtained for initial cancer diagnosis and follow-up.[89,90] However, in the future, individual images can be obtained for body composition analysis to minimize radiation exposure. Indeed, we are aware that single CT scans are specifically performed as part of routine clinical practice (coding, billing, and reporting in medical records) in some centers around the world. This method takes little time and exposes patients to less radiation than a chest X-ray.

CT imaging has limited utility as a prevalent and repeatable technique to measure body composition in critically ill patients due to the radiation dose involved and the necessity of transferring patients out of the ICU.

Additional Methods

Dual-energy X-ray absorptiometry (DXA) is one of the most commonly used body composition assessment tools in research and clinical practice. DXA equipment can be used to measure total body lean soft tissue. It can also be used to measure fat-free mass, fat mass, and fat percentage. DXA has been approved as a body composition assessment tool by the GLIM Body Composition Working Group,[30,31] and European and Asian Sarcopenia working groups.[28,29] DXA is also expensive and depends on body thickness, hydration of soft tissue, and device and software versions.[89,91,92] Despite these drawbacks, DXA remains one of the most popular and useful techniques. DXA measures three body compartments at low radiation doses and is recommended for clinical fat mass assessment. However, the validity of DXA for lean soft-tissue assessment is unknown.[93]

D3Cr (Deuterated Creatine) is a new method of measuring functional muscle mass (FMT) independent of lipids and fibrosis in skeletal muscle.[94] A single oral dose of D3Cr is absorbed and diluted in the creatine pool in skeletal muscle. To estimate the mass of muscle, e.g., creatine pool size, a metabolized, and enriched D3Cr shall be determined from one urine sample. This method is closely related to state-of-the-art MRI technology, but it only moderately relates to DXA in older adults.[95,96] Despite its indirect nature, this method is accurate, noninvasive, and safe, however, it necessitates the use of high-performance liquid chromatography (HPC) which limits its clinical use.[97]

■ CONCLUSION

The clinical practice is ever-evolving and health professionals are encouraged to utilize many of the tools discussed above in their settings, and to assess the loss of muscle mass and malnutrition. Muscle loss and malnutrition may go undetected, but screening is the only way to identify at-risk patients; assessment can diagnose the presence and severity of reduced muscle mass and/or malnutrition. This will help in early nutritional intervention which is an important strategy for improving patient outcomes.

■ REFERENCES

1. Lew CCH, Yandell R, Fraser RJL, Chua AP, Chong MFF, Miller M. Association between malnutrition and clinical outcomes in the intensive care unit: a systematic review. JPEN J Parenter Enteral Nutr. 2017;41(5): 744-58.
2. Mogensen KM, Horkan CM, Purtle SW, Moromizato T, Rawn JD, Robinson MK, et al. Malnutrition, critical illness survivors, and postdischarge outcomes: a cohort study. JPEN J Parenter Enteral Nutr. 2017: 148607117709766.
3. Havens JM, Columbus AB, Seshadri AJ, Olufajo OA, Mogensen KM, Rawn JD, et al. Malnutrition at intensive care unit admission predicts mortality in emergency general surgery patients. JPEN J Parenter Enteral Nutr. 2018;42(1):156-63.
4. Herridge MS, Tansey CM, Matté A, Tomlinson G, Diaz-Granados N, Cooper A, et al. Functional disability 5 years after acute respiratory distress syndrome. N Engl J Med. 2011;364(14):1293-304.
5. Parry SM, El-Ansary D, Cartwright MS, Sarwal A, Berney S, Koopman R, et al. Ultrasonography in the intensive care setting can be used to detect changes in the quality and quantity of muscle and is related to muscle strength and function. J Crit Care. 2015;30(5):1151.e9-1151.e14.
6. Jolliet P, Pichard C, Biolo G, Chioléro R, Grimble G, Leverve X, et al. Enteral nutrition in intensive care patients: a practical approach. Clin Nutr. 1999;18(1):47-56.
7. White JV, Guenter P, Jensen G, Malone A, Schofield M. Consensus statement: Academy of Nutrition and Dietetics and American Society for Parenteral and Enteral

Nutrition: Characteristics recommended for the identification and documentation of adult malnutrition (undernutrition). JPEN J Parenter Enteral Nutr. 2012;36(3):275-83.
8. Kondrup J, Ramussen HH, Hamberg O, Stanga Z; Ad Hoc ESPEN Working Group. Nutritional risk screening (NRS 2002): a new method based on an analysis of controlled clinical trials. Clin Nutr. 2003;22(3):321-36.
9. Maciel LRMA, Franzosi OS, Nunes DSL, Loss SH, Dos Reis AM, Rubin BA, et al. Nutritional risk screening 2002 cut-off to identify high-risk is a good predictor of ICU mortality in critically ill Patients. Nutr Clin Pract. 2019;34(1):137-41.
10. Kondrup J. Nutrition risk screening in the ICU. Curr Opin Clin Nutr Metab Care. 2019; 22(2):159-61.
11. Kondrup J, Allison SP, Ellia M, Vellas B, Plauth M. ESPEN guidelines for nutrition screening 2002. Clin Nutr. 2003;22(4):415-21.
12. McClave SA, Taylor BE, Martindale RG, Warren MM, Johnson DR, Braunschweig C, et al. Guidelines for the provision and assessment of nutrition support therapy in the adult critically ill patient: Society of Critical Care Medicine (SCCM) and American Society for Parenteral and Enteral Nutrition (A.S.P.E.N). JPEN J Parenter Enteral Nutr. 2016;40(2):159-211.
13. Ferguson M, Capra S, Bauer J, Banks M. Development of a valid and reliable malnutrition screening tool for adult acute hospital patients. Nutr Rev. 1999;15(6):458-64.
14. Skipper A, Coltman A, Tomesko J, Charney P, Porcari J, Piemonte TA, et al. Position of the Academy of Nutrition and Dietetics: malnutrition (undernutrition) screening tools for all adults. J Acad Nutr Diet. 2020;120(4):709-13.
15. Anthony PA. Nutrition screening tool for hospitalized patients. Nutr Clin Pract. 2008;23(4):373-82.
16. Guigoz Y, Vellas B, Garry PJ. Assessing the nutritional status of the elderly: the mini nutritional assessment as part of the geriatric evaluation. Nutr Rev. 1996;54(1):S59-65.
17. Detsky AS, McLaughlin JR, Baker JP, Johnston N, Whittaker S, Mendelson RA, et al. What is subjective global assessment of nutritional status? JPEN J Parenter Enteral Nutr. 1987;11:8-13.
18. Erdim A, Aktan AÖ. Evaluation of perioperative nutritional status with subjective global assessment method in patients undergoing gastrointestinal cancer surgery. Turk J Surg. 2017;33(4):253-7.
19. Raguso CA, Maisonneuve N, Pichard C. Subjective Global Assessment (SGA): evaluation and follow-up of nutritional state. Rev Med Suisse Romande. 2004;124(10):607-10.
20. Bector S, Vagianos K, Suh M, Duerksen DR. Does the Subjective Global Assessment Predict Outcome in Critically Ill Medical Patients? J Intensive Care Med. 2016; 31(7):485-9.
21. Heyland DK, Dhaliwal R, Jiang X, Day AG. Identifying critically ill patients who benefit the most from nutrition therapy: the development and initial validation of a novel risk assessment tool. Crit Care. 2011;15(6):R268.
22. Jeong DH, Hong SB, Lim CM, Koh Y, Seo J, Kim Y, et al. Comparison of accuracy of NUTRIC and modified NUTRIC scores in predication 28-day mortality in patients with sepsis: single center retrospective study. Nutrients. 2018;10(7):911.
23. Mendes R, Policarpo S, Fortuna P, Alves M, Virella D, Heyland DK; Portuguese NUTRIC Study Group. Nutritional risk assessment and cultural validation of the modified NUTRIC score in critically ill patients—a multicenter prospective cohort study. J Crit Care. 2017; 37:45-9.
24. Cederholm T, Jensen GL, Correia MITD, Gonzalez MC, Fukushima R, Higashiguchi T, et al. GLIM Core Leadership Committee, GLIM Working Group. GLIM criteria for the diagnosis of malnutrition—a consensus report from the global clinical nutrition community. Clin Nutr. 2019;38(1):1-9.
25. Jensen GL, Cederholm T, Correia MITD, Gonzalez MC, Fukushima R, Higashiguchi T, et al. GLIM criteria for the diagnosis of malnutrition: a consensus report from the global clinical nutrition community. J Parenter Enter Nutr. 2019;43:32-40.

26. Cederholm T, Jensen GL, Correia MITD, Gonzalez MC, Fukushima R, Higashiguchi T, et al. GLIM criteria for the diagnosis of malnutrition—a consensus report from the global clinical nutrition community. J Cachexia Sarcopenia Muscle. 2019;10(1):207-17.
27. Prado CM, Ford KL, Gonzalez MC, Murnane LC, Gillis C, Wischmeyer PE, et al. Nascent to novel methods to evaluate malnutrition and frailty in the surgical patient. JPEN J Parenter Enteral Nutr. 2023;47(Suppl 1):S54-S68.
28. Cruz-Jentoft AJ, Bahat G, Bauer J, Boirie Y, Bruyère O, Cederholm T, et al; Writing Group for the European Working Group on Sarcopenia in Older People 2 (EWGSOP2), and the Extended Group for EWGSOP2. Sarcopenia: revised European consensus on definition and diagnosis. Age Ageing. 2019;48:16-31.
29. Chen LK, Woo J, Assantachai P, Auyeung TW, Chou MY, Iijima K, et al. Asian Working Group for Sarcopenia: 2019 consensus update on Sarcopenia diagnosis and treatment. J Am Med Dir Assoc. 2020;21:300-7. e2.
30. Barazzoni R, Jensen GL, Correia MITD, Gonzalez MC, Higashiguchi T, Shi HP, et al. Guidance for assessment of the muscle mass phenotypic criterion for the Global Leadership Initiative on Malnutrition (GLIM) diagnosis of malnutrition. Clin Nutr. 2022;41(6):1425-33.
31. Compher C, Cederholm T, Correia MITD, Gonzalez MC, Higashiguch T, Shi HP, et al. Guidance for assessment of the muscle mass phenotypic criterion for the Global Leadership Initiative on Malnutrition diagnosis of malnutrition. J Parenter Enteral Nutr. 2022;46(6):1232-42.
32. Bruyère O, Beaudart C, Reginster JY, Buckinx F, Schoene D, Hirani V, et al. Assessment of muscle mass, muscle strength and physical performance in clinical practice: an international survey. Eur Geriatric Med. 2016;7:243-6.
33. Santos LP, Gonzalez MC, Orlandi SP, Bielemann RM, Barbosa-Silva TG, Heymsfield SB; COCONUT Study Group. New prediction equations to estimate appendicular skeletal muscle mass using calf circumference: results from NHANES 1999-2006. J Parenter Enter Nutr. 2019;43:998-1007.
34. Tresignie J, Scafoglieri A, Pieter Clarys J, Cattrysse E. Reliability of standard circumferences in domain-related constitutional applications. Am J Hum Biol. 2013;25(5):637-42.
35. Gonzalez MC, Mehrnezhad A, Razaviarab N, Barbosa-Silva TG, Heymsfield SB. Calf circumference: cut off values from the NHANES 1999-2006. Am J Clin Nutr. 2021;113(6):1679-87.
36. Ishida Y, Maeda K, Nonogaki T, Shimizu A, Yamanaka Y, Matsuyama R, et al. Impact of edema on length of calf circumference in older adults. Geriatr Gerontol Int. 2019;19(10):993-8.
37. Cruz-Jentoft AJ, Baeyens JP, Bauer JM, Boirie Y, Cederholm T, Landi F, et al. Sarcopenia: European consensus on definition and diagnosis: report of the European working group on sarcopenia in older people. Age Ageing. 2010;39(4):412-23.
38. Bohannon RW. Hand-grip dynamometry predicts future outcomes in aging adults. J Geriatr Phys Ther. 2015;18(5):465-70.
39. Roberts HC, Denison HJ, Martin HJ, Patel HP, Syddall H, Cooper C, et al. A review of the measurement of grip strength in clinical and epidemiological studies: towards a standardised approach. Age Ageing. 2011;40(4):423-9.
40. Vaz M, Thangam S, Prabhu A, Shetty PS. Maximal voluntary contraction as a functional indicator of adult chronic undernutrition. Br J Nutr. 1996;76(1):9-15.
41. Webb AR, Newman LA, Taylor M, Keogh JB. Hand grip dynamometry as a predictor of postoperative complications reappraisal using age standardized grip strengths. J Parenter Enteral Nutr. 1989;13:30-3.
42. Klidjian AM, Archer TJ, Foster KJ, Karran SJ. Detection of dangerous malnutrition. J Parenter Enteral Nutr. 1982;6:119-21.
43. Mahalakshmi VN, Ananthakrishnan N, Kate V, Sahai A, Trakroo M. Handgrip strength and endurance as a predictor of postoperative morbidity in surgical patients: can it serve as a simple bedside test? Int Surg. 2004;89:115-21.

44. Newman AB, Kupelian V, Visser M, Simonsick EM, Goodpaster BH, Kritchevsky SB, et al. Strength, but not muscle mass, is associated with mortality in the health, aging and body composition study cohort. J Gerontol A Biol Sci Med Sci. 2006;61:72-7.
45. Kerr A, Syddall HE, Cooper C, Turner GF, Briggs RS, Sayer AA. Does admission grip strength predict length of stay in hospitalised older patients? Age ageing. 2006;35:82-4.
46. Gale CR, Martyn CN, Cooper C, Sayer AA. Grip strength, body composition, and mortality. Int J Epidemiol. 2007;36:228-35.
47. Chen CH, Ho C, Huang YZ, Hung TT. Handgrip strength is a simple and effective outcome predictor in esophageal cancer following esophagectomy with reconstruction: a prospective study. J Cardiothorac Surg. 2011;6:98.
48. Allard JP, Keller H, Jeejeebhoy KN, Laporte M, Duerksen DR, Gramlich L, et al. Malnutrition at hospital admission-contributors and effect on length of stay: a prospective cohort study from the Canadian Malnutrition Task Force. JPEN J Parenter Enter Nutr. 2015;40(4):487-97.
49. Allard JP, Keller H, Teterina A, Jeejeebhoy KN, Laporte M, Duerksen DR, et al. Lower handgrip strength at discharge from acute care hospitals is associated with 30-day readmission: a prospective cohort study. Clin Nutr. 2016;35(6):1535-42.
50. McNicholl T, Dubin JA, Curtis L, Mourtzakis M, Nasser R, Laporte M, et al. Handgrip Strength, but Not 5-Meter Walk, Adds Value to a Clinical Nutrition Assessment. Nutr Clin Pract. 2019;34(3):428-35.
51. Norman K, Stobäus N, Gonzalez MC, Schulzke JD, Pirlich M. Hand grip strength: Outcome predictor and marker of nutritional status. Clin Nutr. 2011;30(2):135-42.
52. Sultan P, Hamilton MA, Ackland GL. Preoperative muscle weakness as defined by handgrip strength and postoperative outcomes: A Systematic Review. BMC Anesthesiol. 2012;12(1):1-10.
53. Gonzalez MC, Correia MITD, Heymsfield SB. A requiem for BMI in the clinical setting. Curr Opin Clin Nutr Metab Care. 2017;20(5):314-21.
54. Earthman CP. Body composition tools for assessment of adult malnutrition at the bedside: a tutorial on research considerations and clinical applications. J Parenter Enter Nutr. 2015;39(7):787-822.
55. Goodpaster BH, Stenger VA, Boada F, McKolanis T, Davis D, Ross R, et al. Skeletal muscle lipid concentration quantified by magnetic resonance imaging. Am J Clin Nutr. 2004;79(5):748-54.
56. van Zijl PCM, Brindle K, Lu H, Barker PB, Edden R, Yadav N, et al. Hyperpolarized MRI, functional MRI, MR spectroscopy and CEST to provide metabolic information in vivo. Curr Opin Chem Biol. 2021;63:209-18.
57. Looijaard WGPM, Stapel SN, Dekker IM, Rusticus H, Remmelzwaal S, Girbes ARJ, et al. Identifying critically ill patients with low muscle mass: agreement between bioelectrical impedance analysis and computed tomography. Clin Nutr. 2020;39:1809-17.
58. Gonzalez MC, Barbosa-Silva TG, Heymsfield SB. Bioelectrical impedance analysis in the assessment of sarcopenia. Curr Opin Clin Nutr Metab Care. 2018;21(5):366-74.
59. da Silva BR, Gonzalez MC, Cereda E, Prado CM. Exploring the potential role of phase angle as a marker of oxidative stress: a narrative review. Nutrition. 2021;93:111493.
60. Denneman N, Hessels L, Broens B, Gjaltema J, Stapel SN, Stohlmann J, et al. Fluid balance and phase angle as assessed by bioelectrical impedance analysis in critically ill patients: a multicenter prospective cohort study. Eur J Clin Nutr. 2020;74:1410-9.
61. Stellingwerf F, Beumeler LFE, Rijnhart-de Jong H, Boerma EC, Buter H. The predictive value of phase angle on long-term outcome after ICU admission. Clin Nutr. 2022;41(6):1256-9.
62. Jung YW, Hong N, Kim CO, Youm Y, Choi JY, Rhee Y. The diagnostic value of phase angle, an integrative bioelectrical marker, for identifying individuals with dysmobility syndrome: the Korean Urban-Rural Elderly Study. Osteoporos Int. 2021;32(5):939-49.

63. Di Vincenzo O, Marra M, Di Gregorio A, Pasanisi F, Scalfi L. Bioelectrical impedance analysis (BIA)-derived phase angle in sarcopenia: a systematic review. Clin Nutr. 2021;40:3052-61.
64. Norman K, Stobäus N, Pirlich M, Bosy-Westphal A. Bioelectrical phase angle and impedance vector analysis—clinical relevance and applicability of impedance parameters. Clin Nutr. 2012;31(6):854-61.
65. Dittmar M. Reliability and variability of bioimpedance measures in normal adults: effects of age, gender, and body mass. Am J Phys Anthropol. 2003;122(4):361-70.
66. Bosy-Westphal A, Danielzik S, Dörhöfer RP, Later W, Wiese S, Müller MJ. Phase angle from bioelectrical impedance analysis: population reference values by age, sex, and body mass index. J Parenter Enter Nutr. 2006;30(4):309-16.
67. Tillquist M, Kutsogiannis DJ, Wischmeyer PE, Kummerlen C, Leung R, Stollery D, et al. Bedside ultrasound is a practical and reliable measurement tool for assessing quadriceps muscle layer thickness. JPEN J Parenter Enteral Nutr. 2014;38(7):886-90.
68. Campbell IT, Watt T, Withers D, England R, Sukumar S, Keegan MA, et al. Muscle thickness, measured with ultrasound, may be an indicator of lean tissue wasting in multiple organ failure in the presence of edema. Am J Clin Nutr. 1995;62(3):533-9.
69. Gruther W, Benesch T, Zorn C, Paternostro-Sluga T, Quittan M, Fialka-Moser V, et al. Muscle wasting in intensive care patients: ultrasound observation of the M. quadriceps femoris muscle layer. J Rehabil Med. 2008;40(3):185-9.
70. Mourtzakis M, Wischmeyer P. Bedside ultrasound measurement of skeletal muscle. Curr Opin Clin Nutr Metab Care. 2014;17(5):389-95.
71. Reid CL, Campbell IT, Little RA. Muscle wasting and energy balance in critical illness. Clin Nutr. 2004;23(2):273-80.
72. Sabatino A, Regolisti G, Bozzoli L, Fani F, Antoniotti R, Maggiore U, et al. Reliability of bedside ultrasound for measurement of quadriceps muscle thickness in critically ill patients with acute kidney injury. Clin Nutr. 2017;36(6):1710-5.
73. Arbeille P, Kerbeci P, Capri A, Dannaud C, Trappe SW, Trappe TA. Quantification of muscle volume by echography: comparison with MRI data on subjects in long-term bed rest. Ultrasound Med Biol. 2009;35(7):1092-7.
74. Puthucheary ZA, Rawal J, McPhail M, Connolly B, Ratnayake G, Chan P, et al. Acute skeletal muscle wasting in critical illness. JAMA. 2013;310(15):1591-600.
75. Fetterplace K, Deane AM, Tierney A, Beach LJ, Knight LD, Presneill J, et al. Targeted full energy and protein delivery in critically ill patients: a pilot randomized controlled trial (FEED Trial). JPEN J Parenter Enteral Nutr. 2018;42(8):1252-62.
76. Puthucheary ZA, Phadke R, Rawal J, McPhail MJ, Sidhu PS, Rowlerson A, et al. Qualitative Ultrasound in Acute Critical Illness Muscle Wasting. Crit Care Med. 2015;43(8):1603-11.
77. Turton P, Hay R, Welters I. Assessment of peripheral muscle thickness and architecture in healthy volunteers using hand-held ultrasound devices; a comparison study with standard ultrasound. BMC Med Imag. 2019;19(1):69.
78. Stock MS, Thompson BJ. Echo intensity as an indicator of skeletal muscle quality: applications, methodology, and future directions. Eur J Appl Physiol. 2021;121(2):369-80.
79. Popuri K, Cobzas D, Esfandiari N, Baracos V, Jägersand M. Body composition assessment in axial CT images using FEM-based automatic segmentation of skeletal muscle. IEEE Trans Med Imag. 2016;35(2):512-20.
80. Cespedes Feliciano EM, Popuri K, Cobzas D, Baracos VE, Beg MF, Khan AD, et al. Evaluation of automated computed tomography segmentation to assess body composition and mortality associations in cancer patients. J Cachexia Sarcopenia Muscle. 2020;11:1258-69.

81. Ahn H, Kim DW, Ko Y, Ha J, Shin YB, Lee J, et al. Updated systematic review and meta-analysis on diagnostic issues and the prognostic impact of myosteatosis: a new paradigm beyond sarcopenia. Ageing Res Rev. 2021;70:101398.
82. Xiao J, Caan BJ, Cespedes Feliciano EM, Meyerhardt JA, Peng PD, Baracos VE, et al. Association of low muscle mass and low muscle radiodensity with morbidity and mortality for colon cancer surgery. JAMA Surg. 2020;155(10):942-9.
83. Lee CM, Kang J. Prognostic impact of myosteatosis in patients with colorectal cancer: a systematic review and meta-analysis. J Cachexia Sarcopenia Muscle. 2020;11:1270-82.
84. Aleixo GFP, Shachar SS, Nyrop KA, Muss HB, Malpica L, Williams GR. Myosteatosis and prognosis in cancer: systematic review and meta-analysis. Crit Rev Oncol Hematol. 2020;145:102839.
85. Elliott JA, Doyle SL, Murphy CF, King S, Guinan EM, Beddy P, et al. Sarcopenia: prevalence, and impact on operative and oncologic outcomes in the multimodal management of locally advanced esophageal cancer. Ann Surg. 2017;266(5):822-30.
86. Miljkovic I, Vella CA, Allison M. Computed tomography-derived myosteatosis and metabolic disorders. Diabetes Metab J. 2021;45(4):482-91.
87. Findlay M, White K, Brown C, Bauer JD. Nutritional status and skeletal muscle status in patients with head and neck cancer: impact on outcomes. J Cachexia Sarcopenia Muscle. 2021;12(6):2187-98.
88. Martin L, Hopkins J, Malietzis G, Jenkins JT, Sawyer MB, Brisebois R, et al. Assessment of computed tomography (CT)-defined muscle and adipose tissue features in relation to short-term outcomes after elective surgery for colorectal cancer: a multicenter approach. Ann Surg Oncol. 2018;25(9):2669-80.
89. Prado CMM, Heymsfield SB. Lean tissue imaging: a new era for nutritional assessment and intervention. JPEN J Parenter Enteral Nutr. 2014;38(8):940-53.
90. Prado CM, Cushen SJ, Orsso CE, Ryan AM. Sarcopenia and cachexia in the era of obesity: clinical and nutritional impact. Proc Nutr Soc. 2016;75(2):188-98.
91. Sutter T, Duboeuf F, Chapurlat R, Cortet B, Lespessailles E, Roux JP. DXA body composition corrective factors between Hologic Discovery models to conduct multicenter studies. Bone. 2021;142:115683.
92. Van Loan MD, Keim NL, Berg K, Mayclin PL. Evaluation of body composition by dual energy X-ray absorptiometry and two different software packages. Med Sci Sports Exerc. 1995;27(4):587-91.
93. Sheean P, Gonzalez MC, Prado CM, McKeever L, Hall AM, Braunschweig CA. American Society for Parenteral and Enteral Nutrition Clinical Guidelines: the validity of body composition assessment in clinical populations. J Parenter Enter Nutr. 2020;44(1):12-43.
94. Evans WJ, Hellerstein M, Orwoll E, Cummings S, Cawthon PM. D3-Creatine dilution and the importance of accuracy in the assessment of skeletal muscle mass. J Cachexia Sarcopenia Muscle. 2019;10(1):14-21.
95. Clark RV, Walker AC, Miller RR, O'Connor-Semmes RL, Ravussin E, Cefalu WT. Creatine (methyl-d3) dilution in urine for estimation of total body skeletal muscle mass: accuracy and variability vs. MRI and DXA. J Appl Physiol. 2018;124:1-9.
96. Zhu K, Wactawski-Wende J, Ochs-Balcom HM, LaMonte MJ, Hovey KM, Evans W, et al. The association of muscle mass measured by D3-creatine dilution method with dual energy X-ray absorptiometry and physical function in postmenopausal women. J Gerontol A Biol Sci Med Sci. 2021;76(9):1591-9.
97. Heymsfield SB, Prado CM, Gonzalez MC, Cederholm T, Jensen GL, Barazzoni R, et al. Response to "Lean body mass should not be used as a surrogate measurement of muscle mass in malnourished men and women: comment on Compher et al." J Parenter Enter Nutr. 2022;46(7):1500-1.

CHAPTER 6

Nutrition in Inflammatory Bowel Disease

Ritu Sudhakar, Kirandeep Kaur

INTRODUCTION

Inflammatory bowel disease (IBD) is a chronic inflammatory, relapsing, and remitting disease of the digestive tract. Ulcerative colitis (UC) and Crohn's disease (CD) are the two common types of IBD.[1] The incidence of IBD is on the rise worldwide, with a high incidence and prevalence of UC and CD in industrialized countries.[2] However, recent evidence shows a worrying change in the disease trends as the prevalence of IBD is increasing even in countries initially thought of as having low incidence, i.e., developing nations like Southeast Asian countries and India.[3,4]

The exact pathophysiology of IBD remains unknown, however, multifactorial etiologies are involved, including interactions between genetic, environmental, and immunological factors. Several factors such as reduced oral food consumption, malabsorption, chronic loss of proteins and blood, and intestinal dysbiosis, can be attributed to malnutrition among IBD patients. Management guidelines recommend that the nutritional status of IBD patients should be periodically evaluated, especially during hospitalization with complications or prior to surgery. Various malnutrition assessment tools are available for use, of which the SaskIBD-NR is a tool specifically designed for IBD patients.[5,6] Micronutrient and vitamin deficiencies, especially anemia, are common even among clinically well IBD patients. Therefore, supplementation and prompt nutritional interventions should be provided to reduce the risk associated with nutritional deficiencies.[7]

Diet may play both a causal and a therapeutic role in IBD, with dietary recommendations forming an integral part of therapy in every aspect of IBD, right from management of active disease to hospitalization and pre- and postsurgical management.[2]

Dietary recommendations are one of the most frequently asked questions by IBD sufferers.[8] Many types of diets are promoted to manage IBD, including oral diets and enteral and parenteral nutrition (PN).[9]

Healthcare professionals involved in the management of IBD should be provided with adequate knowledge of the various nutritional tools, that identify patients at risk of preoperative malnutrition, from both objective and subjective points of view. A specialist IBD dietician should ideally lead the healthcare team on all aspects of nutritional care of IBD patients. The role of an IBD specialist dietician in the context of an IBD patient begins with assessing the nutritional status at the time of diagnosis, during flare-ups, hospital admissions, and pre- and postoperatively Adequate nutritional support keeping in mind, disease activity, current nutritional status, food tolerance, and feeding mode (oral, enteral, or parenteral) should be provided as part of IBD care.

This chapter focuses on two major nutritional aspects, namely assessment of malnutrition and nutritional management in three scenarios, i.e., active IBD, hospitalization, and surgery.

PATHOPHYSIOLOGY OF INFLAMMATORY BOWEL DISEASE

There has been unprecedented progress in understanding of the pathogenesis of IBD, however many aspects remain elusive. As genetics accounts for only 30–40% of disease occurrences, the focus has shifted toward identifying other triggers that may impact disease risk and trajectory.[7] Based on research, there seems to be a complex interaction between genetics, environmental factors, microbial flora, and immune responses that work in tandem to cause IBD.

Figure 1 shows a diagrammatic representation of the interactions of various factors that contribute to the development of IBD.

Luminal gut microbiota can cause chronic intestinal inflammation in genetically susceptible hosts. Inflammation leads to the production of antigens and adjuvants, which trigger pathogenic or protective immune responses. Environmental triggers are considered to be important for the initiation or reactivation of disease expression.[10] One of the most important environmental triggers in IBD is diet, which not only influences factors such as the gut microbiome and immune responses but also contributes toward the reduction of IBD-related symptoms.

The following section elaborates on the multifaceted role of dietary factors and their influence on IBD symptoms.

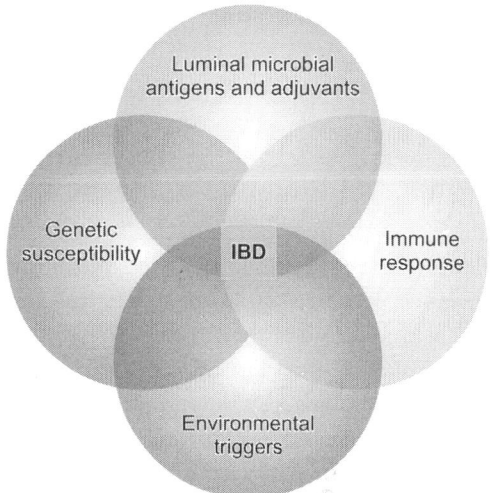

Fig. 1: Interaction of various factors that play a role in inflammatory bowel disease (IBD).[10]
Source: Adapted from Sartor RB. Mechanisms of Disease: pathogenesis of Crohn's disease and ulcerative colitis. Nat Clin Prac Gastroenterol Hepatol. 2006;3(7):390-407.

Diet and Microbiome in IBD

Diet plays an integral role in the development of IBD, and continues to act as a mediator of intestinal inflammation once the disease is established. Dietary habits are known to affect the onset of IBD through their role in an individual's microbial composition.[2,11] Diet can shape the microbiota composition and activity and impact host–microbe interactions. For example, a high-protein diet and red meat intake can result in increased production of bacterial metabolites, such as ammonia, indoles, phenols, and sulfide, that may harm the gut.[2]

In contrast, bacterial fermentation of nondigestible carbohydrates results in the formation of short-chain fatty acids (SCFAs), which are the energy source for host epithelial cells. These SCFAs act as signaling molecules with anti-inflammatory, immunomodulatory, and antioxidative properties. Fat can affect the microbiome by releasing and converting bile salts and altering the microbiota composition.[2]

Dietary Antigens and their Role in Triggering Inflammatory Responses

Studies have shown that saturated fats activate innate receptors and trigger inflammatory cascades. Westernization of the Indian diet is considered one of the primary reasons for the increasing prevalence of IBD in India. Westernized diets are known for their ability to cause intestinal inflammation, leading to colitis, due to their high-fat content.[2,7] The EPIC-IBD study showed that the highest quintile of dietary intakes of n-6 PUFA (linoleic acid) increased the odds of developing UC (OR = 2.49, 95% CI = 1.23–5.07), whereas the highest quintile of dietary intakes of n-3 PUFA (docosahexaenoic acid) was associated with decreased odds of developing UC (OR = 0.32; 95% CI = 0.006–0.97).[7]

High levels of food additives and preservatives also contribute to the increasing prevalence of IBD. A large multinational prospective cohort study (N = 116,087) published in the British Medical Journal showed that a higher intake of ultraprocessed foods is associated with an increased risk of IBD. People who consumed fried food (≥1 serving per day), especially ultra-processed foods, showed the highest risk of IBD. The intake of legumes, white meat, unprocessed red meat, starchy foods, dairy, fruits, and vegetables was not associated with IBD.[11]

Dietary additives, poorly digestible plant polysaccharides, and non-nutrient components are major contributors to the prevalence of IBD. It has been hypothesized that the ever-increasing prevalence of IBD is proportional to the availability of commercialized foods.[2] High-sodium diets are also implicated in the development of IBD due to their role in triggering gut inflammation and increasing intestinal permeability. Dietary phosphate, another emerging food additive used in fast foods and meat, exacerbates colitis, and increases disease activity.[12] Preclinical studies have found that polysaccharides used as emulsifiers, coating agents, stabilizers, or bulking agents can cause dysbiosis and thinning of the mucosal layer and can be implicated in the development of UC and UC-associated colonic cancers.[11,12] Other products like aluminum (used in processed foods and packaging), titanium dioxide (a food pigment that confers a white color), and bisphenol A (a chemical used for food packaging) have been implicated in the exacerbation or risk of developing IBD.[12]

Rapid urbanization trends and globalization culture have increased the availability of distinct food variants, which has spurred dietary changes among Indians.[13] There has been a 1.7-fold and 1.5-fold increase in salt and sugar intake over the last 2 decades. Consumption of snacks and crackers has increased by 9% and snacks and confectionery has increased by 15% in the last 6 years. All these new eating habits might be contributing to the increasing incidence of IBD in India.[14]

Dietary Components that Reduce the Risk of IBD

Emerging evidence suggests that the anti-inflammtory effects of vitamin D may reduce the risk of developing IBD. Similarly, dietary fiber is known to protect against the development of IBD due to its conversion into SCFAs (acetate, butyrate, and propionate). SCFAs are known to play an immunomodulatory role, thus reducing the risk of IBD. Studies show that intake of

24.3 g of dietary fiber per day (highest quintile) in CD patients was associated with a 41% lower risk of exacerbation compared to the lowest quintile of intake (HR = 0.59, 95% CI = 0.3–0.90).[7]

MALNUTRITION AND NUTRITIONAL DEFICIENCIES IN IBD

Malnutrition is a major complication of IBD and is the most important factor responsible for weight loss among patients. A multifactorial etiology contributes toward an impaired nutritional status.[15]

> Data suggest that malnutrition may affect approximately 65–75% of patients with CD and 18–62% of patients with UC.[15]

- Suboptimal energy intake
- Increased basal energy expenditure
- Malabsorption
- Gastrointestinal nutrient loss

Medications: Certain medications affect the absorption and utilization of micronutrients. Glucocorticoids can interfere with the absorption and utilization of calcium, phosphorus, and zinc. They are also related to impaired metabolism of vitamins C and D. Long-term use of glucocorticoids is associated with loss of bone density, deterioration of bone structure, osteoporosis, and increased risk of fractures. Sulfasalazine is a folic acid antagonist and long-term therapies are associated with anemia and hyperhomocysteinemia. Cholestyramine can interfere with the absorption of fat-soluble vitamins, iron, and B_{12} vitamin, and the main side effect is steatorrhea due to impaired absorption of fats.[15]

Malnutrition in IBD patients can result in several adverse clinical outcomes such as higher mortality rate, increased length of stay in the hospital, surgery, infection rate, and even thromboembolic events than those without nutritional deficiencies.[5,15]

Undernutrition in patients with postoperative conditions has also been associated with increased complications, such as infections such as pneumonia and sepsis, anastomotic leakage and breakdown, prolonged hospitalization, and even increased mortality.

Malnutrition causes significant weight loss, and in children, it is a major cause of growth retardation.[15]

The etiology of malnutrition is multifactorial as illustrated in **Flowchart 1**.

Malnutrition among IBD patients can be recognized early in the disease course by various signs and symptoms such as altered body composition, protein–energy malnutrition, and various micronutrient deficiencies. The severity of malnutrition depends on disease activity and duration, extent of disease, and magnitude of the inflammatory response mediated by proinflammatory cytokines (interleukins 1 and 6, tumor necrosis factor, etc.), which together can lead to catabolism and malnutrition. All of these represent clinical concerns among patients with IBD and adequate assessment of nutritional status can be the key toward better patient outcomes.[5]

Assessment of Malnutrition for Patients with Active IBD

Clinicians play a role in objectively assessing the diets of patients presenting with IBD and ensuring adequate eating habits to prevent malnutrition and maintain or reach optimal nutritional status.[16]

> Studies have shown that 20–70% of IBD patients are malnourished.[17]

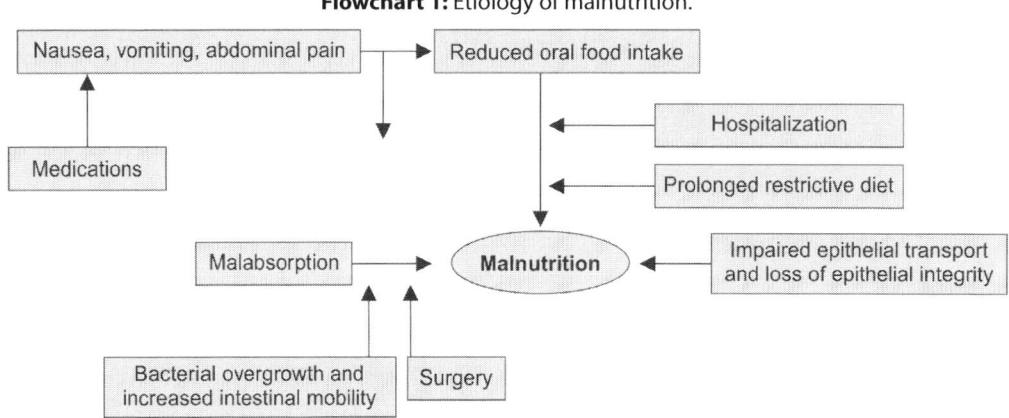

Flowchart 1: Etiology of malnutrition.

Source: Adapted from Sartor RB. Mechanisms of disease: Pathogenesis of Chron's disease and ulcerative colitis. Nat Clin Pract Gastroenterol Hepatol. 2006;3(7):390-407.

Patients with IBD are at a high risk for malnutrition, and hence, need screening and subsequent assessment and management. The European Society for Clinical Nutrition and Metabolism (ESPEN) guidelines on clinical nutrition in IBD place great emphasis on the increased risk of malnutrition among patients with IBD and the need to assess malnutrition early. However, there is no gold standard for assessing nutritional status among patients with IBD.[17] Many methods can be used to assess nutritional status in routine clinical practice.

Body mass index (BMI): This is a basic anthropometric technique that can be used, but it is not accurate in IBD patients since they have altered body composition.[18] Studies show that approximately 41.5% of people with IBD who are sarcopenic present with normal BMI and, therefore may not be identifiable by normal measures.[5]

Bioelectrical impedance analysis (BIA): It is a simple, fast, noninvasive, and effective method to estimate body composition. It is based on two physical principles, resistance (Rz), and reactance.[16,18]

Dual-energy X-ray absorptiometry (DEXA): DEXA scans provide information on bone mineralization.[15,18] Both, BIA and DEXA are considered the gold standard for measuring body composition.

Other methods to measure body composition include total body electrical conductivity (TOBEC) and infrared interactomes.

Screening tools/tests for malnutrition:
- Malnutrition Universal Screening Tool (MUST)
- *Nutritional Risk Screening (NRS):* For critically ill patients
- Mini Nutritional Assessment (MNA)
- Subjective global assessment (SGA)
- SaskIBD-NR tool

Currently, existing nutrition screening tools may be of limited use in patients with IBD because they use BMI and weight loss as key measures. The MUST has not been tested and validated in the patients with IBD. The SGA is the gold standard for assessing malnutrition; however, it does not assess if patients are avoiding particular foods and or food groups, which forms the crux of malnutrition assessment for IBD.[6]

The SaskIBD-NR tool is a validated tool that evaluates four components of malnutrition in IBD patients, viz., gastrointestinal symptoms, weight loss, anorexia, and food restrictions, and can help identify patients who are at nutritional risk and who would thereby benefit from counseling by a dietician. It considers the risk of malnutrition due to reduced food intake and avoidance of specific food groups, which are very common among patients with IBD. The advantages of this tool are given in the following text.[6]

Box 1 provides the questions included in the SaskIBD-NR tool.

Box 2 elaborates the European Crohn's and Colitis Organization (ECCO) 2022 recommendations for the nutritional assessment of IBD patients.

Malnutrition is one of the most important complications of IBD, influencing not only the nutritional status, but also the management of the condition and quality of life; however it remains under-recognized and underdiagnosed. Assessment of malnutrition and deficiencies is the first step toward initiating prompt dietary recommendations which in turn could improve outcomes for IBD patients.[6]

Nutritional Deficiencies and their Implications in Patients with IBD

A significant difference in body composition has been observed between IBD patients and their healthy counterparts. Studies have shown that patients with CD develop malnutrition over a period of time, while those with UC often present with a precipitous nutritional deficiency at hospitalization or at the onset of a severe acute flare. Low muscle mass is associated with an increased need for surgery, poor postsurgical outcomes, and osteopenia.[5]

The types of deficiencies depend on many factors, such as disease localization and extension, disease activity, alimentation,

---

BOX 1: Questions in the SaskIBD-NR tool.

1. Have you experienced nausea, vomiting, diarrhea, or poor appetite for >2 weeks?
2. Have you lost weight in the last month without trying?
3. If YES, how much weight have you lost?
4. Have you been eating poorly because of a decreased appetite?
5. Have you been restricting any foods or food groups?

Scoring system:
Total score: 0–2 = low risk, 3–4 = medium risk, ≥5 = high risk
1. No symptoms = 0, 1–2 symptoms = 1, ≥3 symptoms = 2
2. No = 0, unsure = 1, yes = see answer 3
3. <5 lbs = 0, 5–10 lbs = 1, 10–15 lbs = 2, >15 lbs = 3
4. No = 0, yes = 2
5. No = 0, yes = 2

BOX 2: Recommendations for nutrition assessment of IBD patients in clinical practice: European Crohn's and Colitis Organization (ECCO) 2022.[19]

- Nutritional assessment for all IBD patients to be done by a dietitian in addition to standard screening for micronutrient deficiencies
- BMI should NOT be used as a tool to indicate body composition abnormalities
- Body composition analysis should additionally be undertaken in IBD patients undergoing imaging for disease assessment
- Hand grip strength and waist circumference measures can be used to monitor body composition abnormalities
- Patients diagnosed with malnutrition should be referred to the dietitian for dietary assessment to identify and manage eating patterns and nutritional intake

(BMI: body mass index; IBD: inflammatory bowel disease)

TABLE 1: Micronutrient deficiencies in inflammatory bowel disease (IBD).[15]

Micronutrient	Main symptoms of deficiency	Diagnosis
Iron	Anemia, fatigue, sleeping disorders, restless legs syndrome, attention deficit, discontentment, agitation, female infertility	Transferrin saturation <16% and serum (S) ferritin <30 ng/mL
Calcium	Decreased bone density, hyperparathyroidism, hypertension, and muscle spasms	Bone density scan S. calcium <8.5 mg/dL
Selenium	Cardiomyopathy and cartilage degeneration	S. selenium <70 µg/L
Zinc	Poor wound healing	S. zinc <75 µg/L
Magnesium	Fatigue	S. magnesium <1.41 mEq/L
Vitamin B_9	Megaloblastic anemia, increased risk of colonic dysplasia, hyperhomocysteinemia	S. folate <2.5 ng/mL
Vitamin B_{12}	Megaloblastic anemia, peripheral neuropathy	S. B_{12} <200 pg/mL
Vitamin D	Abnormal bone metabolism	S. 25OHD <15 ng/mL
Vitamin A	Poor wound healing, night blindness, xeropthalmia	S. retinol <30 µg/dL
Vitamin K	Abnormal bone metabolism	S. phylloquinone <1.2 ng/mL

Source: Adapted from Scaldaferri F, Pizzoferrato M, Lopetuso LR, Musca T, Ingravalle F, Sicignano LL, et al. Nutrition and IBD: Malnutrition and/or Sarcopenia? A Practical Guide. Gastroenterol Res Pract. 2017;2017:8646495.

nutritional support, and medication used for IBD as elaborated in **Table 1**.[15] Alterations in the body composition, especially the ratio between fat mass (FM) and lean mass or fat-free mass, commonly occur in IBD. These alterations in body composition may impact the disease course, response to treatment, surgical outcomes, and quality of life.[5] A systematic review revealed that approximately 60% of IBD patients have decreased muscle mass compared to healthy subjects.

Protein-energy malnutrition is most common among IBD patients and can be attributed to inflammation, diarrhea, and inadequate dietary intake.[5]

Micronutrient Deficiencies in IBD: Vitamin A to Zinc

Micronutrient and vitamin deficiencies are common in IBD patients, even among those who look clinically well, and preventions of those deficiencies are important to avoid clinical complications.[15,20] Multiple mechanisms are involved in the development of micronutrient deficiencies among patients with IBD which could be related to disease symptoms (diarrhea, anorexia), pharmacotherapy, and disease-related complications (bowel resection).

The most observed deficiencies in IBD patients are B vitamins, vitamins A, D, E, K, and C; minerals like iron, calcium, magnesium; and trace elements like zinc, selenium, copper, chromium, and manganese.[7]

Iron-deficiency

Anemia is the most common systemic complication and extraintestinal manifestation in IBD, with a prevalence of 9–74%. Iron-deficiency anemia in IBD patients develops because of decreased intake or intestinal absorption and continuous or recurrent blood loss, while anemia of chronic disease in IBD patients is caused due to the inflammatory process. Other causes of anemia in IBD patients are vitamin B_{12} deficiency, folic acid deficiency, or toxic effects of medications like sulfasalazine and thiopurines.[7]

Anemia can negatively impact the quality of life of IBD patients, increases the cost of hospitalization and health care, and reduces the ability to work. Hence, prompt diagnosis and adequate management of iron-deficiency are a must among IBD patients.[7]

Calcium and Vitamin D Deficiency

Osteoporosis and low bone mass are very common among IBD patients of both sexes. Corticosteroid exposure, extensive bowel resection, lack of physical activity, chronic inflammation, and a deficiency of calcium, vitamin D, and other micronutrients can be contributing factors.[5]

Prevalence of calcium deficiency is about 10 and 13% in CD and UC patients, respectively, while up to 70 and 40% of CD and UC patients present with low levels of vitamin D.[5]

Vitamin D and calcium deficiency can be attributed to:[5]
- Reduction in the intestinal absorptive surface after extensive bowel resection
- A restrictive diet that excludes milk and milk products
- Binding of calcium to free fatty acids in the intestine

Folic Acid and Vitamin B_{12} Deficiency

Studies have estimated that 28% of CD patients and 8.8% of UC patients suffer from folic acid deficiency. Potential determinants of folate deficiency are inadequate intake, malabsorption due to surgical resection or fistulas, and certain medications such as methotrexate and sulfasalazine, which potentially inhibit folate absorption. Folic acid deficiency inadvertently leads to anemia, and therefore assessing folate status should be part of the nutritional assessment.[7]

Assessment of malnutrition and nutritional deficiencies form the first part of screening IBD patients. This should be followed by prompt initiation of adequate dietary recommendations depending on current nutritional status, disease severity, and tolerance.

NUTRITIONAL TREATMENT OF INFLAMMATORY BOWEL DISEASE[9]

Patients with IBD are becoming increasingly aware of the role that diet has to play in triggering, exacerbating or relieving IBD symptoms. Although many different diets (other than EEN) are promoted to be beneficial for IBD, evidence and supporting data is sparse.[8]

Diets for IBD patients include oral diets and enteral diets as shown in **Flowchart 2**.

Exclusive Enteral Nutrition

As the name suggests, exclusive enteral nutrition (EEN) is delivery of all the required calories and nutrients through consumption of a liquid formula either orally or through a feeding tube into the gut. The European Society of Gastroenterology, Hepatology and Nutrition (ESPGHAN) and ECCO recommend EEN as the first line of therapy in children with active luminal CD. In fact, the clinical remission rates of IBD patients on EEN are comparable to those on corticosteroid therapy, making it one of the most widely studied and replicated dietary intervention used in the management of pediatric CD.[21-23]

Exclusive enteral nutrition has demonstrated a large number of benefits, including mucosal healing, weight gain, linear growth (in children), improved bone turnover and an improved quality of life.[9]

Elemental, semielemental, and polymeric formulations have all been used

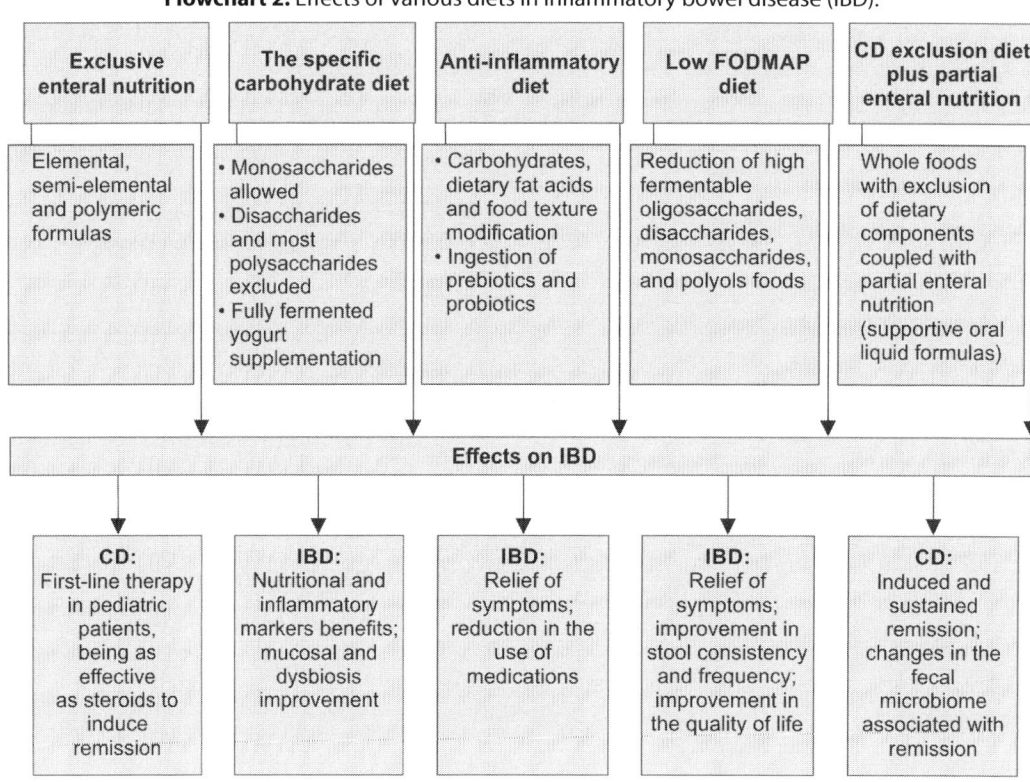

Source: de Castro MM, Pascoal LB, Steigleder KM, Siqueira BP, Corona LP, Ayrizono M, et al. Role of diet and nutrition in inflammatory bowel disease. World J Experimental Med. 2021;11(1):1-16.

with same efficacy for EEN and it has been established by various studies to be able to drive CD into remission.[21,22]

In fistulizing Crohn's disease, EEN acts as a short-term bridge therapy to anti-TNF or surgery and helps in improving nutrition and reducing inflammation. It is preferred in surgical candidates who are at high risk of getting infections.[16]

Though its benefits have been well established for adult CD patients, it is still unclear as to how EEN produces the benefits that it does. However, the possible benefits of EEN on IBD patients could be through the exclusion of antigenic load from the diet, mediated via immunomodulation, restoration of gut mucosal barrier integrity, changes in gut microbiome, reduction of intestinal inflammation and improvement of nutritional status. The EEN protocols need to be followed for 6-8 weeks to be effective in bringing about remission, although the inflammatory markers are likely to begin falling as early as 1-2 weeks post-therapy initiation.[21,24]

The limitation of EEN are usually its acceptance and adherence in the long run, as it involves exclusion of all foods and drinks. Only water is allowed beyond the formula-based diet. Taste fatigue, social incompatibility and deprivation from real food makes it a difficult dietary intervention to follow.

Its role in UC is emerging but we need more data to emphasize its benefits.

> **BOX 3:** Exclusive enteral nutrition (EEN) paradox.[25]
> - EEN is an exciting therapeutic tool in treatment of active CD. But it contains dietary components which are usually implicated as triggers of IBD–emulsifiers like maltodextrin, is low on fiber, reduces diversity of intestinal microbiota below pretreatment levels, causes a decline in number of presumably protective gut bacterial species (*Bifidobacterium* Spp. and *Faecalibacterium prausnitzil*) and leads to decreased concentrations of fecal SCFAs.
> - It is suggested that the bowel rest induced by EEN facilitates mucosal healing by limiting the activity of pathogenic microbes.[25]

A randomized clinical trial showed evidence of synergistic effects of EEN and medical therapy for IBD. They found that EEN was better than TPN in acute severe UC and that there was a lower steroid failure with EEN (25% vs. 43%) **(Box 3)**.[26]

Elimination or Exclusion Diets in IBD

Elimination or exclusion diets can be the cause or the therapy for IBD, with certain dietary components being known to exacerbate or trigger IBD symptoms. On the other hand, some dietary components are known to reduce inflammation. Eliminating the proinflammatory dietary components from the diet is the first logical step toward reducing disease activity.[7]

Elimination diets are based on the principle of excluding or reducing certain dietary components like carbohydrates, gluten, dairy products (lactose), etc., and they offer following benefits:[7]
- Microbiome and mucosal cytokine modulation
- Reduction in gastrointestinal symptoms among patients with IBD by treating superimposed maldigestion
- Improved quality of life.

Whole-food Restricted Diets

These involve dietary restrictions or elimination of specific foods. Calorie and nutritional requirements are met by consuming whole foods rather than manufactured enteral or parenteral feeds. Studies have demonstrated benefits of whole foods in IBD patients in terms of disease activity and prolonged time to relapse.[7]

Low FODMAP Diet

The Low Fermentable Oligo-, Di-, Monosaccharides and polyols Diet or the low FODMAP diet is a well-known dietary approach to control IBD-related symptoms such as abdominal pain, bloating, increased flatulence, and diarrhea.[7]

Exclusions include highly fermentable oligosaccharides, disaccharides, and monosaccharides (foods containing lactose and fructose) as well as polyols (mannitol and sorbitol) **(Box 4)**.

The low FODMAP diet consists of initially eliminating foods high in FODMAPs for 6–8 weeks. Once symptom resolution is observed, the patients are guided on methods to gradually reintroduce high FODMAP foods into the diet, with an aim to determine individual tolerance to specific FODMAPs.[8]

This diet is very restrictive, but studies have shown that successful implementation and adherence can be highly effective in managing IBS-like symptoms.[8] However, many recent studies demonstrate that the low FODMAP diet does not treat IBD and does not result in a reduction in inflammation. Also, this diet is shown to have a negative impact on the microbiome due to the reduced intake of complex carbohydrates that cause fermentation resulting in the disappearance of several bacterial groups. Hence, it is important

> **BOX 4:** Restrictions and allowances of a low FODMAP (Low Fermentable Oligo-, Di-, Monosaccharides and polyols) diet.[8]
>
> *Restrictions:*
> - Wheat, barley, rye
> - Apples, blackberry, canned fruit, date, dried fruit, grapefruit, mango, nectarine, pear, peach, plum, prune, watermelon
> - Avocado, beetroot, cauliflower, cabbage, garlic, leek, mushroom, onion, pea, shallot, snow pea, sweet corn, sweet potato
> - Breaded meats, processed meat containing high fat and sugar
> - Bean, cashew, chickpea, lentil, pistachio, soybean
> - Cow, goat, sheep, condensed, and evaporated milk, butter milk, soy milk (from soybean), soft cheese, and cream
> - Coconut water, green tea, rum, soft drinks, sports drinks, white tea
> - Milk chocolate, sweeteners ending in "-ol," honey.
>
> *Allowances:*
> - Gluten-free foods, oat, rice, quinoa
> - Banana, blueberry, cantaloupe, clementine, grape, kiwi, lemon, lime, mandarin, melons (variety), orange, passion fruit, pineapple, raspberry, strawberry
> - Alfalfa, bean sprout, bell pepper, bokchoy, broccoli ($\leq$1/2 cup), brussels sprout ($\leq$2 sprouts), carrot, corn, cucumber, eggplant, green bean, kale, lettuce, potato, spinach, spring onion (only green top), squash, tomato, turnip, zucchini
> - Almond ($\leq$10 nuts), chia seed, nut butter, macadamia, peanut, pecan, pumpkin seed, walnut
> - Lactose-free yogurt and milk; almond, coconut, rice, or soymilk (from soy protein); hard and low-lactose cheese
> - Fruit and vegetable juice made with allowed food (limit to 1/2 cup satatime), wine (5 fl oz), vodka, gin (1.5 fl oz)
> - Brown sugar, dark chocolate, maple syrup, golden syrup, stevia

that such diets be prescribed to only those patients with inactive IBD and experience functional symptoms without inflammation and that this diet is recommended only for a short period, followed by periodical food rechallenges to establish patient tolerance of each FODMAP group.[7]

Patient-directed Elimination Diet

This dietary pattern differs from diets which exclude proinflammatory foods and instead focuses on personalized elimination strategies, based on food intolerances.[7]

Defined Diets

Defined diets can be described as dietary regimens prescribed based on an underlying "theory" of how food interacts with the body.

There are several defined diets promoted to reduce intestinal inflammation and related medical conditions associated with IBD.[7]

Several popular defined diets being used to alleviate symptoms related to IBD are elaborated below.

Specific carbohydrate diet (SCD): The specific carbohydrate diet is based on the theory that the absorption of complex carbohydrates is limited as compared to simple carbohydrates. The incomplete absorption of complex carbohydrates results in bacterial overgrowth and intestinal injury. The diet recommends elimination of complex carbohydrates and processed foods. **Box 5** elaborates the foods allowed and restricted in a SCD diet.[7]

Trials have demonstrated a marked improvement in clinical and inflammatory

> **BOX 5:** Restrictions and allowances of specific carbohydrate diet (SCD).[7,8]
>
> *Restrictions:*
> - Grains, yams, potatoes, corn
> - Canned fruits and vegetables
> - Smoked, canned and processed meats
> - Milk
> - Chickpeas, soybean
> - Instant tea, coffee, soybean milk, beer
> - Chocolate
> - Margarine
> - Corn syrup
>
> *Allowed:*
> - Fresh fruits and vegetables
> - Unprocessed meat
> - Lentils, split peas
> - Saccharin, honey
> - Xylitol and sorbitol (moderate use)
> - Lactose-free (home-made) yoghurt and cheeses

markers in patients with mild-to-moderate disease. Another study has also shown mucosal healing associated with SCDs among IBD patients.[7]

Though evidence with respect to studies is limited and majority of the studies are conducted on pediatric populations with CD; results seem promising. This diet has the potential to contribute toward vitamin D deficiency, therefore, adequate steps in terms of supplementation have to be considered.[8]

CD-TREAT diet: The CD-TREAT is an individualized food-based diet, with therapeutic effects similar to EEN, based on simple nutrient composition and a mechanism of action involving the gut microbiome, with an aim to induce remission in CD. It recreates EEN by excluding certain dietary components like gluten, lactose and alcohol and matching of others like macronutrients, vitamins, minerals and fiber, by using ordinary food. Better palatability, higher satiety and fewer gastrointestinal side effects are the benefits that CD-TREAT offers in comparison to EEN.[27]

Semivegetarian diet (SVD): This diet was developed in Japan with an aim to maintain remission of CD by diet. It was specifically designed to increase the number of beneficial bacteria in the gut, on the basis of the epidemiological evidence showing that a Western-style diet can trigger or exacerbate IBD. A small nonrandomized study in Japan where subjects were recommended a traditional Japanese food was conducted and patients were followed up to 2 years. 94% of patients in the semivegetarian diet group-maintained remission versus 33% of the control group. The diet was found to be highly effective in preventing the relapse of CD, but it is difficult to reproduce the diet outside Japan.[28]

Anti-inflammatory diet: This diet was developed on the basis of the hypothesis that certain carbohydrates provide a substrate to pathogenic bacteria. Correction of dysbiosis through diet is the principle underlying this plan.[30]

The anti-inflammatory diet (IBD-AID) diet consists of five components:[29]
1. Restricted consumption of specific carbohydrates like lactose, refined or processed complex carbohydrates.
2. Consumption of prebiotics, probiotics and foods that are rich in components that can restore the balance of intestinal microbiota such as soluble fiber, leek, onions, fermented foods.
3. Reduced intake of total fat and saturated fatty acids and increased intake of omega-3 rich foods.
4. Overall dietary pattern review to identify intolerance and malnutrition and deficiencies.
5. Modification of food texture such as cooked, homogenized, and ground to improve nutrient absorption.

Paleolithic diet or the stone-age diet: The theory behind the paleolithic diet is that the human digestive tract has still not evolved to handle modern diets that are derived through agriculture and manufacturing processes. Based on this, the paleo diet consists of lean, nondomesticated meats, nuts, and other noncereal plant foods.[8]

Autoimmune protocol diet: This is an extension of the paleolethic diet, and it focuses on avoidance of refined sugars and gluten and emphasizes on lean protein, fresh and nutrient dense foods with more fiber. It emphasizes on preparation and consumption of fresh foods which are nutrient dense like bone broth, fermented foods and highlights the importance of sleep hygiene and stress management. Foods to be eliminated are grains, legumes, nightshades (tomatoes, potatoes, eggplant and peppers), dairy, eggs, nuts and seeds, processed oils and sugars, and food additives.[30]

Other Diets

Mediterranean Diet

Mediterranean diets are known for their anti-inflammatory effects. However, apart from a small study that investigated the effect of this diet on the microbiome, no studies have tested the diet in patients with IBD.[7]

CD-exclusion Diet

This is a combination of PEN (partial enteral nutrition) and the exclusion diet. Specific dietary components that can cause disruption of intestinal mucous layer or those that cause dysbiosis are excluded. The diet was developed by a group in Israel, based on the theory that Western diets are associated with dysbiosis, increased intestinal permeability and impaired innate immunity **(Table 2).**[31]

TABLE 2: CD exclusion diet regimen.[31]

Time period	Food choices
0–6 weeks	• Daily mandatory food to provide 50% of the calculated energy intake – 150–200 g of chicken breast, two eggs, two potatoes, two bananas, and one apple • Complete liquid formula (Modulen, Nestlé, Vevey, Switzerland) to provide the remaining 50% of energy
7–12 weeks	• Increase in allowed and mandatory foods • Less demanding dietary restrictions • Complete liquid formula reduced to provide 25% of calculated energy intake
13 weeks onward	• No specific diet implemented • Excluded proinflammatory foods: Alcohol, animal fat, dairy, gluten, processed meats, coffee, food additives particularly emulsifying agents and maltodextrins

Partial Enteral Nutrition

This type of diet was developed as an alternative to EEN. Partial enteral nutrition is administered as 50% EN and 50% unrestricted diet. PEN with unrestricted diet vs. EEN when compared, EEN was found to be more superior which confirmed the principle of exclusivity.[32]

However, for optimization of PEN approach, a 12-week study, compared EEN with specific CD exclusion diet (CDED) along with PEN in a pediatric population and demonstrated a higher patient acceptability rate with CDED + PEN and a clinical response rate not significantly different in the two regimens.[33]

The CD exclusion diet plus PEN (CDED + PEN) is a dietary regimen and it involves intake of whole foods with exclusion of certain dietary components. It is often used in children and adults with active IBD.

TABLE 3: Partial enteral nutrition (PEN) diets.[9]

	Allowed	Restrictions
Week: 0–6	Polymeric formula providing 50% of calories	Gluten, dairy products, gluten-free baked goods and breads, animal fat, processed meats, products containing emulsifiers, canned goods, and all packaged products with an expiration date
Week: 7–12	• Fixed portion of whole-grain bread, small amounts of nuts, fruits, legumes, and vegetables are allowed. Up to 18–20 g of fiber per day is allowed • Liquid formula providing 25% of calories	

It consists of supportive oral liquid formulae, and comprises two phases lasting 12 weeks. It is often used in children and adults with active IBD.[9]

Table 3 describes the regimen in detail. Studies conducted on PEN demonstrated nearly 50% reduction in CD relapse rates compared to regular diets.[9]

Pre- and Probiotics in the Management of IBD

The gut and its microbiota play a very important role in the pathogenesis of IBD and dysbiosis is known to promote inflammation and thus exacerbate or increase the risk of developing the condition. The logical answer to this hypothesis was an intervention strategy consisting of pre and probiotics to treat dysbiosis and thus mitigate the risk of development and or relapse of IBD.[7]

Prebiotics

Prebiotics undergo fermentation to form SCFAs and lactate, thereby lowering the luminal pH and resulting in the growth of *Firmicutes*, *Bifidobacteria*, and *Lactobacillus*, but impeding the proliferation of *Bacteroidetes* and *Clostridium difficile*. Prebiotics have also been proposed to promote integrity of the intestinal barrier and modulate inflammatory responses. Examples of prebiotics include inulin and oligofructose. Though there are few published RCTs on the impact of prebiotics on CD patients, no concrete evidence has been found on its clinical benefits in IBD.[7]

Probiotics

These are live microbial food ingredients that can alter the gut microflora and thus confer health benefits to the host. The myriad benefits of probiotics among IBD patients include their impact on reducing inflammation, improving barrier function, potentially inhibiting the growth of harmful bacteria and promoting growth of beneficial ones. Very few studies show any evidence on the benefits of probiotic supplementation on IBD patients. Three low-quality studies showed effectiveness of some probiotics in prevention of CD relapse postsurgery.[7]

We have many guideline-based nutritional recommendations for patients with IBD [Asian Working Group 2019, ESPEN 2020, International Organization for the Study of Inflammatory Bowel Diseases (IOIBD)].[34,35] All these recommend the following:

- Patients with IBD should receive adequate calories, proteins, and fats in their diet. The calorie and protein requirement of a patient with IBD in remission is similar to that of a healthy individual. However, the protein requirement is increased in a patient with active disease.
- Patients should be screened for macro- and micronutrient deficiency including calcium, phosphate, magnesium, iron, folic acid, vitamin D and vitamin B_{12}

- in an appropriate clinical context and supplemented accordingly.
- Increased intake of fruits and vegetables and optimum low-fat dairy (lactose-free dairy if intolerant to lactose)
- To avoid products with maltodextrins, emulsifiers, and thickeners (carboxymethylcellulose and polysorbate-80), artificial sweeteners, red meats/processed meat, food additives (carrageenans, titanium dioxide and other nanoparticles)
- Reduced consumption of palm oil, coconut oil and dairy fats (myristic acid) and avoid trans fats. Increase consumption of omega-3 fats.
- Exclusion diets cannot be recommended to achieve remission in active CD patients, even if the patient has individual intolerances.
- Reduction of insoluble fiber is recommended only in case of presence of strictures.

MALNUTRITION IN HOSPITALIZED PATIENTS WITH IBD

Malnutrition is very common in hospitalized IBD patients, with prevalence ranging from 20 to 70%.[23] Malnutrition in a hospitalized IBD patient is still a growing field of interest; however, there is enough evidence to prove that underdiagnosis of malnutrition in these cases can have significant negative clinical impact including:[36]

- Greater length of hospital stay
- Higher readmission rates after discharge
- Greater need for emergent surgery
- Greater rates of complications and post-opportunistic infections
- Increased mortality

There are various reasons for hospitalized IBD patients to be malnourished like drug interactions, reduced oral intake, malabsorption, gastrointestinal nutrient loss, surgical resections, bacterial overgrowth in the small intestine, chronic dehydration, metabolic bone disease, etc. **(Fig. 2)**.[36]

Evidence suggests that identifying malnutrition among hospitalized IBD patients and introducing nutritional interventions can improve patient outcomes as a whole.[36]

NUTRITIONAL INTERVENTION AND SUPPORT FOR HOSPITALIZED IBD PATIENTS

Nutritional assessment and therapy should begin within 24 hours of hospital admission, especially in patients who are assessed as positive for malnutrition risk.[36] There are several aspects involved in the decision of the optimal feeding route for IBD patients, especially since artificial nutrition in IBD can be complex and involve many patient-related factors such as the ability of the patient to eat, the absorptive capacity of the GI tract, the nutritional status of the patient, and the therapeutic goals (supportive care, treatment of malnutrition, induction of remission, maintenance of remission).[37] The decision will also be based on the type of formula used in earlier studies, and the dietary modulation of the intestinal immune response in IBD along with potential clinical implications.

Nutritional Supplementation for Hospitalized or Critically Ill IBD Patients

Medical nutrition for critically ill IBD patients includes oral nutrition supplements (ONS), enteral nutrition [exclusive enteral nutrition/partial enteral nutrition and parenteral nutrition peripheral (PPN)/Total (TPN)].[36]

Oral Nutrition Supplements

Oral nutrition supplements is the first step; but generally, these are just a minor

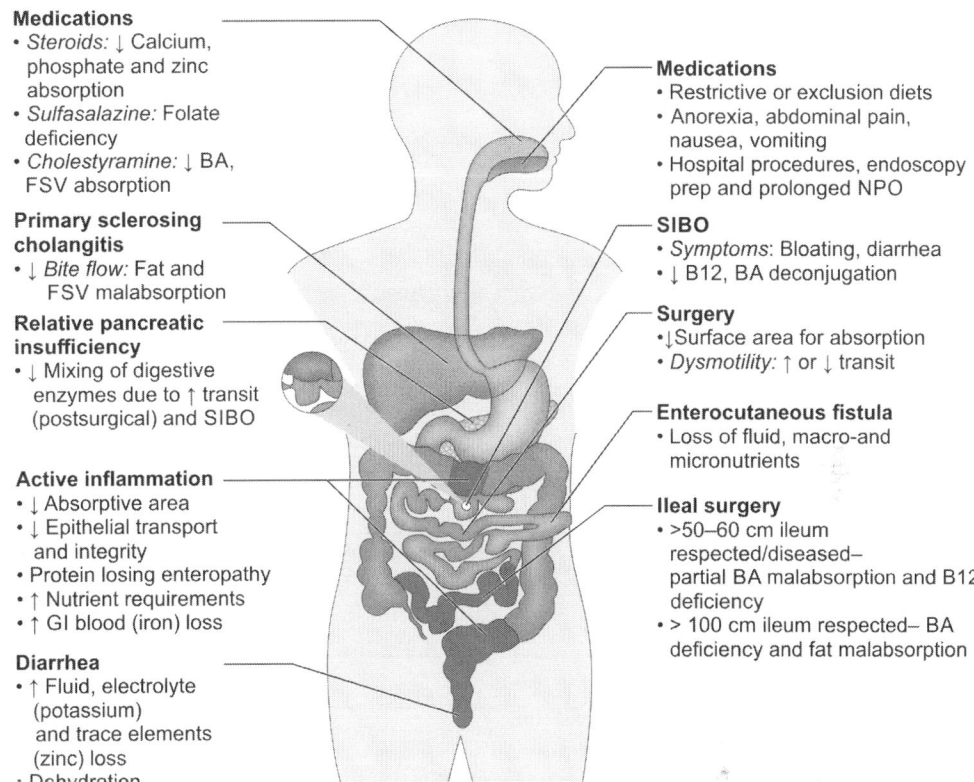

Fig. 2: Multifactorial mechanisms of malnutrition among hospitalised IBD patients.[36] (B12: Vitamin B_{12}; BA: bile acids; GI: gastrointestinal; FSV: fat soluble vitamins A, D, E, K; NPO: nil per os; SIBO: small intestinal bacterial overgrowth)
Source: Chiu E, Oleynick C, Raman M, Bielawaska B. Optimizing inpatient nutrition care of adult patients with inflammatory bowel disease in 21st century. Nutrients. 2021;13(5):1581.

supportive therapy used in addition to normal food. ONS when used as a supplementary intake can provide up to 600 kcal/day without compromising normal food intake in adults.[7]

Oral nutrition supplementation is a safe and feasible route of nutrient administration and is preferred over tube feeding. Advantages include lower cost, maintenance of epithelial barrier integrity, immune modulation, beneficial effects on microbiome, avoidance of intravenous (IV) access related complications.[36]

However, many IBD patients cannot tolerate ONS due to symptoms like vomiting, nausea, and anorexia.[36]

Enteral Nutrition

Enteral nutrition is indicated in patients who cannot meet their nutritional needs through the oral route but have a sufficiently functioning gastrointestinal tract to ensure macro and micronutrient absorption.[36]

The ESPEN defines EN as "comprise all forms of nutritional support that imply the use of dietary foods for special medical purposes" independent of the route of application.

Enteral nutrition can be effectively used as a supplementary means of nutritional intake (supplemental EN) among patients who can eat and drink to some extent. In such patients, nutrients can be infused slowly, at a controlled rate to reduce intolerance that is associated with bolus feeding. The best way to use supplemental EN is overnight as it will not interfere with spontaneous day time oral intake.[36]

In the recent years, comparative studies between elemental, semi-elemental and polymeric formulae show no difference in the efficacy.[38,39]

Enteral nutrition in hospitalized IBD patients is aimed at treating malnutrition and prevent further complications. Evidence also points to its benefits as primary therapy for CD related inflammation. Adults with CD have been observed to benefit with exclusive EN in terms of disease remission.[36]

Nutrition in Hospitalized IBD Patients with Complications

Enteral nutrition: Enteral nutrition can be effectively used in CD patients with partial bowel obstruction due to intestinal stricture, especially if enteral access can be obtained distally to the stricture. In some cases, with partial bowel obstruction, even if the stricture cannot be bypassed, slowly delivered liquid nutrition can be tolerated.[36]

In CD patients who present with complications that may require surgery, there seems to be emerging evidence of the benefits of preoperative enteral nutrition to restore nutritional status. Studies show:[36]

- 1–2 weeks of preoperative EN was associated with significant reduction in postoperative wound and anastomotic complications (compared to no preoperative nutritional interventions).[40]
- 2 weeks of preoperative EN given to malnourished presurgery IBD patients led to similar postoperative outcomes as compared to no EN to their well-nourished presurgery counterparts.[41]
- EN provided to presurgical CD patients with intra-abdominal abscess showed statistically significant improvements in serum hemoglobin and albumin levels along with a decline in inflammatory markers and a low risk of needing surgery.[42]

Parenteral Nutrition

Malnourished patients who are meeting less than 50–60% of their nutritional requirements through oral or enteral routes can be initiated on PN.[36]

Traditionally the delivery of PN has always been through the central route as it allows for administration of a concentrated, high osmolarity solution that can completely meet the patients nutritional and fluid requirement.[36]

Parenteral nutrition can be of two types: Peripheral PN and total PN.

1. *Periheral parenteral nutrition:* It involves the infusion of fluids through a peripheral vein to expedite initiation of nutritional therapy to malnourished, hospitalized IBD patients who may have to endure long periods of fasting or NPO or suboptimal nutrient intake in preparation for hospital-related procedures or due to bowel obstruction. In fact, for a short-term restriction of oral intake in a malnourished IBD patient, PPN can be a logical intervention.[36]

Many disadvantages have also been associated with the use of PPN, such as:[36]
- The exclusive use of PPN may not fully be able to meet the nutritional needs of patients mainly due to osmolarity constraints.
- High vigilance required to ensure feeding complications like volume overload, metabolic derangements, etc.

- Constant monitoring is required to prevent risk of venous injuries like infiltration, phlebitis, or thrombophlebitis.
- To be used cautiously in case of comorbidities such as cirrhosis, liver, kidney, and heart failure
- Cannot be used for more than 10–15 days

2. *Total parenteral nutrition:* Total parenteral nutrition, also called central PN or CPN is indicated in patients in whom the duration of PN therapy is anticipated to be more than 10 days. TPN is indicated in:[36,37]
   - Crohn's disease patients with short bowel syndrome resulting in severe malabsorption of nutrients and or fluid loss which cannot be managed by the enteral route.
   - Patients with several surgeries or with obstructed bowel where there is no possibility of placement of a feeding tube beyond the obstruction.
   - Patients with significant malabsorption, intractable vomiting, high output or proximal fistula, ileus, uncontrolled, severe gastrointestinal bleeding, anastomotic leak.
   - In case peripheral access is not feasible or contraindicated, those with severe malnutrition, fluid restrictions and or with metabolic derangements.

Total parenteral nutrition is a way to achieve bowel rest, correct nutritional deficiencies, and eliminate dietary antigens that can stimulate the mucosal immune system in IBD patients.[22]

Achieving remission rate greater than 80% and avoiding surgical treatment are considered the initial effects of TPN, but delayed relapse is commonly developed after cessation of TPN.[43] Studies showed that there were no significant differences between TPN and EN with respect to the remission rate.[44]

Disadvantages of TPN:
- TPN is rather expensive, with higher chances of infection and thromboembolism due to venous catheter and hepatobiliary complications, being considered independent risk factors.[45,46]
- TPN is not found to be effective in treating patients with severe UC.[37]

Complications of TPN: Numerous potential complications of TPN have been noted including mechanical, gastrointestinal, infectious, metabolic, vascular, biliary, and mechanical issues that can contribute toward mortality and morbidity.[7]

Bowel Rest

This is the most extreme form of an elimination diet, wherein the patient is given total bowel rest, based on the hypothesis that it can help reduce mechanical trauma, intestinal secretions, and the diet-related antigen stimuli. Concomitant TPN with bowel rest was also evaluated to offset malnutrition due to increased requirements of protein and calories secondary to intestinal inflammation. Interestingly, bowel rest failed to show efficacy in colonic disease. Studies demonstrated that 43% of colonic CD and all patients with severe UC still needed surgery despite bowel rest.[7]

In contrast to the promising data from descriptive studies, subsequent controlled trials of bowel rest failed to show efficacy over oral intake for UC or CD. After these studies, the use of total bowel rest as therapy for IBD has been limited primarily to patients who suffer from high output fistulas or short bowel syndrome.[7]

Retrospective studies show that more than 50% of hospitalized IBD patients are kept NPO, and 25% of such orders were deemed unnecessary. Another common dietary prescription among such patients is clear liquid diets. These dietary prescriptions among hospitalized IBD patients are a cause of concern, since periods of fasting or being NPO or being on a clear liquid diet could increase the risk of malnutrition and leading to consequences like longer duration of healing and increased hospital stay.[23]

Optimizing Nutritional Therapy in Hospitalized Patients

Evidence-based guidelines recommend that enteral feeding in the form of formulae or liquids should always take preference over feeding via the parenteral route unless it is completely contraindicated. If oral feeding is not possible, feeding the patient through a nasogastric or nasoenteric tube should be considered. Enteral nutrition should be considered in patients with a functional gastrointestinal tract but who are unable to swallow safely. Supplementary PN to enteral nutrition is recommended in special situations where the absorption of nutrients from the gut is compromised.[34]

The approach to nutrition support in hospitalized IBD patients: The ESPEN 2020 suggests that ONS is the first line when MNT is indicated in IBD patients. EN is used only if oral feeding is insufficient. Formulae or liquid forms of EN always takes preference over PN, unless EN is completely contraindicated. EEN is known to be effective in inducing remission especially among children and adolescents with active CD.

Nasal tubes or percutaneous access can be used for EN in IBD. Standard EN formulations can be used for EEN or supportive EN.

Parenteral nutrition is indicated only if ONS and EN are still insufficient to manage nutritional requirements or when the bowel is dysfunctional or obstructed or in case of complications like anastomotic leak or high output intestinal fistula.[34]

Chiu E et al. have proposed an algorithm **(Flowchart 3)** for nutritional support in hospitalized IBD patients.

Other recommendations:[34]
- For CD patients, every effort should be made to prevent dehydration to minimize the risk of thromboembolism.
- For CD patients with distal fistula and low output, EEN can be provided, while for those with proximal fistula or very high output, nutritional support in the form of partial or TPN can be given.
- For CD patients with nutritional deprivation over many days, standard precautions should be taken to prevent refeeding syndrome.

The ESPEN 2020 nutritional recommendations for IBD patients with complications can be summarized as follows:[34]
- IBD patients with severe diarrhea or a high-output jejunostomy or ileostomy should be monitored for fluid output and sodium levels should be assessed, based on which input can be calculated and adapted; taking into consideration food intolerance that may lead to increased fluid output.
- For patients with high-output stomas, PN can be considered.
- In CD patients with intestinal strictures or stenosis along with obstructive symptoms, a diet with modified texture or distal EN can be recommended.
- CD patients treated with sequestrants (cholestyramine) have a minimal additional risk of fat malabsorption, and therefore may not need differences in nutrition therapy compared to other patients with CD.
- IBD patients with hyperoxaluria may have fat malabsorption and counseling of these patients is important.

Flowchart 3: Proposed algorithm for nutritional support in hospitalized inflammatory bowel disease patients.

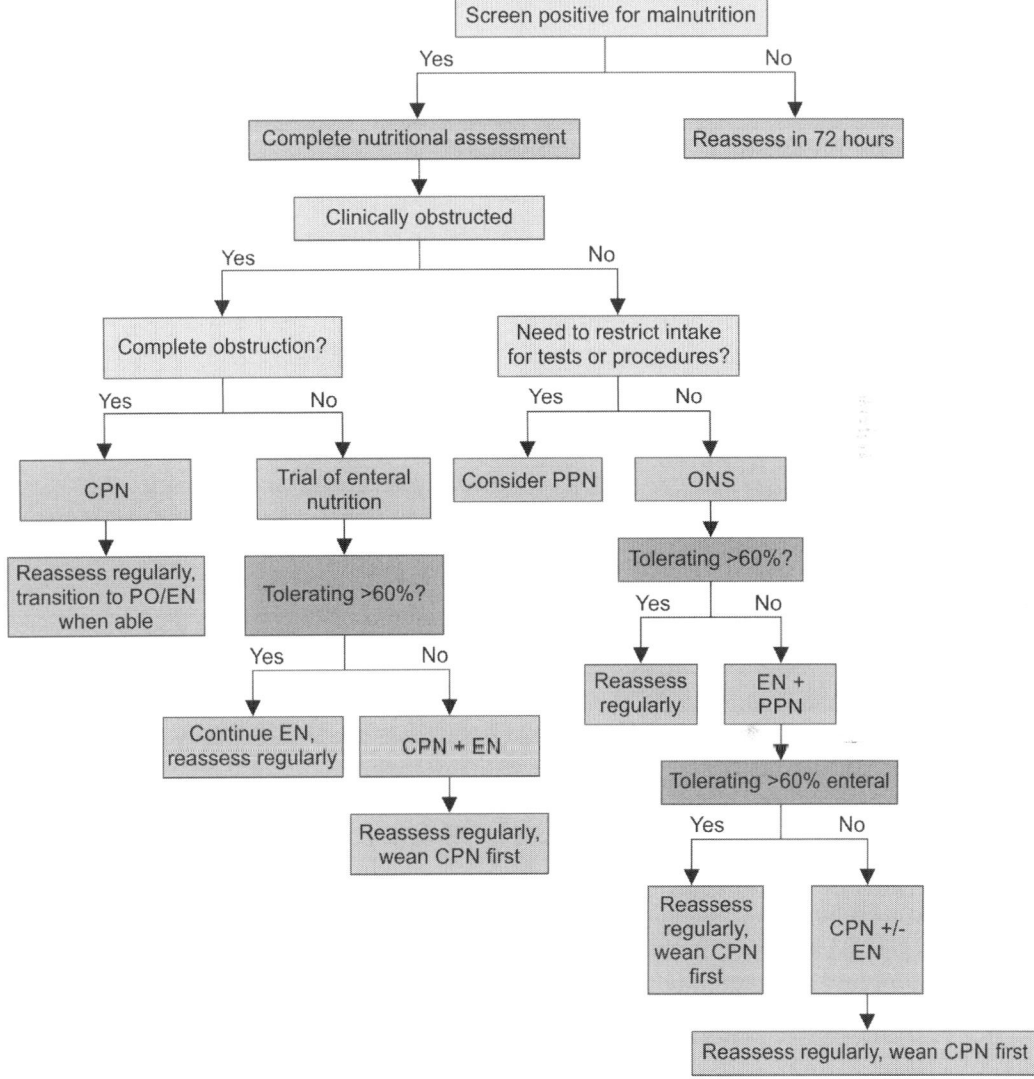

(CPN: central parenteral nutrition; EN: enteral nutrition; ONS: oral nutritional supplement; PO: per os; PPN: peripheral parenteral nutrition)
Source: Chiu E, Oleynick C, Raman M, Bielawska B. Optimizing inpatient nutrition care of adult patients with inflammatory bowel disease in the 21st century. Nutrients. 2021;13(5):1581.

NUTRITIONAL THERAPY FOR PRE- AND POSTSURGICAL IBD PATIENTS

The last few decades have seen a great increase in the availability of therapeutic armamentarium to manage IBD, leading to a decrease in hospitalizations; yet surgery rates remain high.[47] In IBD, surgery represents an essential part of the management spectrum and is indicated for clinical intractability, complications, and neoplasms, and is considered an option in CD patients with isolated ileal disease.[17,48]

Evidence shows that the risk for surgery in a CD patient is approximately 50% during a disease duration of 10 years, while 40% of UC patients requiring hospitalization will ultimately require proctocolectomy. Aggressive disease is known to predispose patients to multiple surgeries, with prevalence data suggesting that 35% of people who require one resection will require a second one within 10 years. The reason why surgery rates are so high is still controversial, but it is postulated that certain molecular mechanisms underlie progression from inflammation to fibrosis which could be the cause of structural damage such as stricture formation, which can be treated only surgically. Postsurgery complications are highly prevalent in IBD and it is evident that nutritional status is one of the major predictors of surgical outcomes.[47,48]

Presurgery Malnutrition

In IBD patients, various factors contribute to the deterioration of nutritional status, such as reduced food intake, increased intestinal losses, malabsorption of nutrients, increased nutritional needs associated with systemic inflammation, and iatrogenic factors (e.g., surgery and medications) which leads to catabolism and sarcopenia.[17,48]

Malnutrition, being a modifiable risk factor for adverse outcomes of surgery, prompt identification and subsequent early nutritional interventions are critical.[48]

According to the ESPEN guidance (2020), the classification of IBD patients at risk of severe malnutrition should include the following criteria:[49]

- Weight loss between 10 and 15% in 6 months
- BMI: 18.5 kg/m^2
- Subjective global assessment grade C
- NRS 5 and serum albumin <3 g/dL (with no evidence of kidney or liver dysfunction).

The Global Leadership Initiative on Malnutrition

The Global Leadership Initiative on Malnutrition (GLIM) represents a new consensus for the diagnosis of malnutrition in CD. It includes three phenotypical criteria (weight loss, low BMI, and reduced muscle mass) and two etiological criteria (reduced food intake or absorption, and increased disease burden or inflammation). If a patient met at least one phenotypical criterion and one etiological criterion, malnutrition was diagnosed. Only one phenotypical criterion for this grade needed to be met to grade a patient's nutritional severity. Details of the GLIM are as follows:[50]

- Weight loss:
  - *Moderate malnutrition:* A nonvolitional weight loss of 5–10% within the past 6 months, or 10–20% beyond 6 months.
  - *Severe malnutrition:* A nonvolitional weight loss of >10% within the past 6 months, or >20% prior to the past 6 months.
- *BMI*:
  The BMI cut-offs for malnutrition risk:
  - *Moderate malnutrition:* <20 kg/m^2 if <70 years, and <22 kg/m^2 if ≥70 years
  - *Severe malnutrition:* A BMI of <18.5 kg/m^2 for those aged <70 years, and <20 kg/m^2 for those aged ≥70 years.
- *Reduced muscle mass*: The FFMI cut-offs for malnutrition risk were <17 kg/m^2 for men and <15 kg/m^2 for women.
- *Reduced food intake or absorption:* Defined as an intake of 50% or less of energy requirements for >1 week, or any reduction for >2 weeks.

- *Increased disease burden or inflammation:* Chronic or recurrent mild-to-moderate inflammation was likely to be associated with malignant disease or any disease that was considered chronic or recurrent.

Nutritional Support for Presurgical IBD Patients

Optimizing nutritional status during the preoperative period contributes to better surgical outcomes. Based on this, guidelines recommend early initiation of nutritional therapy in patients who are unable to eat for >7 days prior to surgery or find it difficult to maintain an oral intake above 60–75% of nutritional needs for >10 days.[48]

In the setting of malnutrition, IBD surgery can be delayed for about 7–10 days to allow for nutritional interventions, keeping in mind the severity of the patient's condition. In an emergency situation, postsurgical nutritional interventions, EN or PN, should be initiated immediately, especially if the patient is unable to resume a full diet within 7 days after surgery. **Box 6** shows the nutrient recommendations for presurgery IBD patients.[36]

A summary of recommendations is mentioned below.[36,48,49]

- Initially, nutritional management is based on increasing caloric intake, which may or may not include oral nutritional supplements. ONS over and above oral nutrition is the first choice of optimizing malnutrition preoperatively.

> **BOX 6:** Nutrient recommendations for presurgery IBD patients.[36]
>
> *ESPEN recommends:*
> - Energy intake = 25–30 kcal/day
> - Protein = 1.5 g/kg/day

(ESPEN: European Society for Clinical Nutrition and Metabolism; IBD: inflammatory bowel disease)

- Choice of nutritional therapy will depend on the current clinical condition and the nutritional status of the patient. Both EN and PN interventions are known to help ameliorate the risk of presurgical malnutrition.
- EN is preferred over PN in most cases, but if EN does not supply more than 60% of the energy needs, PN can be supplemented in case of patients experiencing severe gastrointestinal symptoms such as diarrhea, vomiting, absence of access, and bowel obstruction.[48] The ESPEN recommends initiation of EN if calorie needs cannot be met with ONS alone. Elemental, semielemental or polymeric formulae can be used.
- EEN is shown to lower the risk of postsurgical complications. The British Society of Gastroenterology Consensus, recommend EEN for a minimum period of 4–6 weeks, to reduce symptoms and improve the healing conditions of the intestinal mucosa.
- PN can be considered in specific situations where EEN is not possible. Preoperative use of PN shows a general trend toward improvement in postoperative outcomes. The purpose of TPN in the preoperative period is restoration of energy and protein storage, reduction and/or correction of micronutrient deficiencies, in addition to preventing postsurgical malnutrition in patients at nutritional risk. The duration of TPN in the preoperative period may vary from 5 to 90 days. Most studies show 7–14 days as an ideal duration for total PN in the preoperative period.
- A combination of EEN and TPN should be considered in patients who need nutritional support of more than 60% for the daily needs that cannot be achieved by EEN alone. For example, in patients

with severe and chronic malnutrition associated with CD, with strictures and episodes of partial small bowel obstruction. A recent systematic review (2019) found that EEN is more favorable than TPN, due to the lower incidence of complications and bacterial translocation, preservation of gastrointestinal function, and lower cost.
- However, EEN optimization can be slower than TPN, which should always be considered when planning the time to perform abdominal surgical procedures, on a case-to-case individual basis. Fiorindi et al. (2020) demonstrated the benefits of perioperative nutrition (reduction in fasting duration and increase intake of carbohydrates during the preoperative stage), regardless of nutritional status. These strategies collaborate with an observed reduction of postoperative complications.

According to the British Society of Gastroenterology (2019), presurgical correction of anemia is also an important consideration as it is associated with a reduction in risk of intra-abdominal sepsis, intestinal obstruction, anastomotic dehiscence, pneumonia, and other infections in the postsurgical period. Oral or intravenous iron supplementation is preferred over blood transfusion.[49]

The algorithm for nutritional interventions in pre- and postsurgical IBD patients is shown in **Flowchart 4**.

Protocol for enhanced recovery after surgery (ERAS) recommends the following without compromising surgical outcomes:
- A 6-hour and 2-hour preoperative fasting for liquids, with a carbohydrate-based drink (12% maltodextrin associated or not with proteins) with a volume of 400 mL and 200 mL, respectively.
- 8 hours for solid foods

Enhanced recovery after surgery is contraindicated in certain cases like severe gastroesophageal reflux, pyloric stenosis, gastroparesis, and intestinal obstruction.

Evidence suggests that drinks with high carbohydrate concentration administered 2–3 hours before surgery can improve the patient's nutritional status in the postoperative setting, accelerate recovery, and decrease the length of hospital stay.[49]

In case of pre-planned surgeries, where patients are well-nourished, prehabilitation can be adopted using the ERAS protocol to minimize the risk. A study conducted by Fiorindi C et al. (2020) demonstrated significant improvement in weight, BMI, lean mass in well-nourished CD and UC patients who were prehabilitated prior to surgery. UC and CD patients exposed to the ERAS protocol showed good compliance and had similar mean time to resumption of oral intake. Patients also had an extremely low incidence of postoperative complications.[17]

Guidelines recommend initiation of postoperative EN within 24 hours of surgery for patients who are malnourished and those who cannot reach at least 60% of their nutritional requirement orally with an aim to reduce morbidity and mortality rates.[49]

Clearly, this may not be possible due to the occurrence of postoperative ileus. A study conducted by Nakeeb et al. (2009) demonstrated benefits to patients when nutritional supplements were taken orally (200 mL twice a day), until normal feeding is achieved.[49]

In the postoperative period, a hyperproteic diet is recommended to achieve the required protein goal.[49]

Ideal Duration of Continued Nutritional Support in the Postoperative Period

To date, there seems to be no consensus on the ideal duration of time, postsurgery, required to continue nutritional support. However, some studies recommend that nutritional

Flowchart 4: Algorithm for nutritional interventions in pre- and postsurgical IBD patients: ESPEN 2020.[49]

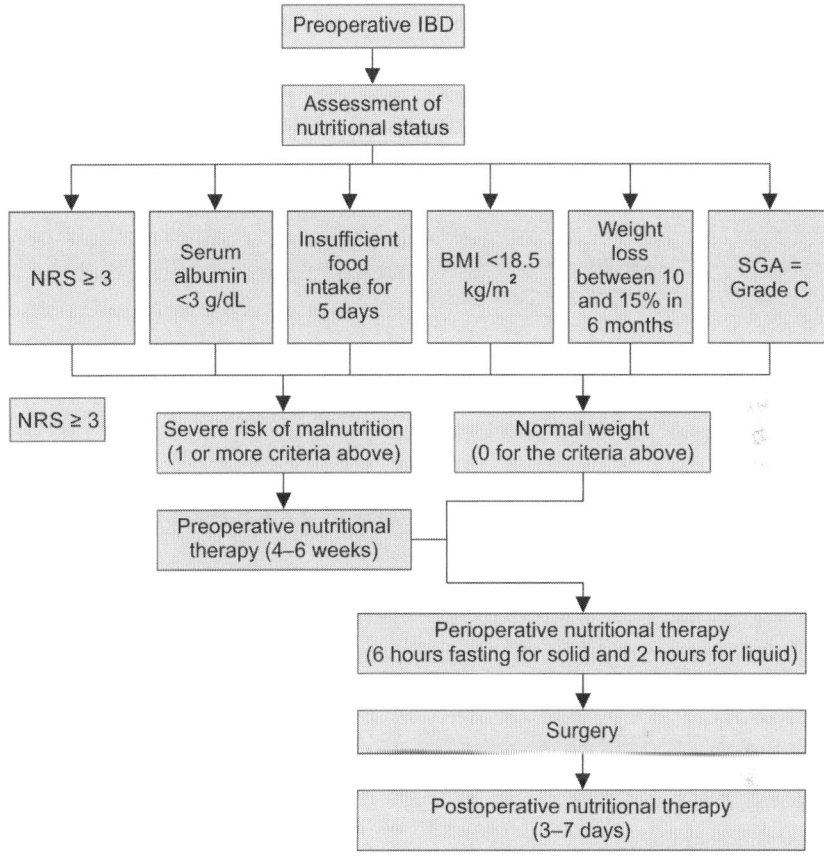

(BMI: body mass index; ERAS: enhanced recovery after surgery; ESPEN: European Society for Clinical Nutrition and Metabolism; IBD: inflammatory diseases; NRS: Nutritional Risk Screening; SGA: subjective global assessment)

therapy between 3 and 10 days (with 7 days being the most common) can greatly benefit in the recovery of nutritional status and quality of life of patients with malnutrition. In eutrophic patients, the evidence is not so clinically relevant.[49]

Immunonutrition

Some studies demonstrated the benefits of immune nutrition with glutamine, arginine, omega-3 fatty acids, and RNA help reduce overall complications when used pre-, peri- and postoperatively. According to the International Anesthesia Research Society (2018), both nourished and malnourished patients should use immune nutrition, mainly in the pre- and perioperative period. The recommended duration of immunonutrition for patients with adequate weight is of at least 7 days.[49]

Malnourished patients need weekly evaluation with serum albumin (>3 g/dL) often being recommended as a marker for a better decision with respect to the duration of use. In elective surgeries, nutritional supplementation should be recommended.

In cases of emergency surgery (severe acute colitis and severe CD with septic or obstructive complications), nutritional optimization should be postponed, due to increased mortality with delayed surgery ESPEN (2020). Nutritional assessment according to the criteria for defining malnutrition serves as a screening tool for preoperative nutritional optimization. Benefits of nutritional care is clearly seen as important not only in the perioperative period but also after surgery and for better postoperative outcomes.[49]

Nutritional Support for IBD Patients Postostomy

Ileostomies and colostomies are the most common forms of stoma created to enable fecal contents to be discharged into an external pouch from the ileum or colon, respectively. Complications of an ostomy include high and/or loose stool output, constipation, blockage, wind, and odor. Dietary interventions are critical for IBD patients postostomy to ensure adequate nutritional status and well-being.[51]

Aims of dietary management:[52]
- To prevent stoma blockage
- To promote healing of the stoma wound
- To minimize unpleasant gastrointestinal upsets like flatulence, diarrhea, odors and constipation.

POSTCOLOSTOMY DIET MANAGEMENT

Early feeding postsurgery is encouraged as it can accelerate the return of bowel function and improve rehabilitation. The diet should progress from a liquid to a low-residue diet and should be high in protein, energy, and micronutrients to promote healing. Salt intake should be monitored along with adequate fluid intake to prevent dehydration. Gradual introduction of new foods is important to identify offending foods and control obstruction.[52]

POSTILEOSTOMY DIET MANAGEMENT

In this procedure, the use of the entire large intestine, rectum, and anus are temporarily bypassed to rest the system in order to allow for healing before joining them back together. This procedure causes a reduction in fat, bile acid and vitamin B_{12} absorption and greater losses of electrolytes. Nutritional requirements for such patients will vary depending on the health of the remaining portion of the bowel, current diagnosis and individual health and the aim of diet therapy is to optimize diets to compensate for these losses.

A high energy, high protein diet, low in insoluble fiber is suggested postoperatively. High-fiber foods should be avoided for at least 4 weeks postsurgery. Recommended foods postsurgery are:[52]
- *Apples:* High in pectin
- *Oats:* Rich in oligosaccharides
- *Spinach and parsley:* Natural deodorizing properties
- *Lean meats and egg whites:* Rich source of protein
- *Liver, eggs, fish:* Good sources of vitamin B_{12}

Diet should also provide an adequate amount of fluids, especially in hot weather.

STEP WISE MANAGEMENT OF CARE POSTILEOSTOMY[52]

First postoperative phase: 1–3 months postsurgery is a phase which is associated with massive diarrhea and limited absorption.

Recommendations: IV or TPN immediately before and for approximately 5 days postsurgery to allow for bowel rest. If diarrhea is >2 L/day, TPN can be used, with gradual increase to avoid refeeding syndrome.

Second postoperative phase: 4–12 months post-surgery is a phase when absorption improves, weight gain begins, and diarrhea is reduced.

Recommendations: PN may be slowly reduced and EN can begin at a slow, continuous rate according to stomal or stool output.

Energy requirement is high, approximately 40–60 kcal/kg/day and protein requirement is 1.2–1.5 g/kg/day. In case of weight loss >1 kg/week or if diarrhea persists (>600 g/day), TPN may need to be restarted.

Third postoperative phase: 18–24 months postsurgery is a phase when total parenteral nutrition could be discontinued, especially when fluid intake is up to 7 L/day and energy intake is sufficient to ensure the desired weight goal. This is a phase when bowel adaptation begins, and oral diet is tolerated.

Recommendations: Six small meals in the proportion of carbohydrates 60%, protein 20%, fats 20% with a limit of 40 g medium-chain triglycerides (MCT). **Tables 4 and 5** can be referred to for foods that provide relief from commonly experienced issues after an ostomy.

If colon is completely resected, diet may need to be 30–40% fat, 20% protein, and 40–50% carbohydrates. Jejunostomy feeding may need to be used as supplementation and oxalate restriction may not be required. PN can be reduced either by decreasing the number of days of PN infusion per week or volume across the week.

Supplementation of zinc, potassium, liquid magnesium, oral calcium, manganese, iron, selenium, vitamins, and other nutrients may be needed. Extra vitamin K may be

TABLE 4: Foods that can cause intolerance.[52]

Stoma obstructive	Odor producing	Increased/loose stool diarrhea	Gas producing
Apple peels, raw cabbage, celery, Chinese vegetables, whole corn kernels, popcorn, coconuts, dry fruits, mushrooms, oranges, nuts, pineapple, fruits with skin and seeds	Baked beans, asparagus, broccoli, cabbage, cod liver oil, eggs, fish, garlic, onions, peanut butter, strong cheeses, some vitamins	Alcoholic beverages, whole grains, bran cereals, cooked cabbage, fresh fruits, green leafy vegetables, milk, prunes, apple and prune juice, raisins, raw vegetables, spices	Alcoholic beverages, carbonated drinks, beans, soy, cabbage, cauliflower, dairy products, chewing gum, milk, nuts, onions, radishes

Source: Adapted from Akbulut G. Nutrition in stoma patients: A practical view of dietary therapy. International J Hematol Oncol. 2011;32(4):061-6.

TABLE 5: Foods that provide relief.[52]

Constipation relief	Odor control	Loose stool control	Reducing flatulence	Color changes
Coffee (warm, hot), cooked fruits and vegetables, fresh fruits, fruit juices, water, mild laxatives	Buttermilk, cranberry juice, orange juice, parsley, tomato juice, yoghurt, peppermint oil	Applesauce, unripe bananas, boiled rice, peanut butter, tapioca, toast, white bread, potatoes, pasta, crackers, boiled rice, weak tea, marshmallows, jellies	Fennel tea, cranberry juice, buttermilk, peppermint oil	Asparagus, beets, food colors, iron pills, licorice, strawberries, tomato sauces

Source: Adapted from Akbulut G. Nutrition in stoma patients: A practical view of dietary therapy. International J Hematol Oncol. 2011;32(4):061-6.

> **BOX 7:** General healthy eating guidelines for ostomy patients.[52]
> - A healthy balanced diet and supplements if needed, to ensure adequate intake of macro- and micronutrients
> - A low-fiber/low-residue diet is recommended postostomy
> - New foods to be added one at a time to observe their effects
> - Eating at regular intervals to reduce incidence of flatulence
> - Thorough chewing of foods to improve tolerance and absorption
> - Avoidance of dairy in case of lactose intolerance

Source: Adapted from Akbulut G. Nutrition in stoma patients: a practical view of dietary therapy. International J Hematol Oncol. 2011;32(4):061-6.

needed for patients on antibiotics. Lactose- and oxalate-restricted diets may be needed for an extended period. Alcoholic beverages and caffeine should be avoided. Fluids should be consumed in between meals rather than with meals to reduce dumping. In case of osmotic diarrhea, a reduction in simple carbohydrates and increase in complex carbohydrates may be needed.[52]

Box 7 describes some general healthy eating guidelines in ostomy patients.

CONCLUSION

Malnourished and active IBD patients present with metabolic stress, with a deficit in macro- and micronutrients, muscle catabolism and increased basal metabolic rate. The screening of nutritional status, performed at diagnosis, hospitalization and during the preoperative period, is of significant importance to identify patients who need nutritional optimization.

Diet may play a causal as well as a therapeutic role in IBD, with dietary recommendations forming an integral part of therapy.

Oral nutrition should be the first choice of nutritional support with or without the use of nutrition supplement formulae. PN has to be resorted to in conditions where oral feeding is contraindicated (in the presence of intestinal obstruction or ischemia, fistula, or bleeding).

Nutritional support can be performed exclusively or in an associated way, depending on the nutritional severity of the patient with IBD. The reduction of complications in the perioperative period is not only associated with adequate surgical technique, but also with adequate nutritional support and clinical preparation before surgery. Therefore, a dietician with a focus in IBD has an important role in the multidisciplinary team, at all stages of treatment for the optimization of the nutritional status of a surgical patient.

REFERENCES

1. Ray G. Inflammatory bowel disease in India – Past, present and future. World J Gastroenterol. 2016;22(36):8123-36.
2. Shivashankar R, Lewis JD. The Role of Diet in Inflammatory Bowel Disease. Curr Gastroenterol Rep. 2017;19(5):22.
3. Jain M, Venkataraman J. Inflammatory bowel disease: An Indian perspective. Indian J Med Res. 2021;153(4):421.
4. Abhirami NR, Laksmi VV, Deepitha AM. A Review on Prevalence of Inflammatory Bowel Disease in India. 2022;12(6):219-23.
5. Balestrieri P, Ribolsi M, Guarino MPL, Emerenziani S, Altomare A, Cicala M. Nutritional Aspects in Inflammatory Bowel Diseases. Nutrients. 2020;12(2):372.
6. Haskey N, Peña-Sánchez JN, Jones JL, Fowler SA. Development of a screening tool to detect nutrition risk in patients with inflammatory bowel disease. 2018;27(4):756-62.
7. Ananthakrishnan AN. Nutritional Management of Inflammatory Bowel Diseases A Comprehensive Guide. Cham Springer International Publishing; 2016.

8. Knight-Sepulveda K, Kais S, Santaolalla R, Abreu MT. Diet and Inflammatory Bowel Disease. Gastroenterol Hepatol (N Y). 2015;11(8):511-20.
9. de Castro MM, Pascoal LB, Steigleder KM, Siqueira BP, Corona LP, Ayrizono M, et al. Role of diet and nutrition in inflammatory bowel disease. World J Exp Med. 2021;11(1):1-16.
10. Sartor RB. Mechanisms of disease: Pathogenesis of Crohn's disease and ulcerative colitis. Nat Clin Pract Gastroenterol Hepatol. 2006;3(7):390-407.
11. Narula N, Wong ECL, Dehghan M, Mente A, Rangarajan, S, Lanas, F, et al. Association of ultra-processed food intake with risk of inflammatory bowel disease: prospective cohort study. BMJ. 2021;374:n1554.
12. Roser M, Ritchie H, Rosado P. Food Supply. Our World in Data; 2013.
13. Marion-Letellier R, Amamou A, Savoye G, Ghosh S. Inflammatory Bowel Diseases and Food Additives: To Add Fuel on the Flames! Nutrients. 2019;11(5):1111.
14. Misra A, Singhal N, Sivakumar B, Bhagat N, Jaiswal A, Khurana L. Nutrition transition in India: Secular trends in dietary intake and their relationship to diet-related non-communicable diseases. J Diabetes. 2011;3(4):278-92.
15. Scaldaferri F, Pizzoferrato M, Lopetuso LR, Musca T, Ingravalle F, Sicignano LL, et al. Nutrition and IBD: Malnutrition and/or Sarcopenia? A Practical Guide. Gastroenterol Res Pract. 2017;2017:8646495.
16. Damas OM, Garces L, Abreu MT. Diet as Adjunctive Treatment for Inflammatory Bowel Disease: Review and Update of the Latest Literature. Curr Treat Options Gastroenterol. 2019;17(2):313-25.
17. Fiorindi C, Luceri C, Dragoni G, Piemonte G, Scaringi S, Staderini F, et al. GLIM Criteria for Malnutrition in Surgical IBD Patients: A Pilot Study. Nutrients. 2020;12(8):2222.
18. Casanova MJ, Chaparro M, Molina B, Merino O, Batanero R, Dueñas-Sadornil C, et al. Prevalence of Malnutrition and Nutritional Characteristics of Patients with Inflammatory Bowel Disease. J Crohns Colitis. 2017;11(12):1430-9.
19. Halmos E. Nutrition assessment of IBD patients [Review of Nutrition assessment of IBD patients]. ECCO; 2016.
20. Montgomery SC, Williams CM, Maxwell PJ. Nutritional Support of Patient with Inflammatory Bowel Disease. Surg Clin North Am. 2015;95(6):1271-9.
21. Green N, Miller T, Suskind D, Lee D. A Review of Dietary Therapy for IBD and a Vision for the Future. Nutrients. 2019;11(5):947.
22. Yoon H, Yang SK, So H, Lee KE, Park SH, Jung SA, et al. Development, validation, and application of a novel tool to measure disease-related knowledge in patients with inflammatory bowel disease. Korean J Intern Med. 2019;34(1):81-9.
23. Palchaudhuri S, Albenberg L, Lewis JD. Diet Recommendations for Hospitalized Patients with Inflammatory Bowel Disease: Better Options than Nil Per Os. Crohns Colitis 360. 2020;2(4):otaa059.
24. Ashton JJ, Gavin J, Beattie RM. Exclusive enteral nutrition in Crohn's disease: Evidence and practicalities. Clin Nutr. 2019;38(1):80-9.
25. Sahu P, Kedia S, Vuyyuru SK, Bajaj A, Markandey M, Singh N, et al. Randomised clinical trial: exclusive enteral nutrition versus standard of care for acute severe ulcerative colitis. Aliment Pharmacol Ther. 2021;53(5):568-76.
26. Day AS. The impact of exclusive enteral nutrition on the intestinal microbiota in inflammatory bowel disease. AIMS Microbiol. 2018;4(4):584-93.
27. Svolos V, Hansen R, Nichols B, Quince C, Ijaz UZ, Papadopoulou RT, et al. Treatment of Active Crohn's Disease with an Ordinary Food-based Diet that Replicates Exclusive Enteral Nutrition. Gastroenterology. 2019;156(5):1354-67.
28. Chiba M, Abe T, Tsuda H, Sugawara T, Tsuda S, Tozawa H, et al. Lifestyle-related disease in Crohn's disease: Relapse prevention by a semi-vegetarian diet. World J Gastroenterol. 2010;16(20):2484-95.

29. Shafiee NH, Manaf ZA, Mokhtar NM, Raja Ali RA. Anti-inflammatory diet and inflammatory bowel disease: what clinicians and patients should know? Intest Res. 2021;19(2):171-85.
30. Konijeti GG, Kim N, Lewis JD, Groven S, Chandrasekaran A, Grandhe S, et al. Efficacy of the Autoimmune Protocol Diet for Inflammatory Bowel Disease. Inflamm Bowel Dis. 2017;23(11):2054-60.
31. Szczubełek M, Pomorska K, Korólczyk-Kowalczyk M, Lewandowski K, Kaniewska M, Rydzewska G. Effectiveness of Crohn's Disease Exclusion Diet for Induction of Remission in Crohn's Disease Adult Patients. Nutrients. 2021;13(11):4112.
32. Johnson T. Treatment of active Crohn's disease in children using partial enteral nutrition with liquid formula: a randomised controlled trial. Gut. 2006;55(3):356-61.
33. Levine A, Wine E, Assa A, Sigall Boneh R, Shaoul R, Kori M, et al. Crohn's Disease Exclusion Diet Plus Partial Enteral Nutrition Induces Sustained Remission in a Randomized Controlled Trial. Gastroenterology. 2019;157(2):440-50.
34. Levine A, Rhodes JM, Lindsay JO, Abreu MT, Kamm MA, Gibson PR, et al. Dietary Guidance From the International Organization for the Study of Inflammatory Bowel Diseases. Clin Gastroenterol Hepatol. 2020;18(6):1381-92.
35. Forbes A, Escher J, Hébuterne X, Kłęk S, Krznaric Z, Schneider S, et al. ESPEN guideline: Clinical nutrition in inflammatory bowel disease. Clin Nutr. 2017;36(2):321-47.
36. Chiu E, Oleynick C, Raman M, Bielawska B. Optimizing Inpatient Nutrition Care of Adult Patients with Inflammatory Bowel Disease in the 21st Century. Nutrients. 2021;13(5):1581.
37. Yamamoto T, Nakahigashi M, Shimoyama T, Umegae S. Does preoperative enteral nutrition reduce the incidence of surgical complications in patients with Crohn's disease? A case-matched study. Colorectal Dis. 2019;22(5):554-61.
38. Sood A, Ahuja V, Kedia S, Midha V, Mahajan R, Mehta V, et al. Diet and inflammatory bowel disease: The Asian Working Group guidelines. Indian J Gastroenterol. 2019;38(3):220-46.
39. Narula N, Dhillon A, Zhang D, Sherlock ME, Tondeur M, Zachos M. Enteral nutritional therapy for induction of remission in Crohn's disease. Cochrane Database Syst Rev. 20181;4(4):CD000542.
40. Costa-Santos MP, Palmela C, Torres J, Ferreira A, Velho S, Ourô S, et al. Preoperative enteral nutrition in adults with complicated Crohn's disease: Effect on disease outcomes and gut microbiota. Nutrition. 2020:70S:100009.
41. Zheng X, Peng X, Xie X, Lian L, Wu X, Hu J, et al. Enteral nutrition is associated with a decreased risk of surgical intervention in Crohn's disease patients with spontaneous intra-abdominal abscess. Rev Esp Enferm Dig. 2017;109(12):834-42.
42. Greenberg GR, Fleming CR, Jeejeebhoy KN, Rosenberg IH. Controlled trial of bowel rest and nutritional support in the management of Crohn's disease. Gut. 1988;29:1309-15.
43. Richman E, Rhodes JM. Review article: evidence-based dietary advice for patients with inflammatory bowel disease. Aliment Pharmacol Ther. 2013;38(10):1156-71.
44. Triantafillidis JK, Papalois AE. The role of total parenteral nutrition in inflammatory bowel disease: current aspects. Scand J Gastroenterol. 2013;49(1):3-14.
45. Egberg MD, Galanko JA, Barnes EL, Kappelman MD. Thrombotic and Infectious Risks of Parenteral Nutrition in Hospitalized Pediatric Inflammatory Bowel Disease. Inflammatory Bowel Diseases. 2018;25(3):601-9.
46. Bischoff SC, Escher J, Hébuterne X, Kłęk S, Krznaric Z, Schneider S, et al. ESPEN practical guideline: Clinical Nutrition in inflammatory bowel disease. Clin Nutr. 2020;39(3):632-53.
47. Stoner PL, Kamel A, Ayoub F, Tan S, Iqbal A, Glover SC, et al. Perioperative Care of

Patients with Inflammatory Bowel Disease: Focus on Nutritional Support. Gastroenterol Res Pract. 2018;2018:7890161.

48. Rocha R, de J Santos G, Santana G. Influence of nutritional status in the postoperative period of patients with inflammatory bowel disease. World J Gastrointest Pharmacol Ther. 2021;12(5):90-9.

49. da Silva ISM, Cambi MPC, Magro DO, Kotze PG. Perioperative Nutritional Optimization in Inflammatory Bowel Diseases: When and How? J Coloproctol. 2021;41(03): 295-300.

50. Lim HS, Kim SK, Hong SJ. Food Elimination Diet and Nutritional Deficiency in Patients with Inflammatory Bowel Disease. Clin Nutr Res. 2018;7(1):48.

51. Mitchell A, Perry R, England C, Searle A, Atkinson C. Dietary management in people with an ileostomy: a scoping review protocol. JBI Database System Rev Implement Rep. 2019;17(2):129-36.

52. Akbulut G. Nutrition in Stoma Patients: A Practical View of Dietary Therapy. International Journal of Hematology and Oncology. 2011;21(1):61-6.

SECTION 2: Planning and Nutritional Interventions

7. **Indirect Calorimetry in Critical Illness**
   Sanjith Saseedharan

8. **Macronutrients in Critical Illness: Nutrition Backbones for Survival and Recovery!**
   Varsha M Asrani

9. **Micronutrient Physiology and Requirements in Critical Illness**
   Ranil Jayawardena

10. **Probiotics, Prebiotics, Synbiotics, and Postbiotics**
    B Ravinder Reddy

11. **Mechanical and Metabolic Complications of Parenteral Nutrition**
    Subhankar Paul, Rajesh Pande

CHAPTER 7

Indirect Calorimetry in Critical Illness

Sanjith Saseedharan

■ INTRODUCTION

Personalized medicine or individualization of care has been holding great promise and there is no more striking example than the use of indirect calorimetry (IC) in the determination of resting energy expenditure (REE). This is all the more important in critical illness. Critical illness is a pathological state, which has similar characteristics across individuals; however, the intensity of the response varies between individuals. Central to all of this is a drop in the skeletal muscle mass and skeletal muscle weight, which contributes to prolonged duration of stay, and increased length on mechanical ventilation with far-reaching implication on morbidity and also mortality. In fact, the body fights hard to maintain homeostasis so that the vitals and organs systems can keep working in clockwork precision. The provision of optimal energy supply to the critically ill patient, thus, becomes vital in the optimization of patient outcomes. What is known is that both underfeeding and overfeeding are known to adversely affect clinical outcomes.[1] This not only requires the help of nutritional support teams but also requires the actual measurement of the energy expenditure (EE) by the use of IC. This requires a correct understanding of the method of measurements, the potential confounders, and limitations to use this to the potential advantage for patients. Needless to say, IC is the gold standard in the measurement of EE, especially over the phases of critical illness and the disease process. With the advent of the new generation of IC machines and devices, the process of measuring EE and thus delivery of the optimal energy to the patient has become even more easy, cost effective, less labor intensive, and can be performed by any individual with a very short-learning curve.[1,2]

■ WHY IS THIS REQUIRED?

Indirect calorimetry is a monitoring tool used to measure EE in order to optimize the delivery of energy in critically ill patients. In the absence of IC, simple weight predictive equations or equations based on weight, height, age, gender, etc., are used to estimate the EE. In fact, this can be extremely inaccurate in obese individuals since their lean body mass may be different from what their actual body weight would be. However, there are multiple studies demonstrating that use of predictive equations are very inaccurate (with deviation of estimated EE by up to 60%) and can potentially lead to poor outcomes due to underfeeding and overfeeding. In fact, studies that have looked at EE using VCO_2 values derived from some ventilators alone have also been proven inferior to the use of IC.[3-5] Importantly,

Zusman et al. demonstrated a U-shaped relationship between the proportion of energy delivered compared to that measured by REE and mortality. The results indicated best survival when around 70% REE was provided.[6] This makes it imperative to measure the exact REE using indirect calorimeter. Importantly, various disease states would have very varying REE.

Sepsis is said to be a hypermetabolic state. However, what is known is that there a substantial variation in the REE and seems to vary based on the degree of response by the body. Importantly, though there is a hyperdynamic state there is bound to be mitochondrial failure and hence reduced consumption of oxygen which may thus alter the REE. Very similar to this a trauma, the patient will have variable REE dependent on the organ involved. For example, an abdominal trauma has much higher REE as compared to a limb injury. In fact in traumatic brain injury, the REE can vary both in duration and degree. Burns patient are known to have an increase in the metabolism by almost 100% and thus EE, which varies widely depending on the degree of burn which can persist all along the healing period which may be as much as 12 months. Cancer patients are unique as these may have a hypermetabolic, a normometabolic, or a hypometabolic state which are all physiological adaptations to the tumor burden and inflammation. Cirrhotic and renal failure patients are unique due to the anabolic resistance, and weight changes that occur due to fluid accumulation (ascites) making predictive equations essentially inaccurate. Hence, the predictability of REE is impossible with most illness more so in patients with critical illness and multi-organ insufficiency which thus requires a formal measurement making the use of IC imperative.

PRINCIPLES OF INDIRECT CALORIMETRY

Every energy-producing reaction oxygen is consumed and CO_2 is produced in proportion to the EE. This is the basic principle of IC in a rather basic sense. The following terminology is important to understand the principles of IC. VO_2 is the measurement of oxygen consumption and VCO_2 is the measured carbon dioxide, both of which are measured from the respiratory gas using a metabolic module and gas analyzers in the indirect calorimeter device. Both these gases are influenced by metabolism to meet energy requirements. Carbohydrates, proteins, and fats also called macronutrients are oxidized in the presence of oxygen and converted to carbon dioxide, water, and heat. This process is proportional to the EE. The equation called as the abbreviated "Weirs equation" is then used to calculate the EE. The ratio of VCO_2/VO_2 is called the respiratory quotient (RQ), which represents the net substrate oxidation. This is usually between 0.7 and 1.2 and values outside of this range in patients should trigger further questioning on the adequacy of measurements. An RQ ≥ 1.0 indicates lipogenesis; complete oxidation of glucose generates a RQ value of 1.0, while a RQ of 0.7 is indicative of a mixed substrate oxidation. However, RQ alone cannot pinpoint which substrates are oxidized. Total energy expenditure (TEE) is the energy required by the human body to go about performing the daily functions. This TEE has three parts, viz., the basal metabolic rate (BMR) or basal energy expenditure (BEE), the thermic effect of food [TEF; also known as diet-induced thermogenesis (DIT)], and the energy cost of physical activity-induced energy expenditure (AEE), i.e., TEE = BMR + DIT + AEE. As the name suggests, AEE is the most variable part of the equation as it depends on the physical exertion or exercise that the person is performing. Our critically ill patients do not perform heavy active exercises and hence the impact is limited in critically ill patient. IC measures the REE which is 50–75% of the TEE and represents the energy required to maintain the cardiac, respiratory, secretary, cellular systems, and basal metabolic tone. Practically speaking, this is the mandatory EE in maintaining the vital activities. Most IC systems use the abbreviated Weirs equation to calculate EE, expressed as: REE (kcal/day) = $(3.94 \times VO_2) + (1.1 \times VCO_2) \times 1{,}440$ where VO_2 and VCO_2 are expressed in L/min and 1,440 is the number of minutes in a day.[7,8]

METHODS OF PERFORMANCE ON INDIRECT CALORIMETRY

There are four methods in which IC can be done.

1. *Total collection systems:* In this system, the entire expired gas is collected in a flexible bag or a rigid system, also called as "mixing chamber".

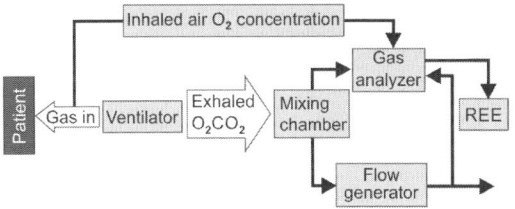

2. *Open circuit indirect systems:* There are two types of these systems. One of these is the ventilated open-circuit systems where a subject breathes into a container through which air is drawn, and the other is expiratory collection systems where a subject inspires from the atmosphere and expires via a nonreturn valve into a measurement unit.

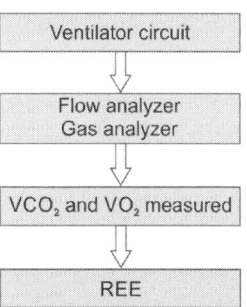

The difference between both the above methods is the fact that the open-circuit indirect systems would require very sensitive and accurate measurements of the exhaled gas flows which poses technical difficulties including the requirement of a fast and accurate sensor whereas the mixing chamber technique eliminates this measurement.

3. *Confinement systems:* Patient is placed in an airtight chamber of known volume. Oxygen consumption and carbon dioxide production are estimated from changes in the concentrations of these gases in a chamber air over time.

4. *Closed circuit systems:* This consists of a sealed respiratory gas circuit in which gaseous concentrations are measured over time.

OVERVIEW OF CONVENTIONAL DEVICES

Most devices used for measuring EE via IC in the hospital-based clinical settings are based on the open-circuit indirect system. All devices that are used in the measurement have quick response oxygen (e.g., paramagnetic) and carbon dioxide (e.g., infrared) sensors and an accurate gas analyzer that measures oxygen and carbon dioxide and their changes in extremely minute amounts (up to 0.001%). These machines are also equipped with flow and volume measuring devices. At the time of writing this chapter, the Q-NRG® and E-sCOVX® (GE Healthcare, Helsinki, Finland) are the most widely used machines/devices used for IC. Here, it is important to note that the Q-NRG® is a new-generation indirect calorimeter, which has been made after the ICALIC investigators (from the ESPEN and ESICM) got together in a multicenter study.[9] Presently, this is the only device that has been tested against mass spectrometry (MAX300-LG, Extrel, Pittsburgh, USA)[10,11] and has demonstrated good accuracy in both, spontaneously breathing patients and mechanically ventilated patients up to an FiO_2 of 75%. In comparison to all other calorimeters, this device has better reactivity, portability, is battery-powered, and does not need any warmup time.[12]

The Q-NRG® requires a single-use flowmeter, which is placed in series in the patient circuit (in ventilated patients) to measure ventilatory parameters. Two sampling lines from the machine are connected to patient circuit and ventilator outlet for the measurement of inspired/expired gases. Importantly and rather cleverly, the machine is equipped with a dynamic micromixing chamber (2 mL), which reduces time for the stabilization of gas concentrations. The proportion of sampled (usually around 0.015% of the minute ventilation) gas in the mixing chamber is proportional to the minute ventilation. This helps in reducing the VO_2 and VCO_2 variability using which the measurements of REE is done using the Weirs equation.

In spontaneously breathing patients, a canopy is used which has a constant flow to create an outward flow through the canopy which dilutes the exhaled gases, which allows the calculation of VO_2 and VCO_2.

While the E-sCOVX® (GE Healthcare, Helsinki, Finland) needs a metabolic module and paramagnetic sensor for O_2 measurement and infrared sensor for CO_2 using which the module samples the oxygen and carbon dioxide on a breath-by-breath basis to calculate the VO_2 and VCO_2 using the flow sensor. However, this module needs the patient to be mechanically ventilated with a compatible ventilator and needs a warmup time of 30 minutes.

ALTERNATIVE METHODS TO INDIRECT CALORIMETRY

Simple predictive weight-based equations are the most commonly used methods in the absence of IC, Fick's principle (uses cardiac output, blood gases and hemoglobin along with the insertion of a Swan Ganz catheter), using simple equations to calculate EE based on VCO_2 derived from mechanical ventilator, double-labeled water method using nonradioactive isotope, simple-motion sensor devices, and use of DEXA (dual-energy X-ray absorptiometry) scans and BIA (bioelectrical impedance analysis). All these methods are fraught with many disadvantages. Apart from all of them being inaccurate in comparison to IC, some of them (e.g., the Fick's method) need insertion of a pulmonary artery catheter and thus makes in invasive. Double-labeled water method is time consuming and expensive, motion sensors have not been extensively studied in clinical practice, while devices like BIA have a problem with hydration status changes that occur in intensive care unit (ICU). Hence, IC thus remains the gold standard in the estimation of EE. In the absence of IC, it is recommended to use simple weight-based predictive equations, viz., 20 kcal/kg/day for the first 7 days followed by 25 kcal/kg/day after 7 days.

HOW FREQUENTLY SHOULD THE ENERGY EXPENDITURE MEASUREMENT BE DONE?

As per the results of the TICACOS study, there was significant variability in the measured REE. Hence, it is recommended to measure REE at least once if the patient is going to be in the ICU for <5 days and in case the patient is going to stay for >5 days, then it is important to conduct the measurement at least twice to thrice per week.[13] IC should also be done when the condition of the patient changes.

LIMITATIONS AND CONFOUNDERS IN THE USE OF INDIRECT CALORIMETRY

- *FiO$_2$:* Stability of FiO$_2$ is very important for an accurate measurement of the VO$_2$. Hence, when there are excessive flow demands as in the presence of high positive end-expiratory pressure (PEEP) (usually >12) or high minute ventilation, there is greater FiO$_2$ variability, unstable expiratory flow characteristics, and thus error in the measurement. Performance of IC at high FiO$_2$ (70% FiO$_2$) is also inaccurate. All these fluctuations can be reduced by the introduction of a mixing chamber which is a dry chamber between the ventilator outlet and the humidifier.
- *Leak:* The entire system should have no leak and hence in the presence of a leaking endotracheal tube cuff, bronchopleural fistula, intercostal drainage, etc. There is a loss of gas and hence an underestimation of the VO$_2$ and VCO$_2$ and thus, the REE and hence in such situations, it is not advisable to rely on REE derived from the indirect calorimeter.
- *Steady state conditions:* Measurements of gas exchange are to be performed in a steady state and in equilibrium. The steady-state period (STS) is defined as a period of low VO$_2$ and VCO$_2$ variations, of <10%. Most of the commercially available indirect calorimeters tend to get to the steady state within 15–30 minutes. Once the steady state is achieved, then measurements of only 4 minutes are needed to be averaged to determine the EE. Hence, it is advisable to perform the reading for at least 2 hours after a change in mechanical ventilation settings. This is also the reason that the reading should not be done after feeding in the case of intermittent feeing, after a physiotherapy session, during or recently following fever, after or during any anxiety or pain-provoking procedures or during or after a change of vasoactive medications. It is advisable to maintain a gap of at least 2 hours before conducting a measurement of EE.
- *Extracorporeal therapies:* It is advisable to perform IC around 2 hours after an intermittent hemodialysis session. At the time of writing this chapter, there is no sufficient data to either refute or support the use of IC during continuous renal replacement therapies or extracorporeal membrane oxygenator use though experts recommend against its use pending more data.[11]
- *Evidence in the subject:* Ticacos was prospective, randomized, single-center, pilot clinical trial comprising 130 mechanically ventilated patients to determine whether nutritional support guided by repeated measurements of resting energy requirements improves the outcome of critically ill patients. Tight calorie control guided by apparently decreased hospital stay and found an improvement in 60-day survival in the per-protocol

study in the isocaloric group (57.9% vs. 48.1%, P = 0.023).[14] Another randomized control trial found that personalized nutrition using IC-derived energy provision could reduce the rate of nosocomial infection.[15] Another interesting study used tracers to study the protein and glucose metabolism along with immunity and inflammation in critically ill patients fed with an individualized measured energy target. The results of this study indicated that such a practice (of individualizing energy provision) improved immunity, less systemic inflammation and demonstrated a trend to less muscle mass loss.[16] All the three studies indicate the reduction in morbidity and length of stay which will thus reduce cost. In a recent meta-analysis and systematic review of four trials, which included data up to January 2021 demonstrated lower 28-day mortality was found when isocaloric IC-guided nutrition was compared with (hypocaloric) feeding protocols using predictive equations.[17]

Another recent systematic review and metanalysis of eight randomized controlled trials (using the largest number of patients till date; n = 911) showed that the use of IC reduced short-term mortality. However, there was no difference in the duration of mechanical ventilation, length of stay in ICU or hospital, or increased incidence of adverse events or mortality.[18] This is in sharp contrast to another recent meta-analysis a year ago (2020), where they did not find any superiority over the use of predictive equations. Here, it is important to point out that the latter meta-analysis had only four trials and much lesser number of patients and did not include the most recent data.[19] What is clear is that there are beneficial effects in the use of IC in guided nutrition in critically ill patients. Major societies like the American Society of Parenteral and Enteral Nutrition have suggested that IC be used to determine energy requirements, when available and in the absence of variables that affect the accuracy of measurement and there is a strong consensus that EE should be done by IC in critically ill patients, especially those who are mechanical ventilated.[20]

CONCLUSION

In the era of evidence-based medicine and personalization of patient care, it is important to prescribe nutrition as per individual patient requirements (very similar to the fact that we would not prescribe a vasopressor without knowing the blood pressure). IC remains the gold standard in the measurement of EE (and hence the prescription of energy), which is very important for global patient care. Predictive equations are a very inaccurate option in this regard. Even with the limited evidence for the use of IC attributed to its rather less widespread use across countries it is important to set and guide nutritional goals based on the right measurement of energy expenditure. Recent developments in technology should help in increasing the use of IC. Routine use of IC along with a feeding protocol should be a standard of care to optimize nutrition.

REFERENCES

1. De Waele E, Honore PM, Malbrain M. Does the use of indirect calorimetry change outcome in the ICU? Yes it does. Curr Opin Clin Nutr Metab Care. 2018;21(2):126-9.
2. Delsoglio M, Achamrah N, Berger MM, Pichard C. Indirect Calorimetry in Clinical Practice. J Clin Med. 2019;8(9):1387.
3. Saseedharan S, Chada RR, Kadam V, Chiluka A, Nagalla B. Energy expenditure in COVID-19 mechanically ventilated patients: A comparison of three methods of energy estimation. JPEN J Parenter Enteral Nutr. 2022;46(8):1875-82.

4. De Waele E, Opsomer T, Honoré PM, Diltoer M, Mattens S, Huyghens L, et al. Measured versus calculated resting energy expenditure in critically ill adult patients. Do mathematics match the gold standard? Minerva Anestesiol. 2015;81(3):272-82.
5. Zusman O, Kagan I, Bendavid I, Theilla M, Cohen J, Singer P. Predictive equations versus measured energy expenditure by indirect calorimetry: A retrospective validation. Clin Nutr (Edinburgh, Scotland). 2019;38(3):1206-10.
6. Zusman O, Theilla M, Cohen J, Kagan I, Bendavid I, Singer P. Resting energy expenditure, calorie and protein consumption in critically ill patients: a retrospective cohort study. Crit Care (London, England). 2016;20(1):367.
7. Weir JB. New methods for calculating metabolic rate with special reference to protein metabolism. J Physiol. 1949;109(1-2):1-9.
8. Hickmann CE, Roeseler J, Castanares-Zapatero D, Herrera EI, Mongodin A, Laterre PF. Energy expenditure in the critically ill performing early physical therapy. Intensive Care Medicine. 2014;40(4):548-55.
9. Oshima T, Berger MM, De Waele E, Guttormsen AB, Heidegger CP, Hiesmayr M, et al. Indirect calorimetry in nutritional therapy. A position paper by the ICALIC study group. Clin Nutr. 2017;36:651-62.
10. Oshima T, Ragusa M, Graf S, Dupertuis YM, Heidegger CP, Pichard C. Methods to validate the accuracy of an indirect calorimeter in the in-vitro setting. Clin Nutr ESPEN. 2017;22:71-5.
11. Delsoglio M, Dupertuis YM, Oshima T, van der Plas M, Pichard C. Evaluation of the accuracy 457 and precision of a new generation indirect calorimeter in canopy dilution mode. Clin Nutr. 2020;39(6):1927-34.
12. Oshima T, Dupertuis YM, Delsoglio M, Graf S, Heidegger C-P, Pichard C. In vitro validation of indirect calorimetry device developed for the ICALIC project against mass spectrometry. Clin Nutr ESPEN. 2019;32:50-5.
13. Achamrah N, Delsoglio M, De Waele E, Berger MM, Pichard C. Indirect calorimetry: The 6 main issues. Clin Nutr. 2021;40(1):4-14.
14. Singer P, De Waele E, Sanchez C, Ruiz Santana S, Montejo JC, Laterre PF, et al. TICACOS international: A multi-center, randomized, prospective controlled study comparing tight calorie control versus Liberal calorie administration study. Clin Nutr. 2021;40(2):380-7.
15. Heidegger CP, Berger MM, Graf S, Zingg W, Darmon P, Costanza MC, et al. Optimisation of energy provision with supplemental parenteral nutrition in critically ill patients: a randomised controlled clinical trial. Lancet. 2013;381(9864):385-93.
16. Berger MM, Pantet O, Jacquelin-Ravel N, Charrière M, Schmidt S, Becce F, et al. Supplemental parenteral nutrition improves immunity with unchanged carbohydrate and protein metabolism in critically ill patients: The SPN2 randomized tracer study. Clin Nutr. 2019;38(5):2408-16.
17. Pertzov B, Bar-Yoseph H, Menndel Y, Bendavid I, Kagan I, Glass YD, et al. The effect of indirect calorimetry guided isocaloric nutrition on mortality in critically ill patients—a systematic review and meta-analysis. Eur J Clin Nutr. 2022;76(1):5-15.
18. Duan JY, Zheng WH, Zhou H, Xu Y, Huang HB. Energy delivery guided by indirect calorimetry in critically ill patients: a systematic review and meta-analysis. Crit Care. 2021;25(1):88.
19. Tatucu-Babet OA, Fetterplace K, Lambell K, Miller E, Deane AM, Ridley EJ. Is energy delivery guided by indirect calorimetry associated with improved clinical outcomes in critically ill patients? A systematic review and meta-analysis. Nutr Metab Insights. 2020;13:1178638820903295.
20. Singer P, Blaser AR, Berger MM, Alhazzani W, Calder PC, Casaer MP, et al. ESPEN guideline on clinical nutrition in the intensive care unit Clin Nutr. 2019;38(1):48-79.

CHAPTER 8

Macronutrients in Critical Illness: Nutrition Backbones for Survival and Recovery!

Varsha M Asrani

INTRODUCTION

The significance of nutrition therapy in critical illness has garnered considerable attention in recent years, as evidenced by a surmountable surge in clinical trials and guidelines.[1,2] Despite this, there is debate and conflicting information posing a challenge toward the translation of the evidence base to clinical-based practices. It has been more apparent and acceptable that critical illness accounts for the variability of phases associated with modifications in physiology and metabolic regulation. This variability now highlights the gaps in current practices and indications for therapeutic advances and interventions of more tailored nutritional therapy in our patients.[3,4]

IRONY OF ACADEMIC MEDICINE

The prevailing paradigm of associating malnutrition, which was historically termed to be associated with protein-energy malnutrition, is now prevalent to a significant extent in acute disease—a condition also known as disease-related malnutrition (DRM) in many countries and is primarily caused by a significant reduced intake leading to a deficiency in calories and protein.[5] As known, when unaddressed, this can result in the onset of significant malnutrition that contributes to adverse outcomes in critically ill patients. The evolving culture of academic medicine alludes to the fact that this problem (malnutrition) is persistent and highly prevalent in acute hospitals, of both developed or developing countries, but little is being done to address the problem. Decades of documentation have not persuaded hospital administrators to seriously modify their policies for nutrition provision, prompting the need for high-quality prospective clinical trials within large-scale populations to demonstrate whether improved nutrition can actually improve clinical outcomes or shorten hospital stays. Unfortunately, the modern intensive care unit (ICU) is heading toward a nutrition research laboratory.[6] Irrespectively, the interim solution to the problem remains adhering to this paradigm, while it is reasonable to infer that the provision of enteral or parenteral nutrition to patients who are unable or unwilling to consume food orally may impede the advancement toward malnourishment.[6]

METABOLIC HIERARCHY IN CRITICAL ILLNESS

Much so recently, it has been recognized that critical illness follows a variable state of metabolic (dys)regulation that may be hierarchical depending on the phase of the illness. Professor Graham Hill, in his article published in 1998, eloquently describes the metabolic response to stress in acute injury and critical illness.[7] His thoughts, even at the time, emphasize that the accurate

CHAPTER 8 | Macronutrients in Critical Illness: Nutrition Backbones for Survival and Recovery!

quantification of the developing physiological changes and adaptation in addition to the understanding of their etiology have been the product of much work by researchers over the past 60 years.[7] These learnings are vitally important to intensivists and surgeons even today due to the new plethora of metabolic modulators that constantly evolve and subject clinical practice to jeopardy. Sadly, even today, ascertaining the importance of nutrition balance and metabolic hierarchy remains suboptimal in clinical practice, predominantly from a clinician's perspective. It is imperative that clinicians dive deeper into the understanding of the utilization of nutrients across the spectrum of critical illness, which may not only improve ICU care and outcomes during ICU stay but potentially adds value to the post-ICU care journey of patients.[8]

The relevance of post-ICU care is much emphasized in today's practice considering that outcomes are not just limited to mortality and ICU length of stay but functional outcomes in patients followed by the ICU journey.

Nevertheless, critical illness is complicated by a plethora of triggers after any stress or injury which generates a multitude of metabolic, hormonal, and immunological responses. The ability of the human body to cope with such responses depends on the preexisting body composition and habitus that enables one to adapt and emerge. However irrespective, these alterations in metabolic dysregulation following an injury or insult position the body into a housekeeping mechanism known as "autophagy". The process of self-destruction of unwanted cellular debris and toxic compounds allows the body to establish a sense of stability following a significant event. Early shock, hemodynamic instability, and massive trauma or hemorrhage, or any insult to the body's physiological processes need to sustain the process of autophagy to allow a survival mechanism to occur. As expected, substrate utilization at this point is maximized following an exhaustion of glycogen stores in the first 3-4 days of illness—also known as the *"ebb"* phase, subsequently followed by the breakdown of lean body mass (LBM) or muscle tissue from nonglucose sources, i.e., *catabolism*, which sustains further to adapt and to fight for survival, also known as the *"flow"* phase (**Fig. 1**). As a result, insulin resistance, deficits in organ perfusion, and a metabolic catchup prevails, and these conditions often multiply if additional metabolism functions are pushed beyond the body's ability to cope with this physiological burden. The impact of overfeeding and underfeeding with regard to macronutrients will be discussed in sections below. Finally, a stable and third phase, also known as *"anabolism"* phase sets in eventually to allow for recovery, stable gut function and absorption, tissue resynthesis, and eventually the ability to move from intensive care therapies. The various phases, so far, have no specific, objective biomarker to allude to the targeted nutrition as yet. Hence, guidelines and recommended best practices offer an interim pathway to attend to targeted nutrition and achieve positive outcomes.

ENERGY IN CRITICAL ILLNESS—POWERING THROUGH THE SPECTRUM OF UNCERTAINTY

In critical illness, the determination of energy requirements is one of the most significant challenges and is of vital importance as prescribed targets are used to guide nutrition delivery. Predictive equations are the commonly used tools that estimate energy expenditure (EE) derived from simple

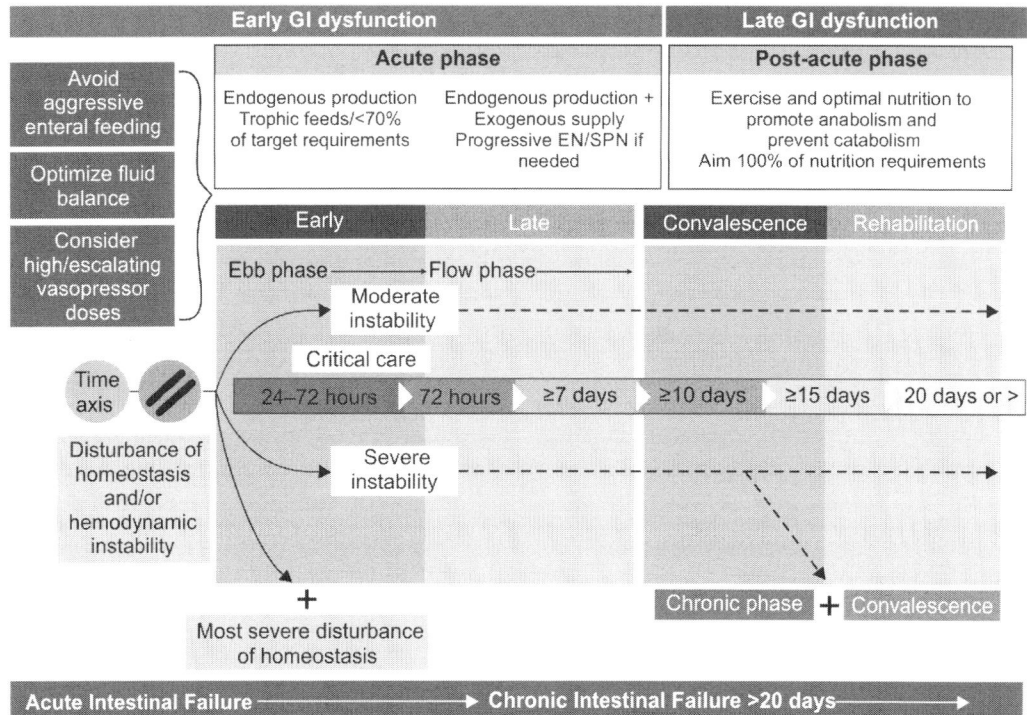

Fig. 1: The spectrum of the acute (Ebb and Flow) and the post-acute phases in critical illness. (GI: gastrointestinal; EN: enteral nutrition; SPN: supplemental parenteral nutrition)
Source: Adapted and modified from Elke et al.[9]

calculations of measurements that can be easily obtained at the bedside, however over the past 5 decades, an evolution of science-based medicine reiterates that these are rather suboptimal and fail to provide a clear and objective understanding of EE in critical illness. Their lack of precision may lead us to consequences of under- or overfeeding our patients. Simultaneously, the evolving evidence confirms the accuracy of measured EE using indirect calorimetry (IC), which is also recommended by practice guidelines and experts.[1,2] As stated in the literature, it is challenging to prescribe for something we cannot measure.[3,10] These inaccuracies precipitate in the most vulnerable populations such as the severely unwell, elderly frail cohorts and malnourished populations with chronic comorbidity.[11,12] Despite this, predictive equations continue to be widely used in the majority of the global ICUs. Hence, ICUs globally are subjected to long-term iatrogenic malnutrition and underfeeding in the absence of an accurate EE measurement. Using IC not only measures the precise energy requirements in patients, but also measures energy delivery in longitudinal studies to address barriers in ICU nutrition administration. Given the availability of new validated IC devices, longitudinal IC measures should be the new standard of care for ICU and post-ICU nutrition delivery.[3,10] IC is a step further in nutrition practice that caters to personalized medicine by delivering optimal nutrition at every phase of critical illness. The initial stage of critical illness, usually within the first 3-4 days to a week, is marked by metabolic changes suggesting a pathophysiological cascade. These changes include inflammation, heightened energy consumption, insulin resistance, and a catabolic response that triggers the utilization of stored energy sources such as hepatic glycogen (glucose), fat (free-fatty acids), and eventually muscle (amino acids). The process of providing nourishment to patients in the ICU differs significantly from that of individuals who are in good health.[13] Nutrition therapy can limit the endogenous energy production process during the initial stages of critical illness. As a result, it is suggested that a gradual escalation of nutrition intake over a period of days should be implemented to avoid excessive feeding. This recommendation is supported by previous research.[1,14,15] The aforementioned concept is exemplified by the correlations observed between the proportion of caloric goal attained during the initial phase of ICU admission and the quantification of EE as determined by IC. Zusman and Weijs have discovered U-shaped associations indicating that an energy intake of 70-80% of the measured EE is optimal, while both lower and higher intakes are linked to elevated mortality rates.[16,17]

Large-scale studies conducted over the past few years (PERMIT)[18] (TARGET)[19] have not necessarily been able to highlight the importance of aggressive rather targeted feeding compared to hypocaloric feeding. The results of these two large-scale randomized controlled trials (RCTs) indicate that there were no significant variations in pertinent clinical endpoints among patients who received low, normal, or high-caloric intake during the initial phase of their stay in the ICU. The endpoints in these two studies suggesting no differences between the groups indicated a "missing" factor in the trial methodologies. In saying that it was a worthwhile effort highlighting the gap which suggests that it is still a mystery of potential alterations across the spectrum of ICU stages that alters nutritional requirements—something we might still be unaware of! It is important to consider that the protein intake remained consistent across all study arms during these trials. These two major trials demonstrated conflicting results compared with other studies, which raise the question of "how were the energy requirements calculated"?[18,19] The use of predictive equations over IC to estimate EE potentially limits the methodology as an inaccurate step in the first place. This obviously contributes to time phases where patients are subjected to overfeeding and underfeeding. Besides, differences and variability between caloric intake, timing of prescribing or escalating energy requirements, phases of critical illness, and undoubtedly the protein delivery are factors that may confound the end outcomes of any study. In saying so, importance of protein should be a key factor when hypocaloric and standard groups for energy delivery are compared. The administration of energy requirements is mainly a fine art of balance, where aggressive nutrition or sustained caloric deficit needs correction from day 3 to 4 onwards, unless gastrointestinal (GI) dysfunction persists and the trajectory of nutrition care changes. It is recommended to use an objective measure to estimate EE, e.g., IC, while accepting a caloric deficit in the first 3-4 days of ICU admission to allow for autophagy to occur that acts as a protective mechanism in critical illness.[1]

Nevertheless, refeeding syndrome, a condition that involves electrolyte shifts in response to the reintroduction of nutrition after a period of starvation, also justifies the gradual increase of macronutrients in the acute phase of critical illness. It has been demonstrated that limiting caloric intake to 500 kcal/day or <50% of the recommended daily intake for a period of 2–3 days is necessary in order to avoid mortality associated with refeeding syndrome.[20-22] Refeeding syndrome has been discussed in detail in Chapter 38.

PROTEIN IN CRITICAL ILLNESS: BUILDING AWAY BLOCK-BY-BLOCK

In the acute stages of critical illness, when the stress response escalates, the coalescence of immunomodulatory factors rises rapidly to support the recovery process.[23] Catabolic breakdown of lean muscle tissue is an involuntary mechanism to support this process, which acts as a protein precursor the sudden increase in requirements.[24] Clinical guidelines from ASPEN/SCCM recommend protein delivery of between 1.2 and 2 g/kg/day,[2] despite which the evidence still remains controversial based on the assumption that optimal protein will attenuate skeletal muscle wasting and improve clinical outcomes, after augmentation in conditions with higher requirements (i.e., burns, obesity, and multitrauma). The recommendations for higher protein requirements are predominantly based on limited RCTs, observational data and expert opinion.[2] Although some observational data indicates that higher protein delivery is associated with improved survival.[17,25-28] Contradictory to this, higher protein delivery during ICU admission has less observed benefits,[29,30] rather contributing to adverse effects (increased urea production and muscle wasting)[24,31] as were observed in small-scale observational studies. Besides, very high-protein requirement (2.2 g/kg/d) has been associated with adverse outcomes particularly in high-risk patients (EFFORT trial).[32] This variability in evidence that is used to support guidelines reflects the paucity of high-quality trials investigating the role of protein provision on clinical outcomes. RCTs comparing higher to lower protein doses have shown no benefit, which also indicate the possibilities of inadequately designed trials and underpowered studies to ascertain an impact on outcomes such as mortality.[30,31,33,34] The route of providing protein may well be important to consider as it is possible that intravenous amino acids may metabolize differently from whole protein molecules via the GI tract provided by enteral feeding.[35] Similarly, a smaller study[34] demonstrated that higher levels of amino acids showed smaller improvements, although not for mortality or length-of-stay.[34] Findings of many such studies may have unadjusted confounding factors that must be interpreted with caution.[36] Besides, the phase of critical illness, route of protein administration, study duration, protein kinetics, and nitrogen balance are additional factors to consider during critical illness. Other observational studies have observed a beneficial effect of protein[3] of 1.2 g/kg associated with lower mortality, yet this was observed in nonseptic patients and patients without overfeeding syndrome. However, the studies also showed an improved outcome when energy provision was lower, hence this concept may allude to lower energy but higher protein delivery, provided these patients are not high-risk. However, testing this in large-randomized trial would be a next step.[17,28] A similar outcome was observed in two studies evaluating early protein delivery (>0.7–0.8 g/kg/day vs. ≤0.7–0.8 g/kg/day) that showed an increased survival[28] and a lower 6-month mortality.[37] Both studies were retrospective in nature with an early versus late-protein (before and after day 3) provision method suggesting the timing may be relevant when introducing protein in critical illness. Contradictorily, the EPaNIC trial evaluated cumulative protein dose in a post hoc secondary analysis, where early delivery of protein was associated with delayed ICU discharge. The study had a shift in the perception of energy and protein delivery in critically ill but of note was based in patients receiving early and late PN.[38] Protein dosages based on guideline recommendations have been prescribed for critically ill patients as part of clinical practice; however, the actual administration is still insufficient. Studies using higher protein dosages compared to lower targets and early versus late administration have not showed significant differences in muscle function modalities. A study showed that the delivery of protein bypassing the stomach is known to have minimal impact, although muscle protein synthesis can be hampered.[39] The evidence on muscle protein kinesis and absorption needs to be further investigated in acute stages of critical illness with an aim to assess changes in muscle mass. Until we explore the evolvement at a cellular level, we may not have the accurate answers from clinical trials per se. Other markers of protein, such as prealbumin, have not necessarily nailed the problem just yet[40,41] and it is being investigated in clinical trials as a risk marker for nutritional status (prealbumin ≤0.10 g/L considered as an indicator of severe nutritional risk, 0.11–0.15 g/L as mild-to-moderate risk, and >0.15 g/L as no risk).[42-44] Not to mention, in order to determine the best suitable protein delivery amount and timing for critically ill patients, data from prospective and randomized studies is still crucial. To better understand the effect of protein dose and timing on clinical outcomes in critical illness, adequately powered RCTs are urgently required. Recent systematic reviews support the evidence on inconsistencies in observational trials on higher protein intake and outcomes in critical illness.[45] In addition to the dose, type, timing, and protein kinesis, the interactions with exercise and rehabilitation are equally important to understand the relationship of protein metabolism in critical illnesses. Irrespective, ideal energy delivery should be managed in such studies by ensuring that it is constant in both the intervention and control groups.

POST-ICU NUTRITION: A NON-NEGOTIABLE INTERVENTION IN CRITICAL ILLNESS

Although the focus of ICU studies has largely been during the first week of ICU admission, the transition toward post-ICU care or ward settings has been a neglected piece of the puzzle. The complexity of ICU status and the weeks of care leads to a half-baked nutrition intervention that needs a continuity of care through their follow-up in the post-ICU state. The post-intensive care syndrome (PICS) highlights the gaps that occur in the absence of suboptimal post-ICU care. One of the major gaps emphasizes protein provision as part of long-term nutrition interventions. The importance of individualized nutrition and nutrition in the post-ICU period is growing. The status of pre, during, and post-ICU is a significant aspect to the overall recovery trajectory; hence, nutrition in these cohorts should not be evaluated as isolated time periods but rather be considered as a spectrum of care across the entire ICU-to-hospital-community stay, with an aim to evaluate long-term functional outcomes.[46,47] Similar to personalized medicine, personalized nutrition in critical care is a puzzle

ENERGY AND PROTEIN IN CLINICAL PRACTICE: PRESCRIBED VERSUS DELIVERED—ARE WE GETTING THIS RIGHT?

A crucial aspect for clinicians to take into account is that patients may not receive to the prescribed energy and protein dosage. A retrospective analysis of a large study from Australia, New Zealand, and international databases encompassing 17,154 patients (ANZ: n = 2,776 vs. international n = 14,378) from 923 ICUs indicated that protein delivery was substantially below the estimated prescriptions, and the results were similar between the regions [0.6 (0.4) g/kg/day vs. 0.6 (0.4) g/kg/day; $P = 0.849$] with a mean ± standard deviation of 56 ± 30% and 52 ± 30% of the intended aim, respectively.[48] Barriers to nutrition provision, unnecessary stops to enteral nutrition for medical procedures, late initiation of nutritional therapy, and GI dysfunction are common factors that associate with low-protein provision. Based on the existing evidence, there is recommendation toward gradual implementation of nutrition therapy including energy and protein during the acute stages of critical illness.[8]

The determination of energy requirements is a crucial aspect in avoiding detrimental consequences of both inadequate and excessive food intake. Nevertheless, the ideal quantity of energy provision is still a topic of debate within academic circles. Variability in EE is observed across various stages of critical illness. During the initial stages of critical illness, a considerable amount of energy substrate is attributed to the nutritional status and endogenous energy production. IC is a method used to measure the resting energy expenditure (REE). Due to the limited physical activity of ICU patients, their REE is expected to approximate their total energy expenditure (TEE). There is a notable discrepancy between predictive formulas and IC in calculating REE, which can result in deviations of up to 1,000 kcal/day from the true EE.[49] Nevertheless, the effect on mortality observed the TICACOS-II trial may not be plausible due to the possible lack of statistical power.[50]

The current understanding of IC lacks consideration for the internal generation of energy that cannot be suppressed by external feeding or insulin, which is commonly observed during the initial stage of critical illness. As of yet, a dependable method for evaluating this output at the patient's bedside has not been established. Hence, it can be concluded that IC continues to be the favored approach for evaluating energy requirements, provided that the initial stage of elevated endogenous energy generation has been resolved.[10] In cases where IC is not accessible, it has been observed that VCO_2 measurements (where kcal/24 h = VCO_2 × 8.19) are marginally more precise than predictive formulas.[1] Secondly, irrespective of the route of administration, the amount of macronutrients administered during early stage of critical illness may worsen the outcome. Enhanced autophagy by nutrient restriction for 1 week may be one of the underlying mechanisms. Autophagy is a cellular housekeeping system clearing damaged organelles and toxic protein aggregates to preserve cell integrity.[51,52] In saying so, critically ill patients may survive after being briefly underfed. However, the amount of underfeeding (trophic to 70% of EE) to aim for during the first week of critical illness is unknown and may vary by case. Underfeeding after the first week of critical illness has not been investigated explicitly and was even reported to result in no difference in outcomes. The initial trophic versus full enteral feeding in acute lung injury trial (EDEN) demonstrated no statistically significant difference in clinical outcomes, including ventilator-free days, among patients with acute lung injury who were provided with trophic versus full enteral feeding for the first 6 days of mechanical ventilation. However, patients receiving trophic enteral feedings experienced fewer episodes of feeding intolerance, despite receiving fewer medications to treat intolerance.[53] Future studies investigating ICU admission to hospital discharge are needed to determine if prolonged underfeeding in critically sick patients affects recovery, function, and cognition, although it is known that in hospitalized patients, malnutrition is linked to increased morbidity, mortality, and healthcare costs.[54-56] Based on the understanding that significantly less is frequently delivered, at least 70% of projected or measured energy should be aimed during the first week of sickness in the absence of definitive evidence.

In light of maintaining the <70% needs within the acute phase of critical illness, it is important to account for the non-nutritive calories that contribute to the additional energy load which may shift the target toward aggressive feeding rather than hypocaloric feeding as recommended. Propofol, a commonly used sedative in the ICU, is formulated in a 10% lipid emulsion that contributes 1.1 kcal/mL. Propofol is often administered in the early phases of critical illness as a common sedative, particularly in ventilator-dependent patients. Its rapid onset and short half-life have advantages over other sedative agents, and it has been proven useful when patient trajectory is moving toward de-sedation and extubation.[57] However, its high calorific load can significantly contribute to caloric intake and add to complications of overfeeding for patients who receive concurrent enteral or parenteral nutrition therapy. In order to avoid potential overfeeding, some clinicians have empirically decreased the infusion rate of the nutrition therapy, which also may have detrimental effects since protein intake may be inadequate. Propofol contributes to 5-24% of total caloric intake when combined with EN or PN.[57] Likewise, it is imperative to ensure that aggressive feeding is avoided in the early phase of critical illness, but also accounting for other nonnutritive calories other than propofol, e.g., 5% dextrose IV fluids. Aggressive feeding in the early phase of acute illness can lead to a high metabolic demand that can trigger the onset of bowel ischemia. While all guidelines favor EN, they do not explicitly address the important combinations of various modalities that may contribute to a dysfunctional gut in response to critical illness, which itself may hinder the initiation of enteral feeding in the first instance.[58] In addition, fluid balance and optimizing vasotherapy have an advantage toward maintaining global perfusion and hemodynamic parameters, but an imbalance (excess or suboptimal) in fluid administration or escalating vasopressor dosing can contribute to gut failure in the setting of an aggressive feeding regimen, which often leads to detrimental effects in these patients **(Fig. 2)**.[59-61] Hence, the aim should be to meet protein and energy targets in the early acute phase of critical illness (days 1-3) and increasing it to 1.2-1.5 g/kg day 3 onward alongside targeted energy requirements to meet 100% of the goal requirements preferably using IC as the gold standard **(Fig. 2)**.[1]

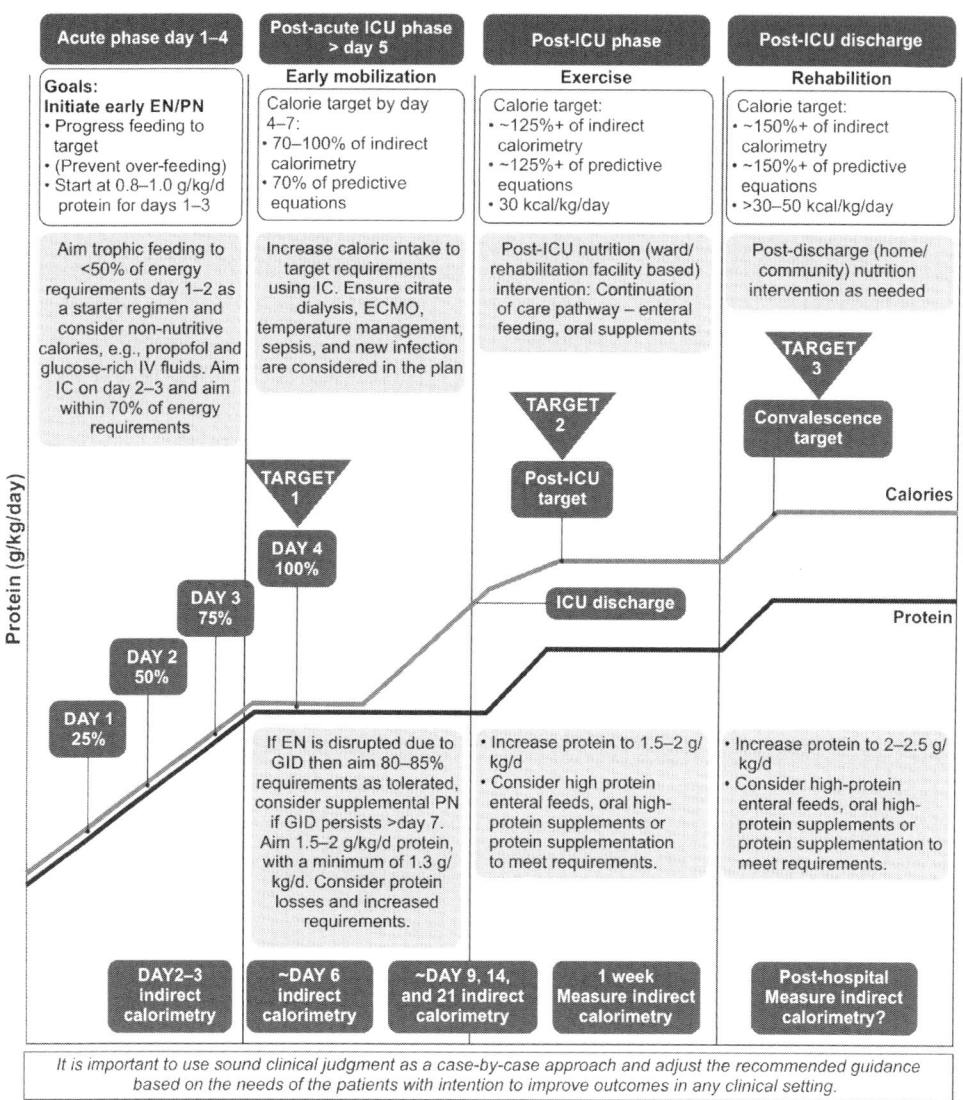

Fig. 2: A practical guide to delivering energy and protein during critical illness and recovery. (ECMO: extracorporeal membrane oxygenation; EN: enteral nutrition; GID: gastrointestinal dysfunction; IC: indirect calorimetry; ICU: intensive care unit; PN: parenteral nutrition)

Early acute phase of ICU: Aim for energy and protein to be gradually increased by 25% every day to target 1 on day 4. Target 1 is 1.3 g/kg/day protein and less than 70% of estimated calories or 100% of indirect calorimetry.*
Chronic critical illness and general wards following ICU release: Target 2. Target 2 calls for 30 kcal/kg/day of calories and 1.5–2.0 g/kg/day of protein.*
Post-ICU: Aim caloric aim (150% of predictive equations or 35 kcal/kg/day) and protein intake of 2.0–2.5 g/kg/day after hospitalization.*
Account for non-nutritive calories—propofol and glucose-rich fluids.
*It is important to use sound clinical judgment on a case-by-case approach to adjust the recommended guidance based on the needs of the patients with an intention to improve outcomes in any clinical settings outlined above.
Source: Adapted and modified from Singer et al.[1]; Wischmeyer[3]; De Waele et al.[10]

With the growing accessibility of bedside body composition measurements, a greater number of studies have been carried out to evaluate protein requirements. In recent times, international guidelines have suggested the evaluation of LBM as a means to establish protein targets for patients who are overweight or obese.[1] Predictive formulas do not offer the same precision to that of an objective measure, particularly with a varied body composition, altering requirements and increased physiological nutrition needs. The estimation of LBM, or muscle mass, can be improved through the use of dual-energy X-ray absorptiometry, CT, or MRI scans. Nevertheless, the implementation of these techniques at the patient's bedside is rather challenging and the cost is prohibitive, rendering them unsuitable for regular repetition.[62]

Recent focus on the bioelectrical impedance analysis (BIA) presents a cost-effective and feasible approach for evaluating LBM among patients in the ICU, particularly with the masking effect of edema in these patients. Hence, BIA has the capability to evaluate the surplus of extracellular water and make necessary adjustments to avoid overestimating LBM.[62,63] Bedside ultrasonography can serve as an alternative method for evaluating LBM; however, it is subject to greater variability based on the operator's proficiency. Hence, there is a wide area to explore ahead, not only with the levels of protein administration and delivery but also evaluating its outcomes in a tailored and objective manner.[64]

CONCLUSION AND THE WAY FORWARD

There is light at the end of the tunnel, and it is what we hope to see eventually when we prescribe macronutrients: Energy and protein—for our patients. Questions still remain, debates still exist, and recommendations are still followed in the interim.[65,66] We seek answers on the exact dosing, timing, route, and metabolic alterations to tailor our nutrition approaches, although to a greater extent we have attempted to dive deeper and deeper over decades. The intricate interplay between acute metabolic alterations, inflammatory response, and dietary intake during the initial stages of critical illness is multifaceted. Recent findings indicate that gradual administration of both protein and calorie intake during the initial stage is crucial in avoiding excessive feeding and elevated caloric consumption while addressing refeeding syndrome. Following this period of 4-7 days, it is imperative to maintain a nutrition of target energy and protein requirements in order to prevent any additional loss of muscle mass and function. Following discharge from the ICU, there is a significant gap in knowledge regarding the precise metabolic profile and nutritional requirements of ICU survivors, necessitating further investigation. Limited data indicates suboptimal nutritional practices among patients who have been discharged from the ICU and those who are currently in the hospital ward with a prolonged recovery period ahead. Additionally, there is a pressing need for research on nutritional and metabolic interventions, such as anabolic and anticatabolic agents, in the context of recovery. The focus on a biomarker to evaluate autophagy and readiness for macronutrient uptake will determine the subjectiveness of prescribing based on an "ICU days" approach. It is recommended to refrain from initiating early energy overfeeding, despite the absence of specific targets. The utilization of IC has the potential to provide valuable guidance for determining energy targets subsequent to the initial phase. The evaluation of LBM through BIA or ultrasound is necessary for the appropriate determination of personalized protein dosage. The adaptation of nutrition therapy to the various stages of the disease and recovery is imperative. In order to effectively combat the negative long-term outcomes associated with ICU stays and facilitate the restoration of our patients' quality of life, it is imperative that we carefully consider the optimal delivery of nutrition and metabolic therapies throughout all stages of illness. It is essential that we prioritize the provision of appropriate nutrition to each patient at the appropriate time. Considerable strides need to be taken in the scientific community toward attaining this objective. We need a novel, robust, and thorough way to evolve our thinking; might be the next step toward designing our trials, thus seeking answers to specific question/s to unsolve the mystery.

REFERENCES

1. Singer P, Blaser AR, Berger MM, Alhazzani W, Calder PC, Casaer MP, et al. ESPEN guideline on clinical nutrition in the intensive care unit. Clin Nutr. 2019;38(1):48-79.
2. Taylor BE, McClave SA, Martindale RG, Warren MM, Johnson DR, Braunschweig C, et al. Guidelines for the provision and assessment of nutrition support therapy in the adult critically ill patient: Society of Critical Care Medicine (SCCM) and American Society for parenteral and enteral nutrition (ASPEN). Crit Care Med. 2016;44(2):390-438.
3. Wischmeyer PE. Tailoring nutrition therapy to illness and recovery. Crit Care. 2017;21(Suppl 3):316.
4. Preiser J. The stress response of critical illness: Metabolic and hormonal aspects, 1st edition. The University of Edinburgh: Springer (Cham) International Publishing; 2016.
5. Cardenas D, Ochoa JB. A paradigm shift in clinical nutrition. Clin Nutr. 2023;42(3):380-3.
6. Hoffer LJ, Bistrian BR. Nutrition in critical illness: A current conundrum. F1000Res. 2016;5:2531.
7. Hill AG, Hill GL. Metabolic response to severe injury. Br J Surg. 1998;85(7):884-90.
8. Lambell KJ, Tatucu-Babet OA, Chapple L, Gantner D, Ridley EJ. Nutrition therapy in critical illness: A review of the literature for clinicians. Crit Care. 2020;24(1):35.
9. Elke G, Hartl WH, Kreymann KG, Adolph M, Felbinger TW, Graf T, et al. Clinical Nutrition in Critical Care Medicine – Guideline of the German Society for Nutritional Medicine (DGEM). Clin Nutr ESPEN. 2019;33:220-75.
10. De Waele E, Jonckheer J, Wischmeyer P. Indirect calorimetry in critical illness: A new standard of care? Curr Opin Crit Care. 2021;27(4):334-43.
11. Reeves MM, Capra S. Predicting energy requirements in the clinical setting: Are current methods evidence based? Nutr Rev. 2003;61(4):143-51.
12. Frankenfield DC, Coleman A, Alam S, Cooney RN. Analysis of estimation methods for resting metabolic rate in critically ill adults. JPEN J Parenter Enteral Nutr. 2009;33(1):27-36.
13. Arabi YM, Casaer MP, Chapman M, Heyland DK, Ichai C, Marik PE, et al. The intensive care medicine research agenda in nutrition and metabolism. Intensive Care Med. 2017;43(9):1239-156.
14. Bendavid I, Singer P, Theilla M, Themessl-Huber M, Sulz I, Mouhieddine M, et al. NutritionDay ICU: A 7 year worldwide prevalence study of nutrition practice in intensive care. Clin Nutr. 2017;36(4):1122-9.
15. Reignier J, Van Zanten ARH, Arabi YM. Optimal timing, dose and route of early nutrition therapy in critical illness and shock: The quest for the holy grail. Intensive Care Med. 2018;44(9):1558-60.
16. Zusman O, Theilla M, Cohen J, Kagan I, Bendavid I, Singer P. Resting energy expenditure, calorie and protein consumption in critically ill patients: A retrospective cohort study. Crit Care. 2016;20(1):367.
17. Weijs PJ, Looijaard WG, Beishuizen A, Girbes AR, Oudemans-van Straaten HM.

Early high protein intake is associated with low mortality and energy overfeeding with high mortality in non-septic mechanically ventilated critically ill patients. Crit Care. 2014;18(6):701.
18. Arabi YM, Aldawood AS, Haddad SH, Al-Dorzi HM, Tamim HM, Jones G, et al. Permissive underfeeding or standard enteral feeding in critically ill adults. N Engl J Med. 2015;372(25):2398-408.
19. Chapple LS, Summers MJ, Bellomo R, Chapman MJ, Davies AR, Ferrie S, et al. Use of a high-protein enteral nutrition formula to increase protein delivery to critically ill patients: A randomized, blinded, parallel-group, feasibility trial. JPEN J Parenter Enteral Nutr. 2021;45(4):699-709.
20. Olthof LE, Koekkoek WACK, van Setten C, Kars JCN, van Blokland D, van Zanten ARH. Impact of caloric intake in critically ill patients with, and without, refeeding syndrome: A retrospective study. Clin Nutr. 2018;37(5):1609-17.
21. Doig GS, Simpson F, Heighes PT, Bellomo R, Chesher D, Caterson ID, et al. Restricted versus continued standard caloric intake during the management of refeeding syndrome in critically ill adults: A randomised, parallel-group, multicentre, single-blind controlled trial. Lancet Respir Med. 2015;3(12):943-52.
22. van Zanten ARH. Nutritional support and refeeding syndrome in critical illness. Lancet Respir Med. 2015;3(12):904-5.
23. Wolfe RR. Underappreciated role of muscle in health and disease. Am J Clin Nutr. 2006;84(3):475-82.
24. Puthucheary ZA, Rawal J, McPhail M, Connolly B, Ratnayake G, Chan P, et al. Acute skeletal muscle wasting in critical illness. JAMA. 2013;310(15):1591-600.
25. Nicolo M, Heyland DK, Chittams J, Sammarco T, Compher C. Clinical outcomes related to protein delivery in a critically ill population. JPEN J Parenter Enteral Nutr. 2016;40(1):45-51.
26. Compher C, Chittams J, Sammarco T, Nicolo M, Heyland D. Greater protein and energy intake may be associated with improved mortality in higher risk critically ill patients: A multicenter, multinational observational study. Crit Care Med. 2017;45(2):156-63.
27. Allingstrup MJ, Esmailzadeh N, Wilkens Knudsen A, Espersen K, Hartvig Jensen T, Wiis J, et al. Provision of protein and energy in relation to measured requirements in intensive care patients. Clin Nutr. 2012;31(4):462-8.
28. Bendavid I, Zusman O, Kagan I, Theilla M, Cohen J, Singer P. Early administration of protein in critically ill patients: A retrospective cohort study. Nutrients. 2019;11(1):106.
29. Casaer MP, Mesotten D, Hermans G, Wouters PJ, Schetz M, Meyfroidt G, et al. Early versus late parenteral nutrition in critically ill adults. N Engl J Med. 2011;365(6):506-17.
30. Allingstrup MJ, Kondrup J, Wiis J, Claudius C, Pedersen UG, Hein-Rasmussen R, et al. Early goal-directed nutrition versus standard of care in adult intensive care patients: The single-centre, randomised, outcome assessor-blinded EAT-ICU trial. Intensive Care Med. 2017;43(11):1637-47.
31. Doig GS, Simpson F, Bellomo R, Heighes PT, Sweetman EA, Chesher D, et al. Intravenous amino acid therapy for kidney function in critically ill patients: A randomized controlled trial. Intensive Care Med. 2015; 41(7):1197-208.
32. Heyland DK, Patel J, Compher C, Rice TW, Bear DE, Lee ZY, et al. The effect of higher protein dosing in critically ill patients with high nutritional risk (EFFORT protein): An international, multicentre, pragmatic, registry-based randomised trial. Lancet. 2023;401(10376):568-76.
33. Fetterplace K, Deane AM, Tierney A, Beach LJ, Knight LD, Presneill J, et al. Targeted full energy and protein delivery in critically ill patients: A pilot randomized controlled trial (FEED trial). JPEN J Parenter Enteral Nutr. 2018;42(8):1252-62.
34. Ferrie S, Allman-Farinelli M, Daley M, Smith K. Protein requirements in the critically ill. JPEN J Parenter Enteral Nutr. 2016;40(6):795-805.

35. Di Girolamo F, Situlin R, Biolo G. What factors influence protein synthesis and degradation in critical illness? Curr Opin Clin Nutr Metab Care. 2017;20(2):124-30.
36. Casaer MP, Van den Berghe G. Comment on "Protein requirements in the critically ill: A randomized controlled trial using parenteral nutrition". JPEN J Parenter Enteral Nutr. 2016;40(6):763.
37. Koekkoek WAC, van Setten CH, Olthof LE, Kars JCN, van Zanten ARH. Timing of PROTein INtake and clinical outcomes of adult critically ill patients on prolonged mechanical VENTilation: The PROTINVENT retrospective study. Clin Nutr. 2019;38(2):883-90.
38. Casaer M, Wilmer A, Hermans G, Wouters P, Mesotten D, Van den Berghe G. Role of disease and macronutrient dose in the randomized controlled EPaNIC trial, a post-hoc analysis. Am J Respir Crit Care Med. 2013.
39. Chapple LS, Gassel RJJ, Rooyackers O. Protein metabolism in critical illness. Curr Opin Crit Care. 2022;28(4):367-73.
40. Arabi YM, Aldawood AS, Al-Dorzi HM, Tamim HM, Haddad SH, Jones G, et al. Permissive underfeeding or standard enteral feeding in high- and Low-Nutritional-risk critically ill adults. Post hoc analysis of the PermiT trial. Am J Respir Crit Care Med. 2017;195(5):652-62.
41. Altun K, Kalin BS, Sert AI, Çelebi NK, Bıçak EA, Cengiz R, et al. Every time prealbumin may not be an indicator for prognosis in critically ill patients. Clin Sci Nutr. 2022;4(2):40-5.
42. Shenkin A. Serum prealbumin: Is it a marker of nutritional status or of risk of malnutrition? Clin Chem. 2006;52(12):2177-9.
43. Mears E. Outcomes of continuous process improvement of a nutritional care program incorporating serum prealbumin measurements. Nutrition. 1996;12(7):479-84.
44. Arabi YM, Al-Dorzi HM, Tamim H, Sadat M, Al-Hameed F, AlGhamdi A, et al. Replacing protein via enteral nutrition in a stepwise approach in critically ill patients: A pilot randomized controlled trial (REPLENISH pilot trial). Clin Nutr ESPEN. 2021;44:166-72.
45. Arabi Y, Al-Dorzi H, Sadat M. Protein intake and outcome in critically ill patients. Curr Opin Clin Nutr Metabol Care. 2020;23(1):51-8.
46. van Zanten ARH, De Waele E, Wischmeyer PE. Nutrition therapy and critical illness: Practical guidance for the ICU, post-ICU, and long-term convalescence phases. Crit Care. 2019;23(1):368.
47. Ridley EJ, Parke RL, Davies AR, Bailey M, Hodgson C, Deane AM, et al. What happens to nutrition intake in the Post–Intensive care unit hospitalization period? an observational cohort study in critically ill adults. JPEN J Parenter Enteral Nutr. 2019;43(1):88-95.
48. Ridley EJ, Peake SL, Jarvis M, Deane AM, Lange K, Davies AR, et al. Nutrition therapy in australia and New Zealand intensive care units: An international comparison study. JPEN J Parenter Enteral Nutr. 2018;42(8):1349-57.
49. De Waele E, van Zanten ARH. Routine use of indirect calorimetry in critically ill patients: Pros cons. Crit Care. 2022;26(1):123.
50. Singer P, Anbar R, Cohen J, Shapiro H, Shalita-Chesner M, Lev S, et al. The tight calorie control study (TICACOS): A prospective, randomized, controlled pilot study of nutritional support in critically ill patients. Intensive Care Med. 2011;37(4):601-9.
51. Vanhorebeek I, Gunst J, Derde S, Derese I, Boussemaere M, Güiza F, et al. Insufficient activation of autophagy allows cellular damage to accumulate in critically ill patients. J Clin Endocrinol Metab. 2011;96(4):E633-45.
52. Masiero E, Agatea L, Mammucari C, Blaauw B, Loro E, Komatsu M, et al. Autophagy is required to maintain muscle mass. Cell Metab. 2009;10(6):507-15.
53. The National Heart, Lung, and Blood Institute Acute Respiratory Distress Syndrome (ARDS) Clinical Trials Network. Initial trophic vs full enteral feeding in patients with acute lung injury: The EDEN randomized trial. JAMA: J Am Med Assoc. 2012;307(8):795-803.
54. Lim SL, Ong KCB, Chan YH, Loke WC, Ferguson M, Daniels L. Malnutrition and its impact on cost of hospitalization, length of

stay, readmission and 3-year mortality. Clin Nutr. 2012;31(3):345-50.
55. Ruiz AJ, Buitrago G, Rodríguez N, Gómez G, Sulo S, Gómez C, et al. Clinical and economic outcomes associated with malnutrition in hospitalized patients. Clin Nutr. 2019; 38(3):1310-6.
56. Isabel TD, Correia M, Waitzberg DL. The impact of malnutrition on morbidity, mortality, length of hospital stay and costs evaluated through a multivariate model analysis. Clin Nutr. 2003;22(3):235-9.
57. Dickerson RN, Buckley CT. Impact of propofol sedation upon caloric overfeeding and protein inadequacy in critically ill patients receiving nutrition support. Pharmacy. 2021;9(3):121.
58. Asrani VM, Brown A, Bissett I, Windsor JA. Impact of intravenous fluids and enteral nutrition on the severity of gastrointestinal dysfunction: A systematic review and meta-analysis. J Crit Care Med (Targu Mures). 2020;6(1):5-24.
59. Asrani VM, McArthur C, Phillips ARJ, Bissett I, Windsor JA. Conservative fluid resuscitation and aggressive enteral nutrition: A potentially lethal combination in patients with critical illness. ANZ J Surg. 2021;91(7-8):1333-4.
60. Reignier J, Plantefeve G, Mira JP, Argaud L, Asfar P, Aissaoui N, et al. Low versus standard calorie and protein feeding in ventilated adults with shock: A randomised, controlled, multicentre, open-label, parallel-group trial (NUTRIREA-3). Lancet Respir Med. 2023.
61. Reignier J, Boisramé-Helms J, Brisard L, Lascarrou JB, Ait Hssain A, Anguel N, et al. Enteral versus parenteral early nutrition in ventilated adults with shock: A randomised, controlled, multicentre, open-label, parallel-group study (NUTRIREA-2). Lancet. 2018;391(10116):133-43.
62. Moonen HPFX, Van Zanten ARH. Bioelectric impedance analysis for body composition measurement and other potential clinical applications in critical illness. Curr Opin Crit Care. 2021;27(4):344-53.
63. Moonen HPFX, van Zanten FJL, Driessen L, Driessen L, de Smet V, Slingerland-Boot R, et al. Association of bioelectric impedance analysis body composition and disease severity in COVID-19 hospital ward and ICU patients: The BIAC-19 study. Clin Nutr. 2021;40(4):2328-36.
64. Hermans AJH, Laarhuis BI, Kouw IWK, Van Zanten ARH. Current insights in ICU nutrition: Tailored nutrition. Curr Opin Crit Care. 2023;29(2):101-7.
65. Ridley EJ, Chapple LS. Nutrition in critical illness—research is worth the EFFORT. The Lancet. 2023;401(10376):527-8.
66. Ridley EJ, Rice TW. NUTRIREA-3: Where to next? Lancet Respir Med. 2023.

CHAPTER 9

Micronutrient Physiology and Requirements in Critical Illness

Ranil Jayawardena

INTRODUCTION

Micronutrients, including essential vitamins and trace elements, play crucial physiological roles within the human body, particularly in the context of critical illness. They have important functions at both the cellular and the molecular levels. Impaired energy metabolism, often observed in critical illness, is closely associated with mitochondrial dysfunction, resulting in physical impairment. Numerous studies have demonstrated the indispensability of specific vitamins such as B, C, and E, as well as minerals like selenium and zinc, in ensuring optimal mitochondrial function.[1] Furthermore, it has been found that cells of the immune system rely on certain micronutrients to function optimally through different stages of the immune response. Vitamins A, B, C, E, B_6, B_{12}, folate, zinc, iron, copper, and selenium are a few examples of these micronutrients.[2] Moreover, the pathophysiology of several critical illnesses, including acute respiratory distress syndrome, ischemia–reperfusion injury, and sepsis-induced multiorgan dysfunction, is closely associated with oxidative stress-mediated cell damage. Micronutrients with antioxidant properties have been identified as potential agents capable of mitigating the detrimental effects of excessive oxidative stress. In particular, the antioxidant properties of vitamins A, C, and E, along with the trace elements selenium and zinc, have been extensively discussed.[3] Furthermore, in critical illnesses, the adequate availability of micronutrients such as Fe, folic acid, and vitamin B_{12} is crucial for erythropoiesis, the red blood cell production process. These deficits are the cause of anemia, which is extremely common in people with critical illnesses. Additionally, persistent functional iron deficiency can contribute to iron dysmetabolism, where reduced iron availability adversely affects the functioning of vital organs.[4] When considered collectively, the evidence highlights the importance of micronutrients in critical illnesses, particularly in energy metabolism, immune response modulation, oxidative stress regulation, and erythropoiesis.

PREVALENCE OF MICRONUTRIENT DEFICIENCY IN PATIENTS WITH CRITICAL ILLNESS

It has been widely reported that protein and energy malnutrition are highly prevalent in cases of critical illness. Moreover, deficiencies in various micronutrients have been observed in patients with critical illnesses, significantly impacting the disease prognosis. Vitamin D deficiency, in particular, is highly prevalent among critically ill patients, with a prevalence range of 40-70% reported in observational studies and further deterioration of vitamin D levels during intensive care unit (ICU) stays.[5] Similarly, in the context of critically ill coronavirus disease 2019 (COVID-19) adult patients, a study found that 82% had low vitamin C levels.[6] Additionally, a multicenter, prospective cohort study involving critically ill children revealed an 11% prevalence of thiamine deficiency, with new cases developing during the ICU stay.[7] Several micronutrient deficiencies have also been reported. For example, a case–control study on critically ill children with sepsis found a significantly higher prevalence of vitamin A deficiency in the study group compared to the control group (58.8% vs 12.2%; $p <0.001$). Moreover, vitamin A deficiency was associated with septic shock, with an unadjusted odds ratio (OR) of 3.297 [95% confidence interval (CI) 1.169–9.300; $p = 0.024$].[8] Similar to vitamin deficiencies, mineral deficiencies are also common in critical illnesses. An observational study involving 269 ICUs found that nearly 80% of critically ill patients infected with COVID-19 had low Zn levels.[9] Additionally, critically ill patients show a notable incidence of iron deficiency, with estimates indicating rates of up to 40% at the time of ICU admission.[10] However, it is worth noting that functional iron deficiency may have short-term advantages against invading microbes.

REQUIREMENTS OF DIFFERENT MICRONUTRIENTS

Thiamine

A recent systematic review examining the supplementation of thiamine has yielded mixed findings. The included studies utilized thiamine doses ranging mainly from 100 to 500 mg/day, administered for a duration of 3 days until discharge. One notable positive outcome was a 42% reduction in the development of ICU delirium observed in the thiamine-supplemented group compared to the placebo groups. Nevertheless, the data regarding mortality did not demonstrate promising results. A pooled analysis of seven randomized controlled trials (RCTs) revealed no statistically significant difference in mortality between the groups ($n = 1,005$; OR 1.03; 95% CI 0.77–1.36). Similarly, thiamine use did not show a significant reduction in the length of hospital stay (LOS), length of ICU stays, or length of mechanical ventilation.[11] Administration of intravenous (IV) thiamine 200 mg every 12 hours for 4 days or until ICU discharge along with vitamin C (1.5 g every 6 hours for 4 days or until ICU discharge) and hydrocortisone (50 mg every 6 hours for 7 days or until ICU discharge followed by a taper over 3 days) is effective in preventing progressive organ dysfunction, including acute kidney injury, and reducing the mortality of patients with severe sepsis and septic shock.[12] Additionally, Blakeslee and Hyrkäs reported in their review that the early administration of IV thiamine in doses of 200–500 mg two to three times daily resulted in improved lactate clearance among adults with septic shock.[13] IV thiamine is low-cost and safe; therefore, administration of 200–300 mg/day for at-risk patients and 100 mg/day for all critically ill patients should be considered.[14]

Vitamin B Combination

In a small RCT involving critically ill COVID-19 patients, the administration of a low-dose of vitamin B cocktail did not result in significant improvements in clinical or biochemical parameters. However, an analysis of the 30-day mortality rates revealed a slight decrease in the intervention group compared to the control group, although the difference was not statistically significant (83.3% vs 96.1%, $p = 0.07$).[15]

Vitamin C

Shrestha et al. conducted a systematic review and meta-analysis, encompassing 53 studies with a total of 352,395 critically ill patients. Their primary objective was to assess the impact of vitamin C on various outcomes, including LOS, 28/30-day mortality, ICU mortality, and renal safety. A subanalysis of the RCTs within this study ($n = 27$) did not identify any favorable impact of vitamin C on the LOS. However, there was a small yet significant reduction in the length of ICU stay observed among the vitamin C group compared to the placebo/standard of care group in the RCTs (mean difference −0.70; 95% CI −1.39 to −0.02; $n = 1,712$; $I^2 = 86\%$; $p = 0.04$). No significant relationship was found between hospital mortality outcomes and ICU mortality. The administration of vitamin C supplements did not result in adverse renal events.[16] In a recent systematic review and meta-analysis conducted by Lee et al., the use of IV vitamin C as monotherapy in critically ill patients yielded significant effects. They demonstrated a reduction in overall mortality associated with IV vitamin C supplementation [risk ratio (RR) 0.73; 95% CI 0.60-0.89; $p = 0.002$]. Subgroup analysis further indicated a similar beneficial effect, particularly among critically ill patients at high risk of mortality.[17] Another review showed that vitamin C supplementation reduced the duration of mechanical ventilation by an average of 14% ($p = 0.00001$). However, it is important to note that there was substantial heterogeneity among the studies. In five trials involving 471 patients who required ventilation for >10 hours, a dosage of 1-6 g/day of vitamin C led to an average reduction in ventilation time by 25% ($p < 0.0001$).[18] Cosupplementation of thiamine and vitamin C exhibited a significant decrease in the Sequential Organ Failure Assessment (SOFA) score [weighted mean difference (WMD) −0.73; 95% CI −1.29-0.17; I^2 0.0%], but it did not have a significant impact on the mortality rate in critically ill patients.[19] In view of the current evidence, IV vitamin C supplementation can be effective for patients with deficiencies, and it is not associated with serious adverse effects. However, it is worth noting that the European Society for Clinical Nutrition and Metabolism (ESPEN) guideline does not recommend the use of a single, high dose of antioxidant vitamins for critical illness.[20]

Vitamin D

Vitamin D can be obtained from two distinct sources. Firstly, it can be synthesized in the skin through endogenous production under the influence of ultraviolet B radiation, provided there is sufficient liver and renal function. Secondly, it can be acquired through dietary supplements and dietary sources, including both animal- and plant-based foods, as well as fortified products. Despite this, hypovitaminosis D is prevalent not only in the general population but also among critically ill patients. Vitamin D deficiency in critically ill patients has been associated with an increased mortality rate and prolonged hospital stays.[21]

Numerous studies have investigated the supplementation of vitamin D in critically ill patients. In a randomized, double-blind, placebo-controlled, single-center trial conducted in five ICUs, 492 critically ill adult White patients with vitamin D deficiency (≤20 ng/mL) were assigned to receive either oral or nasogastric tube administration of a single dose of 540,000 IU of vitamin D_3, followed by monthly maintenance doses of 90,000 IU for 5 months ($n = 249$), or a placebo ($n = 243$). The administration of high-dose vitamin D_3, compared to a placebo, did not result in a reduction in LOS, hospital mortality, or 6-month mortality.[22] In another extensive randomized, double-blind, placebo-controlled phase III trial involving a large cohort of participants ($n = 1360$), early supplementation with 540,000 IU of vitamin D_3 was examined in critically ill patients who had vitamin D deficiency and were at a heightened risk of mortality. Although the supplementation increased serum vitamin D_3 levels in the intervention group, it did not improve 90-day mortality (23.5% in the vitamin D group vs 20.6% in the placebo group; $p = 0.26$) or other secondary clinical, physiological, or safety endpoints.[23] Nevertheless, no adverse effects were reported with high-dose vitamin D supplementation in critically ill patients with vitamin D deficiency. According to ESPEN guidelines, vitamin D supplementation is recommended for patients with low plasma vitamin D levels (<50 nmol/L), and they further support the administration of a single mega dose of vitamin D (500,000 IU) within a week after admission.

Selenium

Selenium supplementation in critically ill patients exhibits considerable heterogeneity in terms of patient characteristics, supplementation doses, and duration. Jaff et al. conducted an umbrella review that analyzed systematic reviews and meta-analyses of RCTs investigating the effects of Se therapy in critically ill patients. The study included 17 meta-analyses comprising 24 RCTs that met the inclusion criteria. The findings revealed that Se supplementation can significantly reduce the incidence of mortality (RR 0.83; 95% CI 0.71 0.98; $p = 0.024$) and acute renal failure (RR 0.67; 95% CI 0.46–0.98; $p = 0.038$). However, the certainty of the evidence supporting these outcomes was considered to be low. On the other hand, the effects of Se supplementation on the risk of infection ($p = 0.207$), pneumonia ($p = 0.675$), length of ICU stay ($p = 0.876$), LOS ($p = 0.757$), and duration of ventilation ($p = 0.329$) were not statistically significant. Moreover, no significant effects were observed for the risk of infection, pneumonia, length of ICU stay, LOS, and duration of ventilation.[24] In a meta-analysis, there was no significant treatment effect of high-single-dose selenium for mortality (RR 0.95; 95% CI 0.88–1.02; $p = 0.15$), ICU and hospital LOS, renal function, or ventilator days.[25] Consequently, the use of selenium supplementation for critically ill patients remains uncertain.

Zinc

Zinc, an essential trace element, plays a vital role in the formation of metalloenzymes, protein metabolism, RNA conformation, and membrane stabilization. Furthermore, it is integral to cellular growth and replication, rapid epithelialization, wound healing, cellular immunity, and protection against oxidative stress. Critically ill patients with recurrent sepsis have been found to exhibit persistently low serum Zn levels, while surgical sepsis patients with lower serum Zn levels are more susceptible to recurrent sepsis episodes.[26] Despite the well-documented adverse outcomes associated with Zn deficiencies in critical illness, limited interventions have been reported. Noninterventional studies, however, have shown promising effects, as zinc supplementation was linked to reduce inhospital mortality [hazard ratio (HR) 0.48; 95% CI 0.28–0.83; $p = 0.009$) and 30-day mortality (HR 0.51; 95% CI 0.30–0.86; $p = 0.012$) in critically ill patients with acute kidney injury.[27] Similar benefits were observed in critically ill patients with COVID-19 who received zinc sulfate as adjunctive therapy, with lower 30-day mortality (HR 0.52; 95% CI 0.29–0.92; $p = 0.03$).[28] However, a combination of four interventions involving zinc supplementation among critically ill patients yielded a nonsignificant reduction in mortality (RR 0.63; 95% CI 0.25–1.59; $p = 0.33$) and LOS in intensive care (–0.35 days, $p = 0.17$). Consequently, due to the scarcity of clinical data, there is insufficient evidence to support the routine use of high-dose zinc supplementation in critically ill patients.[29]

COMBINATION OF TRACE ELEMENTS AND VITAMINS

A meta-analysis using multitreatment comparison (MTC) revealed that the administration of a combination of different micronutrients, including selenium, zinc, and copper, was ranked as the most efficient in reducing the LOS in the ICU. Additionally, a combination of "selenium, zinc, copper, and vitamin E" was identified as the best treatment for reducing infection risk. Ventilator days were minimized with the administration of "selenium, zinc, and manganese," while LOS was shortened with a combination of "selenium, zinc, and copper."[30]

CONCLUSION

In summary, micronutrient deficiencies are highly prevalent among critically ill patients and are associated with poor health outcomes, including an increased risk of infection, longer hospital stays, and ultimately, higher mortality rates. However, there is no conclusive evidence to support high doses of any micronutrient, especially antioxidant vitamins. Some evidence suggests that thiamine and vitamin D supplementation can be beneficial on a short-term basis. It would be prudent to provide the Dietary Reference Intake (DRI) of micronutrients to prevent deficiencies during chronic illness.

REFERENCES

1. Wesselink E, Koekkoek WAC, Grefte S, Witkamp RF, van Zanten ARH. Feeding mitochondria: Potential role of nutritional components to improve critical illness convalescence. Clinical Nutr. 2019;38(3):982-95.
2. Moore A, Khanna D. The Role of Vitamin C in Human Immunity and Its Treatment Potential Against COVID-19: A Review Article. Cureus. 2023;15(1):e33740.
3. Koekkoek WA, van Zanten AR. Antioxidant Vitamins and Trace Elements in Critical Illness. Nutr Clin Pract. 2016;31(4):457-74.
4. Litton E, Lim J. Iron Metabolism: An Emerging Therapeutic Target in Critical Illness. Crit Care. 2019;23(1):81.
5. Amrein K, Papinutti A, Mathew E, Vila G, Parekh D. Vitamin D and critical illness: What endocrinology can learn from intensive care and vice versa. Endocr Connect. 2018;7(12):R304-R15.
6. Tomasa-Irriguible TM, Bielsa-Berrocal L. COVID-19: Up to 82% of critically ill patients had low Vitamin C values. Nutr J. 2021;20(1):66.
7. Akkuzu E, Yavuz S, Ozcan S, Sincar S, Bayrakci B, Kendirli T, et al. Prevalence and Time Course of Thiamine Deficiency in Critically Ill Children: A Multicenter, Prospective Cohort Study in Turkey. Pediatr Crit Care Med. 2022;23(5):399-404.
8. Zhang X, Yang K, Chen L, Liao X, Deng L, Chen S, et al. Vitamin A deficiency in critically ill children with sepsis. Crit Care. 2019;23(1):267.
9. Gonçalves TJM, Gonçalves SEAB, Guarnieri A, Risegato RC, Guimarães MP, de Freitas DC, et al. Association Between Low Zinc Levels and Severity of Acute Respiratory Distress Syndrome by New Coronavirus SARS-CoV-2. Nutr Clin Pract. 2021;36(1):186-91.
10. Bellamy MC, Gedney JA. Unrecognised iron deficiency in critical illness. Lancet. 1998;352(9144):1903.
11. Santo T Jr, Clark B, Hickman M, Grebely J, Campbell G, Sordo L, et al. Association of Opioid Agonist Treatment With All-Cause Mortality and Specific Causes of Death Among People With Opioid Dependence:

A Systematic Review and Meta-analysis. JAMA Psychiatry. 2021;78(9):979-93.
12. Marik PE, Khangoora V, Rivera R, Hooper MH, Catravas J. Hydrocortisone, Vitamin C, and Thiamine for the Treatment of Severe Sepsis and Septic Shock: A Retrospective Before-After Study. Chest. 2017;151(6):1229-38.
13. Blakeslee PA, Hyrkäs K. Impact of supplemental thiamin on lactate levels in adults with septic shock. Nutr Clin Pract. 2023;38(3):580-601.
14. Amrein K, Oudemans-van Straaten HM, Berger MM. Vitamin therapy in critically ill patients: focus on thiamine, vitamin C, and vitamin D. Intensive Care Med. 2018;44(11):1940-4.
15. Majidi N, Bahadori E, Shekari S, Gholamalizadeh M, Tajadod S, Ajami M, et al. Effects of supplementation with low-dose group B vitamins on clinical and biochemical parameters in critically ill patients with COVID-19: a randomized clinical trial. Expert Rev Anti Infect Ther. 2022:1-7.
16. Shrestha DB, Budhathoki P, Sedhai YR, Mandal SK, Shikhrakar S, Karki S, et al. Vitamin C in Critically Ill Patients: An Updated Systematic Review and Meta-Analysis. Nutrients. 2021;13(10):1364.
17. Lee Z-Y, Ortiz-Reyes L, Lew CCH, Hasan MS, Ke L, Patel JJ, et al. Intravenous vitamin C monotherapy in critically ill patients: a systematic review and meta-analysis of randomized controlled trials with trial sequential analysis. Ann Intensive Care. 2023;13(1):14.
18. Hemilä H, Chalker E. Vitamin C may reduce the duration of mechanical ventilation in critically ill patients: a meta-regression analysis. J Intensive Care. 2020;8:15.
19. Shokri-mashhadi N, Aliyari A, Hajhashemy Z, Saadat S, Rouhani MH. Is it time to reconsider the administration of thiamine alone or in combination with vitamin C in critically ill patients? A meta-analysis of clinical trial studies. J Intensive Care. 2022;10(1):8.
20. Singer P, Blaser AR, Berger MM, Alhazzani W, Calder PC, Casaer MP, et al. ESPEN guideline on clinical nutrition in the intensive care unit. Clin Nutr. 2019;38(1):48-79.
21. Zajic P, Amrein K. Vitamin D deficiency in the ICU: a systematic review. Minerva Endocrinol. 2014;39(4):275-87.
22. Amrein K, Schnedl C, Holl A, Riedl R, Christopher KB, Pachler C, et al. Effect of high-dose vitamin D3 on hospital length of stay in critically ill patients with vitamin D deficiency: the VITdAL-ICU randomized clinical trial. JAMA. 2014;312(15):1520-30.
23. Ginde AA, Brower RG, Caterino JM, Finck L, Banner-Goodspeed VM, Grissom CK, et al. Early High-Dose Vitamin D_3 for Critically Ill, Vitamin D-Deficient Patients. N Engl J Med. 2019;381(26):2529-40.
24. Jaff S, Zeraattalab-Motlagh S, Amiri Khosroshahi R, Gubari M, Mohammadi H, Djafarian K. The effect of selenium therapy in critically ill patients: an umbrella review of systematic reviews and meta-analysis of randomized controlled trials. Eur J Med Res. 2023;28(1):104.
25. Manzanares W, Lemieux M, Elke G, Langlois PL, Bloos F, Heyland DK. High-dose intravenous selenium does not improve clinical outcomes in the critically ill: a systematic review and meta-analysis. Crit Care. 2016;20(1):356.
26. Hoeger J, Simon TP, Beeker T, Marx G, Haase H, Schuerholz T. Persistent low serum zinc is associated with recurrent sepsis in critically ill patients - A pilot study. PLoS One. 2017;12(5):e0176069.
27. Xia W, Li C, Zhao D, Xu L, Kuang M, Yao X, et al. The Impact of Zinc Supplementation on Critically Ill Patients With Acute Kidney Injury: A Propensity Score Matching Analysis. Front Nutr. 2022;9:894572.
28. Al Sulaiman K, Aljuhani O, Al Shaya AI, Kharbosh A, Kensara R, Al Guwairy A, et al. Evaluation of zinc sulfate as an adjunctive therapy in COVID-19 critically ill patients: a two center propensity-score matched study. Crit Care. 2021;25(1):363.
29. Heyland DK, Jones N, Cvijanovich NZ, Wong H. Zinc supplementation in critically ill patients: a key pharmaconutrient? JPEN J Parenter Enteral Nutr. 2008;32(5):509-19.
30. Gudivada KK, Kumar A, Sriram K, Baby J, Shariff M, Sampath S, et al. Antioxidant micronutrient supplements for adult critically ill patients: A bayesian multiple treatment comparisons meta-analysis. Clin Nutr ESPEN. 2022;47:78-88.

CHAPTER 10

Probiotics, Prebiotics, Synbiotics, and Postbiotics

B Ravinder Reddy

"Beneath our superficial differences, we are all of us walking communities of bacteria. The world shimmers, a pointillist landscape made of living beings"
— **Lynn Margulis**

INTRODUCTION

Earth, as a planet, is dominated by microbes. Bacteria were actually the sole "living" beings for the first 3 billion years and played the most pivotal role in the evolution of complex living organisms, including humans, and like earth, humans too are dominated by bacteria.[1] Human Microbiome Project (HMP) and next-generation sequencing (NGS) have demonstrated and characterized the different sets of commensal microbes. The tremendous amount of ongoing pioneering work over the past two decades, using shotgun metagenomic sequencing, has clearly demonstrated the crucial role of the microbiomes in human health and pathogenesis of various diseases.[2] A significant aspect of these homeostatic functions is enabled by the bioactive molecules produced by the gut microbiota. Therefore, modulation of human microbiome offers a potential option in maintaining an optimal health and in managing the various pathological conditions. Diet is the most vital aspect in maintaining a "healthy" microbiome, in addition to various other factors.[3] Additionally, the microbiome can be modulated by probiotics, prebiotics, synbiotics, and postbiotics (PPSP) by consuming functional, fermented, and fortified food and drinks and especially in the form of medications. PPSP regulate the diversity and the composition of symbiotic gut microbiota as well as the production of their metabolites, enhancing their homeostatic roles in metabolism, mucosal immunity, and intestinal barrier functions.

DEFINITIONS

The International Scientific Association for Probiotics and Prebiotics (ISAPP) defines *probiotics* as "live microorganisms which when administered in adequate amounts confer a health benefit."

Prebiotics are defined as nonviable substrates that are selectively used by host microorganisms and confer health benefits. Certain subtypes of dietary carbohydrates, such as cellulose, hemicellulose, lignins, mucins, and pectin fiber, cannot be digested into smaller units due to lack of specific intestinal enzymes. These low-digestible and undigestible carbohydrates undergo fermentation by specific microbiota in the large intestine whose growth and proliferation are thus enabled. In other words, prebiotics generally are the nondigestible components of dietary fiber which act as food for probiotics. However, all dietary fibers are not prebiotics.[4,5]

Synbiotics are a combination of prebiotics and probiotics, resulting in a synergistic beneficial effect. As per ISAPP, synbiotics are defined as "mixture of live microorganisms and substrates selectively utilized by host microorganisms that confer a health benefit."[6]

Postbiotics are compounds with bioactive properties. They include short-chain fatty acids (SCFAs), cell wall fragments, lipopolysaccharides (LPS), enzymes, amino acids, and vitamins. A 2019 consensus statement by ISAPP defines postbiotics as a "preparation of inanimate microorganisms and/or their components that confers health benefits on the host." Postbiotics are thus made up of inactivated microbes, with or without their cell components and with or without their metabolites, all of which result in beneficial effects.[7] Multiple terms referring to nonviable probiotics exist and are used interchangeably—inactivated probiotics, ghost biotics, heat-killed probiotics, paraprobiotics, parapsychobiotics, immunobiotics, and microbial lysate. Inactivated or heat-killed probiotics are termed paraprobiotics.[8]

▪ MECHANISM OF ACTIONS

The beneficial roles of probiotics are due to their effects on establishing, amplification, and proliferation of the beneficial microbiota and modulating the microbial metabolic pathways while moderating the immune responses by molecular mechanisms at the epithelial surfaces (refer to Chapter 3 for immune cells and their different responses and Chapter 42 for the various roles of gut microbiome). The benefits of probiotics include production of antimicrobial peptides such as bacteriocins secreted especially by the genus *Lactobacillus*, inhibiting pathogenic bacterial growth by reducing the pH in the colon by SCFAs—butyrate, lactate, and acetate, by *Lactobacillus* and *Bifidobacterial* species. They reduce the inflammation by inhibiting inflammatory pathways and increasing the release of anti-inflammatory mediators, strengthening the intestinal integrity. Probiotics are involved in modulating systemic and specific mucosal immune responses, stimulate activation of macrophage and natural killer (NK) cells, and lessen the incidence of food allergies. By enabling the production of SCFAs, probiotics play a vital role in proliferation of epithelial cells, act as fuel for colonocytes, and help in absorption of electrolytes and minerals. They regulate glucose metabolism and transport, by producing glucagon-like peptide-1 (GLP-1) and in fatty acid oxidation, regulation of lipid and cholesterol metabolism. They also play a role in satiety by producing peptide YY (PYY) and regulate the gut–brain axis. They are involved in the production of certain B vitamins such as riboflavin, folic acid, and cobalamin, especially by *Lactobacillus* species.[9,10]

Prebiotic sources of dietary fibers are the nondigestible short chains of fructose and galactose molecules, the fructooligosaccharides (FOS) and galactooligosaccharides (GOS). They occur naturally in many plant-based nutrients such as bananas, onions, garlic, asparagus, whole grains, cereals, and legumes, including various beans, lentils, and nuts. These are fermented by *Lactobacillus* and *Bifidobacterium* species to produce SCFAs. In addition to the various metabolic and immunomodulating effects, SCFAs, especially lactate and acetate, act as nutrients and "cross feed" other microbial species such as *Eubacteria* and *Roseburia*, as well as *Faecalibacterium prausnitzii*, which, in turn, produce butyrate. Consumption of prebiotic FOS, including the soluble inulin, enhances the population of beneficial commensals

(*Bifidobacterial* species), and reduction in the proliferation of pathogenic bacteria (*Clostridium perfringens, Escherichia coli,* and *Salmonella*) also enables scavenging of reactive oxygen species (ROS). The resultant antioxidant effects also facilitate colonic smooth muscle function and protect colonic mucosa from the damaging effects of LPS produced by various species of pathogenic gram-negative bacteria. Inulin plays a role in preventing lipid peroxidation and degradation of ascorbic acid.[11,12] *Lactobacillus* and *Bifidobacterium* species, which produce the enzyme β-galactosidase (β-GOS), act on GOS and intensify their own respective growth and proliferation. They induce secretion of interleukin 10 (IL-10), which has multiple effects. They downregulate the activation of T cells and inflammatory mediators [IL-1, IL-6, tumor necrosis factor alpha (TNF-α)] and enhance B cell proliferation and production of antibodies as well as differentiation of regulatory T cells (T_{regs}). Lactulose, a type of synthetic sugar which is commonly used as a laxative and in managing hepatic encephalopathy, also has prebiotic properties. Studies in humans have shown a dose-dependent, person-specific prebiotic effect, with an increase in the percentage of *Bifidobacterium* at a dose of 2 g and above per day, lasting for up to 7 days after stopping lactulose.[13] Resistant starch (RS) is a nondigestible carbohydrate which occurs naturally in various grains, including oats, beans, and legumes. It is fermented in the colon and has prebiotic effect by increasing the number of beneficial microbiota—*Bifidobacterium, Akkermansia,* and *Bacteroidetes* species in the gut.[14] Prebiotics impart several benefits by multiple mechanisms, the chief of which are immunomodulatory effects, improving and strengthening intestinal barrier functions, reducing the population of pathogenic gut bacteria, and enabling the production of SCFAs; they regulate the metabolic pathways of glucose and lipids, including satiety, obesity, and protection from developing fatty liver via its effects on secondary bile acids, insulin resistance, GLP-1, and PYY.

Mechanisms of action of synbiotics can be due to the combined but independent actions of probiotics and prebiotics, termed "complementary" synbiotics. On the other hand, when the microbe within the synbiotic preparation increases in number because of the coadministered prebiotic, then they are termed "synergistic" synbiotics. Complementary synbiotics are commonly used in clinical trials and constitute majority of the commercially available synbiotics. The most successful and a very large, randomized placebo-controlled trial utilized complementary synbiotic-containing *Lactobacillus plantarum* and FOS in rural Indian newborns. The study which enrolled 4,556 infants showed a significant reduction in sepsis and mortality in the treatment group.[15] The beneficial effects of synbiotics are thought to be due to the increase in the survival of probiotics during their upper gastrointestinal transit, thus contributing to the intestinal homeostasis by increasing the quantity of *Lactobacillus* and *Bifidobacterium* species and the positive effects because of their expansion.[16]

Postbiotics are the bioactive substances generated by the metabolic pathways of various probiotic organisms: Organic acids such as SCFAs, lactic acid, acetic acid, B-vitamins, vitamin K and antioxidant enzymes such as glutathione peroxidase, superoxide dismutase, reduced nicotinamide adenine dinucleotide (NADH) peroxidase, as well as microbial cell wall components such as lipoteichoic acid, peptidoglycan, cell surface proteins, and LPS. Postbiotics' benefits occur at the mucosal interface and include antimicrobial, anti-inflammatory effects, immunomodulation, and augmenting intestinal integrity. Systemic benefits include antioxidant, antineoplastic, antiobesogenic, antihypertensive, and hypocholesterolemic effects.[17]

CLINICAL APPLICATIONS

Probiotics, prebiotics, synbiotics, and postbiotics, in the form of medications, are known to modulate the beneficial microbiota and increase their quantity on a short-term basis. Consumption of mainly a plant-based diet along with fermented foods and drinks has the potential for maintaining the long-term diversity and magnitude of healthy commensals.[18]

The predominant clinical benefits of PPSP are enhancing the functions and integrity of various intestinal barriers (described in Chapter 42), regulatory modulation of immune responses, and multiple systemic effects. However, due to the specific populations of the microbiota within the gut and other niches, the effects of PPSP may not be uniform and consistent. The major therapeutic benefits include the antimicrobial actions against various pathogenic organisms, including *Helicobacter pylori*, in decreasing the incidence of diarrhea due to antibiotic usage (*Clostridium difficile*), and other infective causes, including acute gastroenteritis. Various species of *Lactobacillus* (especially *Lactiplantibacillus plantarum, L. acidophilus, Limosilactobacillus reuteri, Lacticaseibacillus rhamnosus, Lactobacillus delbrueckii subsp. bulgaricus, Lacticaseibacillus casie, Lacticaseibacillus paracasei*, and *L. kefir*) and *Bifidobacterium* (*B. longum, B. bifidum, B. lactis*, and *B. infantis*), including the probiotic yeast and *Saccharomyces boulardii*, have shown to reduce the severity and duration of diarrhea and in hastening the regeneration of normal flora. They also reduce opportunistic infections due to candida-associated colonizations. Probiotics are also of benefit in certain autoimmune diseases (such as rheumatoid arthritis, multiple sclerosis, systemic lupus erythematosus, myasthenia gravis, and celiac disease), including inflammatory bowel diseases (IBD), such as Crohn's disease and ulcerative colitis, as well as irritable bowel syndrome (IBS).[19-22]

Routine use of PPSP in critical illness remains inconclusive due to the myriad nature and uniqueness of every critically ill patient. However, a recent systemic review and meta-analysis showed a reduced incidence of infection rates, including ventilatory-associated pneumonia (VAP) and diarrhea. Due to varying nature, etiology, and intensity of critical illness, the effects of probiotics could be specific to the patient as well to the strains and species of probiotics.[23] Another meta-analysis of randomized controlled trials to analyze the safety and efficacy of probiotics and synbiotics showed a reduction in VAP, other hospital-acquired infections, and duration of hospital stay, but without any effect on the overall mortality.[24] Yet, another systemic review of trials from four major databases (PubMed, ScienceDirect, Embase, and Cochrane Systemic Reviews) failed to show beneficial effects of probiotics.[25]

In acute pancreatitis, especially in the initial hyperinflammatory phase, the nature and diversity of gut microbiome play a crucial role in the outcomes. Attempts to alter the gut microbiota with prebiotics and probiotics in the past have been associated with an increase in mortality. However, two recent studies showed that synbiotics as well as probiotics alone showed some benefit in terms of reducing the duration of hospitalization but without any effects on mortality. Another study reported an increase in the tolerance to enteral feeds, when given with soluble fibers.[26]

In surgical patients, gut dysbiosis and an increase in pathogenic microbiota have been associated with an increase in surgical site infections (SSIs), anastomotic leaks, and recurrences of diseases such as IBD and colorectal cancers. Prebiotics and synbiotics have the potential to increase and expand the healthy commensal bacteria, which result in beneficial effects in the surgical patients. Multiple trials, systemic reviews, and meta-analyses showed a significant reduction in SSIs, infections at remote sites (such as urinary tract), incidence of septicemia, abdominal distention, diarrhea, duration of antibiotic usage, and postoperative pyrexia. In addition, perioperative use of synbiotics was associated with increased tolerance to solid foods, reduced hospital stay, and enhanced recovery of intestinal functions. Therefore, short-term use of prebiotics and especially synbiotics are associated with reduction in various postsurgical complications.[27-29]

Additionally, the supplements of PPSP have demonstrated antioxidant effects and antineoplastic properties and have shown to be beneficial in a significant number of other conditions, which include necrotizing enterocolitis in preterm neonates and infants, in autism spectrum disorders, and in hypertensive individuals.[7,10]

CONCLUSION

Our understanding and the options to modulate the microbial commensals by PPSP, including the use of synthetic biotherapeutic molecules, have expanded tremendously due to an enormous amount of clinical and preclinical (animal-model) research. While diet remains the cornerstone in maintaining the quantity and diversity of healthy commensal microorganisms, short-term interventions by PPSP, as supplements, play a key role in managing diverse diseases is a novel therapeutic modality.

REFERENCES

1. Gibbons A. (2016). Microbes in our guts have been with us for millions of years. [online] Available from: https://www.science.org/content/article/microbes-our-guts-have-been-us-millions-years [Last accessed August, 2023].
2. Jovel J, Patterson J, Wang W, Hotte N, O'Keefe S, Mitchel T, et al. Characterization of the gut microbiome using 16S or shotgun metagenomics. Front Microbiol. 2016;7:459.
3. Ogunrinola GA, Oyewale JO, Oshamika OO, Olasehinde GI. The human microbiome and its impact on health. Int J Microbiol. 2020;2020:8045646.
4. Gibson GR, Hutkins R, Sander ME. Expert consensus document: The International Scientific Association for Probiotics and Prebiotics (ISAPP) consensus statement on the definition and scope of prebiotics. Nat Rev Gastroenterol Hepatol. 2017;14:491-502.
5. Roberfroid M, Gibson GR, Hoyles L, McCartney AL, Rastall R, Rowland I, et al. Prebiotic effects: Metabolic and health benefits. Br J Nutr. 2010;104:S1-63.
6. Gomez Quintero DF, Kok CR, Hutkins R. The Future of Synbiotics: Rational Formulation and Design. Front Microbiol. 2022;13:919725.
7. Salminen S, Collado MC, Endo A, Hill C, Lebeer S, Quigley EMM, et al. The International Scientific Association of Probiotics and Prebiotics (ISAPP) consensus statement on the definition and scope of postbiotics. Nat Rev Gastroenterol Hepatol. 2021;18:649-67.
8. Vinderola G, Sanders ME, Salminen S. The concept of postbiotics. Foods. 2022;11(8):1077.
9. Banerjee D, Jain T, Bose S, Bhosale V. Importance of probiotics in human health. In: Rani

V, Yadav UCS (Eds). Functional Food and Human Health. Singapore: Springer; 2018. pp. 539-54.
10. Tegegne BA, Kebede B. Probiotics, their prophylactic and therapeutic applications in human health development: A review of the literature. Heliyon. 2022;8:e09725.
11. Guarino MPL, Altomarc A, Barera S, Locato V, Cocca S, Franchin C, et al. Effects of inulin on proteome changes induced by pathogenic lipopolysaccharide in human colon. PLoS One. 2017;12:e169481.
12. Miene C, Weise A, Glei M. Impact of polyphenol metabolites produced by colonic microbiota on expression of COX-2 and GSTT2 in human colon cells (LT97). Nutr Cancer. 2011:63:653-62.
13. Ruszkowsi J, Witkowsi JM. Lactulose: Patient- and dose-dependent prebiotic properties in humans. Anaerobe. 2019;59:100-6.
14. Masrtinez I, Kim J, Duffy PR, Schlegel VL, Walter J. Resistant starches types 2 and 4 have differential effects on the composition of the fecal microbiota in human subjects. PLoS One. 2010;5(11):e15046.
15. Panigrahi P, Parida S, Nanda NC, Satpathy R, Pradhan L, Chandel DS, et al. A randomized synbiotic trial to prevent sepsis among infants in rural India. Nature. 2017;548(7668):407-12.
16. Pandey KR, Naik SR, Vakil BV. Probiotics, prebiotics, and synbiotics—a review. J Food Sci Technol. 2015;52(12):7577-87.
17. Li HY, Zhou DD, Gan RY, Huang SY, Zhao CN, Shang A, et al. Effects and mechanisms of probiotics, prebiotics, synbiotics, and postbiotics on metabolic diseases targeting gut microbiota: A narrative review. Nutrients. 2021;13:3211.
18. Wastyk HC, Fragiadakis GK, Perelman D, Dahan D, Merrill BD, Yu FB, et al. Gut microbiota-targeted diets modulate human immune status. Cell. 2021;184:4137-53.
19. Sen M. Role of probiotics in health and disease—a review. Int J Adv Life Sci Res. 2019;2(2):1-11.
20. Ghasemian A, Eslami M, Shafiei M, Najafipour S, Rajabi A. Probiotics and their increasing importance in human health and infection control. Rev Res Med Microbiol. 2018;29(4):153-8.
21. Souza M, Barbalho SM, de Alvares Goulart R, de Cássio Alves de Carvalho A. The current and future role of drugs and probiotics in the management of inflammatory bowel disease. J Biosci Med. 2015;3:76-85.
22. Harper A, Naghibi MM, Garcha D. The role of bacteria, prebiotics, and diet in irritable bowel syndrome. Foods. 2018;7(2):13.
23. Alsuwaylihi AS, McCullough F. The safety and efficacy of probiotic supplementation for critically ill adult patients: A systemic review and meta-analysis. Nutr Rev. 2023;81(3): 322-32.
24. Sharif S, Greer A, Skorupski C, Hao Q, Johnstone J, Dionne JC, et al. Probiotics in critical illness: A systemic review and meta-analysis of randomised controlled trials. Crit Care Med. 2022;50(8):1175-86.
25. Naseri A, Seyedi-Sahebari S, Mahmoodpoor A, Sanaie S. Probiotics in critically ill patients: An umbrella review. Indian J Crit Care Med. 2022;26(3):339-60.
26. van den Berg FF, Marja A. Update on the management of acute pancreatitis. Curr Opin Crit Care. 2023;29(2):145-51.
27. Skonieczna-Zydecka K, Kaczmarczyk M, Łoniewski I, Lara LF, Koulaouzidis A, Misera A, et al. A systemic review, meta-regression evaluating the efficacy and mechanisms of probiotics and synbiotics in the prevention of surgical site infections and surgery-related complications. J Clin Med. 2018;7(12):556.
28. Chowdhury AH, Adiamah A, Kushairi A, Varadhan KK, Krznaric Z, Kulkarni AD, et al. Perioperative probiotics or synbiotics in adults undergoing elective abdominal surgery: A systemic review and meta-analysis of randomised controlled trials. Ann Surg. 2022;271(6):1036-47.
29. Amitay EL, Carr PR, Gies A, Laetsch DC, Brenner H. Probiotic/synbiotic treatment and postoperative complications in colorectal cancer patients: Systematic review and meta-analysis of randomised clinical trials. Clin Transl Gastroenterol. 2020;11(12):e00268.

CHAPTER 11

Mechanical and Metabolic Complications of Parenteral Nutrition

Subhankar Paul, Rajesh Pande

INTRODUCTION

Parenteral nutrition (PN) is a form of nutritional support delivered via intravenous (IV) route directly into the bloodstream, bypassing the gastrointestinal (GI) tract. It administers proteins, carbohydrates, fats, vitamins, and minerals in various proportions. Depending upon the constituents it may be total parenteral nutrition (TPN) or partial parenteral nutrition (PPN).[1] Aims of TPN are to prevent and restore nutritional deficits by supplying adequate calories and essential nutrients, allow bowel rest and remove antigenic mucosal stimuli. TPN is used when enteral feeding is either not indicated or tolerated.[2] TPN may be administered via central or peripheral venous access depending on the composition and osmolarity of the solution. Central venous access is commonly preferred over peripheral due to less risk of thrombophlebitis and vascular damage.[3]

As per the European Society for Clinical Nutrition and Metabolism (ESPEN) 2019 guidelines, oral diet is always preferred over enteral nutrition (EN) or PN in critically ill patients who are able to eat. However, if oral intake is not possible, early EN (within 48 hours) should be initiated rather than early PN or delayed EN among critically ill adults. In case of contraindications to oral and EN, PN should be implemented within 3–7 days. Early and progressive PN is recommended over no nutritional therapy in case of contraindications for EN in severely malnourished patients. General contraindications of EN in critically ill patients are uncontrolled shock, uncontrolled hypoxemia, and acidosis, uncontrolled upper GI bleed, gastric aspirate >500 mL/6 h, bowel obstruction, bowel ischemia, abdominal compartment syndrome, and high-output fistula without distal feeding access.[4] American Society for Parenteral and Enteral Nutrition (ASPEN) 2016 guidelines recommend to start hypocaloric PN with adequate protein in high risk, severely malnourished critically ill patients over the first week of intensive care unit (ICU) stay.[5]

Parenteral nutrition is an important therapeutic intervention that can be used in adults, children, and infants in different medical or surgical scenarios. While PN can provide essential nutrients to critically ill patients, it is associated with many risks. Complications of PN can be classified into mechanical, infectious, metabolic, and nutritional. However, recently published CALORIES and NUTRIREA-2 studies have dismissed many myths regarding PN-related complications. These studies demonstrated that by using appropriate preventive measures and monitoring a marked reduction in PN related complications could be achieved.[6,7]

Complications of PN include:
- Vascular access device (VAD)-related complications
- Infectious complications
- Metabolic complications.

VASCULAR ACCESS DEVICE-RELATED COMPLICATIONS

The mechanical complications related to vascular access for TPN are catheter migration, arrhythmia, lumen occlusion, catheter dislocation, rupture of external tract, and venous thrombosis.[8] Site of insertion may determine thrombosis. Among central venous access, subclavian and femoral vein have the lowest and highest risks of symptomatic thrombosis, respectively. However, there has been a higher incidence of pneumothorax with subclavian than jugular-vein or femoral-vein catheterization. Using USG placement for central venous catheter (CVC) and ensuring that the tip is placed at the cavoatrial junction reduces the incidence of thromboembolic complications.[9]

Peripheral PN is associated with a higher incidence of thrombophlebitis which depends upon the composition of the PN solution as well as the mechano-physical properties of the access catheter. The risk exponentially increases when the osmolality of the PN solution is >900 mOsmol/L.[10,11] Cyclical feeding over continuous infusion, elective cannula changes, use of stronger polyurethane catheters with larger internal diameter over fine-bore, 15-cm silicone catheters are some of the suggested measures for decreasing rate of phlebitis. Pharmacological preventive measures such as synergistic use of heparin and hydrocortisone, topical glyceryl trinitrate patches and gels with nonsteroidal anti-inflammatory drugs (NSAIDs) over the cannula insertion site have been suggested for reducing thrombophlebitis events.[12-15]

Peripherally inserted central catheters (PICC) lines were reported to have higher rates (up to 5%) of thromboembolic events among hospitalized patients. In a multicentric study over 50,000 patients on home PN, thrombosis rate of 0.23 per 1,000 catheter days was reported. Tunneled catheters, e.g., Hickman's or port-a-cath are recommended for home PN delivery who require this for 3 months or more. With appropriate care, these lines can even be maintained for years.[16,17]

For CVC-related thrombosis, ESPEN guidelines recommend:
- Ultrasound-guided insertion
- Use of a VAD with the smallest caliber needed for the patient
- Positioning the tip of the central VAD in the junction of superior vena cava and the right atrium.[18]

However, after the Pronovost study, widespread implementation of guidelines on care, diagnosis, and therapy of complications of CVCs access in PN patients, and the introduction of nutrition support teams, the incidence of PN-related complications has markedly reduced.[19]

Another crucial safety issue related to PN delivery is Y-site compatibility of various IV drugs during PN therapy. Administering PN and medications at the Y-site is not recommended, but may be unavoidable in ICU setting when many IV drugs and fluids are to be infused simultaneously in critically ill patients. In a study of in vitro physicochemical compatibility of 1:1 contact between PN and medications, incompatibility was reported with following medications at tested concentrations—after 1 hour: pantoprazole (0.8 mg/mL), esomeprazole (0.8 mg/mL), albumin (200 mg/mL) and after 4 hours: amoxicillin (50 mg/mL) plus clavulanic acid (10 mg/mL), cefepime (100 mg/mL). ASPEN recommends use of in-line filters for PN delivery to reduce potential harms due to particulates and microprecipitates, microorganisms and air emboli. In-line filters are recommended for high-risk critically ill patients (immune-suppressed or neonates, infants, and children).[1,3]

INFECTIOUS COMPLICATIONS[18-22]

Infections related to CVC and PN solution can present with serious intravascular catheter-related infections. Published literature on this subject has used the terms central line-associated bloodstream infection (CLABSI) and catheter-related bloodstream infection (CRBSI) interchangeably. CLABSI is a surveillance definition from the Centers for Disease Control and Prevention (CDC) and is defined by a laboratory-confirmed bloodstream infection (BSI) in a patient with a central line >48 hours from symptom onset and unrelated to an infection from another site. However, CRBSI is a clinical definition which requires specific laboratory testing criteria that more thoroughly identifies the catheter as the primary source of the BSI.

A recent systematic review has demonstrated that PN gives rise to BSI of 0.38–4.58 episodes per 1,000 catheter days. Another study reported PN to be an independent risk factor for developing CLABSI (95% CI: 2.20–3.19, odds ratio: 2.65). Subclavian-vein catheterization is associated with a lower risk of BSI than jugular or femoral venous catheterization. Tunneled catheters and implanted venous access devices are associated with lower incidence of CLABSI. The most common organisms identified for CRBSI include coagulase-negative *Staphylococci*, *Staphylococcus aureus*, *Klebsiella pneumoniae*, and *Candida*. Subcutaneous tract and exit site infections of PICC, pocket infections of implanted ports, and fungal CRBSI must be managed with central line removal along with appropriate antimicrobial therapy.

Investigators have demonstrated that it is possible to decrease CRBSI in ICU to "near zero" infection rate by introducing a checklist approach in managing CVC lines. Various international guidelines recommend Bundled approaches for CVC insertion and maintenance for preventing CRBSIs like **(Table 1)**, staff education,

TABLE 1: Bundled approach for preventing CRBSI.

Insertion bundle for CVC	*Maintenance bundle for CVC*
• WHO recommended hand hygiene before insertion • Maximal sterile barrier precautions • Strict aseptic technique • Best insertion site according to individual patient characteristics—avoid femoral site in obese adults • Skin preparation with >0.5% chlorhexidine with 70% alcohol • Place a sterile, transparent, semipermeable dressing over the insertion site • For patients ≥18 years, chlorhexidine impregnated dressing for short-term nontunneled catheters	• Strict adherence to hand hygiene • Scrub the access port or hub with friction immediately prior to each use with an appropriate antiseptic (chlorhexidine, povidone iodine, an iodophor, or 70% alcohol) • Use of only sterile devices to access CVCs • Immediately replacement of wet, soiled, or dislodged dressings • Routine dressing changes using aseptic technique donning sterile gloves—gauze dressings at least every 2 days and semipermeable dressings at least every 7 days • Chlorhexidine bath for ICU patients over 2 months of age • For patients ≥18 years, chlorhexidine impregnated dressing for short-term nontunneled catheters • Change administration sets for continuous infusions not more frequently than every 4 days, but at least every 7 days; for blood products or fat emulsions change tubing every 24 hourly, for propofol infusion change tubing every 6–12 hourly or when the vial is changed

(CRBSI: catheter-related bloodstream infection; CVC: central venous catheter; ICU: intensive care unit; WHO: World Health Organization)

training, and quality improvement projects, prompt removal of unnecessary CVCs, various supplemental strategies, e.g., use of antimicrobial impregnated catheters, and antiseptic impregnated caps for access ports.

METABOLIC COMPLICATIONS OF PARENTERAL NUTRITION

Metabolic complications of PN can be classified into acute (due to nutritional deficiency states, or nutrition excess) and chronic (long-term) metabolic complications.[23] Incidence of metabolic complications is much more in patients who are severely malnourished, have organ dysfunction, no supervision by a nutrition support team, or when physicians do not perceive PN as a powerful adjunct therapy and instead use it as urgent and "life-saving".[3,23]

- *Clinically relevant acute metabolic complications:* These are life-threatening functional disturbances either due to nutrient deficiencies or excess.
- *Complications due to nutrient deficiencies:* Failure to administer a balanced and adequate amount of macro- and micronutrients may lead to short- or long-term nutrient deficiencies. Nutrient requirements of critically ill patients are often difficult to estimate precisely in presence of multiple risk factors such as extremes of age (infants, children, and elderly), poor nutritional status, disease severity, etc. Among the acute deficiencies, there are two deserve special emphasis:
  1. *Hypoglycemia* due to changes in secretion, sensitivity, or administration of insulin, sudden discontinuation of high-glucose infusion rate, etc.)
  2. *Hypophosphatemia [as in refeeding syndrome (RFS) and may be lethal]:* Phosphate has many important metabolic roles in our body such as formation of DNA/RNA, adenosine triphosphate, 2,3-DPG, and plays an important role in phagocytosis, chemotaxis, platelet aggregation, and nervous system conduction pathway. Hypophosphatemia manifests as arrhythmias, constipation, paresthesia, muscular weakness, hypotonia, confusion, convulsions, or coma. Hence, serum phosphate concentrations must be corrected prior to initiating TPN and monitored throughout this therapy.[24]

- *Metabolic complications from overfeeding:* Overfeeding represents a metabolic burden where continued overloading leads to organ dysfunction. Major examples are: Hyperglycemia, azotemia (protein/amino-acid overload), hypercalcemia, and hypertriglyceridemia.

   Hyperglycemia is the most common complication (up to 50% incidence rate) after initiating TPN. Oxidation rate of dextrose is reduced in the elderly, metabolically stressed patients (e.g., critically ill patients with sepsis or organ failure), patients with diseases that alter insulin's effects (e.g., diabetes and acute pancreatitis), reduced central and peripheral sensitivity to insulin, and in patients receiving medications that alter glucose metabolism (e.g., corticosteroids, catecholamine vasopressors, tacrolimus, etc.). Uncontrolled hyperglycemia can cause fluid and electrolyte disturbances, or hyperglycemic hyperosmolar syndrome, and increased susceptibility to infection. Hyperglycemia encountered during TPN is independently linked with higher mortality rates, infection, organ dysfunction, and increased length of hospital stay. ASPEN guidelines suggest to maintain blood glucose levels between

140 and 180 mg/dL. Hyperglycemia must be treated appropriately with planned intermittent insulin doses or a continuous inulin infusion, especially in critically ill patients.[4,23]

Hypertriglyceridemia is another common complication of TPN, particularly in patients receiving lipid emulsions. High levels of triglycerides may result in pancreatitis, coagulopathy, and other complications. The use of lipid emulsions containing a lower concentration of soybean oil and a higher concentration of medium-chain triglycerides (MCTs), olive oil, and fish oil have been shown to reduce the incidence of hypertriglyceridemia, length of ICU stay, duration of mechanical ventilation, and mortality in critically ill patients in some studies with low statistical precision.[3,25]

High doses of protein intake exceeding patient's requirements may lead to high levels of nitrogen-waste such as urea and creatinine, hypertonic dehydration, and metabolic acidosis.[3]

Careful patient evaluation and planning a stepwise increment of nutrient amounts along with frequent monitoring of biochemical parameters are the only effective way of prevention of overfeeding.

- *Refeeding syndrome:*[26,27] RFS is a potentially life-threatening acute metabolic complication that may occur when a prolonged malnourished patient is started on PN or EN. It is characterized by a rapid transcellular shift of fluid and electrolytes that can lead to low serum concentrations of predominately intracellular ions, e.g., phosphate, potassium, magnesium, and abnormalities in glucose metabolism leading to thiamine deficiency, dysnatremia, and water imbalance.

In critically ill patients, RFS can have serious consequences, involving cardiorespiratory, endocrinal, and neurological complications. Key pathophysiology is depicted in **Flowchart 1**. Refeeding hypophosphatemia is one of the key mechanisms resulting in cardiac dysfunction, respiratory failure, hematologic, endocrine, and neuromuscular dysfunction, and thus can be potentially fatal. Other electrolyte abnormalities such as hypokalemia, hypomagnesemia, and hypocalcemia are also common and have disastrous consequences.

Critically ill patients who are chronic alcoholics, have a low body mass index (BMI), anorexia nervosa, or anorexia bulimia, on high-dose corticosteroids, severe burns, sepsis, or trauma or have been malnourished for a prolonged period with little or no oral intake for several days are usually at a higher risk of developing RFS.

For preventing RFS, intensivists first need to identify the high-risk category patients. All patients should have a complete blood and urinary laboratory evaluation before initiation of TPN to obtain baseline data, organ dysfunction, and to identify and correct preexisting electrolyte abnormalities. Initiation of PN should be done gradually with close monitoring of clinical conditions and serum electrolytes. During the early phase (initial 3–5 days) of PN, stepwise increments in macronutrients are delivered until estimated nutrient requirements are met. Adequate protein and calories are to be provided as per patient's metabolic needs, without exceeding them. The frequency of biochemical monitoring depends upon

CHAPTER 11 | Mechanical and Metabolic Complications of Parenteral Nutrition

Flowchart 1: Schematic diagram showing pathophysiology of refeeding syndrome.

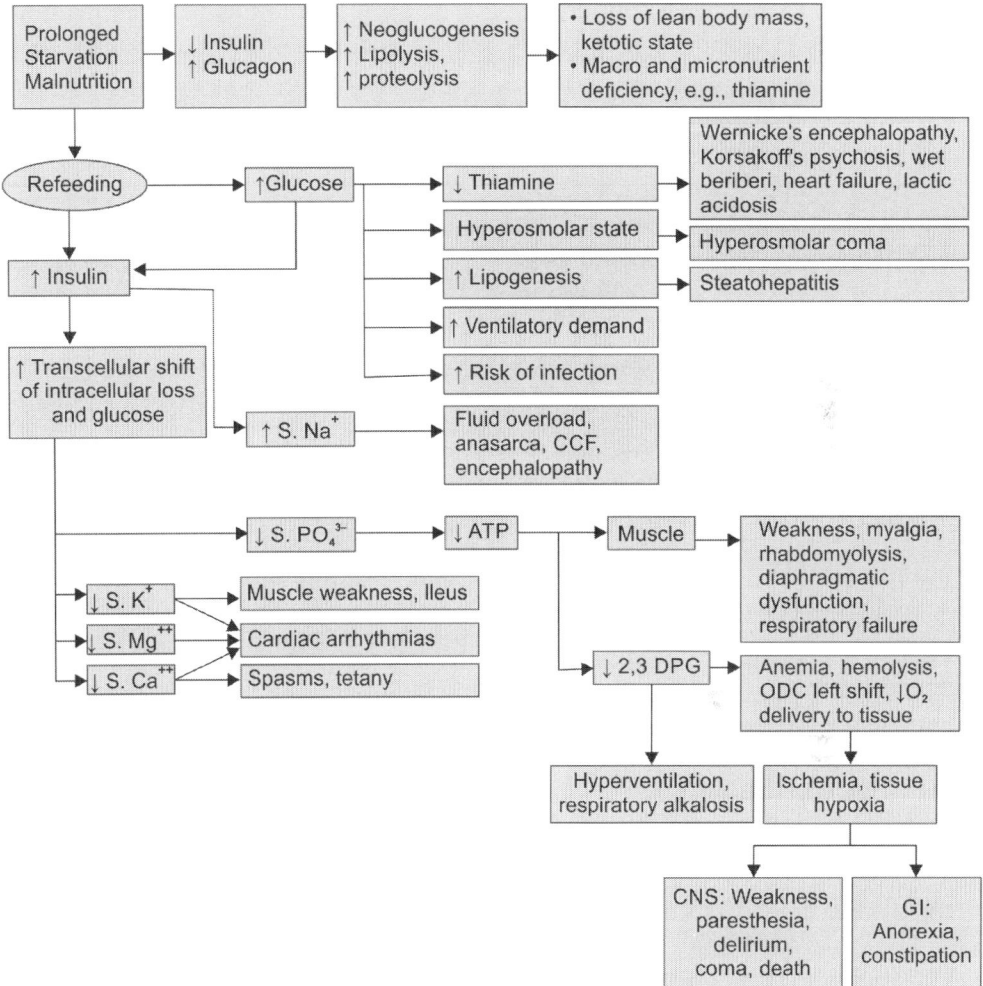

(ATP: adenosine triphosphate; CCF: congestive cardiac failure; CNS: central nervous system; DPG: diphosphoglycerate; GI: gastrointestinal; ODC: oxygen dissociation curve; S.: serum)

the patient's clinical or nutritional status and the stage of PN.

If RFS is suspected or diagnosed, prompt intervention is necessary. Management strategies include serial monitoring of serum electrolyte levels, and early aggressive corrective measures as needed, and reducing or temporarily stopping nutrition support until severe electrolyte imbalances are corrected.

- *Long-term metabolic complications*: Metabolic complications due to long-term use of TPN are mainly hepatobiliary complications and bone disease as discussed next.

HEPATOBILIARY COMPLICATIONS[28,29]

Factors responsible for excessive PN-related liver injury are high levels of glucose and phytosterols (in plant-based lipid emulsions), deficiency of essential fatty acids, taurine, and hypermagnesemia. PN-related hepatotoxicity is mainly seen with long-term use and may be due to either steatosis or cholestasis. Long-term PN may lead to biliary complications such as biliary sludge, cholelithiasis, and acalculous cholecystitis. About 15–30% adults on long-term PN develop end-stage liver disease (ESLD) which is more likely due to cholestasis.

- *Hepatic steatosis:* Hepatic steatosis is a frequent complication of long-term use of TPN manifested as elevation of plasma aminotransferases, hepatic enlargement, and altered echotexture of liver parenchyma on ultrasonography. It is mainly caused by overfeeding, especially with glucose. The measures to limit hepatic steatosis include limiting the calory delivery as per the requirement of the patient, lowering the carbohydrate load and cyclic PN (TPN period followed by no IV feeding for 6–8 hours).
- *Cholestatic liver disease:* Cholestatic liver disease is a serious complication of TPN, which may progress to cirrhosis and even liver failure. It is more frequently observed among children and neonates treated with TPN. Exact etiology is unknown, but main contributing factors are:
  - Decrease in enterohepatic cycle of bile acids (short bowel syndrome and fistulas) leading to depletion of bile acids and increase in lithogenicity of bile.
  - Bacterial overgrowth with portal endotoxemia (e.g., in blind loop) leading to production of hepatotoxic secondary bile acids in small bowel (especially lithocholic acid) and directly increases intrahepatic cholestasis.
  - *Glucose overfeeding:* Decreases fatty acid oxidation in liver leading to accumulation of re-esterified fatty acids in hepatocytes (liver steatosis). De novo synthesis of fatty acids from exogenous glucose may also play a role.
  - Products of lipid peroxidation
  - *Phospholipid part of lipid emulsion:* Content and composition of phospholipids can be responsible for liver injury connected with PN.
  - Decreased motility of gallbladder (GB)
  - Lack of vitamin E

  Clinical jaundice, hyperbilirubinemia, and increases in γ-glutamyl transferase and alkaline phosphatase are apparent in serum. On histopathology, cholestasis associated with periportal and portal infiltration, extensive fibrosis, and finally cirrhosis can be seen.

  Preventive strategies for cholestatic hepatic dysfunction include—decreasing the amount of macronutrients especially glucose, providing cyclic PN, promoting some oral/EN, type of amino acids provided, e.g., taurine, changing lipid composition, etc. may prove beneficial. Progression to ESLD due to TPN in short bowel syndrome may be an indication for both liver and intestinal transplantations.
- *Cholelithiasis and acalculous cholecystitis:* GB stasis during TPN and increased lithogenicity of bile are important factors for developing gallstones or GB sludge with subsequent cholecystitis. Providing small amounts of oral or EN and administration of cholecystokinin to stimulate GB contraction have been proposed as prevent measures.

METABOLIC BONE DISEASE[30]

Patients on long-term home PN have reported both osteoporosis and osteomalacia. Bone diseases related to PN are associated with reduction of bony calcium (also apparent in bone histopathology) and increased urinary calcium excretion, increased serum alkaline phosphatase, bony pain, and fractures. Proposed etiological factors are:
- Low intake of calcium, vitamin D, and phosphate
- Lack of magnesium in TPN
- Prolonged immobilization with demineralization of bones
- Excessive amino acids (especially sulfur containing) in TPN
- Aluminum contamination
- Vitamin D toxicity
- Use of heparin or corticosteroids in some patients

There are no proven preventive strategies for this complication. However, adequate intake of calcium, magnesium phosphate, and vitamin D intake in proper dosage along with active and passive physiotherapy seem to be useful.

CONCLUSION

Total parenteral nutrition is a complex therapy with many mechanical and metabolic risks associated with vascular access, improper nutritional composition, and lack of monitoring and supervision. Optimizing the management of PN is essential to prevent complications and improve patient outcomes. Appropriate initiation and monitoring of PN, appropriate catheter selection and care, use of lipid emulsions containing a lower concentration of soybean oil and a higher concentration of MCTs, glycemic control, and other evidence-based strategies can help to prevent complications of PN in critically ill patients. Individualizing nutritional assessment and delivery with close collaboration between ICU physicians, pharmacists, and nutritionists can optimize PN management, reduce complications, and improve patient outcomes.

REFERENCES

1. Berger MM, Pichard C. Development and current use of parenteral nutrition in critical care—an opinion paper. Crit Care. 2014;18:478.
2. Preiser JC, van Zanten AR, Berger MM, Biolo G, Casaer MP, Doig GS, et al. Metabolic and nutritional support of critically ill patients: consensus and controversies. Crit Care. 2015;19:35.
3. Cotogni P. Management of parenteral nutrition in critically ill patients. World J Crit Care Med. 2017;6(1):13-20.
4. Singer P, Blaser AR, Berger MM, Alhazzani W, Calder PC, Casaer MP, et al. ESPEN guideline on clinical nutrition in the intensive care unit. Clin Nutr. 2019;38(1):48-79.
5. McClave SA, Taylor BE, Martindale RG, Warren MM, Johnson DR, Braunschweig C, et al. Society of Critical Care Medicine; American Society for Parenteral and Enteral Nutrition. Guidelines for the Provision and Assessment of Nutrition Support Therapy in the Adult Critically Ill Patient: society of Critical Care Medicine (SCCM) and American Society for Parenteral and Enteral Nutrition (ASPEN). JPEN J Parenter Enteral Nutr. 2016;40(2):159-211.
6. Harvey SE, Parrott F, Harrison DA, Bear DE, Segaran E, Beale R, et al. Trial of the route of early nutritional support in critically ill adults. N Engl J Med. 2014;371(18): 1673-84.
7. Reignier J, Boisramé-Helms J, Brisard L, Lascarrou JB, Ait Hssain A, Anguel N, et al. Enteral versus parenteral early nutrition in ventilated adults with shock: a randomised, controlled, multicentre, open-label,

parallel-group study (NUTRIREA-2). Lancet. 2018;391(10116):133-43.
8. Hartl WH, Jauch KW, Parhofer K, Rittler P; Working group for developing the guidelines for parenteral nutrition of The German Association for Nutritional Medicine. Complications and monitoring—Guidelines on Parenteral Nutrition, Chapter 11. Ger Med Sci. 2009;7:Doc17.
9. Parienti JJ, Mongardon N, Mégarbane B, Mira JP, Kalfon P, Gros A, et al. Intravascular Complications of Central Venous Catheterization by Insertion Site. N Engl J Med. 2015;373(13):1220-9.
10. Bayer-Berger M, Chiolero R, Freeman J, Hirschi B. Incidence of phlebitis in peripheral parenteral nutrition: effect of the different nutrient solutions. Clin Nutr. 1989;8(4):181-6.
11. Messing B, Leverve X, Rigaud D, Krummel Y, Botta D, Latarget J, et al. Peripheral venous complications of a hyperosmolar (960 mOsm) nutritive mixture: The effect of heparin and hydrocortisone. A multicenter double-blinded random study in 98 patients. Clin Nutr. 1986;5(1):57-61.
12. Madan M, Alexander DJ, Mellor E, Cooke J, McMahon MJ. A randomised study of the effects of osmolality and heparin with hydrocortisone on thrombophlebitis in peripheral intravenous nutrition. Clin Nutr. 1991;10(6):309-14.
13. Wright A, Hecker JF, Lewis GB. Use of transdermal glyceryl trinitrate to reduce failure of intravenous infusion due to phlebitis and extravasation. Lancet. 1985;2(8465):1148-50.
14. Payne-James JJ, Bray MJ, Kapadia S, Rana SK, McSwiggan D, Silk DB. Topical nonsteroidal anti-inflammatory gel for the prevention of peripheral vein thrombophlebitis. A double-blind, randomised, placebo-controlled trial in normal subjects. Anaesthesia. 1992;47(4):324-6.
15. Cowl CT, Weinstock JV, Al-Jurf A, Ephgrave K, Murray JA, Dillon K. Complications and cost associated with parenteral nutrition delivered to hospitalized patients through either subclavian or peripherally-inserted central catheters. Clin Nutr. 2000;19(4):237-43.
16. Moureau N, Poole S, Murdock MA, Gray SM, Semba CP. Central venous catheters in home infusion care: outcomes analysis in 50,470 patients. J Vasc Interv Radiol. 2002;13(10):1009-16.
17. Pronovost P, Needham D, Berenholtz S, Sinopoli D, Chu H, Cosgrove S, et al. An intervention to decrease catheter-related bloodstream infections in the ICU. N Engl J Med. 2006;355:2725-32.
18. Pittiruti M, Hamilton H, Biffi R, MacFie J, Pertkiewicz M. ESPEN Guidelines on Parenteral Nutrition: central venous catheters (access, care, diagnosis and therapy of complications). Clin Nutr. 2009;28:365-77.
19. Loveday HP, Wilson JA, Pratt RJ, Golsorkhi M, Tingle A, Bak A, et al. Epic 3: National evidence-based guidelines for preventing healthcare-associated infections in NHS hospitals in England. J Hosp Infect. 2014; 86(Suppl 1):S1-S70.
20. Lorente L, Villegas J, Martín MM, Jiménez A, Mora ML. Catheter-related infection in critically ill patients. Intensive Care Med. 2004;30:1681-4.
21. Ruiz-Santana S, Saavedra P, León C. "Near zero" catheter-related bloodstream infections: turning dreams into reality. Crit Care Med. 2012;40:3083-4.
22. Peredo R, Sabatier C, Villagrá A, González J, Hernández C, Pérez F, et al. Reduction in catheter-related bloodstream infections in critically ill patients through a multiple system intervention. Eur J Clin Microbiol Infect Dis. 2010;29:1173-7.
23. Sobotka L, Camilo ME. Basics in clinical nutrition: Metabolic complications of parenteral nutrition. e-SPEN, the Eur e-J Clin Nutr Metabol. 2009;3(4):e120-2.
24. Wong GJY, Pang JGT, Li YY, Lew CCH. Refeeding Hypophosphatemia in Patients Receiving Parenteral Nutrition: Prevalence, Risk Factors, and Predicting Its Occurrence. Nutr Clin Pract. 2021;36(3):679-88.

25. Edmunds CE, Brody RA, Parrott JS, Stankorb SM, Heyland DK. The effects of different IV fat emulsions on clinical outcomes in critically ill patients. Crit Care Med. 2014;42:1168-77.
26. Khan LU, Ahmed J, Khan S, Macfie J. Refeeding syndrome: a literature review. Gastroenterol Res Pract. 2011;2011:pii: 410971.
27. van Zanten AR. Nutritional support and refeeding syndrome in critical illness. Lancet Respir Med. 2015;3(12):904-5.
28. Angelico M, Della Guardia P. Hepatobiliary complications associated with total parenteral nutrition. Aliment Pharmacol Ther. 2000;14(Suppl 2):54.
29. Guglielmi FW, Boggio-Bertinet D, Federico A, Forte GB, Guglielmi A, Loguercio C, et al. Total parenteral nutrition-related gastroenterological complications. Digest Liver Dis. 2006;38(9):623-42.
30. Buchman AL, Moukarzel A. Metabolic bone disease associated with total parenteral nutrition. Clin Nutr. 2000;19(4):217-31.

SECTION 3

Enteral Nutrition in Critical Illness

12. **Enteral Nutrition in Critical Illness: Physiological Benefits and Beyond**
    Krishnan Sriram, Chitra Mahesh

13. **Gastrointestinal Disturbances in Critically Ill Patients**
    Ganshyam Jagathkar, Radha Reddy Chada

14. **Enteral Access: Device and Selection**
    Srinivas Samavedam, Arun Kumar

15. **Initiation, Maintenance, and Progression of Enteral Feeds**
    Urvi Shukla, Arti Bhalerao, Anuja Phalle

16. **Monitoring and Management of Complications of Enteral Nutrition**
    Deven Juneja, Anjali Mishra

Enteral Nutrition in Critical Illness: Physiological Benefits and Beyond

Krishnan Sriram, Chitra Mahesh

INTRODUCTION

Nutrition therapy has been declared as a basic global human right.[1] Not every clinical situation in critical care requires parenteral nutrition (PN). There is a need to encourage clinicians to follow an aggressive approach to enteral or oral nutrition. This is possible with the availability of access devices and easy-to-use protocols. This chapter will explain the physiological and other benefits associated with enteral nutrition (EN), emphasizing real world pragmatic approach. The term "enteral nutrition" will be used with the understanding that the oral route will be used wherever possible. The opinions expressed are supported by evidence-based recommendations of major societies, which can be sourced for detailed references.

GENERAL PHYSIOLOGICAL BENEFITS OF ENTERAL NUTRITION

The benefits of EN in critical illness have been recognized for decades and supported by prospective randomized trials,[2,3] especially attenuation of the stress response, metabolic rate, and decreased secretion of counter-regulatory hormones including cortisol and catecholamines. EN is the only known modality known to have this beneficial effect; no pharmacological intervention has ever shown any significant and sustained clinical benefit. Better glycemic control with well-accepted benefits is also understandable.[4] Polymeric enteral formulas are designed to contain carbohydrates and proteins that assure that digested end products are formed at variable intervals, thus avoiding surges. This contrasts with PN where glucose and amino acids are infused continuously. The nutrients delivered into the gut have the benefit of first passing through the portal system into the liver for optimal metabolism. Enhanced visceral blood flow due to EN[5] facilitates absorption of nutrients aided by the direct effects of EN on normalization of the endocrine, paracrine, and neurocrine functions of gastrointestinal (GI) peptides. These effects are—EN helps to maintain anti-inflammatory vagal tone.[6] EN decreases gastric stress ulceration. EN increases intestinal contractility, which, in turn, facilitates aboral transmission of bacteria. EN releases trophic hormones, such as gastrin, bombesin, and motilin, and increase in release of secretory immunoglobulin A (IgA).[7] The positive effects and benefits of EN on gut mucosa, lymphoid tissue, intestinal microbiota, and GI function in general will be discussed further, all resulting in a decrease of morbidity and costs in critically ill patients.

Gut Mucosa and Lymphoid Tissue

Avoidance of enteral feeding and dependence on PN adversely affect the gut mucosal barrier and gut-associated lymphoid tissue (GALT).[8] Animal studies from decades ago have convincingly shown loss of intestinal mucosa when EN was withheld, resulting in increased permeability. Increased permeability was confirmed by bacterial translocation to mesenteric lymph nodes. Human studies have subsequently confirmed that when EN is not administered, small intestinal mucosal thickness, villous height, and crypt depth decrease, with an increase in intestinal permeability.[9] Translocation involves not only bacteria, but also viruses, fungi, and toxins. Translocation is at least partly responsible for the systemic inflammatory responses. EN exerts anti-inflammatory effects through bile acid metabolism and microbiota. EN suppresses tumor necrosis factor alpha (TNF-α) production by CD4+ T cells in addition to improving the dysregulation of T-helper cells.[10]

Gut-associated lymphoid tissue is the largest lymphoid organ in the body. Over two-thirds of immune cells reside in the GI tract. GALT is responsible for both local and systemic immunity, a decline of which occurs rapidly within 5 days of disuse of the intestinal tract. The encouraging fact is that EN will attenuate mucosal atrophy and limit translocation. EN improves gut function and improves the immune responses in several clinical situations.

Healing of GI Anastomosis

Intensivists and clinical nutritionists are often faced with the hesitation of surgeons to initiate early enteral feeding in postoperative patients with GI and colonic anastomosis. This is an age-old practice that warrants change. There is now two decades of research to support the safety of early postoperative EN and avoidance of routine nasogastric decompression. A strongly worded title of a randomized multicenter trial concluded that allowing normal food at will after major GI surgery does not affect morbidity.[11]

Enteral nutrition increases GI anastomotic strength due to increased collagen synthesis and mucosal healing. Early enteral or oral feeding improves anastomotic strength, and thereby decreases procedure-related complications including anastomotic leaks.[12]

Enhanced recovery after surgery (ERAS) protocols encourage clinicians to abandon unproven practices regarding postoperative resumption of oral or enteral feeding,[13] further supported by current (2022) and previous (2016) versions of guidelines from the American Society for Parenteral and Enteral Nutrition (ASPEN) and Society for Critical Care Medicine.[14,15]

Gut Microbiota

Preservation of normal gut microbiota is an important benefit of EN. The term "microbiota" includes bacteria (aerobic, anaerobic, potentially pathogenic, and commensals), viruses, and phages. A normal gut microbiome helps to minimize gut dysmotility. Among various other benefits, gut flora also helps glucose homeostasis.[16] Gut bacteria are good sources of some vitamins, biotin, and vitamin K.[17]

The normal microbiome is altered by several factors, including critical illness itself with associated vasoactive medications, stress ulcer prophylaxis, and other interventions.[18] Antibiotics, low intestinal perfusion, lack of prebiotics, and other factors produce dysbiosis with detrimental sequelae. Maintaining a normal gut microbiome both in health and illness depends heavily on oral and EN.[19]

Fiber

Fiber, both soluble and insoluble, is an important component of diet. Whereas insoluble fibers (e.g., soy polysaccharide) add to the bulk of stools, soluble fibers (e.g., fructose oligosaccharides, methylcellulose, pectin, and guar) get fermented in the colon, thanks to inherent bacteria present in the colon, into short-chain fatty acids (SCFAs) (acetoacetic, butyric, and propionic acids). SCFAs stimulate colonocytes and aid in absorption of water and, especially sodium. Scientific enteral formulas available in India are formulated with a variety of mainly soluble fibers, such as inulin, fructose oligosaccharides, gum arabic, guar gum, and resistant maltodextrins. Although traditionally, dietary fiber is considered inert in terms of energy balance, fermentation of fiber does help in providing some calories, highly beneficial for patients with short gut syndrome.[20] Each gram of soluble fiber can be expected to provide 2 kcal, a significant source of additional energy intake in patients with short bowel and intact colon.

The routine addition of fiber to EN has been questioned and we are cautioned to not use fiber in critically ill patients, especially those with impaired motility and risk of bowel ischemia. For stable medical and surgical intensive care unit (ICU) patients, the ASPEN 2009 guidelines do recommend the use of soluble fiber but not with the intention of decreasing diarrhea.

Protein Accretion and Sarcopenia

Improved nitrogen balance with enteral feeding has been known for many years. PN, on the other hand, results in accumulation of mainly fat in the muscle.[21,22] Some amino acids are metabolized to a great extent in the splanchnic tissues, indicating that the requirement for these amino acids is greater when administered enterally rather than parenterally. It is relatively easy to provide more protein of different compositions via EN, fulfilling a requirement that an optimal combination of proteins is beneficial for clinical outcomes.[23]

Although visceral protein levels are no longer used to diagnose malnutrition, increasing levels by optimal EN is beneficial. Protein kinetics of peripheral muscles and utilization of nutrients are better with EN when compared to the parenteral route.[24]

Ambulating patients on EN for physiotherapy is easier than those on PN, as the devices used for access can be placed "on hold" with ease. Exercises including weight training are an important method of diminishing or even reversing sarcopenia in critical illness. Additional proteins can be administered enterally with the current recommendations of reaching higher targets of up to 2 g/kg/day. Reversal of sarcopenia is an important aim of nutritional therapy.

OTHER ORGAN SYSTEMS

Enteral nutrition increases renal blood flow and has been shown to decrease renal injury.[25] Fluid balance in renal failure is easier to control with EN than with intravenous fluids, as high concentration renal-specific enteral formulas can be used.

Enteral nutrition avoids the adverse effects of PN on the liver, such as steatosis, cholestasis, and cholelithiasis. EN minimizes liver injury and improves survival after hemorrhagic shock. Hepatic stress response is blunted with EN, resulting in higher serum levels of synthesized proteins, and a decrease of acute-phase proteins. EN is preferentially indicated in diverse conditions of hepatic failure including alcoholic hepatitis, cirrhosis, and transplantation. Oral supplements are strongly recommended and improve nutritional status and liver functions, decrease complications, and prolong survival.[26]

Access

Obtaining access for EN delivery is generally easy and can be performed by physicians, healthcare extenders such as physician assistants or advanced practice nurses, and dietitians.[27] Protocols for maintaining patent access are also easily practiced and enforced. Physicians are quite adept at obtaining advanced methods of access, such as gastrostomy or jejunostomy. These procedures can be done at the bedside, or in procedure suites, by surgeons, intensivists, gastroenterologists, and intervention radiologists. In comparison, PN requires expert skills in central venous access, strict maintenance of these lines, and frequent changes of peripheral venous access sites to avoid thrombophlebitis.

Fluid Balance

Maintenance of fluid balance is easier with EN. The free water content of commercially available enteral formulations will list the amount of free water in a specific volume, say in 100 mL of the formula. This may vary between 750 and 850 mL, depending on the concentration and caloric density. Additional free water can be administered via the feeding route to make up the water intake. When powdered formulations are used, the amount of added water is known in advance. Volume-based feeding (ordering volume per 24 hours rather than per hour) is therefore easier with its known advantages, including better delivery of planned requirements and glycemic control.[28]

CONTINUOUS VERSUS INTERMITTENT SCHEDULES

Nutrition therapy for critically ill patients, enteral or parenteral, is invariably on a continuous basis. This facilitates maintenance of fluid balance, hemodynamic stability, and glucose homeostasis. However, this does not fit into normal circadian rhythms. Continuous provision of nutrition may result in hepatic steatosis. To obviate this, the enteral feeding regimen can be adjusted to intermittent or cyclical. Other adjustments in medications, e.g., insulin dosing and timing, will also need to be modified. This facility of adjusting rates and timing is a unique and beneficial feature of EN. Improved muscle protein synthesis is an additional benefit of intermittent enteral feeding.

Disruptions in normal circadian patterns of feeding may also affect the gut microbiome, which in turn is influenced by nutrients presented to the intestinal lumen and mucosa.[29] Catabolic and anabolic metabolism of all macronutrients is affected by exposure to light or darkness. It is impossible to make these appropriate changes in delivery of PN.

Modular Adjustments and Additives

Scientific enteral formulas contain macronutrients in accepted proportions. However, certain conditions may require addition of a specific module. Addition of protein powder is often recommended if a high protein formula is not available. Fiber may be added to or given through feeding tubes. Chyle leaks form a unique set of problems where the fat content of enteral feeds needs to be modified. This might require minimizing long-chain fatty acids and substituting with medium-chain fatty acids, which are not absorbed through the lymphatic system, while carbohydrates and proteins can be liberally administered.[30] These variations in administration of modular components of macronutrients are possible only with EN. Carnitine and glutamine are examples of additives that can be added to EN formulas.

Electrolyte Corrections

Enteral feeding offers a unique and natural method of correcting electrolyte imbalances. Hyponatremia, if confirmed to be due to diminished intake, can be corrected by adding NaCl to the formula. (The Na content of scientific enteral formulations is noted in milligrams and generally not in mEq. 1 g or 1,000 mg of NaCl contains 17.5 mEq of elemental Na. 1 g or 1,000 mg of elemental Na is equivalent to 34.5 mEq of Na.) Hypernatremia can be corrected by simultaneous administration of free water at a rate not to exceed the enteral formula flow rate. Potassium, in elixir forms, can be used to correct hypokalemia. If parenteral forms of phosphate are not readily available, oral preparations of Na or K phosphate can be added to the enteral formula.

Micronutrients

Multiple trace element admixtures and multivitamin preparations specific for PN are not readily available in many Asian countries. Shortage of these even in more advanced countries occurs, often requiring efforts by clinicians to optimize delivery enterally. Micronutrients are an important component of nutrition therapy and an urgent need to sensitize clinicians regarding this matter has been publicized.[31] Micronutrients can be administered orally or via the intragastric route even if EN goals are not met, provided the duodenum and proximal jejunum are accessible and functional. With the understanding of the importance of thiamine in critical illness, the enteral route, along with EN, offers a unique opportunity for ease of cost-effective administration, especially if thiamine as a single pharmaceutical is not available for parenteral use. Toxicity is rare. There are innate systems by which trace elements are not even absorbed if the levels are adequate.[32]

■ INFECTIOUS COMPLICATIONS

Decreasing infections, with attendant cost benefits, is an important reason why EN is preferred. PN, on the other hand, is recognized as an etiologic factor in both bacterial and fungal infections, due to the vascular access devices as well as the infusate itself. The decrease of infectious complications with EN is especially remarkable in postsurgical patients.[33] Fungal infections may occur as a complication of PN, but not with EN.

Refeeding Syndrome

Refeeding syndrome (RFS) is increasingly recognized as a complication of both enteral and PN therapies, even in obese patients. The exact incidence has been reported to be as high as 48%, although one cannot be sure of this figure as criteria for making the diagnosis have varied. With increasing awareness of RFS and preemptive correction of electrolyte abnormalities, the incidence of RFS may decrease.

In addition to decrease in serum levels of potassium (K), magnesium (Mg), and phosphorous (P), signs and symptoms of thiamine deficiency are all recognized as components of RFS.[34]

The question is whether EN is less of a risk of RFS when compared to PN. Except for very high glucose levels after initiation of PN, the rate of infusion does not need urgent revisions. EN is initiated at low rates and advanced only when tolerance and other factors have been considered. This fits in with the measures recommended to prevent RFS, suggesting that one of the physiologic benefits of EN is a decreased incidence of RFS, although there are no publications to date to confirm this.

Dysglycemia

The maintenance of glucose levels within specified range (e.g., 110–140 mg/dL) and minimizing glycemic variability are standard approaches in critical illness. EN offers a unique opportunity for maintenance of glucose levels by various means available to the intensivist. Basal and supplemental insulin regimens can be altered, depending on the schedule of enteral feeding (continuous, intermittent, or cyclical). Unlike PN where dextrose is infused directly into the venous system, carbohydrates in EN are of various types with different glycemic indices. Some are more favorable in diabetic-specific and renal-specific enteral formulas and require digestion before absorption as simple sugars.[35] Oral antidiabetic medications are generally not administered to ICU patients, especially in patients on PN with hyperglycemia, but can be selectively used with EN, with a decreased risk of hypoglycemia when compared to insulin.

Hyperglycemia with PN requires the use of insulin, by means of a separate insulin drip, or long-acting subcutaneous insulin. Addition of insulin directly to the PN infusate should be done only by trained pharmacists under sterile conditions, following strict procedural protocols. This is not possible or safe in all hospitals.[36]

OTHER ENDOCRINE SYSTEMS

Early EN has been shown in small studies to benefit thyroid hormone levels in critically ill patients.[37] The mechanism is not clear, although one can surmise that the selenium content of enteral products may be responsible. Selenium has been closely involved with the production of active thyroid hormone. The same study also demonstrated that EN positively affects the levels of testosterone with its known anabolic effects.

DRUG-ENTERAL NUTRIENT INTERACTIONS

The enteral route used for EN offers a unique opportunity to administer medications. Several pharmacologic agents are available only for parenteral route. Intramuscular and subcutaneous injections are best avoided in critically ill patients. Bleeding into muscles and hematomas may occur in patients who have hypocoagulability either due to the disease process itself or intentionally as part of the treatment plan. In such cases, medications can be administered orally or enterally. In addition to cost savings, the time spent by nursing and pharmacy staff is also minimized. EN should be held for at least 30 minutes prior to and after administration of medications. Dosage adjustments may be needed due to crushing of tablets or adherence of the medication to tubing.

The list of potential drug-nutrient interactions and side effects is too long for this chapter. The examples include zinc loss with angiotensin-converting enzyme inhibitors and angiotensin II receptor antagonists, hypomagnesemia with proton pump inhibitors, and vitamin B_{12} deficiency with metformin, to name a few. Detailed information can be obtained from the package insert from the manufacturer or from internet sources and excellent reviews.[38]

PSYCHOLOGICAL BENEFITS

In addition to the benefits of EN in easily definable physiological parameters, satisfaction of patients and their caregivers should be considered. It has been well accepted for decades that oral or enteral feeding improves the psychosocial aspects of cancer patients. Although one may assume that is logical that quality of life improves with EN, reviews have suggested that this may not always be the case.[39]

COST-EFFECTIVENESS

Enteral nutrition is less expensive than PN, with the cost of access devices and products being a fraction of the cost of the latter. The maintenance of access routes involving nursing time is also to be considered. Budget-impact studies have clearly confirmed the economic benefits of EN.[40] Clinicians' responsibilities do not end with discharge from the ICU. Continuing optimal EN postdischarge results in reduced overall costs, emphasizing the importance of EN in the continuum of care.[41]

CONCLUSION

We have summarized the current information on the benefits of EN based on earlier research as well as more recent studies. Physiological benefits shown in earlier animal models have been confirmed in human clinical trials. The availability of various kinds of enteral access devices and availability of clinicians skilled in obtaining and maintaining access for optimal delivery of nutrients have all improved patient care and survival. This has been aided by our better understanding of metabolic requirements, fluid status, and acid–base and electrolyte abnormalities, many of which can be managed by the enteral route. Cost-effectiveness of EN is a major benefit in the management of critically ill patients.

REFERENCES

1. Cardenas D, Correia MITD, Ochoa JB, Hardy G, Rodriguez-Ventimilla D, Bermúdez CE, et al. Clinical nutrition and human rights: An international position paper. Nutr Clin Pract. 2022;37:534-44.
2. Moore FA, Moore EE, Jones TN, McCroskey BL, Peterson VM. TEN versus TPN following major abdominal trauma—reduced septic mortality. J Trauma. 1989;29:916-23.
3. Kudsk KA, Croce MA, Fabian TC, Minard G, Tolley EA, Poret HA, et al. Enteral versus parenteral feeding. Effects on septic morbidity after blunt and penetrating abdominal trauma. Ann Surg. 1992;215:503-13.
4. Magnusson J, Tranberg KG, Jeppson B, Lunderquist A. Enteral versus parenteral glucose as the sole nutritional support after colorectal resection: A prospective randomized comparison. Scan J Gastroenterol. 1989;24:539-49.
5. Bengmark S, Gianotti L. Nutritional support to prevent and treat multiple organ failure. World J Surg. 1996;20:474-81.
6. Pavlor VA, Tracey KJ. The vagus nerve and the inflammatory reflex-linking immunity and nutrition. Nat Rev Endocrinol. 2012;28(12):743-54.
7. McClave SA, Heyland DL. The physiologic response and associated clinical benefits from provision of early enteral nutrition. NCP. 2009;24:305-15.
8. Khan J, Iiboshi Y, Nezu R, Chen K, Cui L, Yoshida H, et al. Total parenteral nutrition increases uptake of latex beads by Peyer's patches. JPEN J Parenter Enteral Nutr. 1997;21:31-5.
9. Buchman AL, Moukarzel AA, Bhuta S, Belle M, Ament ME, Eckhert CD, et al. Parenteral nutrition is associated with intestinal morphologic and functional changes in humans. JPEN J Parenter Enteral Nutr. 1995;19:453-60.
10. Xio F, Gao X, Hu H, Le J, Chen Y, Shu X, et al. Exclusive enteral nutrition exerts anti-inflammatory effects through modulating microbiota, bile acid metabolism, and immune activities. Nutrients. 2022;14:4463.

11. Lassen K, Kjave J, Fetveit T, Tranø G, Sigurdsson HK, Horn A, et al. Allowing normal food at will after major gastrointestinal surgery does not affect morbidity: A randomized multicenter trial. Ann Surg. 2008;247:721-9.
12. Osland E, Yunus RM, Khan S, Memon MA. Early versus traditional postoperative feeding in patients undergoing resectional gastrointestinal surgery: A meta-analysis. JPEN J Parenter Enteral Nutr. 2011;35(4):473-87.
13. Gianotti L, Sandini M, Ramagnoli S, Carli F, Ljungqvist O. Enhanced recovery programs in gastrointestinal surgery: Actions to promote nutritional and metabolic care. Clin Nutr. 2019;39:2014-24.
14. McClave SA, Taylor BE, Martindale RG. Guidelines for the provision and assessment of nutrition support therapy in the adult critically ill patient, American Society for Parenteral and Enteral Society (ASPEN) and Society for Critical Care Medicine (SCCM). JPEN J Parenter Enteral Nutr. 2016;40:159-211.
15. Compher C, Bingham AL, McCall J, Patel J, Rice TW, Braunschweig C, et al. Guidelines for the provision of nutrition support therapy in the adult critically ill patient: The American Society for Parenteral and Enteral Nutrition. JPEN J Parenter Enteral Nutr. 2022;46:12-41.
16. Albers DJ, Levine M, Gluckman B, Ginsberg H, Hripcsak G, Mamykina L. Personalized glucose forecasting for type 2 diabetes using data assimilation. PLoS Comput Biol. 2017;13:e1005232.
17. Cresci GA (Ed). Gut microbiome in the critically ill. Nutrition support for the critically ill: A guide to practice, 2nd edition. New York: CRC Press; 2015. pp. 169-83.
18. Yelin KB, Flett C, Merakou P, Mehrotra P, Stam J, Snesrud E, et al. Genomic and epidemiological evidence of bacterial transmission from probiotic capsule to blood in ICU patients. Nat Med. 2019;25:1728-32.
19. Sharif S, Greer A, Skorupski C, Hao Q, Johnstone J, Dionne JC, et al. Probiotics in Critical Illness: A Systematic Review and Meta-Analysis of Randomized Controlled Trials. Crit Care Med. 2022;50:1175-85.
20. Matarese LE, O'Keefe SJ, Kandl HM, Bond G, Costa G, Abu-Elmagd K. Short bowel syndrome: Clinical guidelines for nutritional management. Nutr Clin Pract. 2005;40:493-502.
21. Casaer MP, Langouche L, Coudyzer W, Vanbeckevoort D, De Dobbelaer B, Güiza FG, et al. Impact of early parenteral nutrition on muscle and adipose tissue compartments during critical illness. Crit Care Med. 2013;41:2298-309.
22. Sriram K, Sauper AJ, Mizock BA. Body composition and parenteral nutrition: Where's the beef? Crit Care Med. 2013;41(10):2439-41.
23. Burrin DG, Davis TA. An optimal combination of proteins is beneficial for clinical outcomes. Curr Opin Clin Nutr Metab Care. 2004;7:79-87.
24. Harrison LE, Hochwald SN, Heslin MJ, Berman R, Burt M, Brennan MF. Early postoperative enteral nutrition improves peripheral muscle kinetics in upper gastrointestinal cancer surgery patients undergoing complete resection: A randomized trial. JPEN J Parenter Enteral Nutr. 1997;21:202-7.
25. Mouser JF, Hak EB, Kuhl DA, Dickerson RN, Gaber LW, Hak LJ. Recovery from ischemic acute renal failure is improved with enteral compared with parenteral nutrition. Crit Care Med. 1997;25:1748-54.
26. Plauth M, Cabre E, Riggio O, Assis-Camilo M, Pirlich M, Kondrup J, et al. ESPEN Guidelines on enteral nutrition: Liver Disease. Clin Nutr. 2006;25:285-94.
27. Pash E. Enteral nutrition: Options for short term access. Nutr Clin Pract. 2018;33:170-6.
28. Prest PJ, Justice J, Bell N, McCarroll R, Watson CM. A volume-based feeding protocol improves nutrition delivery and glycemic control in surgery trauma intensive care unit. JPEN J Parenter Enteral Nutr. 2020;44(5):880-8.
29. Gutierrez Lopez DE, Lashinger LM, Weinstock GM, Bray MS. Circadian rhythms and the gut microbiome synchronize the host's metabolic response to diet. Cell Metab. 2021;33:873-87.

30. Sriram K, Meguid RA, Meguid MM. Nutritional support in adults with chyle leaks. Nutrition. 2016;32:281-6.
31. Blaauw R, Osmond E, Sriram K, Ali A, Allard JP, Ball P, et al. Parenteral provision of micronutrients to adult patients: An expert consensus paper. JPEN J Parenter Enteral Nutr. 2019;43(Suppl 1):S5-23.
32. Berger MM, Shenkin A, Schweinlin A, Amrein K, Augsburger M, Biesalski HK, et al. ESPEN micronutrient guideline. Clin Nutr. 2022;41(6):1357-424.
33. Petrov MS, van Santvoort HC, Besselink MG, van der Heijden GJ, Windsor JA, Gooszen HG. Enteral nutrition and the risk of mortality and infectious complications in patients with severe acute pancreatitis—a meta-analysis of randomized rials. Arch Surg. 2008;143:1111-7.
34. Silva JSV, Seres D, Sabino K, Berdahl GJ, Citty SW, Cober MP, et al. ASPEN consensus recommendations for refeeding syndrome. Nutr Clin Pract. 2020;35:178-95.
35. Patel VN, Dijk G, Malarkey B, Brooke JR, Whelan K, MacLaughlin HL, et al. Glycemic response to a renal-specific oral nutritional supplement in patients with diabetes undergoing hemodialysis: A randomized cross over trial. JPEN J Parenter Enteral Nutr. 2021;45:267-76.
36. Sriram K, Blaauw R. Addition of insulin to parenteral nutrition is not universally safe. JPEN J Parenter Enteral Nutr. 2019; 43:13.
37. Brown RO, Dickerson RN. Drug-nutrient interactions. In: Cresci GA (Ed). Nutrition Support for the Critically Ill: A Guide to Practice, 2nd edition. New York: CRC Press; 2015. pp. 313-27.
38. Chourdakis M, Kraus MM, Tzellos T, Sardeli C, Peftoulidou M, Vassilakos D, et al. Effect of early compared with delayed enteral nutrition on endocrine function in patients with traumatic brain injury: An open-labeled randomized study. JPEN J Parenter Enteral Nutr. 2012;36:108-16.
39. Bozzetti F. Quality of life and enteral nutrition. Curr Opin Clin Nutr Metab Care. 2008;11:661-5.
40. Sulo S, Feldstein J, Partridge J, Schwander B, Sriram K, Summerfelt WT. Budget impact of a comprehensive nutrition-focused quality improvement program for malnourished hospitalized patients. Am Health Drug Benefits. 2017;10(5):262-70.
41. van Zanten ARH, De Waele E, Wischmeyer PE. Nutrition therapy and critical illness. Practical guidance for the ICU, post-ICU, and long-term convalescence phases. Crit Care. 2019;23:368.

CHAPTER 13

Gastrointestinal Disturbances in Critically Ill Patients

Ganshyam Jagathkar, Radha Reddy Chada

INTRODUCTION

Multiple gastrointestinal (GI) problems may occur in critically ill patients. Shock is often one of the key risk factors for these problems, since it substantially lowers splenic perfusion linked to intestinal dysmotility, alters the tolerance to enteral nutrition, and causes anatomical and functional alterations in the GI tract.[1-3] Critically ill patients typically have GI dysfunction, which is linked to worse clinical outcomes.[4] Drug usage that alters motility is a significant additional factor.[3] Constipation, an increase in gastroesophageal reflux, and higher prevalence of delayed gastric emptying are all potential effects of opioid-induced GI problems.[1]

In practice, evaluation of mechanical and physiological GI function in critically ill patients is sometimes challenging and is typically restricted to clinical symptoms, physical examination, and what are essentially improved input-output metrics. It is typically adequate to examine the functional integrity of the GI tract and how well or poorly it is functioning in the specific patient based on the overall impression from clinical observations and laboratory testing.[5] There is evidence that the existence of GI symptoms in critically ill patients impacts the prognosis, although it is noteworthy that there is a large variation in the reported incidence of symptoms among the few studies that have been conducted.[4] This is triggered, at least in part, by the absence of a consensus on what constitutes a substantial GI symptom as well as differences in how failed GI function is evaluated. This issue is exacerbated by the lack of any reliable tests that can be used to assess the GI functionality and performance. Studies have reported that approximately 60% of intensive care patients will have at least one GI symptom during their stay[6,7] and among those with multiple symptoms, GI bleeding or absent bowel sounds is associated with increased morbidity and mortality. Pathophysiological mechanisms and multi-faceted clinical presentation of GI dysfunction is presented in **Figure 1**.[5]

The European Society of Intensive Care Medicine (ESICM) Working Group on Abdominal Problems has published recommendations on terminology, definitions, and management of GI disturbances in the critically ill population.[6] These definitions and terminology are used in the following discussions on GI problems of critical care patients.

ACUTE GASTROINTESTINAL INJURY

Acute gastrointestinal injury (AGI) is the malfunctioning of the GI tract in critically ill patients because of their acute illness. Its severity is evaluated similarly to how acute

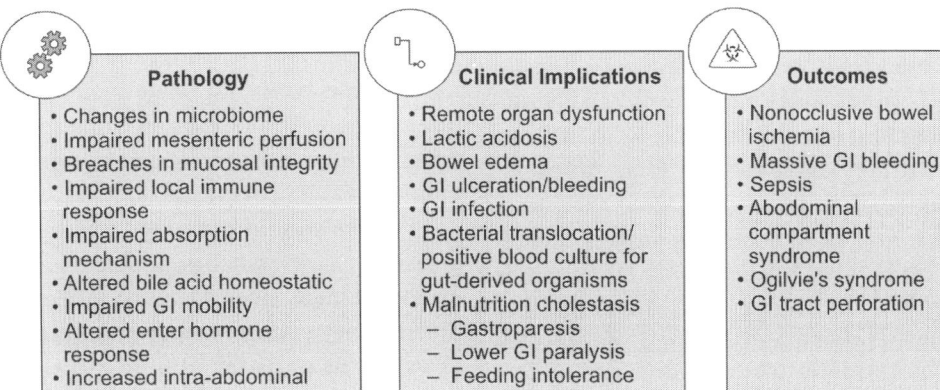

Fig. 1: Pathophysiological mechanisms and multi-faceted clinical presentation of gastrointestinal (GI) dysfunction.[4]

TABLE 1: Gastrointestinal (GI) dysfunction.[6]

	Definition	Example
Grade I (risk of developing gastrointestinal dysfunction or failure)	The function of the GI tract is partially impaired, expressed as GI symptoms related to a known cause and perceived as transient	Nausea/vomiting in the immediate postoperative period, absent bowel sounds after abdominal surgery
Grade II (gastrointestinal dysfunction)	The GI tract is not able to perform digestion and absorption adequately to satisfy the nutrient and fluid requirements of the body. There are no changes in general condition of the patient related to GI problems	Gastroparesis with high gastric residuals, diarrhea, grade I intra-abdominal hypertension (IAP 12–15 mm Hg), visible blood in gastric content or stool, feeding intolerance*
Grade III (gastrointestinal failure)	Loss of GI function, where restoration of GI function is not achieved despite interventions and the general condition is not improving	Persistent feeding intolerance, GI paralysis, bowel dilatation, grade 2 IAH (IAP 16–20 mm Hg), and bowel ischemia
Grade IV (gastrointestinal failure with severe impact on distant organ function)	AGI has progressed to become directly and immediately life-threatening with worsening of MODS and shock	Bowel necrosis, abdominal compartment syndrome (IAP >20 mm Hg), and hemorrhagic shock from GI bleeding

*Feeding intolerance is present if at least 20 kcal/kg/day cannot be given via enteral route within 72 hours of attempted feeding.
(AGI: acute gastrointestinal injury; IAH: intra-abdominal hypertension; IAP: intra-abdominal pressure; MODS: multiorgan dysfunction score)

kidney injury is assessed as enumerated in **Table 1**.[6] In addition, AGI may be further defined as primary or secondary: primary AGI is associated with primary disease or direct injury to organs of the GI system, while secondary AGI results from a host response in critical illness without primary pathology of the GI system.

DIARRHEA

The passing of three or more loose or liquid stools (Bristol Stool Chart 5, 6, or 7) with total mass >250 g or total volume >250 mL/day constitutes diarrhea.[8,9] The reported incidence of diarrhea on critical care units varies from 2 to 95% and has proven difficult to establish with certainty. Diarrhea is estimated to occur in approximately 15–18% of critically ill patients who receive enteral nutrition, compared to only 6% of such patients who do not receive enteral nutrition.[10,11] Critical care patients had a mean diarrheal frequency of 6.4%, according to 2011 multi-center Spanish research.[12] Patients who experience diarrhea may experience complications such as malabsorption, electrolyte imbalance, skin breakdown, dehydration, infection, necessity for patient isolation, cost of stool tests to rule out *Clostridium difficile*, and prolonged stay in the intensive care unit (ICU).[13-16] Further, concomitant psychological stressors to the patient include compromised dignity and increased nurse workload with associated costs.[17,18]

Risk Factors for Diarrhea[14,19]

- Enteral nutrition (odds ratio: 4.1)
- Antibiotic therapy
- Increasing ICU length of stay
- Hyperglycemia
- Hypoalbuminemia
- Elevated white cell count
- *Clostridium difficile* infection.

Management[20]

The mainstay of therapy is symptomatic management with maintenance of appropriate fluid status and electrolyte balance to prevent secondary deterioration (e.g., renal dysfunction).[9,21,22] A fecal collection system (e.g., Flexiseal™) reduces the risk of perianal skin damage and bedsores and can be used if the stool is type 7.[23] The addition of soluble fiber to enteral feeding solutions prolongs transit time and may alleviate symptoms although evidence is weak.[9,22,24-26]

A cause should be sought and treated if possible (e.g., prokinetics, antibiotics, inflammatory bowel disease, malabsorption).[13] The routine sending of stool cultures is rarely of value for patients admitted to the ICU. Instead, stool should be sent for analysis of *C. difficile* endotoxin and culture for pathogens considered if results are negative and diarrhea is persistent. Routine stool culture will identify *Salmonella*, *Campylobacter*, and *Shigella* species. If there is clinical suspicion of other pathogens the laboratory should be notified, and local guidelines are implemented. The examination of stool samples for ova and parasites (e.g., for *Giardia*, *Cryptosporidium*, *Cyclospora*, and *Entamoeba histolytica*) may be appropriate if the patient has a history of foreign travel or immunosuppression. Testing for these is done by collecting three samples sent for analysis at least 24 hours apart since parasite excretion may be intermittent. Where *C. difficile* is isolated, appropriate medical management is essential. Specific dosing depending on local policies, with oral or enteral nutrition can be considered.[13]

VOMITING (EMESIS)

Any visible regurgitation of gastric contents, regardless of the amount, constitutes vomiting.[6] Outside of the critical care unit, vomiting is typically defined as the oral expulsion of GI contents caused by contractions of the gut and abdominal wall muscles. However, in ICU patients, these involuntary and muscular contractions are not noticeable. Therefore, in the ICU population, vomiting and regurgitation should be considered together. Additionally, in the absence of physical obstruction, impaired gastric emptying is the likely etiology.[27] In contrast to conscious patients outside the critical care environment, the sensation of nausea is less of an issue than any regurgitation that may occur, as patients are often sedated or anesthetized within the ICU. Hence, the role of commonly used antiemetics is reduced, as they are only likely to be of value in conscious patients or where forceful emesis is occurring.[6]

GASTROINTESTINAL DYSMOTILITY

Gastrointestinal motility is a natural defense mechanism, and it is considered a crucial factor in preventing bacterial overgrowth together with gastric acidity.[28] However, in critically ill patients, it can be affected by factors including ischemia, analgesic drugs, adrenergic agents, dehydration, and preexisting diseases such as diabetes.[29,30] GI dysmotility is a serious challenge in the ICU. While dysmotility can manifest as anything from modest symptoms like delayed gastric emptying-related nausea to complete gut failure with ileus being the most common form of dysmotility in the ICU.[31] Typically, ileus is suspected when a patient exhibits abdominal distention, nausea, vomiting, absence of stools, or flatus. Dilated bowel is frequently noted on imaging. ICU patients typically experience GI dysmotility or ileus for a number of reasons, such as surgical conditions, systemic inflammation, electrolyte imbalances, an increase in intracranial pressure, and the administration of several antimotility drugs. Nearing 50% of ventilated patients have antral hypomotility, decreased gastric emptying, and weakened migrating motor complexes, which causes a number of issues, not the least of which is a decreased capacity to tolerate enteral nutrition.[32,33] Hypomotility can usefully be divided into gastroparesis and intestinal motor inhibition; though obviously these can, and often do, coexist in the same patient.

GASTROPARESIS

Gastrointestinal failure has been variously defined as "gastroparesis and intestinal ileus", or "gastrointestinal hemorrhage". It is common with an incidence of 18%.[34] Gastroparesis is impaired gastric emptying without physical obstruction and can be assessed by the quantity of gastric aspirate obtained over a set period.[35] Assuming that gastric juice is generated at a rate of about 1 L/day, the volume that is not aspirated may be used to determine how much gastric juice passes past the pyloric sphincter.[36]

Intestinal Motor Inhibition

Intestinal motor inhibition refers to disruption of the basic patterns of propulsion seen in the small and large bowel. These are controlled primarily by integrated reflex circuits in the enteric nervous system, the activity of the interstitial cells of Cajal (the "pacemakers" of the bowel), and the smooth muscle cells themselves.[37] Modulation of motility by the autonomic nervous system and endocrine messengers provides fine tuning of propulsive activity. In critical illness, any or all these systems can become disrupted, and restoration of normal function can be very difficult.

CONSTIPATION

Constipation outside of a critical care setting denotes uneasy or infrequent bowel motions with hard stool and/or painful defecation.[37,38] Although it is important to keep in mind that physiological stool frequency can vary from one to two evacuations per day to one evacuation every third or fourth day, clinical indications include the lack of stool for three or more consecutive days without mechanical obstruction. There may or may not be bowel sounds. Due to sedation, it might be difficult to diagnose the symptom of difficulties passing stools in the majority of critically ill patients. However, it has been noted that infrequent bowel movements (nondefecation) are a common problem in the critically ill and may be caused by GI dysmotility.[39] The phrase "paralysis of the lower GI tract" has been proposed due to the possibility that these symptoms may not be expressed by patients receiving critical care.[40] This is the inability of the bowel to pass stool due to impaired peristalsis. Adverse symptoms associated with infrequent bowel movements, or constipation, may include abdominal distention, pain, restlessness, poor tolerance of enteral feeding, confusion, and intestinal obstruction with nausea, vomiting and risk of pulmonary aspiration.[33,41] It may also be associated with raised intra-abdominal pressure, which can impact on respiratory function. Abdominal distention associated with constipation may be associated with bacterial overgrowth.[42] Because of variations in its definition, studies have revealed that the incidence of constipation among patients hospitalized to critical care units varies between 15 and 83%.[10,40,43,44] Patients stand the risk of bowel perforation due to intestinal pseudo-obstruction, which can occasionally be caused by severe GI dysmotility.[45,46] Constipation is frequently accompanied by gastroparesis and ileoparesia, manifestations that delay and complicate the start of enteral feeding,[2,44] making it more difficult to achieve the nutritional adequacy.

Management of Hypomotility

Initial supportive therapy choices and goal-directed specialized therapies can be used for management. These proposals are based on Herbert & Holzer's suggested unified standard approach from 2008.[47] Drugs lowering GI motility (e.g., opioids, sedatives, and catecholamines) should be ceased whenever feasible, and conditions hindering peristalsis (e.g., hypokalemia and hyperglycemia) should be treated. Due to their delayed onset of action, laxative medications must either be used prophylactically or initiated early to be effective.

GASTROINTESTINAL BLEEDING

The macroscopic presence of blood as hematemesis or melena can be used to demonstrate blood loss into the lumen of the GI tract. Most ICU patients experience asymptomatic but endoscopically visible GI tract mucosa damage throughout their stay, whereas a lesser percentage,[48] or 5–25%, experience clinically visible GI tract bleeding.[48,49] Clinically, important bleeding, defined as overt bleeding requiring blood transfusion or causing hemodynamic instability, occurs in 1.5–4% of ventilated patients.[48,50,51] Stress ulceration of the upper GI tract begins within hours of the onset of critical illness. Most overt GI bleeding is caused by either gastric or esophageal ulceration.[52]

Management

The patient's hemodynamic condition is what dictates how GI bleeding is initially managed. Urgent endoscopy should be done if the patient is unstable, and bleeding locations should be controlled either by adrenaline injection, clipping, banding, or injection of sclerosant.[53] Interventional radiology should be investigated, and, in rare circumstances, a laparotomy may be necessary if bleeding cannot be managed endoscopically. Endoscopy is still the best course for therapy if the patient is hemodynamically stable, but with less urgency. Any nasogastric feeding would need to be halted during the active management of GI bleeding, but it should be resumed as soon as clinically recommended.

ABDOMINAL HYPERTENSION AND COMPARTMENT SYNDROME

Definition

- Intra-abdominal hypertension (IAH) is present if the intra-abdominal pressure (IAP) is found to be 12 mm Hg or more in at least two separate measurements 1-6 hours apart, or if the mean of IAP measurements over 24 hours is 12 mm Hg or more (provided at least four measurements are made).[54-56]
- Abdominal compartment syndrome (ACS) is defined as a sustained increase in IAP to 20 mm Hg or greater, again in at least two separate measurements 1-6 hours apart, with new onset organ failure.[54]

Management of Abdominal Hypertension

Intermittent monitoring of IAP should be done if IAF/ACS is suspected. IAH and compartment syndrome patients will need parenteral nutrition till they recover. To prevent additional GI and pulmonary edema in these patients, fluid delivery needs to be closely controlled.

CONCLUSION

Acute GI injury is categorized I-IV according to severity and might be primary or secondary. The therapy of diarrhea tries to determine a cause and reduce any downstream physiological effects. Diarrhea is a frequent and perhaps inevitable complication of critical care. Treatment for hypomotility might be challenging since the etiology is complicated and multifactorial. Differentiating between upper and lower GI paralysis enables for more focused treatments, and the most successful methods often involve a multimodal strategy that includes prokinetics and laxatives when necessary. In critical illness, GI ulceration is frequent and can result in substantial GI bleeding. Endoscopic management is the gold standard. It is debatable how assistance suppression should be used and when in relation to endoscopy. IAP measurement ought to be done. If conservative treatments are ineffective, surgical intervention is the only option when there is a suspicion of IAH or ACS. Resuming appropriate mode of nutrition intervention during and after any of the GI disturbances should be the primary goal to prevent malnutrition and its adverse outcomes.

REFERENCES

1. Chappell D, Rehm M, Conzen P. Opioid-induced constipation in intensive care patients: relief in sight? Crit Care. 2008; 12:161.
2. López-Herce J. Gastrointestinal complications in critically ill patients: what differs between adults and children? Curr Opin Clin Nutr Metab Care. 2009;12:180-5.
3. Nassar Jr AP, Silva FMQ, Cleva R. Constipation in intensive care unit: incidence and risk factors. J Crit Care. 2009;24:630, e9-e12.
4. Reintam Blaser A, Poeze M, Malbrain ML, Björck M, Oudemans-van Straaten HM, Starkopf J; Gastro-Intestinal Failure Trial Group. Gastrointestinal symptoms during the first week of intensive care are associated with poor outcome: a prospective multicentre study. Intensive Care Med. 2013;39(5):899-909.

5. Reintam Blaser A, Preiser JC, Fruhwald S, Wilmer A, Wernerman J, Benstoem C, et al. Gastrointestinal dysfunction in the critically ill: a systematic scoping review and research agenda proposed by the Section of Metabolism, Endocrinology and Nutrition of the European Society of Intensive Care Medicine. Crit Care. 2020;24:224.
6. Reintam Blaser A, Malbrain ML, Starkopf J, Fruhwald S, Jakob SM, De Waele J, et al. Gastrointestinal function in intensive care patients: terminology, definitions and management. Recommendations of the ESICM Working Group on Abdominal Problems. Intensive Care Med. 2012;38:384-94.
7. Reintam A, Parm P, Kitus R, Kern H, Starkopf J. Gastrointestinal symptoms in intensive care patients. Acta Anaesthesiol Scand. 2009;53(3):318-24.
8. Lankisch PG, Mahlke R, Lübbers H, Lembcke B, Rösch W. Zertifizierte medizinische Fortbildung: Leitsymptom Diarrhö. Dtsch Arztebl. 2006;103:261-9.
9. Wiesen P, Van Gossum A, Preiser JC. Diarrhoea in the critically ill. Curr Opin Crit Care. 2006;12:149-54.
10. Montejo JC. Enteral nutrition-related gastrointestinal complications in critically ill patients: a multicenter study. The Nutritional and Metabolic Working Group of the Spanish Society of Intensive Care Medicine and Coronary Units. Crit Care Med. 1999;27(8):1447-53.
11. Luft VC, Beghetto MG, de Mello ED, Polanczyk CA. Role of enteral nutrition in the incidence of diarrhea among hospitalized adult patients. Nutrition. 2008;24(6):528-35.
12. Izaguirre Guerricagoitia L, Truchuelo Aragón A; Grupo de Investigación de Prevalencia de Diarrea. Prevalence of diarrhea in critical patients units in Spain: a multicenter study. Enferm Intensiva. 2011;22(2):65-73.
13. de Brito-Ashurst I, Preiser JC. Diarrhea in critically ill patients: the role of enteral feeding. JPEN J Parenter Enteral Nutr. 2016;40(7):913-23.
14. Tirlapur N, Puthucheary ZA, Cooper JA, Sanders J, Coen PG, Mooneshinghe SR, et al. Diarrhoea in the critically ill is common, associated with poor outcome, and rarely due to *Clostridium difficile*. Sci Rep. 2016;6:24691.
15. Reintam Blaser A, Deane AM, Fruhwald S. Diarrhoea in the critically ill. Curr Opin Crit Care. 2015;21(2):142-53.
16. Jakob SM, Butikofer L, Berger D, Coslovsky M, Takala J. A randomized controlled pilot study to evaluate the effect of an enteral formulation designed to improve gastrointestinal tolerance in the critically ill patient-the SPIRIT trial. Crit Care. 2017;21(1):140.
17. Heidegger CP, Graf S, Perneger T, Genton L, Oshima T, Pichard C. The burden of diarrhea in the intensive care unit (ICU-BD). A survey and observational study of the caregivers' opinions and workload. Int J Nurs Stud. 2016;59:163-8.
18. Smith CE, Faust-Wilson P, Lohr G, Kallenberger S, Marien L. A measure of distress reaction to diarrhea in ventilated tube-fed patients. Nurs Res. 1992;41(5):312-3.
19. Ferrie S. Managing Diarrhea During Enteral Feeding in ICU. In: Rajendram R, Preedy VR, Patel VB (Eds). Diet and Nutrition in Critical Care. New York: Springer; 2015. pp. 1647-57.
20. Sabol VK, Friedenberg FK. Diarrhea: diagnostic approach to common medical problems in the hospitalized adult. AACN Clin Issues. 1997;8(3):425-36.
21. Pawlowsky SW, Warren CA, Guerrant R. Diagnosis and treatment of acute or persistent diarrhea. Gastroenterology. 2009;136:1874-86.
22. Whelan K, Schneider SM. Mechanisms, prevention, and management of diarrhea in enteral nutrition. Curr Opin Gastroenterol. 2011;27:152-9.
23. Padmanabhan A, Stern M, Wishin J, Mangino M, Richey K, DeSane M; Flexi-Seal Clinical Trial Investigators Group. Clinical evaluation of a flexible fecal incontinence management system. Am J Crit Care. 2007;16(4):384-93.
24. Rushdi TA, Pichard C, Khater YH. Control of diarrhea by fiber-enriched diet in ICU patients on enteral nutrition: a prospective randomized controlled trial. Clin Nutr. 2004;23(6):1344-52.

25. Spapen H, Diltoer M, Van Malderen C, Opdenacker G, Suys E, Huyghens L. Soluble fiber reduces the incidence of diarrhea in septic patients receiving total enteral nutrition: a prospective, double-blind, randomized, and controlled trial. Clin Nutr. 2001;20(4):301-5.
26. Nakao M, Ogura Y, Satake S, Ito I, Iguchi A, Takagi K, et al. Usefulness of soluble dietary fibre for the treatment of diarrhoea during enteral nutrition in elderly patients. Nutrition. 2002;18:35-9.
27. Fauci AS, Braunwald E, Kasper DL, Hauser SL (Eds). Harrison's principles of Internal Medicine, 17th edition. USA: McGraw-Hill Education; 2007.
28. Mesejo A, Juan M, García-Simón M. Enteral access and intestinal function assessment in the critically ill patient. Nutr Hosp. 2007;22(2):37-49.
29. Shimizu K, Ogura H, Hamasaki T, Goto M, Tasaki O, Asahara T, et al. Altered gut flora are associated with septic complications and death in critically ill patients with systemic inflammatory response syndrome. Dig Dis Sci. 2010;56:1171-7.
30. Shimizu K, Ogura H, Asahara T, Nomoto K, Morotomi M, Nakahori Y, et al. Gastrointestinal dysmotility is associated with altered gut flora and septic mortality in patients with severe systemic inflammatory response syndrome: a preliminary study. Neurogastroenterol Motil. 2011;23:330.e157.
31. Evans DC, Martindale RG. Chapter 78: Intestinal Dysmotility of Critical Illness. In: Rajendram R (Ed). Diet and Nutrition in Critical Care, 1st edition. Berlin, Germany: Springer; 2015. pp. 1038-47.
32. Kao CH, ChangLai SP, Chieng PU, Yen TC. Gastric emptying in head-injured patients. Am J Gastroenterol. 1998;93(7):1108-12.
33. Nguyen T, Frenette AJ, Johanson C, Maclean RD, Patel R, Simpson A, et al. Impaired gastrointestinal transit and its associated morbidity in the intensive care unit. J Crit Care. 2013;28(4):537, e511-37.
34. Reintam A, Parm P, Redlich U, Tooding LM, Starkopf J, Köhler F, et al. Gastrointestinal failure in intensive care: a retrospective clinical study in three different intensive care units in Germany and Estonia. BMC Gastroenterol. 2006;6:19.
35. Aswath GS, Foris LA, Ashwath AK, Patel K. Diabetic Gastroparesis. [Updated 2023; Mar 27]. In: StatPearls [Internet]. Treasure Island (FL): StatPearls Publishing; 2023.
36. Stojek M, Jasiński T. Gastroparesis in the intensive care unit. Anaesthesiol Intensive Ther. 2021;53(5):450-5.
37. Fukuda S, Miyauchi T, Fujita M, Oda Y, Todani M, Kawamura Y, et al. Risk factors for late defecation and its association with the outcomes of critically ill patients: a retrospective observational study. J Intensive Care. 2016;4:33.
38. Prat D, Messika J, Avenel A, Jacobs F, Fichet J, Lemeur M, et al. Constipation incidence and impact in medical critical care patients: importance of the definition criterion. Eur J Gastroenterol Hepatol. 2016;28(3):290-6.
39. Chapman MJ, Nguyen NQ, Deane AM. Gastrointestinal dysmotility: evidence and clinical management. Curr Opin Clin Nutr Metab Care. 2013;16(2):209-16.
40. Azevedo RP, Machado FR. Constipation in critically ill patients: much more than we imagine. Rev Bras Ter Intensiva. 2013;25(2):73-4.
41. Patel PB, Brett SJ, O'Callaghan D, Anjum A, Cross M, Warwick J, et al. Protocol for a randomised control trial of methylnaltrexone for the treatment of opioid-induced constipation and gastrointestinal stasis in intensive care patients (MOTION). BMJ Open. 2016;6(7):e011750.
42. Asai T. Constipation: does it increase morbidity and mortality in critically ill patients? Crit Care Med. 2007;35:2861-2.
43. Mostafa SM, Bhandari S, Ritchie G, Gratton N, Wenstone R. Constipation and its implications in the critically ill patient. Br J Anaesth. 2003;91(6):815-9.
44. de Souza Lopes Guerra T, Marshall NG, Mendonça SS. Chapter 18: Constipation in Intensive care. Rajendram R, Preedy VR, Patel VB (Eds). Diet and Nutrition in Critical Care, 1st edition. Berlin, Germany: Springer; 2015. pp. 236-46.

45. Ross SW, Oommen B, Wormer BA, Walters AL, Augenstein VA, Heniford BT, et al. Acute colonic pseudo-obstruction: defining the epidemiology, treatment, and adverse outcomes of ogilvie's syndrome. Am Surg. 2016;82(2):102-11.
46. van der Spoel JI, Oudemans-van Straaten HM, Stoutenbeek CP, Bosman RJ, Zandstra DF. Neostigmine resolves critical illness-related colonic ileus in intensive care patients with multiple organ failure—a prospective, double-blind, placebo-controlled trial. Intensive Care Med. 2001;27(5):822-7.
47. Herbert MK, Holzer P. Standardized concept for the treatment of gastrointestinal dysmotility in critically ill patients—current status and future options. Clin Nutr. 2008;27(1):25-41.
48. Mutlu GM, Mutlu EA, Factor P. GI complications in patients receiving mechanical ventilation. Chest. 2001;119:1222-41.
49. Dobos NM, Warrillow SJ. Gastrointestinal problems in intensive care. Anaesth Intensive Care Med. 2021;22(2):95-100.
50. Cook DJ, Fuller HD, Guyatt GH, Marshall JC, Leasa D, Hall R, et al. Risk factors for gastrointestinal bleeding in critically ill patients. Canadian Critical Care Trials Group. N Engl J Med. 1994;330:377-81.
51. Mayr VD, Dünser MW, Greil V, Jochberger S, Luckner G, Ulmer H, et al. Causes and determinants of outcome in critically ill patients. Crit Care. 2006;10:R14.
52. Siddiqui AH, Farooq U, Siddiqui F. Curling Ulcer. In: StatPearls [Internet]. Treasure Island (FL): StatPearls Publishing; 2023.
53. Barkun AN, Bardou M, Kuipers EJ, Sung J, Hunt RH, Martel M, et al.; International Consensus Upper Gastrointestinal Bleeding Conference Group. International consensus recommendations on the management of patients with nonvariceal upper gastrointestinal bleeding. Ann Intern Med. 2010;152:101-13.
54. Malbrain ML, Cheatham ML, Kirkpatrick A, Sugrue M, Parr M, De Waele J, et al. Results from the international conference of experts on intra-abdominal hypertension and abdominal compartment syndrome. I. Definitions. Intensive Care Med. 2006;32: 1722-32.
55. De Keulenaer BL, De Waele JJ, Powell B, Malbrain ML. What is normal intra-abdominal pressure and how is it affected by positioning, body mass and positive end-expiratory pressure? Intensive Care Med. 2009;35:969-76.
56. Malbrain ML, De laet I, Cheatham M. Consensus conference definitions and recommendations on intra-abdominal hypertension (IAH) and the abdominal compartment syndrome (ACS)—the long road to the final publications, how did we get there? Acta Clin Belg Suppl. 2007;62: 44-59.

CHAPTER 14

Enteral Access: Device and Selection

Srinivas Samavedam, Arun Kumar

INTRODUCTION

Early and timely initiation of nutritional support to a critically ill patient has a pivotal role in management and overall outcome. It is well appreciated that enteral nutrition (EN) is preferred over parenteral route. The 2016 Society for Critical Care Medicine and the American Society for Parenteral and Enteral Nutrition Guidelines for the Provision and Assessment of Nutrition Support Therapy in the adult critically ill patient recommend that early EN should be commenced within 24–48 hours in the critically ill patient who cannot take orally.[1]

Depending on patient's ailment, integrity of gut, functional status of gut, and the expected duration of therapy, decision for EN for short term or longer duration shall be determined. This chapter will review the various options available for enteral feeding.

TYPES OF DEVICES

Enteral access devices often vary with composition and elements of tubing material and size, which by convention are measured using the French (Fr) scale. Many of the feeding tubes that are commercially available are made of polyurethane or silicone. The Fr-size is a measure of the external diameter of a catheter. One Fr unit is equal to 0.33 millimeters. Thus, the larger the Fr, the larger the catheter. Based on the expected duration of use, they are classified as:
- Short-term utility
- Long-term utility.

Short-term Utility[2]

This is the commonly utilized initial feeding modality in intensive care unit (ICU). Short-term refers to placement of tube up to 4–6 weeks. Based on the intended location, they are subclassified as:
- Gastric placement
- Enteric placement
- Dual placement tubes.

Gastric Placement

This group of feeding devices can be via nasal (nasogastric) or oral route (orogastric).

They are placed after measuring length of the tube from the tip of the patient's nose to the earlobe and then to the xiphisternum and inserted through oral cavity. In patients with altered nasal anatomy or nasal trauma, sinusitis, or facial fractures, oral placement is recommended. They could be of either small-bore or large-bore tubes.

Small-bore feeding tube: Commercially available feeding tubes that are intended for enteral feeding usually have a small bore. Commonly available sizes range between 8 and 12 Fr and are color-coded.

They are made of silicone, polyurethane, or could be a mixture of both.

Advantages: They are more soft than that of wide bore counterparts, more pliable, and more patient friendly.

Disadvantages: The small diameter of the tube makes them prone for clogging. Because of the same reason, they pose difficulties in aspirating gastric contents.

Large-bore feeding tube: These tubes are made of polyvinyl chloride and usually more than 14 Fr.

They are primarily meant for the purpose of gastric decompression and lavage. They can still be employed for the purpose of feeding for a short time. However, it is recommended to change the tube to a smaller bore within 5–7 days.

Advantages: Being stiff, it helps in easy placement of the tube, wide bore aids in effective suctioning.

Disadvantages: Not patient friendly as it causes more discomfort, increased risk of aspiration.

Enteric Placement

Passed from oral/nasal route, the intended tip position in the small intestine is at the duodenum or jejunum. The usual length of the tube is 36 inches and tubes up to 45–55 inches are commercially available.

They are of small bore and made of polyurethane or silicone. To aid the performer, these tubes have a temporary metal stylet or guidewire within the lumen so that it makes the tube stiff thereby making the insertion process easy.

Alternatively, some manufacturers of enteric placement tubes have a weighted material at the tip of the tube, common tungsten. The rationale behind is that the weight may help to maintain tube position in the gut.

Dual Placement Tubes

Dual lumen tubes, as the name suggests, the outlet holes of one lumen are positioned in the stomach and the other extends into the small intestine. With dual-lumen tubes, the gastric lumen is often used for either decompression and drainage of the stomach or medication administration. The small-bowel lumen, also called jejunal lumen, is typically used for tube feeding.

Alternatively, a larger-bore nasogastric tube can be placed temporarily in one of the nares which can be employed for gastric decompression and drainage. Through the other nare, a small-bore feeding tube can be inserted for isolated feeding to the small bowel.

Choosing between pyloric and postpyloric positions:[3] Those patients who require tube feeding due to dysphagia, odynophagia, anorexia, and poor oral intake can be initiated on pyloric feeds.

Those set of patients ideal for postpyloric feeding are:
- Intolerance to gastric feed—abdominal pain, distention, nausea, and vomiting
- High risk of aspiration–inability to protect the airway, mechanical ventilation, age >70 years, reduced level of consciousness, poor oral care, inadequate nurse: patient ratio, supine positioning, neurologic deficits, and gastroesophageal reflux.

Although the European Society for Clinical Nutrition and Metabolism (ESPEN) guidelines advocate gastric access as the standard of care to initiate EN, few literature and meta-analysis support postpyloric feeding was able to deliver proportions of the estimated energy requirement and can help to reduce gastric residual volume.

Though there is no mortality benefit with postpyloric feeds, it decreases the incidence of pneumonia. The decision, therefore, has to individualized depending on the provider and the overall condition of the patient.[4]

Placement techniques of short-term use tubes:

- *Blind placement:* Placing oral/nasal feeding tube at the bedside in ICU is a common day-to-day practice. The distal end of tube is placed in stomach or small intestine as desired. Nowadays, tubes with radiopaque line with or without stylet running throughout are commercially available so as to aid visibility. The tip position can be then confirmed radiologically using X-ray. Alternatively, upon a blind placement of tube, the contents are aspirated and based on the volume and color of the aspirate, rough estimate of the tip location can be made as:
  - *Gastric placement:* Usually large volume, either greenish, white- or brown-colored aspirate
  - *Small intestinal placement:* Small volume, bile colored

  Another technique is to use prokinetic agents until contraindicated wherein feeding tube is inserted as per standard protocol to the stomach followed by 10 mg metoclopramide, wait for 10 minutes and advance at 10 cm intervals to a depth of 70–80 cm (10-10-10 technique).

- *Fluoroscopy guided:* The fluoroscopic technique is reliable and expensive, often requiring mobilizing to radiological suite, thereby delaying early initiation of feeding. Moreover, radiation exposure is not negligible when fluoroscopic guidance is used. However, there are increased chances of placement at the desired site using fluoroscopy especially when attempted postpyloric placement.[5]

- *Ultrasound guided:* Placement is performed with a stylet in place, using intermittent saline or water injections that show ultrasonic tube localization. Utilizing point-of-care ultrasound enables real-time insertion of a gastric tube with high sensitivity, in a short time with high first-attempt success rate and limited passage-related complications.[6]

- *Endoscopic technique:* Though placement of feeding using endoscopy is under direct vision and confirms definitive placement, it requires skill and expertise and it is time consuming. Though an available modality, it is generally considered as last resort and isolated studies even suggest us endoscopic placement is inferior to ultrasound-guided placement.[7]

- *Video-assisted real-time placement:* Enteral feeding tubes are placed under direct visualization of anatomical landmarks using Integrated Real Time Imaging System (called IRIS feeding tube). These tubes are equipped with a mini-video camera at the distal tip, allowing real-time visualization on an external portable monitor during tube insertion and thereby potentially eliminating the need for X-ray confirmation after the procedure. Though lacking robust data, studies show a high success rate for gastric placement compared with postpyloric placement.[8]

- *Electromagnetic image-guided placement:* To facilitate tube placement, a receiver unit is positioned on the patient's abdomen over the xiphoid process to direct signal from the electromagnetic tip of the stylet within the tube. The electromagnetic tip traces the path of the tube tip, which is displayed in real time on the monitor. Based on the images seen on the monitor and clinical observations while placing the tube, performing clinician can determine the tip of the feeding tube location, whether the tube is in the gastrointestinal tract or lungs, and, if needed, alter the pathway of the tube during placement to avoid entry into the lungs.[9]

Long-term Utility[10]

Also called as stomal or percutaneous tube, they are usually placed surgically in those patients wherein long-term feeding >4–6 weeks is needed.

Those tubes fall in under this category are classified based on the resting location as:
- Prepyloric tube
- Postpyloric tube.

Prepyloric Tube

Gastrostomy tube, commonly referred to as "G tube" falls into this category. When compared with oral/nasally placed tubes, they are shorter in length and have a larger diameter (12–30 Fr). Hence, they are less prone for tube block for their large diameter. Similar to small bore oral/nasal tubes, they are made of silicone, polyurethane, or could be a mixture of both.

G tubes are further classified as:
- Standard G tube
- Low-profile G tube.

Standard G tube: Gastrostomy tubes are frequently utilized stomal feeding tubes in clinic practice. It comes with 6–10-inch long tube with graded marking over the surface. They have both internal and external retention devices to prevent dislodgment.

The external retention device is usually circular in shape and this firmly sits over the abdomen upon the insertion site. This can be adjusted by the patient for the desired fit.

The internal retention devices are of two types:
1. *Balloon G tubes:* It employs an inflatable balloon for internal retention of the tube. Balloon volume depends on the manufacturer. The balloon is filled with sterile water or normal saline. This requires to be changed at intervals of 3–4 months.
2. *Nonballoon G tubes:* Retention device has a funnel commonly takes shape of that of a mushroom or dome-shaped. They can stay in place for 6–12 months. Frequently used endoscopically percutaneous endoscopic gastrostomy (PEG) tube falls into this category.

They can be of single or double port tubes. The second port in a dual port tube could be utilized for the purpose of administering fluid and/or medication.

Low-profile G tube: Designed as an office-wear device, low-profile G tube comes with a compact, short, and sturdy tube of 12–24 Fr and 0.8–7.0 cm in length. For their ergonomics, they are preferred in pediatric and those active patients. Similar to standard G tube, they come with balloon and nonballoon variants. The most important difference in low-profile G tube when compared with standard G tube is that the external retention device cannot be adjusted as per need. Hence, tube size selection is of utmost importance and change of tube is warranted for fit issues. For this reason, it is advised to employ a stoma measuring device to approximate the length of the tube. Since ideal length is almost not always possible, this has a higher incidence of discomfort to patient, pain, leakage, and related complications.

Postpyloric Tube

This category includes jejunostomy tube (J tube) and gastrojejunostomy tubes (GJ tube).

Utility of these is similar to prepyloric counterparts except that the location of tip is to the small intestine. As per manufacturer recommendations, GJ tubes are of size 14–24 Fr and J tubes of size 5–16 Fr. Rest of the device characteristics are similar to that of G tubes.

Placement techniques of long-term use tubes:
- *Endoscopy-assisted placement*: The technique involves insertion of the gastrostomy tube through the abdominal wall at a point where the stomach and abdominal wall are in the closest contact. At this point there are three commonly used techniques in clinical practice: (i) pull technique, (ii) push (guidewire) technique, and (iii) introducer (Russell) method, of which, the pull technique is commonly into practice. The surgical insights are beyond the scope of this review.
- *Radiological placement*: With fluoroscopy, computed tomography, or ultrasound guidance, and percutaneous radiological gastrostomy can be performed transabdominally with push type A technique (Seldinger) and push type B technique (Peel away sheath). Alternatively, percutaneous transesophageal gastrotubing with image guidance can be used to place esophagostomy when gastrostomy is contraindicated such as massive refractory ascites, hostile abdomen, or massive peritoneal carcinomatosis.[11]
- *Gastropexy*: Gastropexy, the apposition of the anterior stomach wall to the anterior abdominal wall, enhances the safety of a tube gastrostomy. It is typically achieved with suturing, T-fasteners, and a bumper-bolster combination in surgical, radiologic, and endoscopic gastrostomies, respectively. Fibrous adhesions between the stomach and abdominal wall will develop after a while and maintain the gastropexy.[12]

■ COMPLICATIONS[13]
Short-term Utility Tubes
Overall complication rates are less with short-term utility tubes. Common complication is misplacement into the bronchial tree with resulting pneumonitis, pneumonia, and/or pneumothorax if not recognized.

Long-term Utility Tubes
During the procedure:
- Aspiration—when performed in a patient with low Glasgow Coma Scale, excessive administration of sedation, when procedure done upon a full stomach.
- Bleeding—if procedure is performed in the background of coagulopathy.
- Perforation peritonitis—from accidental puncture of bowel. Usually due to inappropriate puncture site/technique.
- Prolonged ileus–secondary to pneumoperitoneum.

Postprocedure:
- Retention device related ulcer—due to unnoticed excessive approximation of internal and external retention device. This may lead to ulceration and bleeding.
- Tube related—when excess length of the tube is kept within, its tip could irritate and cause ulceration of the gastric mucosa.
- Infection—from tube insertion site
- Leakage of contents from stoma—particularly of concern in those on corticosteroids, have diabetes, are severely malnourished, have increased gastric acid secretion, or use hydrogen peroxide to cleanse stoma site infections.
- *Buried bumper syndrome (BBS)*: Here, the internal fixation device migrates alongside the tract of the stoma outside

the stomach. Excessive compression of tissue between the external and internal fixation device of the gastrostomy tube is considered as the main etiological factor leading to BBS. Inability to insert, loss of patency, and leakage around the PEG tube are considered to be a typical symptomatic triad.

- Gastric outlet obstruction—caused by distal migration of the internal bolster into the pylorus or small bowel when the external retention device is excessively loose.
- Inadvertent tube removal—common with standard G tubes
- Formation of fistula—colo-cutaneous fistula
- Tumor seeding.

CONCLUSION

Enteral feeding is the most preferred route of nutritional support in the ICU. Nasogastric tube is the most preferred and commonly used route of feeding in ICU when oral feeding is not feasible or safe. Multiple options are available for such situations. Feeding beyond the pylorus may be beneficial in certain situations. Long-term feeding would need direct gastric access.

REFERENCES

1. Kozeniecki M, Fritzshall R. Enteral nutrition for adults in the hospital setting. Nutr Clin Pract. 2015;30:634-51.
2. Pash E. Enteral nutrition: options for short-term access. Nutr Clin Pract. 2018;33(2):170-6.
3. Kuwajima V, Bechtold ML. Should I start with a postpyloric enteral nutrition modality? Nutr Clin Pract. 2021;36(1):76-9.
4. Zhang Z, Xu X, Ding J, Ni H. Comparison of postpyloric tube feeding and gastric tube feeding in intensive care unit patients: a meta-analysis. Nutr Clin Pract. 2013;28(3):371-80.
5. Miller KR, McClave SA, Kiraly LN, Martindale RG, Benns MV. A tutorial in enteral access in adult patients in the hospitalized setting. JPEN J Parenter Enteral Nutr. 2014;38:282-95.
6. Yaseen M, Kumar A, Bhoi S, Sinha TP, Jamshed N, Aggarwal P, et al. Point-of-care ultrasonography-assisted nasogastric tube placement in the emergency department: a randomized controlled trial. Eur J Emerg Med. 2022;29(6):431-6.
7. Li G, Lin J, Liu Y, Yang Q, Tong Z, Ke L, et al. Ultrasound-assisted versus endoscopic nasojejunal tube placement for acute pancreatitis: A retrospective feasibility study. Gastroenterol Res Pract. 2021;2021:4903241.
8. Slingerland-Boot R, Bouw-Ruiter M, van Manen C, Arbous S, van Zanten A. Video-assisted placement of enteral feeding tubes using the Integrated Real-Time Imaging System (IRIS)-technology in critically ill patients. Clin Nutr. 2021;40(8):5000-7.
9. Hahn M, Byham-Gray L, Samavat H, Roberts S, Brody R. Small-bore feeding tubes placed with an electromagnetic imaging device leads to cost avoidance and decreased time to initiation of enteral nutrition. Nutr Clin Pract. 2023;1-10.
10. Reddick CA, Greaves JR, Flaherty JE, Callihan LE, Larimer CH, Allen SA. Choosing wisely: enteral feeding tube selection, placement, and considerations before and beyond the procedure room. Nutr Clin Pract. 2023;38:216-39.
11. Rajan A, Wangrattanapranee P, Kessler J, Kidambi TD, Tabibian JH. Gastrostomy tubes: Fundamentals, periprocedural considerations, and best practices. World J Gastrointest Surg. 2022;14(4):286-303.
12. Ah-San P, Soon-Teck H, Maetani I. A simple gastropexy for the loop-gastrostomy tube. J Minim Access Surg. 2012;8(4):154-5.
13. Stayner JL, Bhatnagar A, McGinn AN, Fang JC. Feeding tube placement: errors and complications. Nutr Clin Pract. 2012;27(6):738-48.

CHAPTER 15

Initiation, Maintenance, and Progression of Enteral Feeds

Urvi Shukla, Arti Bhalerao, Anuja Phalle

INTRODUCTION

Critically ill patients have physiological and metabolic changes in response to their illness. Though they may be protective, they increase the risk of malnutrition. Several ancient physicians, like Hippocrates and Celsius, prescribed certain foods to their patients in convalescence.[1] Scientific interest in feeding patients started in the first half of the 20th century. Techniques for gastrointestinal (GI) tract access began to improve, and by the 1950s, significant changes in refined feeds developed, such as feeds for astronauts and the production of elementary diets. Over the last 30 years, we have seen a consistent development in enteral nutrition (EN). Special organ-specific diets, improvements in feeding tubes such that they are now thinner and more comfortable, use of calorimetry to decide the requirement of caloric intake, and improved access to the gut via surgical or endoscopic route have all promoted enteral feeding.[2]

Malnutrition is a consequence of acute illness and hospitalization. Almost 40–60% of patients admitted to intensive care units (ICUs) have a severe risk of malnutrition.[3,4] Evidence suggests that critically ill patients with malnutrition (macronutrient and micronutrient deficiency) suffer from increased infectious morbidity, prolonged hospital stay, and increased mortality.[4] Even hospitalized medical and surgical patients without malnutrition are typically subjected to stress resulting in a hypercatabolic state. This is characterized by increased protein breakdown leading to a loss of lean body mass, poor wound healing, and unfavorable outcomes. This breakdown of lean body mass is not entirely suppressed by protein and energy intake. Additionally, there may be extreme degrees of lipid and glucose intolerance. Under these circumstances, providing adequate and optimal nutrition support to the critically ill is a challenge.

GOAL OF NUTRITION SUPPORT

Nutrition support has become a routine and essential part of the care of critically ill patients. The main goal of nutrition support is to provide an optimum amount of nutrients to prevent malnutrition from becoming the leading cause of morbidity and mortality in the disease process. The other goals include:
- Improve nutrition assessment indices
- Prevent single and multiple nutrient deficiencies
- Promote organ integrity and function
- Modify inflammatory response to disease
- Prevent complications associated with nutritional support
- Positively influence the patient outcomes.

Nutrition Assessment

The American Society for Parenteral and Enteral Nutrition (ASPEN) recommends that all patients admitted to ICU should have a nutritional assessment and risk screening. This helps to assess nutritional status and prescribe personalized nutritional interventions. Subjective global assessment (SGA) is a valuable assessment tool developed by the Canadian Malnutrition Task Force. It is a simple bedside test used to diagnose malnutrition and identify those who would benefit most from nutrition care. The assessment includes taking a history of recent intake, weight change, GI symptoms, and a clinical evaluation. SGA has been validated in a variety of patient populations.

"Nutrition Risk Screening 2002" (NRS 2002), the "Malnutrition Universal Screening Tool" (MUST), the "Nutrition Risk in the Critically Ill" score (NUTRIC score) or mNUTRIC (modified NUTRIC) are some of the nutritional risk scores.[5] According to a systematic review of nutritional risk scores, the mNUTRIC score was the most commonly used score. This was followed by NRS 2002 and NUTRIC. The use of risk scoring was associated with better identification of patients with nutrition risk, preexisting malnutrition, better-individualized nutrition therapy, and better achievement of nutritional targets.[5] mNUTRIC is the first nutritional risk assessment score validated across diverse ICU populations. It scores from 0 to 9, with 0 being no risk at all, and 9 being maximum nutrition risk. Patients who score >5 benefits the most from aggressive nutritional therapy.[6] This is a slight modification from the original NUTRIC score that used interleukin-6 (IL-6) as a marker of inflammation. It was observed that very few ICUs monitored IL-6 levels, and hence this variable was dropped from the modified NUTRIC score.[7] Anthropometric measurements such as albumin, pre-albumin levels, and transferrin are acute phase reactants and do not accurately reflect nutritional status in critically ill patients.[8] Specific experimental assessment tools are available but not validated: (A) individual calcitonin levels, C-reactive protein (CRP), interleukin-1, interleukin-6, and citrulline; (B) ultrasound to measure muscle mass and evaluate muscle tissue changes; and (C) computed tomography (CT) scan to assess for adipose deposits.

Determination of Energy Needs

Resting energy expenditure (REE) can be calculated using predictive equations, indirect calorimetry (IC), or simple weight-based formula. More than 200 predictive equations have been tested; however, their accuracy is very low when applied to patients with different characteristics than what they were designed for. They are also inaccurate in obese or underweight patients.

Indirect calorimetry is a gold standard in determining energy expenditure and caloric needs. It helps to monitor nutrition variation over time and to individualize nutrition prescriptions similar to personalized medicine or goal-directed therapy. The latest models of IC are smaller, able to analyze oxygen consumption (VO_2), and carbon dioxide production (VCO_2) on a breath-by-breath basis, and are relatively accurate in critical situations. However, their uptake into ICUs is limited due to costs and awareness. TICACOS study showed that providing nutrition to critically ill patients guided by IC reduced 60-day mortality per protocol analysis.[9] In a systematic review published in 2021,[10] IC-guided therapy significantly reduced short-term mortality, but there were no differences in ICU/hospital length of stay (LOS) and duration of mechanical ventilation. However, the trials enrolled in the review were judged of moderate quality. Even though the European Society of Parenteral and Enteral Nutrition (ESPEN) has now graded a weak recommendation to use IC in guiding nutritional needs, the simple weight-based formula has gained popularity for its simplicity and relative noninferiority, i.e., 25 kcal/kg/day.[11] In patients who have undergone aggressive resuscitation or presented with edema, actual dry or pre-morbid weight may be used to calculate caloric requirements. In obese patients [body mass index (BMI) >30], the adjusted body weight is used to calculate nutritional needs.

Adjusted body weight
= Actual body weight – ideal body weight
× 0.25 + ideal body weight
(Ideal body weight = Male: 49 kg + 6
× number of inches over 5 feet tall
Female: 45 kg + 5 × number of inches
over 5 feet tall)

Process of Enteral Nutrition/Feeds

"Enteral feeding" refers to the nutrition supplied through the GI tract using a tube or stoma. Enteral feed is considered for all hospitalized patients who cannot eat or reach their nutrition goals due to a variety of clinical conditions (Flowchart 1). The use of the GI tract for feeding helps in preserving intestinal mucosal integrity, barrier function, and immunologic function and attenuates the catabolic response.[8] It is preferred over the parenteral route due to its benefits and ease of use. A systematic review and meta-analysis of randomized controlled trails (RCT) suggested that enteral feeding was significantly associated with a reduced number of infections and related complications and reduced ICU LOS compared to parenteral nutrition (PN).[12] Enteral feeding can be 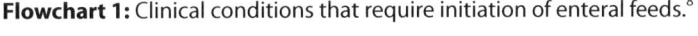 prepyloric or postpyloric.[13]

■ MODES OF ENTERAL FEEDING

Access for the enteral route can be obtained by nasogastric, orogastric, nasoenteric, percutaneous endoscopic gastrostomy (PEG), percutaneous endoscopic gastrojejunostomy, or jejunostomy tubes (Fig. 1). The latter three are short surgical or endoscopic procedures. For EN <30 days, nasogastric or

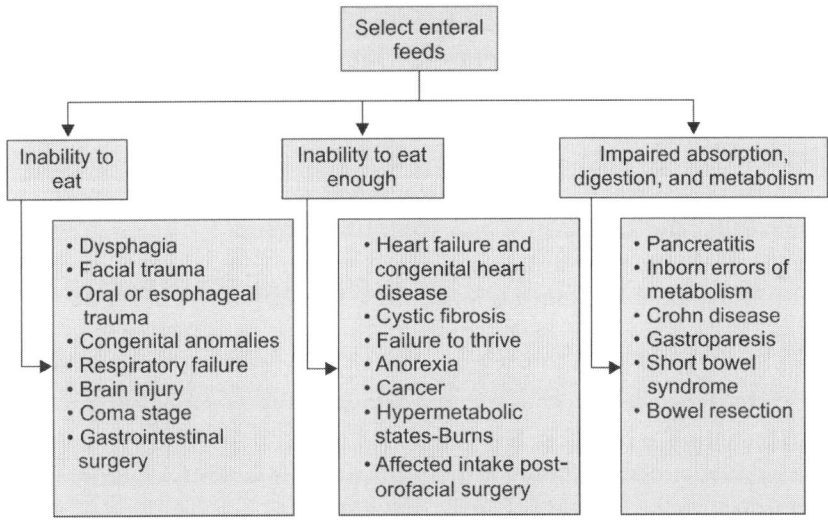

Flowchart 1: Clinical conditions that require initiation of enteral feeds.[8]

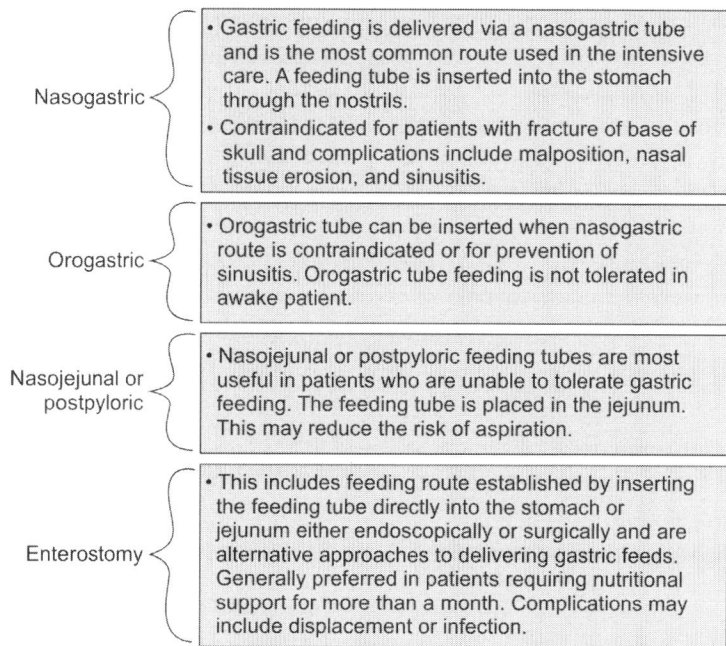

Fig. 1: Describes the various enteral access available for nutrition delivery.

nasoenteric tubes are preferred in patients with a functional GI tract, and gastric feeds are well tolerated. Sometimes, critically ill patients may have gastroparesis causing delays in transit across the pylorus. This may lead to high gastric residual volumes and associated complications such as vomiting, aspiration, and delay in achieving target daily nutrition. However, prepyloric feeding has the advantage of a more physiologic form. The stomach has a tremendous reservoir to tolerate large volumes; it helps in glucose homeostasis and allows flexibility in the composition and manner of tube feeding. Gastric feeding can be a bolus or a continuous infusion. Bolus feeding resembles more physiologic feeding, is associated with peaks and troughs of insulin secretion, and helps in stomach contractility.[14]

Postpyloric feeding is feeding beyond the pylorus, i.e., duodenum, jejunum, or the small intestine (distal to the ligament of Treitz ideally). Tube placement is difficult, making postpyloric feeding uncommon. Postpyloric feeding has a presumed advantage in patients with severe risk of aspiration, patients with emesis, patients who are intolerant of gastric feeding, and those with major surgery or trauma. Postpyloric feeding helps to achieve nutritional targets quickly as it is associated with reduced gastric residual volumes and a sense of better tolerance.[14] However, the incidence of pneumonia with prepyloric and postpyloric feeding was the same. Also, there was no difference in mortality between the two groups.[15]

ENTERAL FEEDING COMPOSITION

Before selecting an enteral formula for feeding a critically ill patient, it is worth knowing the types of enteral formulae, as >100 formulations are available. Selecting the appropriate formula may be confusing at times.[16]

Polymeric Formula

These are also known as standard diets and can be used as a source of nutrition in critically ill individuals with normal GI function. They provide nitrogen as whole protein casein, egg white solids, or soy protein. Carbohydrates are provided as corn syrup, maltodextrins, or glucose oligosaccharides. Fat is usually provided as soya, safflower, or canola oil. These are available in concentrations of 1–2 kcal/mL. Protein content differs from 40 to 100 g/L. Some polymeric formulae may have a combination of soluble and insoluble fiber, and some may be fiber free.

For patients who are hemodynamically unstable and at risk for developing bowel ischemia, the use of fiber-containing formulae should be avoided. Standard formulae do not have enough proteins to meet the increased protein requirements in critically ill patients.[17]

Oligomeric Formula

These are also termed as "elemental" or "semi-elemental diets". Oligomeric diets are predigested and are formulated to require minimal digestion by the GI tract. They provide nitrogen as oligopeptides from partially hydrolyzed whole protein or crystalline amino acids. Carbohydrates tend to be provided as glucose oligosaccharides. Fat is present as 2–4% of total calories as linoleic acid and medium chain triglycerides (MCT) is added to some formulae. Some formulations provide micronutrients such as vitamin C, D, and E, selenium, and omega-3 fatty acids.[17]

Oligomeric formulae may be used in patients with malabsorption, reduced absorptive area post-GI surgery, chyle leak, pancreatic dysfunction, severe malnutrition, and hypoalbuminemia with resultant gut edema and malabsorption or who have shown intolerance to standard feeds.

Immune-modulating Formula

These formulae comprise pharmacologically active substances aiming to modulate the immune response. These are not recommended for routine use in critically ill patients; however, they may have benefits in specific clinical conditions such as surgical patients.[18]

Disease-specific Formula

The disease-specific or organ-specific formulae are available that cater to the unique nutritional needs of patients. Special diets are available for conditions such as liver disease, diabetes, GI conditions, pulmonary disease, renal disease, stress, and immunomodulatory formulae for conditions like sepsis and trauma. **Flowchart 2** demonstrates the nutritional composition of disease-specific formulae.[19]

In a critical care setting, standard diets that are isotonic or near isotonic solutions providing 1–1.5 kcal/mL are considered appropriate and are well tolerated. Immune-modulating formulae may be used in a surgical setting postoperatively. Disease-specific and energy-dense (2 kcal/mL) formulae may be used in a personalized situation where it may benefit managing the electrolyte imbalances and providing nutrition when patients are on volume restrictions.[7]

While prescribing EN therapy, it is essential to consider the time of delivery, delivery route, composition, the ratio of the energy substrate to protein, and associated comorbid conditions and tolerance. Patients on enteral feeding will require regular monitoring of the response to the therapy and tailoring the nutrition therapy if clinical conditions demand.

■ INITIATION OF ENTERAL FEEDS

The oral/enteral route is preferred in all hospitalized and critically ill patients.

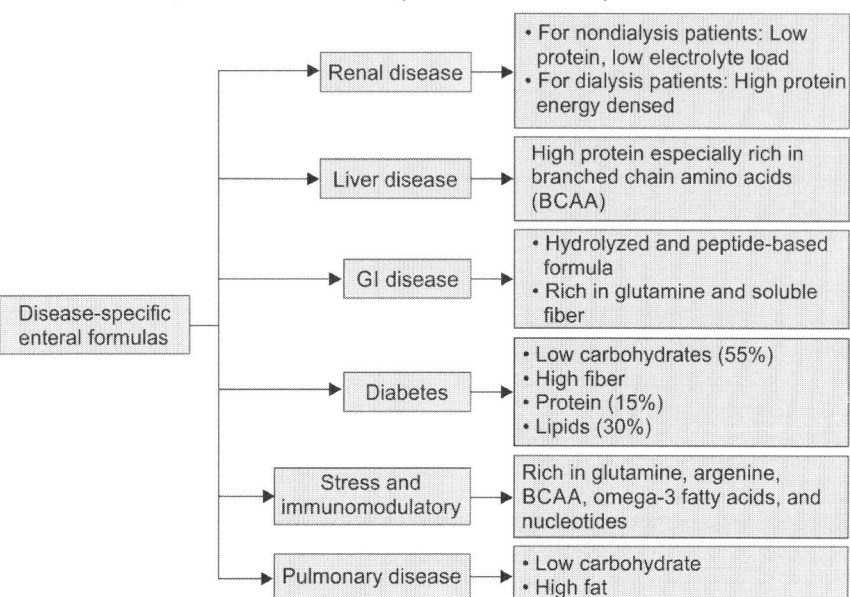

Flowchart 2: Nutritional composition of disease-specific formulae.

EN can be initiated once the appropriate access is established and the patient is hemodynamically stable. The formulation, composition, delivery strategy, and delivery rate are the important factors to be documented when prescribing nutrition.[20,21] There is very sketchy evidence as to the timing of initiation. The most recent guidelines from ASPEN suggest initiating EN for a patient with high nutritional risk or a malnourished patient within 24–48 hours of admission to the hospital. For patients who are morbidly well-nourished or are considered low risk for malnutrition and are expected to resume oral intake, EN can be delayed for 5–7 days. These patients have no recommendations for specialized nutrition therapy.

In ICU patients with shock, early up to target EN may suggest harm. In a French study, 2,410 patients randomized to target (25 kcal/kg) EN early or PN were studied. All these patients were mechanically ventilated and on vasopressor support. EN was associated with a small but significantly higher incidence of bowel ischemia and other GI complications like vomiting. There was no difference in outcomes concerning ventilatory days, ICU LOS, or mortality. The French study focused on the vasopressor dose at which the risk of bowel ischemia would be more evident. It did not necessarily say early target EN was associated with bowel ischemia. In other studies, the incidence of bowel ischemia is <1% of patients with shock. Hence, current recommendations state that vasopressor use is not a contraindication to start EN.[22,23]

Physicians usually start EN when the vasopressor dose and hemodynamic status have stabilized. There is no recommendation as to what constitutes a high dose of vasopressors to withhold EN. Doses up to 17.5 µg norepinephrine equivalent per minute have been tolerated with no sign of bowel ischemia. Assumed risk factors for inducing bowel ischemia include under-resuscitated patients, gut hypoperfusion without overt shock, a lactate level of >2 mmol/L, and a rapid increase of EN to target caloric needs.[24]

In patients who demonstrate signs of early EN intolerance (vomiting and large gastric residual volumes), the quantity of feed needs to be reduced. The amount of EN tolerated before signs of intolerance becomes the new daily target. This may mean they will have an energy-caloric gap that may need to be filled using alternative methods. Forcefully feeding patients to meet energy-caloric targets can lead to harm or increased risk of nonocclusive bowel ischemia. Oren Zusman studied patient outcomes with increasing percentage administered calories (%adcal) to REE, i.e., %adcal/REE.[25] The hazard ratio was 0.98 when administered calories increased from 0 to 70%, i.e., reduced mortality. However, increases above 70% showed a hazard ratio of 1.01, i.e., increasing mortality. Here we suggest that for patients in shock or recovering from the shock, it may be prudent to target hypocaloric feeds.[2,7,22] Increasing protein supplementation and hypocaloric feeding were associated with reduced mortality.[25]

In summary, initiation of EN in critically ill patients should target a caloric intake of 15 kcal/kg/day and a protein intake of 0.8–1 g/kg/day **(Flowchart 3)**. Even hypocaloric feeding (500 kcal/day) with adequate protein (1 g/kg/day protein) intake in the

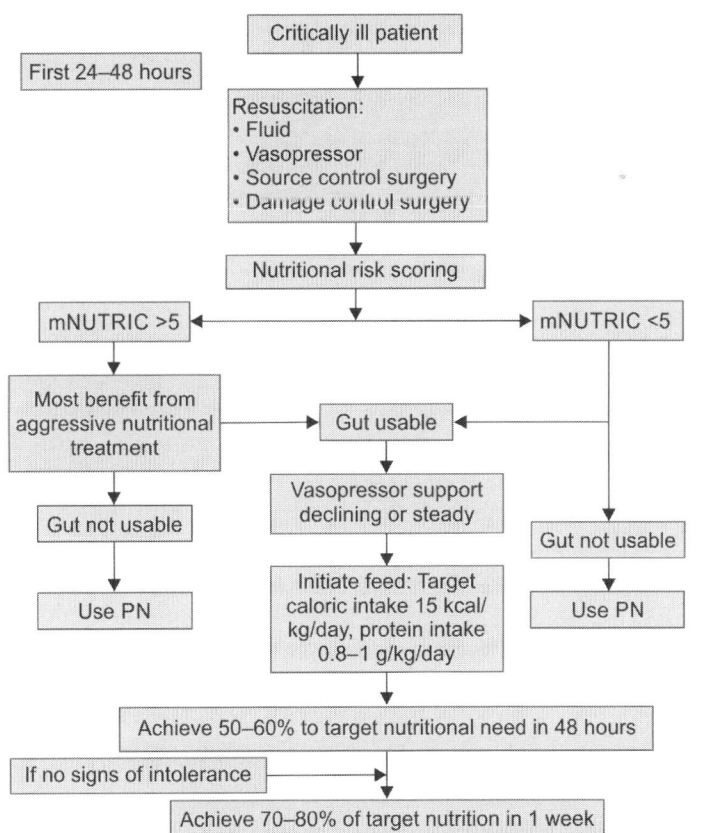

Flowchart 3: Initiation of enteral feeds.

(mNUTRIC: modified Nutrition Risk in Critically Ill; PN: parenteral nutrition) early phase of ICU admission has shown similar outcomes compared to high-energy feeds.[26,27]

Once the acute resuscitation phase is over, which may take 4–5 days, and feed tolerance is established, caloric intake can be increased to target daily requirements. This may not be justified for patients who have mNUTRIC score >5 at ICU admission. These patients have very low or nil metabolic reserve to tolerate hypocaloric feeds in the first week, and supplemental PN may have to be considered.[28]

PROGRESSION AND MAINTENANCE OF ENTERAL FEEDS

Once the critically ill patient has safely crossed the phase of acute resuscitation that usually lasts 0–4 days, EN should be escalated over the next 48 hours to achieve protein-calorie targets. This would include protein of 1.2–2 g/kg/day and an energy target of 25 kcal/kg/day.

Achieving this goal reduces loss of lean body mass, improves functional recovery, and assists with early mobilization.[28]

Enteral nutrition should aim to provide >80% of energy goals except for patients at risk for refeeding syndrome or GI intolerance. Protein calorie deficiencies beyond the 1st week are associated with increased mortality and poor functional outcomes at 3–6 months post-ICU stay.[5]

Minnesota Starvation Study is a landmark study conducted at the end of World War II. It is a seminal study that defines the nutritional needs to recover from severe weight loss or loss of lean body mass following sepsis. It showed that fasting healthy volunteers with significant weight loss needed up to 5,000 kcal/day for 6 months to 2 years to regain lost lean body mass. Maintenance feeds of post-ICU survivors should address this ongoing need for high-calorie protein supplementation to improve functional recovery.[29]

Maintaining and progressing EN to total targeted nutrition need to be done aggressively. Critical illness leads to hypercatabolism and severe protein losses that continue beyond the first 2 weeks. The International Nutrition Survey conducted regularly by the Canadian Critical Care Nutrition group reveals that the average caloric intake for the first 12 days of ICU admission is a poor 1,034 kcal with 47 g of proteins.[30] They found protein-energy deficiency by delivery of hypocaloric feeds continues well into the 2nd week and beyond. Methods to improve EN delivery using prokinetic agents like metoclopramide or erythromycin, or postpyloric feeding have not shown additional benefits in improving delivery of EN. New guidelines recommend abandoning measurement of gastric residual volume (GRV), OR using target GRV >500 mL before feeds are stopped to help improve EN delivery and reduce the incidence of iatrogenic malnutrition.[7]

At discharge from ICU, these patients should continue to get EN targeted for replacing lean body mass and functional recovery. As patients mobilize, their metabolic demands will increase, and energy requirements can exceed 4,000 kcal/day with protein needs of 1.2–2 g/kg/day. This heightened nutrition may have to continue for months to help patients recover to any meaningful life. To reach this target, oral nutritional supplements, and EN must be continued for months.[31]

CONCLUSION

Feeding patients through their critical illness is necessary for survival and ensuring a good quality of life post-ICU care. We need to understand the varying needs of these patients as they travel through their illness, and nutrition delivery should appropriately target various phases of critical illness. Early hypocaloric feeding is acceptable, but the inability to increase feeding in convalescence amounts to negligence and is a potential iatrogenic cause of poor quality of life. We should aim to produce survivors of critical illness and not victims.

REFERENCES

1. Harborview Medical Center. ENTERAL FEEDING GUIDELINES. [online] Available from: http://merinco.vn/Data/upload/files/t%C3%A0i%20li%E1%BB%87u%20c%C3%B4ng%20ty/KANGUROO/Enteral_Feeding_Guidelines.pdf. [Last accessed June, 2023].
2. Bechtold ML, Brown PM, Escuro A, Grenda B, Johnston T, Kozeniecki M, et al. When is enteral nutrition indicated? JPEN J Parenter Enteral Nutr. 2022;46(7):1470-96.
3. Vavruk AM, Martins C, Mazza do Nascimento M. Validation of malnutrition clinical characteristics in critically ill patients. Nutr Clin Pract. 2021;36(5):993-1002.
4. Hejazi N, Mazloom Z, Zand F, Rezaianzadeh A, Amini A. Nutritional assessment in critically ill patients. Iranian J Med Sci. 2016;41(3):171-9.
5. Heyland DK, Dhaliwal R, Jiang X, Day AG. Identifying critically ill patients who benefit the most from nutrition therapy: the development and initial validation of a novel risk assessment tool. Crit Care. 2011;15:1-1.
6. Rahman A, Hasan RM, Agarwala R, Martin C, Day AG, Heyland DK. Identifying critically-ill patients who will benefit most from nutritional therapy: further validation of the "modified NUTRIC" nutritional risk assessment tool. Clin Nutr. 2016;35(1):158-62.
7. McClave SA, Taylor BE, Martindale RG, Warren MM, Johnson DR, Braunschweig C, et al. Guidelines for the provision and assessment of nutrition support therapy in the adult critically ill patient: Society of Critical Care Medicine (SCCM) and American Society for Parenteral and Enteral Nutrition (ASPEN). JPEN J Parenter Enteral Nutr. 2016;40(2):159-211.
8. Elke G, van Zanten AR, Lemieux M, McCall M, Jeejeebhoy KN, Kott M, et al. Enteral versus parenteral nutrition in critically ill patients: an updated systematic review and meta-analysis of randomized controlled trials. Crit care (London, England). 2016;20(1):117.
9. Duan JY, Zheng WH, Zhou H, Xu Y, Huang HB. Energy delivery guided by indirect calorimetry in critically ill patients: a systematic review and meta-analysis. Crit Care. 2021;25:88.
10. Cerra FB, Benitez MR, Blackburn GL, Irwin RS, Jeejeebhoy K, Katz DP, et al. Applied nutrition in ICU patients: a consensus statement of the American College of Chest Physicians. Chest. 1997;111(3):769-78.
11. Hoffer LJ, Bistrian BR. Appropriate protein provision in critical illness: a systematic and narrative review. Am J Clin Nutr. 2012;96(3):591-600.
12. Ahmad A, Duerksen DR, Munroe S, Bistrian BR. An evaluation of resting energy expenditure in hospitalized, severely underweight patients. Nutrition. 1999;15(5):384-8.
13. Jabbar A, McClave SA. Pre-pyloric versus post-pyloric feeding. Clin Nutr. 2005;24(5):719-26.
14. Boulton-Jones JR, Lewis J, Jobling JC, Teahon K. Experience of post-pyloric feeding in seriously ill patients in clinical practice. Clin Nutr. 2004;23(1):35-41.
15. Heyland DK. Canadian Critical Care Clinical Practice Guidelines Committee: Canadian clinical practice guidelines for nutrition support in mechanically ventilated, critically ill adult patients. JPEN J Parenter Enteral Nutr. 2003;27:355-73.
16. Yeh DD, Velmahos GC. Disease-specific nutrition therapy: one size does not fit all. Eur J Trauma Emerg Surg. 2013;39:215-33.
17. Mueller CM, McClave SA, Kuhn JM. The ASPEN adult nutrition support core curriculum. (No Title). 2017.
18. Blaauw R, Du Toit AL. Case Study: Enteral formula: Selecting the right formula for your patient. South African J Clin Nutr. 2017;30(2):39-45.

19. Zadák Z, Kent-Smith L. Basics in clinical nutrition: Commercially prepared formulas. e-SPEN, the European e-Journal of Clinical Nutrition and Metabolism. 2009;4(5): e212-5.
20. Preiser JC, Arabi YM, Berger MM, Casaer M, McClave S, Montejo-González JC, et al. A guide to enteral nutrition in intensive care units: 10 expert tips for the daily practice. Crit Care. 2021;25(1):1-3.
21. Indian Dietetics Association. Nutrition Support in the Critically ill: Enteral Nutrition, Adults. In: Indian Dietetics Association (Ed). Clinical Dietetics Manual, 2nd edition. New Delhi: Elite Publishing House; 2018. p. 135.
22. Reignier J, Boisrame-Helms J, Brisard L, Lascarrou JB, Hssain AA, Anguel N, et al. Enteral versus parenteral early nutrition in ventilated adults with shock: a randomised, controlled, multicentre, open-label, parallel-group study (NUTRIREA-2). Lancet. 2018; 391(10116):133-43.
23. Reintam Blaser A, Starkopf J, Alhazzani W, Berger MM, Casaer MP, Deane AM, et al. Early enteral nutrition in critically ill patients: ESICM clinical practice guidelines. Intensive Care Med. 2017;43:380-98.
24. Singer P, Rattanachaiwong S. Editorial on "enteral versus parenteral early nutrition in ventilated adults with shock: a randomised, controlled, multicentre, open-label, parallel-group study (NUTRIREA-2)". J Thorac Dis. 2018;10(Suppl 9):S974.
25. Zusman O, Theilla M, Cohen J, Kagan I, Bendavid I, Singer P. Resting energy expenditure, calorie and protein consumption in critically ill patients: a retrospective cohort study. Crit Care. 2016;20(1):1-8.
26. Arabi YM, Aldawood AS, Haddad SH, Al-Dorzi HM, Tamim HM, Jones G, et al. Permissive underfeeding or standard enteral feeding in critically ill adults. N Engl J Med. 2015;372(25):2398-408.
27. Arabi YM, Al-Dorzi HM. Trophic or full nutritional support. Curr Opin Crit Care. 2018;24(4):262-8.
28. Wischmeyer PE. Nutrition therapy in sepsis. Crit Care Clin. 2018;34(1):107-25.
29. Keys A, Brožek J, Henschel A, Mickelsen O, Taylor HL. The biology of human starvation (2 vols). Minneapolis: University of Minnesota Press; 1950.
30. Alberda C, Gramlich L, Jones N, Jeejeebhoy K, Day AG, Dhaliwal R, et al. The relationship between nutritional intake and clinical outcomes in critically ill patients: results of an international multicenter observational study. Intensive Care Med. 2009;35:1728-37.
31. Puthucheary ZA, Wischmeyer P. Predicting critical illness mortality and personalizing therapy: moving to multi-dimensional data. Crit Care. 2017;21(1):1-2.

CHAPTER 16

Monitoring and Management of Complications of Enteral Nutrition

Deven Juneja, Anjali Mishra

INTRODUCTION

In the past few decades, numerous studies have been done establishing the superiority of enteral nutrition (EN) over parenteral nutrition (PN). EN plays a significant role in preserving gut integrity (hence reducing antigenic leak and inflammation), mucosal architecture, gut-associated lymphoid tissue, and immune functions.[1] Hence, it is considered safer than PN, but it has its own set of complications. These can be broadly classified as mechanical, gastrointestinal, metabolic, and infectious. Although critically ill cases are most likely to benefit from EN, they are also the ones who may face maximum challenges in tolerating the enteral feeds and suffer from life-threatening metabolic complications on receiving full nutritional support. Hence, the gradual introduction of titrated feeds and prior knowledge of the anticipated complications can greatly aid in the process of prevention, early recognition, and management of these complications. The management of complications associated with enteral feeding depends on the specific complication and its severity. However, there are some general principles that can be followed to prevent and manage these complications.

All patients should be evaluated as potential candidates for enteral feeding, at the earliest, after assessing the gastrointestinal tract function and ruling out the presence of nausea, vomiting, and gastrointestinal dysfunction in the form of ileus or malabsorption. Any recent history of alimentary tract surgery or injury should also be taken into consideration. Any trauma at the site of tube placement, head trauma, or facial bone fracture is a relative contraindication to nasoesophageal tube insertion. The patient's ability to withstand sedation and surgical procedure should be assessed before planning a surgical tube placement. The clotting parameters may be deranged in many critically ill patients, especially in those with underlying renal or liver disease.[2] Hemodynamics play an important role in determining gut perfusion and motility. Compromised intestinal perfusion in hemodynamically unstable patients can result in mucosal injury and exacerbate the loss of gut barrier function. The mesenteric blood flow may be compromised in a hypotensive state which may further contribute to intestinal ischemia.[3] Lastly, the patient's gag reflex, swallowing ability, level of consciousness, and ability to guard the upper airway should be thoroughly assessed as aspiration pneumonia is a serious and potentially fatal complication of enteral feeds, especially in critically ill patients.

It is also important to assess the patient's nutritional and medical status before initiating enteral feeding. This can help to identify any potential risk factors for complications and inform the choice of feeding route, formula, and delivery method. Clinical assessment and screening nutrition assessment are two commonly used methods to evaluate a patient's nutritional status and identify any nutritional deficiencies or risks before formulating the nutritional regimen. The assessment may also involve the use of nutritional screening tools, such as the subjective global assessment (SGA) or the Malnutrition Universal Screening Tool (MUST), to identify patients who may be at risk for malnutrition or who may require further nutritional evaluation. Screening nutrition assessment, on the other hand, is a quick and simple method to identify patients who may be at risk for malnutrition. This method involves the use of simple screening tools, such as the mini nutritional assessment (MNA) or the Nutritional Risk Screening (NRS-2002), to evaluate a patient's nutritional status based on factors such as weight loss, dietary intake, and functional status. Healthcare providers should consider using both methods in combination to ensure a comprehensive evaluation of a patient's nutritional status and to identify any potential metabolic complications that may arise from enteral feeding or other nutritional interventions.[4,5]

Healthcare providers should monitor patients regularly for signs and symptoms of any complications and should ensure proper placement and positioning of the feeding tube to prevent aspiration and tube-related complications. Implementation of an aseptic technique during tube insertion and care to minimize the risk of infection is highly recommended.

COMPLICATIONS OF ENTERAL FEEDING

Mechanical Complications

A significant proportion of hospitalized and even home care patients will require a conduit to deliver enteral feeds. These mechanical complications are generally secondary to these tubes used to deliver enteral feeds. These complications may further be classified as immediate and delayed **(Table 1)**. The immediate complications may occur at the time of tube insertion or immediately after the procedure. These include malposition, local trauma, bleeding and even aspiration if airway is not secure. Delayed complications may develop over a period of time and may include accidental dislodgment, leakage from the tube, and ulceration at the site of insertion

TABLE 1: Mechanical complications associated with enteral feeding.

Type of tubes	Time of complication	Complications	Monitoring
Nasogastric or nasojejunal tubes	Immediate	• Local trauma • Bleeding • Malposition • Perforation	• Correct tube placement • Check chest X-ray
	Late/delayed	• Tube obstruction • Malposition • Accidental dislodgment of tube • Leakage • Erosion and ulceration at the insertion site • Nasogastric tube syndrome	• Tube patency • Check chest X-ray • Marking the exit site • Change in voice, hoarseness • Swelling or pain in neck/pharynx

Contd...

Contd...

Type of tubes	Time of complication	Complications	Monitoring
Percutaneous endoscopic gastrostomy	Acute	• Misplacement • Bleeding • Wound infection • Pneumoperitoneum ileus • Peristomal leakage	• Coagulopathy (INR and platelets) • Site inspection (swelling, redness, pus, bleeding, leak, and dislodgment)
	Chronic	• Gastrocutaneous fistulae • Tube blockage • Peristomal leakage • Dislodgment/removal • Wound infection • Bleeding • Buried bumper syndrome	• Check endoscopy • Patency of tube • Site inspection (swelling, redness, pus, bleeding, leak, and dislodgment)

or its tract.[6,7] Although with the advent of new fine bore soft and flexible tubes made with polyurethane and silicone, the rate of these mechanical complications has reduced. However, the usage of feeding tubes should be limited, ideally 4–6 weeks, depending on patient recovery.

To avoid tube obstruction, warm water should be used to flush the tube after feeding or after aspirating back from it. It is mandatory to ensure that the feeding tubes are flushed intermittently during brief interruptions in cases of continuous drips or infusions. Delivery of thick feeds and certain medications through small-sized tubes may also result in clogging, which can be dislodged by adequate warm saline flushes, with alternating pressure and suction. Although, it is preferable to deliver only liquid medications, viscous medications, and tablets can also be delivered safely after crushing and mixing with water. Tube occlusion can also occur as a result of drug-to-drug interaction causing precipitation of components and changes in formula consistency. Hence, simultaneous administration of multiple medications and enteral formulas should be avoided. There are various mechanical interventions such as endoscopic catheters or braided quid wires which may help to relieve obstruction, but should be used with extreme caution as they may potentially perforate the tube and injure the surrounding structures.[2] Sometimes, replacement of tube is the easiest and most viable option.

Premature tube removal by the patient and dislodgment can be avoided by selecting the right size and marking its exit point at the body, so that any tube migration from its original position can be picked up early. The blind insertion techniques have been a known cause of tube malposition in 0.5–16% of cases resulting in serious complications such as pneumothorax, pleural/pulmonary infusion of feeds, and pulmonary abscess.[8] It is therefore mandatory to check for the tube position immediately after insertion and ensure urgent correction, if needed. Confirming the correct tube placement using the air instillation and auscultation method is an inaccurate and unreliable method, particularly in patients with altered consciousness, diminished gag reflex or any neurological impairment. Hence, radiological verification of the tube is highly recommended. In the case of gastrostomy and enterostomy tubes, leaks into the peritoneal cavity can be checked by using contrast media.[9,10]

Rarely, patients on prolonged nasogastric tube feeding have been reported to develop nasogastric tube syndrome characterized by sudden and life-threatening vocal cord palsy with patients presenting with signs and symptoms of upper airway obstruction.[11] Generally, it is associated with bilateral vocal cord palsy, but cases with unilateral vocal cord palsy have also been reported.[12] It is thought to be secondary to posterior cricoarytenoid muscles paresis due to ulceration and infection. As it may be a life-threatening complication, any change in voice, hoarseness of voice or pharyngodynia, in a patient with nasogastric tube should be carefully investigated.[11,12]

Complications Associated with Percutaneous Endoscopic Gastrostomy

Patients in whom nasogastric or nasojejunal tubes are not feasible or contraindicated, may be fed enterally through percutaneous endoscopic gastrostomy (PEG). Although a relatively safe and minimally invasive procedure, PEG insertion has been reported to be associated with certain acute and chronic complications. Acute complications, defined as occurring within 7 days of the procedure, are usually intervention related and include bleeding, wound infection, pneumoperitoneum and ileus. Those occurring 7 days after the procedure are labeled as chronic complications, these include tube leakage, spontaneous removal, obstruction, recurrent aspiration pneumonia, and buried bumper syndrome, where the internal fixation device migrates and gets lodged between the skin and the gastric wall.

The risk of significant bleeding is low with an incidence of 2.67% and is attributed to local vessel injury and mucosal tears. The European Society of Gastrointestinal Endoscopy considers this procedure as high risk of bleeding and recommends coagulopathy correction before PEG insertion. The recommended threshold for the procedure is an international normalized ratio (INR) <1.5 and a platelet count of ≥50 000/μL.[13]

The incidence of peristomal wound infection after PEG placement is about 3–70% and is largely influenced by placement technique or the patient factors such as immunosuppressive state, steroid therapy, diabetes, malnutrition, or obesity. Apart from standard aseptic precautions of the surgical field, prophylactic antimicrobial therapy (penicillin or cephalosporin-based) 30 minutes before the procedure has been advocated to reduce the incidence of postoperative infections. In cases of potentially fatal infective wounds such as necrotizing fasciitis, surgical debridement with long-term antibiotic coverage may be essential.[14]

Peristomal leakage may be caused by a variety of factors, including improper tube placement, inadequate sealing of the stoma, or irritation of the skin around the stoma. Symptoms of peristomal leakage may include redness, irritation, and inflammation around the stoma, as well as leakage of fluid or stomach contents onto the skin. If left untreated, peristomal leakage can lead to infection, skin breakdown, and other complications. Treatment for peristomal leakage may include repositioning of the feeding tube, application of protective skin barriers or dressings, and use of medications to control inflammation or infection. In some cases, surgical revision of the stoma may be necessary.[6]

Gastrocutaneous fistulae are difficult to manage and occur due to misplacement of PEG or postgastrostomy removal. Clinically, it may present as watery diarrhea or stool around the site of the PEG insertion. Contrast injection aids in establishing the diagnosis. Management is usually conservative that may require PEG removal while awaiting spontaneous closure of fistulae. Surgical intervention including colonic exploration may rarely be required in severe cases.[14]

Gastrointestinal Complications

Gastrointestinal complications such as nausea, vomiting, diarrhea, constipation, and regurgitation are common with enteral feeds. Administering enteral feeds in large boluses, too rapidly or at the wrong temperature, are the usual causes of abdominal discomfort, especially in patients with preexisting gastrointestinal complaints or postsurgical patients.[2] Prior to the initiation of enteral feeds, every effort should be made to address these existing symptoms with antiemetics, prokinetics, and gastroprotectant drugs, as necessary. To prevent reflux and vomiting, the patient should be fed sitting upright at a minimum of 30–45° angle. Intravenous hydration and electrolyte replenishment should be appropriate, if the feeds are held due to nonacceptability. It is important to pay attention to the medications going on with the feeds as concurrent administration of some medications (including antibiotics, analgesics, antacids, oral magnesium or phosphate, and prokinetic agents) can exacerbate gastrointestinal issues that the patient is experiencing.[6]

Diarrhea is one of the most frequent complications of EN and is variably defined by indices such as volume of >200–300 g/day or frequency of more than three to five times in a day.[15] Diarrhea may be classified as infectious or noninfectious and the distinction is important as the treatment may vary. It may be precipitated by several factors including medications, rate of enteral feed administration, infection, poor tolerance to certain feeds and displacement of a feeding tube from the stomach to the small bowel. Some liquid medications containing hypertonic nonabsorbable sugar such as sorbitol can also precipitate diarrhea.[16] High-fat blenderized diets can cause steatorrhea in patients with poor fat digestion and malabsorption syndrome. Liquid diets are low residue and frequently result in soft stools, if not profuse diarrhea.[2] Oral and intravenous broad-spectrum antibiotics also contribute to the growth of diarrhea-causing organisms such as *Clostridium difficile* (*Pseudomembranous enteritis*), *Klebsiella* and *Escherichia coli*.

Compared to intermittent infusion, the incidence of diarrhea is less with continuous infusion. Other factors such as the composition of EN, including the percentage of carbohydrates, lipids and lactose, type of nitrogen source, percentage of dietary fibers, and osmotic pressure may also influence gut motility.[15]

Prolonged diarrhea can result in nutrient deficiency, malnutrition, and increased mortality. It can further cause a loss of effective circulatory volume, electrolyte abnormalities with loss of potassium, chloride, magnesium, and other essential elements, and metabolic acidosis with bicarbonate loss due to the excretion of digestive juices. Persistent diarrhea may also result in the contamination of surgical wounds and development of bed sores.[17] The factors to be considered in the management of feed-associated diarrhea have been summarized in **Box 1**.[18,19]

Other frequently reported complications of enteral feed include abdominal pain, distention, and constipation **(Table 2)**. Constipation can result from prolonged immobilization, decreased bowel motility, lack of fiber intake, impaction, and use of calorie-dense formulas with reduced water content. Prior history of irregular bowel movements and medication history should be thoroughly noted. Changes in the motility pattern, fluid, and fiber intake should also be taken into account. Constipation can often be misdiagnosed as bowel obstruction and needs to be clearly differentiated from the latter. Very often optimal hydration and the

> **BOX 1:** The factors to be considered in the management of feed-associated diarrhea.
> - Maintain a record of bowel frequency, consistency of stool and recent changes in the feeds. Rule out stool incontinence and constipation independent of feeding.
> - A stool culture may be considered to rule out infective etiology.
> - Any significant past medical history of preexisting bowel disease.
> - A planned break or alteration in the feeding schedule including decrease in the delivery rate may help to alleviate the symptoms.
> - Hydration and electrolyte replenishment is of prime importance.
> - Consider modifications to the feed regimens that may subside the symptoms gradually (such as reducing volume or concentration of feeds initially).
> - Addition of commercial mixed (soluble plus insoluble) fiber may help to reduce persistent diarrhea (should be avoided in patients at high risk for bowel ischemia, obstruction, and severe dysmotility).
> - A fermentable soluble fiber (such as insulin, fructooligosaccharides) can be added in the dose of 10–20 g over 24 hours as adjunctive therapy.
> - If malabsorption is suspected, consider switching to small peptide formulations.
> - If the symptoms continue, enteral nutrition should be interrupted and parenteral nutrition should be initiated.

TABLE 2: Nonmechanical complications associated with enteral feeding.

Type of complications	Complications	Monitoring
Gastrointestinal	• Nausea/vomiting diarrhea • Constipation, regurgitation • Abdominal distention or bloating	• Gastric residual volume • Monitor rate, volume, and frequency of feed • Monitor composition of feed • Liver function tests • Electrolytes • Stool color, consistency, and mucus • Infections (*Clostridium difficile*) • Concomitant medications • Frequency and amount of stools • Bowel sound auscultation • Measurement of abdominal girth • Assessment of abdominal distention • Chest X-ray/abdomen
Infectious	• Aspiration pneumonitis • Sinusitis • Peristomal cellulitis • Septic peritonitis • Infective diarrhea	• Gastric residual volume • Correct tube positioning • Bowel sound auscultation • Measurement of abdominal girth • Assessment of abdominal distention • Assessment for airway protection • Neurological status • Level of sedation • Bowel movement • Frequency and amount of stools • X-ray abdomen and sinuses

Contd...

Contd...

Type of complications	Complications	Monitoring
Metabolic	• Hyperglycemia • Hypoglycemia • Dyslipidemias • Dyselectrolytemia • Refeeding syndrome • Underfeeding • Overfeeding • Gut ischemia	• Blood glucose • Serum triglycerides • Serum electrolytes • Electrocardiograph • Intake/output • Calorie count • Protein count • Composition of feed • Nutritional screening • Serum lactates • Abdominal girth • Abdominal X-ray/CT scan

addition of insoluble fibers to the formulas can resolve the problem. However, persistent constipation may require using stool softeners and bowel stimulants.

About 20% of patients on enteral feeds suffer from nausea and vomiting with delayed gastric emptying being the most common cause. Conscious patients may complain of abdominal discomfort and a sense of bloating. In mechanically ventilated patients and those requiring sedation, intermittently interrupting the sedation can be considered. Administering prokinetic drugs, using the low-fat formula and decreasing the delivery rate may also help.[18]

Infectious Complications

Aspiration Pneumonia

Gastroesophageal reflux (GER), induced by gastroparesis, is a frequent cause of aspiration pneumonia. Critically ill patients who aspirate are at high risk for nosocomial pneumonia, which is then associated with an increased hospital stay, cost, and poor outcome. Intensive care unit (ICU) patients often have altered sensorium due to ongoing sedation or neurological diseases, which increases their risk for aspiration. ICU patients with a Glasgow Coma Scale (GCS) score of less than nine and those requiring a high level of sedation are particularly at risk. Tube-fed patients, especially with a lower GCS, are at significantly greater risk of microaspiration and recurrent aspiration.[20]

Whether microaspiration of EN increases the risk of aspiration pneumonia is still controversial. However, some chemical characteristics of the material aspirated influence the risk of developing pneumonia. Aspiration of highly acidic gastric contents may cause acute lung injury which is initially not infective, aspiration pneumonitis, but may potentially predispose the patient to secondary infection because of impaired bacterial clearance. The bacteria in the aspirate are frequently antibiotic-resistant and colonize the oropharynx. This process occurs commonly in patients on mechanical ventilation.[21]

Gastric residual volume (GRV) measurements have traditionally been used to monitor the risk of aspiration in ICU patients. A high GRV has often been used to reduce the rate of infusion or for temporary cessation of feeding. However, a clear cut-off value of GRV that indicates a high risk of aspiration has not been established. The recent guidelines on EN by Society of Critical Care Medicine (SCCM) and the American Society for Parenteral and Enteral Nutrition (ASPEN) published in 2016 do not suggest routine use of GRV for monitoring aspiration risk in ICU patients receiving EN. The guidelines suggest against holding EN for GRVs <500 mL in the absence of clinical signs of feed intolerance. However, GRVs in the range of 200–500 mL may be concerning in some patients and should lead to the implementation of measures and algorithmic approaches to decrease the risk of aspiration. Some alternative strategies can potentially be used to monitor ICU patients receiving EN. These include thorough daily physical examinations (such as bowel sound auscultation, measurement of abdominal girth, and assessment of abdominal distension), evaluating risk factors for aspiration and reviewing abdominal radiologic films and scans, when needed.[19,22]

A stepwise approach is required in patients on enteral feed to reduce the aspiration risk. Good oral care, regular assessment of tolerance and tube position, and the head end of the bed elevation to >30–45° play a key role in prevention of aspiration.[23] Recent guidelines published by the American College of Gastroenterology (ACG) have recommended slower feeding into the stomach and postpyloric feeding (although technically difficult) as a measure for gastroparesis management.[24] An alternative with the placement of a feeding tube into the small bowel, with the tip below the ligament of Treitz, has also been successfully studied. The institutions where small bowel access can easily be attained, the Canadian Clinical Practice Guidelines recommend routine use of small bowel feeding especially in high-risk patients.[25,26] The ASPEN authors, however, advise against the routine use of jejunal feeding and recommend it only for critically ill patients with gastric feed intolerance.[26]

A Japanese study reported that feeding with new formulas that have high viscosity may suppress GER. These formulas, depending on the stomach pH, can change phase from liquid to semisolid and can be administered via smaller-sized tubes as well.[27] An elemental diet formula which has rapid pyloric transit and may potentially reduce aspiration risk, but may lead to a higher risk of diarrhea.[28]

Prokinetic agents have shown some benefits in patients with gastroparesis. The North American Summit recommends prokinetic drugs in cases with more than two major risk factors for aspiration **(Table 3)**.[29] ASPEN and the Canadian Guidelines recommend consideration of metoclopramide to improve motility in

TABLE 3: Risk factors for aspiration defined by the North American Summit.	
Major risk factors	**Other risk factors**
Altered sensorium and decreased level of consciousness	Noncontinuous or intermittent feeding
Previous history of episodes of aspiration	Poor oral care
Persistently high gastric residual volume	Abdominal/thoracic surgery
Delayed gastric emptying	Traumatic injury
Known structural abnormality of the aerodigestive tract or neuromuscular disease	Presence of a nasoenteric tube
Malpositioned feeding tube	Large size and diameter of feeding tube
Persistent vomiting	Advanced age
Endotracheal intubation	Transportation
Supine positioning	Inadequate nursing staff

patients experiencing feed intolerance, as evident by emesis and high GRV. However, routine use of metoclopramide in all patients receiving enteral feed has not been shown to alter the frequency of nosocomial pneumonia or have any mortality benefit. Metoclopramide antagonizes the inhibitory effects of dopamine on gastric contractility and its side effect profile has concerns for dystonias and tardive dyskinesia. Erythromycin promotes gastric emptying by stimulating motilin receptors, however, its use has not been promoted much because of the concern of inducing antibiotic resistance. Cisapride was withdrawn from the market because of the risk of lethal arrhythmias.[23]

Rhinosinusitis

Prolonged presence of nasogastric tube in a particular nostril may impede sinus drainage by blockage of the osteomeatal complex.[30] This may result in sinusitis, which if not promptly recognized and treated, may lead to ascending infection and bone erosion. Hence, it may be prudent to change the side whenever nasogastric tube is being replaced, in patients requiring long-term nasogastric feeding.

Other Infectious Complications

Other infectious complications associated with EN include contamination of feeding formula, peristomal cellulitis, or septic peritonitis. Contamination can be avoided by practicing basic hygiene measures. Commercial liquid diets should be kept under refrigeration and discarded after 2 days and blenderized diets have to be prepared daily. The cleaning and maintenance of devices used for preparation and delivery should be thoroughly checked. Peristomal cellulitis is usually a complication of gastrostomy, esophagostomy, or jejunostomy tubes. This complication can be avoided by making sure that the site is cleaned, and sterile and the tubes are not secured too tightly to the body wall.[2]

Metabolic Complications

Dysglycemias are the most common metabolic complications of EN. Both hypo- and hyperglycemia can occur, particularly in patients with diabetes or impaired glucose tolerance. Enteral feeding solutions may contain high levels of glucose, which can lead to elevated blood glucose (BG) levels and insulin resistance. This can be especially problematic in patients with diabetes, who may require additional insulin to regulate their BG levels. Patients receiving enteral feeding should be closely monitored for signs of hyperglycemia, such as frequent urination, excessive thirst, and blurry vision. Regular BG monitoring and adjustment of the feeding regimen may be necessary to prevent or manage hyperglycemia in these patients. In some cases, the use of specialized enteral feeding solutions with lower levels of glucose or the addition of insulin to the feeding regimen may be necessary to prevent hyperglycemia.[2,31] Continuous, instead of intermittent feeding, may help in reducing glycemic variability.

Refeeding Syndrome

Refeeding syndrome (RFS) is a potentially life-threatening metabolic complication that can occur in patients who have severe muscle wasting due to prolonged starvation, malnutrition or a catabolic disease and are then rapidly given nutrition, often through enteral feeding. The syndrome is characterized by major shifts in electrolytes, fluid balance, and metabolism that can cause a range of symptoms, including cardiac arrhythmias, respiratory failure, seizures, confusion, coma, and even death.

The rapid provision of nutrients, particularly carbohydrates, stimulates insulin release and promotes glucose uptake by cells. This, in turn, leads to a rapid shift of potassium, magnesium, and phosphate ions into the re-expanding intracellular compartment resulting in decrease in serum levels. This phenomenon occurs more rapidly, within hours of initiating PN and may take days with EN.[32,33]

The resulting electrolyte imbalances can cause muscle weakness, cardiac arrhythmias, seizures, and respiratory failure. The shift in metabolism can also cause thiamine (vitamin B_1) deficiency, as it is the co-factor for the enzymes involved in carbohydrate-dependent metabolic pathways. This can lead to neurological symptoms such as confusion, ataxia, peripheral neuropathy and Wernicke's encephalopathy (dry Beri Beri). The cardiovascular compromise may present with tachycardia, hypotension, peripheral edema, lactic acidosis, and fluid overload with LV (left ventricular) heart dysfunction (wet Beri Beri).[34]

To prevent the refeeding syndrome, it is important to allow permissive underfeeding and gradually increase the amount of nutrition provided, monitor electrolyte levels closely, and administer supplements as needed. This can be done through a stepwise approach that gradually increases the number of calories and nutrients, reaching the caloric goals eventually over 3–4 days.[19] Patients at high risk of refeeding syndromes may require more careful monitoring and management to prevent complications **(Box 2)**.[35]

ECG monitoring is recommended in all high-risk patients. In case of severe electrolyte abnormality (K <2.5 mmol/L, Mg <0.5 mmol/L and PO_4 <0.32 mmol/L) 24-hour cardiac monitoring should be done. Electrolyte levels should be checked daily for the first week, and every alternate day in the second week. Thiamine has to be administered at least 30 minutes before nutrition initiation to prevent Wernicke's encephalopathy **(Box 3)**.[36,37] Patients at high risk should be deliberately underfed with a starting rate of 10 kcal/kg every 24 hours.

> **BOX 2:** Patients at risk for refeeding syndrome.
> - Prolonged starvation
> - Chronic alcoholism
> - Postoperative patients
> - Anorexia nervosa
> - Low body mass index (<18.5 kg/m^2) with rapid weight loss
> - Morbid obesity associated with significant weight loss/recent bariatric surgery
> - History of malabsorption syndrome such as cystic fibrosis and inflammatory bowel disease

> **BOX 3:** Treatment strategy for critically ill patients with refeeding syndrome.
> - Correct fluid and electrolyte imbalances, including hypophosphatemia, hypokalemia, and hypomagnesemia.
> - Correct fluid overload and edema, as necessary.
> - Start with low-calorie nutritional support and gradually increase as tolerated. Restriction to 500 kcal over 24 hours during the first 48 hours
> - Calculate the amount of nonnutritional calories and total caloric load from intravenous solutions, propofol, and citrate (used in renal replacement therapy).
> - Gradually increase feeding after 48 hours of caloric restriction in daily steps of 25% of the target until the calorie and nutrition goal is reached
> - Glucose monitoring to maintain normoglycemia. Intravenous insulin for hyperglycemia
> - Thiamine supplementation intravenously 100 mg daily for a minimum of 7–10 days.
> - Monitor for signs of heart failure, arrhythmias, and respiratory failure, and provide appropriate supportive care.
> - Consider the use of enteral or parenteral nutrition, depending on the severity of the patient's condition.

If the BMI is ≤14 kg/m² or prolonged starvation for 14 days, then feeding should be started at a minimal dose of 5 kcal/kg/24 hours.[38]

Gut Ischemia

A dreaded but rare complication of EN is development of feeding related bowel ischemia or nonocclusive bowel ischemia (NOBI). Early clinical features may be nonspecific or patients may present with crampy abdominal pain and bloating. Later on, patients may develop abdominal distention and paralytic ileus. In severe cases, there may be transmural bowel necrosis, which may also progress to septic shock, multiorgan failure and death.[39] The pathophysiology is not clearly understood, but NOBI is generally considered to develop because of increased energy demands in order to absorb intraluminal nutrients from the EN in the state of metabolic stress. Additionally, continued EN in the presence of ileus may lead to bacterial overgrowth leading to further distention and impairment of mucosal perfusion. Generation of intraluminal toxins by the EN may also cause direct mucosal injury and cell death.[3] Hence, it is generally recommended to avoid EN in patients with refractory shock, on high or increasing vasopressor support, and during shock resuscitation.[19]

Other Metabolic Complications

The other metabolic complications associated with EN are dyselectrolyemias, hyperlipidemias, underfeeding, and overfeeding. All these complications may be prevented by careful selection and administration of EN with proper intake/output monitoring and charting the nutritional requirements versus nutritional delivery. A multidisciplinary team approach should be adopted, especially for malnourished and critically ill patients, who are at higher risk of developing these complications.

■ CONCLUSION

The management of complications associated with enteral feeding requires a multidisciplinary approach, close monitoring, and proactive intervention. By following the best practices, the risk of complications can be minimized and safe and effective enteral feeding, even for critically ill patients, can be assured. Consultation with a registered dietitian or healthcare provider is recommended to ensure that the enteral formula is properly balanced and meets the patient's nutritional needs. Healthcare professionals should also educate patients and caregivers about the signs and symptoms of complications and when to seek medical attention.

■ REFERENCES

1. Seres DS, Valcarcel M, Guillaume A. Advantages of enteral nutrition over parenteral nutrition. Therap Adv Gastroenterol. 2013;6(2):157-67.
2. Michel KE. Preventing and managing complications of enteral nutritional support. Clin Tech Small Anim Pract. 2004;19(1): 49-53.
3. Marvin RG, McKinley BA, McQuiggan M. Nonocclusive bowel necrosis occurring in critically ill trauma patients receiving enteral nutrition manifests no reliable clinical signs for early detection. Am J Surg. 2000;179: 7-12.
4. Singer P, Blaser AR, Berger MM, Alhazzani W, Calder PC, Casaer MP, et al. ESPEN guideline on clinical nutrition in the intensive care unit. Clin Nutr. 2019;38:48-79.
5. Hoffmann M, Schwarz CM, Fürst S, Starchl C, Lobmeyr E, Sendlhofer G, et al. Risks in Management of Enteral Nutrition in Intensive Care Units: A Literature Review and Narrative Synthesis. Nutrients. 2020;13(1):82.

6. Adeyinka A, Rouster AS, Valentine M. Enteric Feedings. [Updated 2022 Dec 26]. In: StatPearls [Internet]. Treasure Island (FL): StatPearls Publishing; 2023.
7. McClave SA, Chang WK. Complications of enteral access. Gastrointest Endosc. 2003;58:739-51.
8. Halloran O, Grecu B, Sinha A. Methods and complications of nasoenteral intubation. JPEN J Parenter Enteral Nutr. 2011;35(1):61-6.
9. Levy H. Nasogastric and nasoenteric feeding tubes. Gastrointest Endosc Clin N Am. 1998;8(3):529-49.
10. Sparks DA, Chase DM, Coughlin LM, Perry E. Pulmonary complications of 9931 narrow-bore nasoenteric tubes during blind placement: a critical review. JPEN J Parenter Enteral Nutr. 2011;35(5):625-9.
11. Sofferman RA, Haisch CE, Kirchner JA, Hardin NJ. The nasogastric tube syndrome. Laryngoscope. 1990;100(9):962-8.
12. Nehru VI, Al Shammari HJ, Jaffer AM. Nasogastric tube syndrome: the unilateral variant. Med Princ Pract. 2003;12(1):44-6.
13. Arvanitakis M, Gkolfakis P, Despott EJ, Ballarin A, Beyna T, Boeykens K, et al. Endoscopic management of enteral tubes in adult patients - Part 1: Definitions and indications. European Society of Gastrointestinal Endoscopy (ESGE) Guideline. Endoscopy. 2021;53(1):81-92.
14. Boeykens K, Duysburgh I. Prevention and management of major complications in percutaneous endoscopic gastrostomy BMJ Open Gastroenterol. 2021;8:e000628.
15. Tatsumi H. Enteral tolerance in critically ill patients. J Intensive Care. 2019;7:30.
16. Michel KE, Higgins C. Nutrient-drug interactions in nutritional support. J Vet Emerg Crit Care. 2002;12:163-7.
17. Wiesen P, Van Gossum A, Preiser JC. Diarrhoea in the critically ill. Curr Opin Crit Care. 2006;12:149-54.
18. Bodoky G, Kent-Smith L. Basics in clinical nutrition: Complications of enteral nutrition. e-SPEN, Eur E J Clin Nutr Metabol. 2009;4: e209-e211.
19. McClave SA, Taylor BE, Martindale RG, Warren MM, Johnson DR, Braunschweig C, et al. Guidelines for the Provision and Assessment of Nutrition Support Therapy in the Adult Critically Ill Patient: Society of Critical Care Medicine (SCCM) and American Society for Parenteral and Enteral Nutrition (ASPEN). JPEN J Parenter Enteral Nutr. 2016;40(2):159-211.
20. Metheny NA, Clouse RE, Chang YH, Stewart BJ, Oliver DA, Kollef MH. Tracheobronchial aspiration of gastric contents in critically ill tube-fed patients: frequency, outcomes, and risk factors. Crit Care Med. 2006;34:1007-15.
21. Marik PE. Aspiration pneumonitis and aspiration pneumonia. N Engl J Med. 2001;344:665-71.
22. Montejo JC, Miñambres E, Bordejé L, Mesejo A, Acosta J, Heras A, et al. Gastric residual volume during enteral nutrition in ICU patients: the REGANE study. Intensive Care Med. 2010;36(8):1386-93.
23. Mizock BA. Risk of aspiration in patients on enteral nutrition: frequency, relevance, relation to pneumonia, risk factors, and strategies for risk reduction. Curr Gastroenterol Rep. 2007;9(4):338-44.
24. Camilleri M, Parkman HP, Shafi MA, Abell TL, Gerson L. Clinical guideline: management of gastroparesis Am J Gastroenterol. 2013;108(1):18-38.
25. Heyland DK, Dhaliwal R, Drover JW, Gramlich L, Dodek P; Canadian Critical Care Clinical Practice Guidelines Committee. Canadian clinical practice guidelines for nutrition support in mechanically ventilated, critically ill adult patients. JPEN J Parenter Enteral Nutr. 2003;27:355-73.
26. ASPEN Board of Directors and The Clinical Guidelines Task Force. Guidelines for the use of parenteral and enteral nutrition in adult and pediatric patients. JPEN J Parenter Enteral Nutr. 2002;26(1 Suppl):1SA-138SA. Erratum in: JPEN J Parenter Enteral Nutr. 2002;26(2):144.
27. Kokura Y, Suzuki C, Wakabayashi H, Maeda K, Sakai K, Momosaki R. Semi-solid nutrients for prevention of enteral tube feeding-related complications in Japanese Population: a systematic review and meta-analysis Nutrients. 2020;12(6):1687.

28. Horiuchi A, Nakayama Y, Sakai R, Suzuki M, Kajiyama M, Tanaka N. Elemental diets may reduce the risk of aspiration pneumonia in bedridden gastrostomy-fed patients Am J Gastroenterol. 2013;108(5):804-10.
29. McClave SA, DeMeo MT, DeLegge MH, DiSario JA, Heyland DK, Maloney JP, et al. North American Summit on aspiration in the critically ill patient: consensus statement. JPEN J Parenter Enteral Nutr. 2002;26:S80-5.
30. Adeyemo AA, Fasunla AJ, Adeosun AA, Abdullahi H. Rhinosinusitis; a potential hazard of nasogastric tube insertion. Ann Ib Postgrad Med. 2007;5(1):44-5.
31. McCray S, Walker S, Parrish CR. Much Ado About Refeeding. Pract Gastroenterol. 2004;28:26-44.
32. McKnight CL, Newberry C, Sarav M, Martindale R, Hurt R, Daley B. Refeeding Syndrome in the Critically Ill: a Literature Review and Clinician's Guide. Curr Gastroenterol Rep. 2019;21(11):58.
33. Boot R, Koekkoek KWAC, van Zanten ARH. Refeeding syndrome: relevance for the critically ill patient. Curr Opin Crit Care. 2018;24(4):235-40.
34. Quiming C, Qiu L. Thiamine deficiency (Beriberi) induced polyneuropathy and cardiomyopathy: case report and review of the literature. J Med Cases. 2014;5(5):3018-311.
35. Chen J, Fan C. Prevention and management of refeeding syndrome in patients with chronic critical illness. 2016;19(7):737-9.
36. Friedli N, Stanga Z, Sobotka L, Culkin A, Kondrup J, Laviano A, et al. Revisiting the refeeding syndrome: results of a systematic review. Nutrition. 2017;34:151-60.
37. Zeki S, Culkin A, Gabe SM, Nightingale JM. Refeeding hypophosphataemia is more common in enteral than parenteral feeding in adult in patients. Clin Nutr. 2011;30(3):365-8.
38. Van Zanten A. Nutritional support and refeeding syndrome in critical illness. Lancet Respir Med. 2015;3:904-5.
39. Melis M, Fichera A, Ferguson MK. Bowel necrosis associated with early jejunal tube feeding: a complication of postoperative enteral nutrition. Arch Surg. 2006;141:701-4.

SECTION 4: Parenteral Nutrition in Critical Illness

17. **Parenteral Nutrition: Indications and Formulations**
    Arijit Sardar, Rajesh Pande

18. **Intravenous Access for Parenteral Nutrition**
    Viswanath Atreyapurapu, PC Gupta

19. **Safe Practices in Parenteral Nutrition Therapy**
    Priya Mistry, Gil Hardy

20. **Nutrient–Drug: Interactions and Compatibility**
    T Mohan S Maharaj, Varalakshmi Diwakarla

21. **Fluid and Electrolytes in Critical Illness**
    Bharat Jagiasi, Priya Sonavdekar

CHAPTER 17

Parenteral Nutrition: Indications and Formulations

Arijit Sardar, Rajesh Pande

■ INTRODUCTION

When oral feeding is not possible for many days, nutrition therapy is required to maintain a necessary body composition and normal physical and mental activity. The choice of feeding route whether enteral or parenteral depends on the condition of the patient and function of the gastrointestinal (GI) tract.

Parenteral nutrition (PN) is a method of delivering nutrition intravenously to patients who cannot tolerate or absorb nutrition through their normal digestive tract. It was initially called hyperalimentation, and its use was confined to patients with severe malnutrition, short bowel, or advanced cancer cachexia. It is called total PN, when the entire caloric requirement is met by intravenous nutrition, or supplemental PN, where enteral nutrition (EN) is inadequate or unable to meet the complete energy requirement, and PN is added. The administration of PN requires presence of a central venous catheter or a peripherally inserted central catheter (PICC) line, although low osmolarity PN solutions are now available that can be inserted through a peripheral venous cannula.

■ INDICATIONS

Parenteral nutrition is used in conditions where the enteral route cannot be used. A few common clinical situations where PN is indicated are summarized next.

- *Intestinal failure (IF) or GI failure:* IF has been defined by the European Society for Parenteral and Enteral Nutrition consensus guidelines as a reduction in gut function below the minimum necessary for the absorption of nutrients from the GI tract to maintain health and growth.[1] IF is further classified into three subclasses, such as acute (type 1 IF), prolonged acute (type 2 IF), and chronic (type 3 IF). Acute type 1 IFs are mostly self-limiting temporary conditions and do not require PN. Type 2 and type 3 IFs require PN support for weeks to months, and sometimes even for years. A few examples of acute chronic type 2 IFs are intra-abdominal sepsis, prolonged paralytic ileus, high-output abdominal stomas and fistulas, severe mucositis, and GI dysmotility. Type 3 IFs are mostly chronic and include causes such as extensive small bowel diseases, chronic fistulas, short bowel syndromes, etc.[2]
- *Partial GI disorders:* Partial GI failure may occur where normal GI function is expected to return shortly. Temporarily, PN may be prescribed for individuals with conditions such as acute exacerbations of Crohn disease, ulcerative colitis, intractable nausea, vomiting, and diarrhea.
- *Bowel rest:* Certain conditions require bowel rest for healing, and PN can provide nutrition until the bowel is ready

TABLE 1: American Society for Parenteral and Enteral Nutrition (ASPEN) and the European Society for Clinical Nutrition and Metabolism (ESPEN) recommendations to initiate parenteral nutrition (PN).

Parenteral nutrition	ASPEN recommendations	ESPEN recommendations
Initiation	*Exclusive PN:* • Use only when EN is not possible • Low nutrition risk (NRS 2002 ≤3 or NUTRIC score ≤5): start after 7 days • High nutrition risk (NRS 2002 ≥5 or NUTRIC score ≥5): exclusive PN as soon as possible *Partial or supplemental PN:* • Unable to meet >60% protein requirement by EN • Consider after 7 days in both low and high nutrition risk	*Exclusive PN:* Expected contraindication or intolerance to normal (EN or oral) nutrition up to 3 days: Start PN within 24–48 hours *Partial or supplemental PN:* Less than targeted enteral feeding after 2 days of EN feeding

(EN: enteral nutrition; NRS: Nutrition Risk Screening; NUTRIC: Nutrition Risk in Critically Ill)

to accept EN. It is used in conditions such as esophageal acid corrosions, gut inflammations, and intra-abdominal surgeries where bowel rest is required for proper healing.

- *Cancer and chemotherapy:* Some chemotherapeutic regimens and some GI cancers are known to cause severe GI disturbances in the form of nausea, vomiting, diarrhea, graft versus host diseases, colitis, etc. PN may be used to deliver energy support during such periods when patient is undergoing radiotherapy and chemotherapy.
- *Hypermetabolism or increased nutritional requirements:* Burns, trauma, sepsis, or extensive surgical procedures are a few conditions where metabolic demand is so high that EN alone may not be sufficient to provide energy requirements.
- *Severe malnutrition:* At times, severe malnutrition precludes the possibility of starting EN, and PN or supplemental PN may be used to build up the nutritional status.

INITIATION OF PARENTERAL NUTRITION

Parenteral nutrition can be exclusive, partial, or supplemental. Exclusive PN is indicated when initiation of EN is not possible, or it is contraindicated. Partial or supplemental PN is considered when EN cannot meet the entire energy requirement of an individual.[3] The American Society for Parenteral and Enteral Nutrition (ASPEN) and the European Society for Clinical Nutrition and Metabolism (ESPEN) have given specific indications to initiate PN. **Table 1** summarizes their recommendation to initiate PN.[4,5]

FORMULATIONS

Triple chamber bag: Protein, carbohydrate, and lipid solutions are kept in three separate chambers and premixed by agitation before infusion. These bags can be kept at room temperature and have a longer half-life. Protein chambers typically contain all essential and nonessential amino acids along with electrolytes (sodium, potassium, magnesium, phosphate, chloride, and acetate). Fat chambers typically include soybean oil, olive oil, fish oil, egg lecithin, long-chain triglycerides, or a balanced mixtures of all the components. Electrolytes and micronutrients can be present in the commercially available preparations or added separately to the bag after mixing all three components based on individual needs.

The carbohydrate chamber typically contains dextrose injections of 20–50%.

Single-chamber bag: It does not require mixing before infusion. Readymade bags with protein, carbohydrate, and fat, along with electrolytes and micronutrients are readily available for infusion. Typically, it is unstable at room temperature and has a low-shelf life.

Individual components: Formulations such as dextrose, amino acids, and lipid emulsions are available separately to cater to individual patients' needs.

Table 2 represents recommendations on different components based on ASPEN and ESPEN guidelines[4,5] and **Table 3** provides a comparison of various lipid emulsion solutions available.[6]

TABLE 2: American Society for Parenteral and Enteral Nutrition (ASPEN) and the European Society for Clinical Nutrition and Metabolism (ESPEN) guidelines-based recommendations on different parenteral nutrition (PN) components.

Components	Source	ASPEN recommendations	ESPEN recommendations
Carbohydrate	Dextrose solutions (20–50%) are generally recommended	• Target: 140–180 mg/dL • Targets may vary in different subsets of patients (postcardiovascular surgery or head trauma)	• Minimal requirement: 2 g/kg body weight hyperglycaemia >10 mmol/L should be avoided • Target: 4.5–6.1 mmol/L
Protein	Should contain all essential and semi-essential amino acids	• Dose >1.2 g/kg/day • Parenteral glutamine should not be used routinely	• Dose: 1.3–1.5 g/kg of ideal body weight • Should contain L-glutamine (0.2–0.4 g/kg/day)
Lipid	Different preparations are available: Soybean oil, olive oil, fish oil, and mixed-chain triglycerides	• Limit soybean oil-based preparations up to 100 g/week in the first week • No recommendations for alternative IV lipid emulsions (olive oil or fish oil), as they are not available in the USA	• Provides essential fatty acids to ICU patients • Long-chain and medium-chain triglycerides mixture emulsions are well tolerated • The clinical advantage of long-chain triglycerides is yet to be proven • Olive oil-based preparations are better tolerated • DHA and EPA have beneficial roles over cell membranes and inflammations *Dose:* 0.7–1.5 g/kg over 24 hours
Electrolytes	Na, K, Ca, Mg, Po$_4$, acetate, and chloride are minimally recommended	Standard daily dosing has been recommended for electrolytes	Should be guided by daily monitoring
Micronutrients (vitamins and trace elements)	Both water-soluble and lipid-soluble vitamins and trace elements (copper, chromium, manganese, zinc, and selenium) should be present	Standard daily dosing has been recommended for both vitamins and trace elements	Should contain a daily dose of vitamins and micronutrients

(DHA: docosahexaenoic acid; EPA: eicosapentaenoic acid; ICU: intensive care unit)

TABLE 3: Composition of lipid emulsions (LE).

	Olive oil LE	SMOF LE	Soybean oil LE
Soybean oil g/L	40	60	200
Olive oil g/L	160	50	0
MCT g/L	0	60	0
Fish oil g/L	0	30	0
Egg phospholipids g/L	12	12	12
Glycerol g/L	22.5	25	22.5
pH	7–8	7.5–8.8	7–8
Osmolarity mOsmol/L	270	273	265
a tocopherol mg/L	30	30	30
Major FAs, % by weight			
Oleic	58.3	27.8	22.3
Linoleic	17.7	18.7	53
a Linoleic	2	2.4	8
Arachidonic	0.3	0.5	0.3
EPA	<0.02	2.4	<0.02
DHA	0.23	2.2	0.34

(DHA: docosahexaenoic acid; EPA: eicosapentaenoic acid; MCT: medium-chain triglyceride; SMOF: soybean oil, medium-chain triglycerides, olive oil, and fish oil)

CONCLUSION

Enteral nutrition with good caloric intake in malnourished patients reduces mortality, but many ICU patients are unable to tolerate EN due to hemodynamic instability, paralytic ileus, gut failure, bowel rest or protein-caloric inadequacy as in cancer patients who are in severe catabolic state. Recent guidelines suggest PN initiation in these patients within 24–48 hours. PN can also be used as supplemental nutrition in addition to EN to fulfill the remaining/additional energy and protein requirements. Various formulations are available in the market, but triple chamber bags containing carbohydrates, lipids and proteins along with essential vitamins and trace elements are preferred due to ease of administration and adequate energy and protein content.

REFERENCES

1. Pironi L, Arends J, Baxter J, Bozzetti F, Pelaez RB, Cuerda C, et al. endorsed recommendations: definition and classification of intestinal failure. Clin Nutr. 2015;34:171-80.
2. Fetterplace K, Holt D, Udy A, Ridley E. Parenteral nutrition in adults during acute illness: a clinical perspective for clinicians. Intern Med J. 2020;50(4):403-11.
3. Berger MM, Pichard C. When is parenteral nutrition indicated? J Intensive Med. 2022; 2(1):22-8.
4. Singer P, Berger MM, Van den Berghe G, Biolo G, Calder P, Forbes A, et al. ESPEN Guidelines on Parenteral Nutrition: Intensive Care. Clin Nutr. 2009;28(4):387-400.
5. McClave SA, Taylor BE, Martindale RG, Warren MM, Johnson DR, Braunschweig C, et al. Guidelines for the Provision and Assessment of Nutrition Support Therapy in the Adult Critically Ill Patient: Society of Critical Care Medicine (SCCM) and American Society for Parenteral and Enteral Nutrition (ASPEN). JPEN J Parenter Enteral Nutr. 2016;40(2):159-211.
6. Dai YJ, Sun LL, Li MY, Ding CL, Su YC, Sun LJ, et al. Comparison of Formulas Based on Lipid Emulsions of Olive Oil, Soybean Oil, or Several Oils for Parenteral Nutrition: A Systematic Review and Meta-analysis. Adv Nutr. 2016;7:279-86.

CHAPTER 18

Intravenous Access for Parenteral Nutrition

Viswanath Atreyapurapu, PC Gupta

INTRODUCTION

An appropriate vascular access is vital for patients who are either totally or partially dependent on parenteral nutrition (PN).[1] The choice of vascular access depends on several factors, which include, but are not limited to, expected duration of therapy, PN solution, availability of access sites, and condition of the patient. Ultrasound-guided venous access and confirmation of access tip at the cava-atrial junction using fluoroscopy are now the standard of care.[2] While subclavian vein was the common site of access earlier, we now prefer to use the internal jugular vein (IJV) for central venous access. It is easier to visualize with ultrasound and is associated with fewer complications. The right IJV is preferred over the left since the course of the superior vena cava is straight and shorter. The femoral vein is least preferred since accessing it would limit mobility and it is associated with a higher risk of infective complications. Prevention of infective and thrombotic complications through implementation of evidence-based protocols is the key for the maintenance of intravenous (IV) access.[3] This chapter aims to discuss the importance of IV access for PN and explore various aspects related to its use. The basic venous anatomy of the upper limb is shown in **Figure 1**.

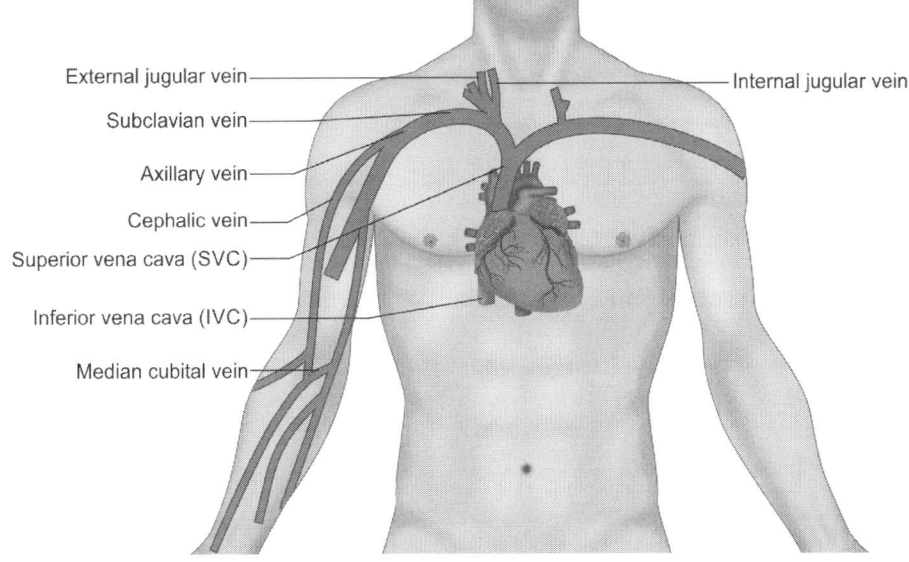

Fig. 1: Anatomy of upper limb veins.

CHOICE OF INTRAVENOUS ACCESS

- *Peripheral vs. central IV access:* Most patients requiring PN need a central venous access that delivers nutrients into the right atrium. PN using a peripheral cannula can be delivered if the duration of therapy is short and a low osmolality solution is used. Though there is no clear cut-off value of osmolality for use of peripheral lines, a central line should be considered if the duration of PN is expected to be more than 4 weeks, osmolality exceeds 900 mOsm/L, pH of the solution is <5 or >9, and for patients on home total parenteral nutrition (TPN).[4] The options for peripheral delivery of PN include short IV cannulas and midline catheters, which are long (20–25 cm) catheters made of silicone or polyurethane. Midline catheter tip is placed in the basilic or axillary vein.[5]

    Availability of peripheral veins and possibility of thrombophlebitis are the key factors to be considered when delivering peripheral PN. The above complication can be prevented by the use of ultrasound guidance, aseptic technique, and use of low osmolality, neutral lipid-based solutions.[1]

- *Central venous access:* Central venous access devices are catheters or devices whose tip is centrally placed. The classification of ventral venous access devices is based on duration of delivery of PN—short-, medium-, or long-term access.

    In patients requiring a short-term access, a single or multiple lumen polyurethane catheter, which is inserted in one of the central veins (neck or groin), is used. These are suitable in hospitalized patients for a limited duration.[6]

    A nontunneled central venous catheter (Hohn catheter) or a peripherally inserted central catheter (PICC) is used for medium term (up to 3 months).

    Hohn catheters are 5–7F single- or double-lumen catheters made of silicone and are around 35 cm in length. Some catheters come with an antimicrobial cuff at the exit site.[7]

    Peripherally inserted central catheter lines are 50–60 cm catheters made of silicone or polyurethane and inserted to arm veins (cephalic, basilic, or brachial veins). Both Hohn catheters and PICC lines are suitable for patients receiving in-hospital or home-based TPN. Though PICC lines have the advantage of low rates of mechanical and infective complications owing to their site of insertion in the arm and being away from oral and nasal secretions, an obvious disadvantage is that the exit position disables one hand, making self-care difficult.

    Options for long-term delivery of PN are cuffed tunneled central catheters **(Fig. 2)** like Hickman and Broviac or

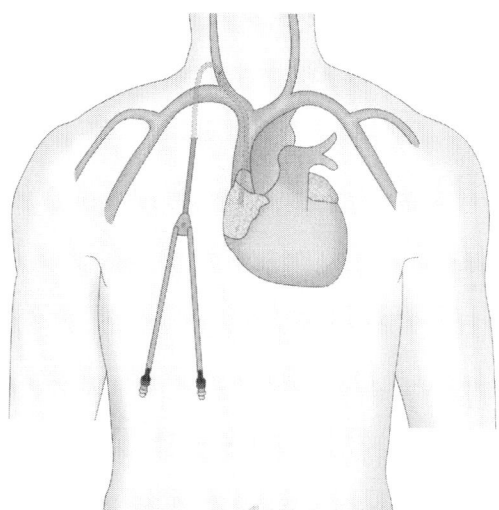

Fig. 2: Double lumen cuffed catheter placed through right internal jugular vein access.

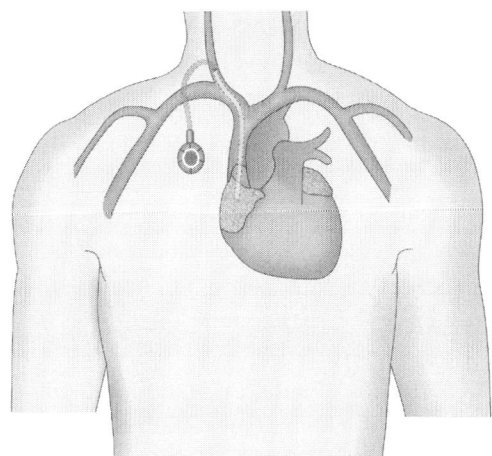

Fig. 3: Port-a-cath. Access via right internal jugular vein.

a totally implantable vascular access device (TIVAD), commonly known as port-a-cath **(Fig. 3)**. The choice between both depends on patient preference, compliance, institutional preference, and the experience of care givers. A tunneled catheter may be preferred for patients requiring continuous PN, while TIVAD may be more appropriate in those requiring intermittent PN.[8]

There are several reports of use of arteriovenous fistula for delivery of PN, with several case series reporting low incidence of sepsis. Though data is limited to recommend their use as a routine, they are of advantage in patients with limited venous access options, those on hemodialysis, or those with recurrent catheter-related sepsis.[9]

INSERTION AND MANAGEMENT OF INTRAVENOUS ACCESS— GENERAL PRINCIPLES[1,3,10]

A proper evidence-based technique is crucial for access function and prevention of complications. A written or typed informed consent should be obtained and it should include intent of the procedure along with possible complications and alternatives. It should be duly signed by the patient (or his/her representative) and the physician in the presence of a witness.

- *Setting:* The procedure should be performed in an operation theater, radiology suite, or an intensive care unit under proper aseptic precautions. Bedside insertion is not recommended unless carried out as an emergency. Ensure all necessary equipment including an ultrasound and fluoroscope are available.
- *Personnel:* The operator and the assistant should be appropriately trained, qualified, and competent to carry out the procedure and be well versed with devices and equipment.
- *Insertion:* Aseptic technique with full sterile barrier technique should be used. Hand hygiene with surgical hand scrub and full body draping should be followed. Skin preparation should be carried out with chlorhexidine-isopropyl alcohol solution and allowed to air dry. Site of insertion is based on the device used (central vs. peripheral).

  Ultrasound should be used for insertion of all catheters. Risk of malposition is higher with left-sided neck catheters compared to right side. High exit site of catheter in the neck is associated with higher rates of infection and it is difficult to take care of insertion site. Femoral catheters should be avoided whenever possible due to higher incidence of infective complications. The ideal position of catheter tip is at the atriocaval junction as it is associated with low rates of mechanical and thrombotic complications. The position of the tip should be ensured ideally with

fluoroscopy during the procedure or with an X-ray in the immediate postprocedure period. Ensure that blood can be aspirated freely from the lumen of the catheter.
- *Securement and dressing*: Most catheters need to be secured to the skin at exit site, which preferably should be done using a stabilization device like Statlock. Routine use of sutures is not recommended due to increased incidence of thrombophlebitis and sepsis. A transparent, sterile, semipermeable dressing allows for observation of exit/access sites.[11]

    In case of a TIVAD, the port is placed subcutaneously in the infraclavicular fossa under local anesthesia. It is important to secure the catheter properly to the port to avoid the risk of detachment and embolization into the pulmonary circulation.
- *Documentation*: It should include details of technique, type and size of the device, position of tip, and flow through lumen(s) along with date, time, and names of operator.

CATHETER MANAGEMENT AND CARE

Maintain an aseptic no-touch technique while handling a catheter by ensuring proper hand hygiene and use of personal protective equipment. Inspect the site of insertion for signs of inflammation, infection, or leakage. Decontaminate the ports and catheter hub with chlorhexidine-propyl alcohol solution before and after accessing the device. Flush the lumens with normal saline to ensure patency of the lumens before use. Dressing should be changed every 7 days or earlier if there is a compromise in the barrier. For port-a-cath, only atraumatic Huber needles should be used to access the port.[6]

COMPLICATIONS AND TROUBLESHOOTING

- *Catheter-related infections*: Catheter-related infections pose a significant risk in patients receiving PN. The clinical features of catheter-related sepsis can range from local erythema or pus discharge to systemic signs like chills, fever, leukocytosis, and shock. The cornerstone for diagnosis of catheter-related blood stream infection (CRBSI) is to obtain paired blood culture samples for quantitative culture—one from the catheter and other from the periphery. Routine use of blood cultures without clinical suspicion of sepsis is not useful.

    If a catheter is infected, it need not be removed if the symptoms are mild. Antibiotics should be started empirically followed by those based on cultures. Antibiotic lock solutions can be given for gram-positive cocci infections for 2 weeks to salvage a long-term device. Pus at the exit site, local abscess, or septic shock warrants prompt removal of the catheter. A temporary catheter can be inserted at a different site while insertion of a long-term catheter should await systemic antibiotic therapy and negative blood cultures.

    In case of persistent systemic infection following catheter removal, transesophageal echocardiography (TEE) or appropriate imaging should be carried out to look for septic emboli, infective endocarditis, or other metastatic infection.

    Use of silicone catheters, single-lumen catheters, and tunneled catheters is associated with lower incidence of catheter-related infections. Following aseptic technique during insertion and handling of catheters as described above is the key to sepsis prevention. Routine use of antibiotic prophylaxis, routine replacement of catheters, in-line filters, or use of heparin is not associated with lowering the risk of infections.[12,13]

- *Thrombosis:* Thrombosis is a potential complication associated with IV access for PN. Injury to the vein wall, thrombogenicity of the catheter material, and a prothrombotic state like malignancy appear to play a role in its pathogenesis. Low-grade evidence suggests that use of silicone or polyurethane catheters, single lumen devices, use of USG guidance, optimal tip positioning, and right-sided catheter placement may reduce the incidence of central vein thrombosis. Prophylactic anticoagulation is not effective against venous thrombosis except in patients with malignancy or previous thrombotic event.

  Management of thrombosis includes catheter removal if it is infected, obstructed, or mispositioned. Local or systemic thrombolysis is used in acute (<24 hours) symptomatic patients. Patients with chronic symptoms are best managed with anticoagulation using low-molecular-weight heparin (LMWH) and oral anticoagulants. In case of venous thrombosis with a functioning catheter, the patient should be started on anticoagulation and the catheter can remain in use.[14,15]

- *Fibrin sheath:* Fibrin sheath can form around the catheter in the vein after the catheter has been in situ for a few weeks. The first indication of a fibrin sheath is often a failure to aspirate through the catheter while infusion could continue uninterrupted. The fibrin sheath can be disrupted or stripped using endovascular techniques.[16]

- *Mechanical issues:* Mechanical issues such as catheter kinking, occlusion, or malfunction can impede the delivery of PN. The most common cause of catheter obstruction is precipitation of lipids, drugs, or contrast materials. Catheters should be flushed and locked with a saline solution when not in use. Heparin flush may be used if recommended by device manufacturers or when catheters are infrequently accessed. Heparin flush immediately before or after lipid infusion can cause lipid precipitation in the lumen and should be interposed with a saline flush. Management of an obstructed catheter includes exchange over a guidewire, removal and replacement, or pharmacological clearance. Clearance should be done using a 10-mL syringe to avoid pressure damage to the catheter. The agents used to clear the catheter based on nature of obstruction are— ethanol for lipids, thrombolytics for clots, sodium hydroxide or hydrochloric acid for drugs, and sodium bicarbonate for contrast media.

  Catheter dislodgement can occur due to accidental pulling or tugging on the catheter, improper securement, or physical activity. Use of appropriate stabilization devices, nursing protocols, dressing, and ensuring catheter cuff is at least 2.5 cm inside the tunnel from exit site ensure proper stability of the catheter.

  External damage to the catheter while changing dressing using scissors or due to solvents like ethanol can be managed using specific repair kits or by exchanging catheter over a guidewire.[1,3]

- *Other complications:* Complications related to any central venous access include pneumothorax, hemothorax, arterial injury, arteriovenous fistula, malposition in pleural or pericardial or abdominal cavity, and chyle leak. An uncommon complication is breakage of catheter or detachment of catheter from port a cath and embolization into the right atrium or pulmonary circulation. These can almost always be retrieved percutaneously using a snare.[17]

CATHETER REMOVAL

Catheter should be removed once it has served its purpose or if indicated due to a complication. Noncuffed catheters can be directly and gently pulled out and hemostasis can be achieved at the exit site with manual pressure for a few minutes. In case of cuffed catheters, the cuff needs to be dissected free from ingrown fibrous tissue under local anesthesia before pulling out the catheter. Similarly, a port-a-cath also needs to be dissected free before it can be removed along with the catheter. It is good to have the patient propped up in bed while removing the catheter to reduce venous pressure and ensure faster hemostasis. A sterile dressing should be secured at the exit site for 24–48 hours.[18]

CONCLUSION

Access for PN is often midline or central venous access. Adherence to use of aseptic techniques and use of ultrasound and fluoroscopy can minimize placement-related complications. Following infection prevention protocols, regular assessment, and prompt intervention are essential in minimizing infective, thrombotic, and mechanical complications.

ACKNOWLEDGMENT

The authors thank Dr Laxmi Gupta for the artwork.

REFERENCES

1. Pittiruti M, Hamilton H, Biffi R, MacFie J, Pertkiewicz M. ESPEN Guidelines on Parenteral Nutrition: Central Venous Catheters (access, care, diagnosis and therapy of complications). Clin Nutr. 2009; 28(4):365-77.
2. Randolph AG, Cook DJ, Gonzales CA, Pribble CG. Ultrasound guidance for placement of central venous catheters: a meta-analysis of the literature. Crit Care Med. 1996;24(12):2053-8.
3. Lappas BM, Patel D, Kumpf V, Adams DW, Seidner DL. Parenteral Nutrition: Indications, Access, and Complications. Gastroenterol Clin North Am. 2018;47(1):39-59.
4. Isaacs JW, Millikan WJ, Stackhouse J, Hersh T, Rudman D. Parenteral nutrition of adults with a 900 milliosmolar solution via peripheral veins. Am J Clin Nutr. 1977;30(4):552-9.
5. Payne-James J, Grimble G, Kapadia S, Silk D. Peripheral parenteral nutrition. J R Soc Med. 1991;84(6):383-4.
6. Ryder M. Evidence-based practice in the management of vascular access devices for home parenteral nutrition therapy. JPEN J Parenter Enteral Nutr. 2006;30(1 Suppl): S82-93, S98-9.
7. Raad I, Davis S, Becker M, Hohn D, Houston D, Umphrey J, et al. Low infection rate and long durability of nontunneled silastic catheters. A safe and cost-effective alternative for long-term venous access. Arch Intern Med. 1993;153(15):1791-6.
8. Staun M, Pironi L, Bozzetti F, Baxter J, Forbes A, Joly F, et al. ESPEN Guidelines on Parenteral Nutrition: Home Parenteral Nutrition (HPN) in adult patients. Clin Nutr. 2009;28(4):467-79.
9. Al-Amin A, Wood J, Atturu G, Gouda MR, Donnellan CF, Burke DA. Use of arteriovenous fistulae for home parenteral nutrition—a review of the literature. J Vasc Access. 2013;14(2):99-103.
10. Kovacevich DS, Corrigan M, Ross VM, McKeever L, Hall AM, Braunschweig C. American Society for Parenteral and Enteral

Nutrition Guidelines for the Selection and Care of Central Venous Access Devices for Adult Home Parenteral Nutrition Administration. J Parenter Enter Nutr. 2019;43(1):15-31.
11. Ullman AJ, Cooke ML, Mitchell M, Lin F, New K, Long DA, et al. Dressing and securement for central venous access devices (CVADs): A Cochrane systematic review. Int J Nurs Stud. 2016;59:177-96.
12. Raad I. Intravascular-catheter-related infections. Lancet. 1998;351(9106):893-8.
13. Siegman-Igra Y, Anglim AM, Shapiro DE, Adal KA, Strain BA, Farr BM. Diagnosis of vascular catheter-related bloodstream infection: a meta-analysis. J Clin Microbiol. 1997;35(4):928-36.
14. Barco S, Atema JJ, Coppens M, Serlie MJ, Middeldorp S. Anticoagulants for the prevention and treatment of catheter-related thrombosis in adults and children on parenteral nutrition: a systematic review and critical appraisal. Blood Transfus Trasfus Sangue. 2017;15(4):369-77.
15. Wall C, Moore J, Thachil J. Catheter-related thrombosis: A practical approach. J Intensive Care Soc. 2016;17(2):160-7.
16. Chang DH, Mammadov K, Hickethier T, Borggrefe J, Hellmich M, Maintz D, et al. Fibrin sheaths in central venous port catheters: treatment with low-dose, single injection of urokinase on an outpatient basis. Ther Clin Risk Manag. 2017;13:111-5.
17. Kornbau C, Lee KC, Hughes GD, Firstenberg MS. Central line complications. Int J Crit Illn Inj Sci. 2015;5(3):170-8.
18. Drewett SR. Central venous catheter removal: procedures and rationale. Br J Nurs. 2000-2001;9(22):2304-15.

CHAPTER 19

Safe Practices in Parenteral Nutrition Therapy

Priya Mistry, Gil Hardy

INTRODUCTION

It is well established that at least one-third of adult patients admitted to hospital are either malnourished or at significant risk of disease-related malnutrition (DRM).[1,2] An estimated 33% of US patients are malnourished upon hospital admission, many undiagnosed, leading to a rapid decline in their nutritional status during hospitalization.[3] Likewise, in Australia/New Zealand, it is estimated that 30–40% of hospital patients are malnourished.[4] In the UK, over 20% of patients in outpatient clinics are at medium to high risk of DRM, with chronic diseases, the elderly, those recently discharged from hospital, and those who are poor or socially isolated most vulnerable nutritionally.[5] The overall cost of DRM has been estimated at around 15% of the total public expenditure on health and social care (GBP 23.5 billion).[6]

Clinical nutrition is a human right according to the Vienna Declaration, endorsed by over 75 international professional societies.[7] Parenteral nutrition (PN) is an important life-saving therapeutic modality that is used in adults, children, and infants for indications related to intestinal failure (IF). Appropriate prescription and use of this complex therapy aim to maximize clinical benefit while minimizing the potential risk of adverse events.

PARENTERAL NUTRITION: INDICATIONS, BENEFITS, AND POTENTIAL RISKS TO PATIENT SAFETY

Parenteral nutrition is a multi-ingredient medicinal product administered intravenously when nutritional requirements cannot be met using the gastrointestinal tract. Comprising over 40 ingredients, it contains macro- and micronutrients needed to sustain life. Indications for PN include inadequate or unsafe oral/enteral nutrition, or a non-functioning, inaccessible or perforated gastrointestinal tract.[8] PN can be used short term in hospital for acute IF or given at home for long-term conditions, e.g., short-bowel syndrome.

Parenteral nutrition is widely regarded, but not unanimously, as a high-risk medicine. Its specialist use may contribute to lack of awareness among healthcare professionals who do not use PN in their daily practice. The World Health Organization (WHO) do not recognize PN as a high-risk medicine;[9] however in the USA, PN is broadly accepted as a high-risk medicine in acute care.[10] Patient safety with regards to PN has been extensively publicized as a key priority at national conferences and through national guidelines.[11,12] In the UK, national reports have highlighted the importance of multidisciplinary nutrition support teams (NST) to ensure the safe prescribing of PN.[8,13] A medication error is defined by the WHO as any preventable event that may cause or lead to inappropriate medication use or patient harm while the medication is in the control of the healthcare professional, patient, or consumer.[14] The European Medicines Agency (EMA) describe a medication error as an unintended failure in the drug treatment process that leads to, or has the potential to lead to harm to the patient.[15] In the UK, the preferred term for a medication error is patient safety incident, which is defined by the National Health Service (NHS) of England and Wales, as any unintended or unexpected incident which could have, or did, lead to harm.[16] Mistakes in prescribing, dispensing, storing, preparation, and administration of medicines are the most common preventable cause of undesired adverse events in medication practice and present a major public health burden.[15] Medication errors related to PN have been recognized as being multifactorial.[17]

Several aspects need to be considered related to the provision of PN. This includes procedures for prescribing or procurement, and complex manufacturing/compounding processes which need consideration of physicochemical stabilities when compounding a multi-ingredient preparation. PN is an ideal medium for bacterial growth, making microbial contamination a risk during compounding and administration. A recent scoping literature review provides a foundation of knowledge on PN-related incidents over the last 20 years.[18] Case studies, cross-sectional observation studies, with a small number of experimental studies were reviewed and analyzed. Case studies, which represented 50% of the 104 articles in this review, were separated into incidents related to microbial contamination, venous access, micronutrients, electrolytes, intravenous lipid emulsion (ILE) toxicity and glycemic control. Actual reported incidents in the observation studies were mainly cross-sectional single-site studies and only provided a snapshot rather than a longitudinal view. A PN-specific prevalence study on a national scale in the USA reported 1,311 PN incidents over 2 years, of which 1.4% caused harm.[19] More recently, a national evaluation of harm associated with patient safety incident reports in England and Wales used a national incident reporting system and found only 54 incident reports in a 5-year period related to PN causing moderate/severe harm or death.[20] They also revealed that contributory factors include patients aged <1 year, dependence on home parenteral nutrition (HPN), comorbidities, and staff errors. This study also confirmed that incidents of all grades of severity occur at all patient ages **(Fig. 1)**.

Parenteral nutrition prescribing, dispensing, compounding, administration, and monitoring are key process stages which will be examined in the following sections to understand which areas present a risk of medication errors, and to propose strategies that should minimize areas of potential patient harm when successfully using PN therapy.

■ PRESCRIBING

Patient factors and comorbidities can have an impact on prescribing the different nutritional components of PN. The metabolism of macro- and micronutrients, fluids and/or electrolytes can be affected by patient's other medical conditions. This may include infection, age (young/elderly), compromised immune system, postoperative complications, complex venous access, diabetes, malnutrition/obesity, heart failure, and kidney or liver disease. This list is not

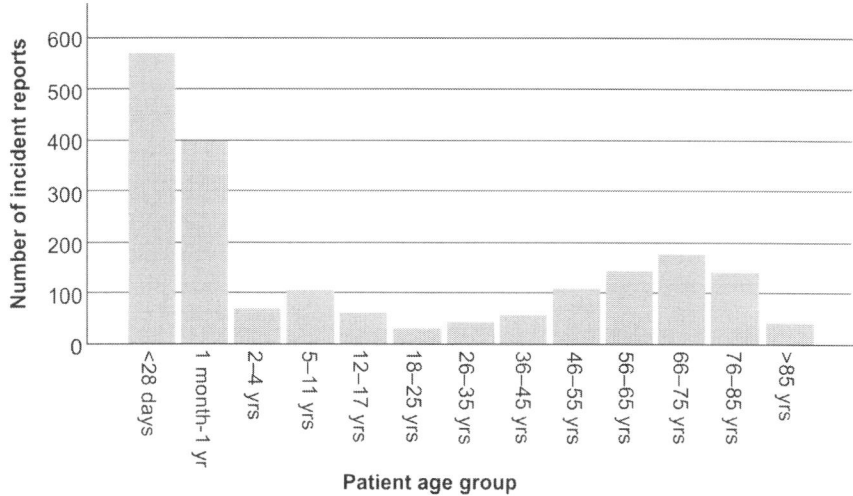

Fig. 1: Breakdown of PN-related incident reports by patient age. (PN: parenteral nutrition)
Source: Reproduced with permission from Mistry P, Fox A, Latter S. National evaluation of harm associated with patient safety incident reports related to the provision of parenteral nutrition to patients, using a national incident reporting system. Nutr Clin Pract. 2023.

exhaustive but provides an insight into the complexity of decision-making which goes into prescribing PN. Patients with heart/kidney disease may have altered metabolism that necessitates more careful monitoring of fluid and sodium requirements. A diabetic patient may require cautious titration of glucose within the PN formulation. Immunocompromised patients or those with ongoing infection may be at a higher risk of catheter-related sepsis. Patients with postoperative complications, e.g., wound dehiscence, fistulae or malnutrition/obesity may have altered macro/micronutrient requirements and need a more patient-specific bespoke PN formulation. Issues related to venous access may cause central venous catheter placement challenging, resulting in peripheral venous access being the only option for PN. This will affect the PN regimen, that should have an upper osmolarity limit of 850 mOsm/L for peripheral PN formulations, as recommended by the European Society for Clinical Nutrition and Metabolism Nutrition (ESPEN).[21] Incorrect route of administration with fatal consequences was highlighted in cross-sectional observation studies and case reports looking at medication errors related to PN.[20,22,23] A critical care patient may be affected by several of these patient factors making prescribing even more challenging.

Concurrent medications are also a key consideration when prescribing PN. Patients on medicines such as diuretics may require careful assessment of their sodium, potassium, magnesium, and fluid requirements. Critical care patients on propofol (formulated in an ILE carrier) may require a reduction in prescribed energy, due to the lipid content. Some intravenous infusions such as antibiotics may be infused in large volumes, or when given throughout the day as repeated doses add up to a large fluid volume. This may require the need for reduced PN volume (and sodium if sodium-containing diluents used) to avoid the risk of overhydration and/or pulmonary/peripheral edema. It is also important to consider pharmaceutical compatibility when patients are having multiple intravenous medications, as most are incompatible with PN. Hence, PN needs dedicated venous access.

In many countries, acute hospitals will have a hospital formulary limiting the availability of PN formulations to three to five multichamber bags (MCB). Furthermore, limited access to inhouse or external aseptic compounding units will affect the ability to prescribe MCB requiring micronutrient or electrolyte additions. For prescribers, this may require additional prescriptions to ensure these needs are met separately. Some aseptic compounding units may be able to manufacture patient specific PN formulations which require determination of individual PN components. In each of these cases, the prescriber needs to be fully aware of available prescribing options and be trained to prescribe the correct dose of PN in the form of MCB, with or without additions, or patient-specific PN with its individual components.

The prescribing platform used for PN can also present as an opportunity to introduce risk of medication errors. Paper prescriptions require manual calculation of PN ingredient doses, provide little support for decision-making around stability matrices, and include errors related to illegibility and transcription. Computerized provider order entry (CPOE) systems may be used for PN prescribing. Studies have demonstrated the impact of technological advances in healthcare systems on PN-related patient safety incidents and demonstrated a reduction in medication errors[18] **(Fig. 2)**. The gold standard has been recognized as an integrated prescribing, compounding and administration system linked to electronic health records and enhanced by clinical decision support (CDS) features.[24] In 2013, a national survey in the USA revealed that only one third of the responding institutions had electronic PN order entry available.[25] There was a clearly demonstrated reduction in incidents related to transcribing or ingredient calculation. However, unintended consequences of electronic prescribing may be sociotechnological or related to

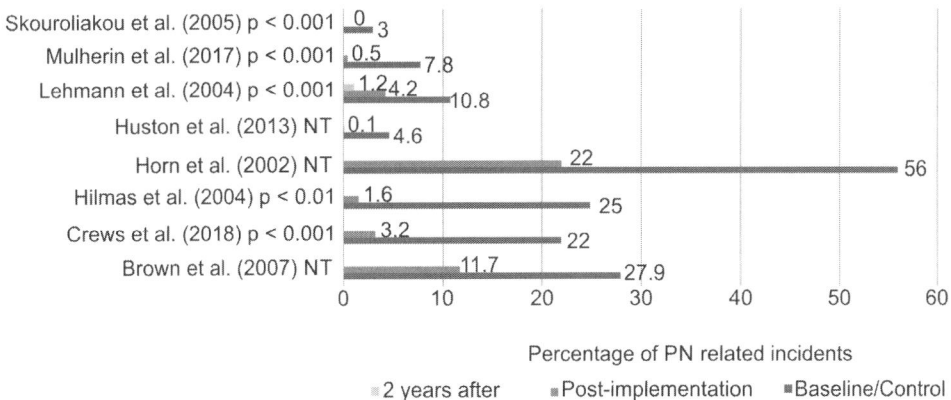

Fig. 2: Summary of results from studies relating to implementation of a computerized PN prescribing tool. (PN: parenteral nutrition)
Source: Reproduced with permission from Mistry P, Smith RH, Fox A. Patient safety incidents related to the use of parenteral nutrition in all patient groups: A systematic scoping review. Drug Saf. 2022;45(1):1-18.

inadequate implementation.[26] A national review of aseptic services in England reported that only 33% of facilities had electronic prescribing systems in clinical areas for aseptically prepared products such as chemotherapy and PN.[27] A recent publication by the UK Department of Health and Social Care recommended that patient safety systems, including barcode technology, decision support, electronic prescribing and medicines administration should ideally be incorporated in product specifications for PN.[28] The European Statement of Hospital Pharmacy (2014) encourages hospital pharmacists to take the lead in developing, monitoring, reviewing, and improving medicine use processes and the use of medicine related technologies.[29]

PARENTERAL NUTRITION DISPENSING AND COMPOUNDING

Procurement is a key area for the hospital pharmacy and governs availability of all medicines to clinicians. Without adequate procurement and management of stock levels, shortages in PN and/or formulation ingredients can impact patient care. Clinical repercussions of shortages in micronutrients and electrolyte salts have been recognized for decades. Zinc shortages between 2012 and 2013 led to its omission in pediatric PN formulations for babies in Texas, resulting in two deaths and six cases of dermatitis.[30] A patient with gastrointestinal dysmotility and substantial drainage losses who required PN, developed a nonanion gap metabolic acidosis secondary to a shortage of both potassium acetate and sodium acetate additives after receiving 11 days of chloride-rich PN.[31] Holcombe et al.[32] describe in detail the full impact of ongoing sterile injectable drug shortages, namely components of PN over a 12-year period. The reasons given for drug shortages included regulatory, natural disasters, voluntary recalls, issues with raw materials, increase in demand, discontinuation, loss of manufacturing site, and quality issues. They describe how ongoing shortages in PN components constitute a risk in the PN-compounding process as it introduces the need to deviate from standard operating procedures. Alterations to a standardized process can lead to medication errors that can adversely affect patient outcomes. A detailed account of PN incident reports due to drug shortages by Storey et al.[19] described 12 incidents related to ILE shortage during a 2-year period. They reported 746 errors in year 1 compared with 602 in year 2 but were not able to demonstrate a statistically significant association between the number of errors and drug shortages. To prepare for shortages the Food and Drug Administration (FDA) and the EMA have introduced medicine shortage catalogs as a platform to share information with hospital pharmacy procurement teams as they happen. Early notifications allow time to initiate actions aimed at preventing supply disruptions from turning into shortages and mitigating the impact of shortages.

The process of compounding in aseptic services is a recognized area of high risk and PN is considered a medium-risk compounded preparation.[33] A PN MCB can require multiple manipulations to make electrolyte and micronutrient additions. A patient-specific PN bag could require 10–20 separate injectable nutrients, combined in a single bag. To ensure strict adherence to protocol and standardized competencies, national standard documents have been advocated by the American Society for Parenteral and Enteral Nutrition (ASPEN).[34] In the UK, the Quality Assurance of Aseptic

Preparation Services Standards Handbook is a vital reference for pharmacy staff, and provides standards for unlicensed aseptic preparation.[35] An analysis of national aseptic compounding incident reports over 4 years in UK hospitals reported 711 incidents in adult PN and 184 in pediatric PN.[36] No incidents reached the patient, but potential harm was assigned for each incident to grade severity. The data suggested that the higher number of errors in adult PN production may be a result of UK practices, where adult PN is prepared at the end of the working day. Errors in transcribing were the most common stage of error for adult PN (13.1%) and pediatric PN (19%). The majority of incidents resulted in negligible clinical outcomes, with 21 (11.7%) major potential outcomes for adults and 15 (2.2%) major potential outcomes for pediatrics. There was a single (0.6%) pediatric PN error with catastrophic potential outcome. No further information was provided about this case, although the authors reported errors with pediatric PN were more likely to be detected in clinical areas during or after administration than other sterile products, recommending the need for robust final checks and release procedures to stop these errors from leaving the production area. They also suggested that the higher proportion of PN incidents in pediatric patients resulting in more serious outcomes may be related to the complexity of the PN regimens, requiring more manipulation or the greater vulnerability of this patient group.

As with electronic prescribing systems, automated compounding systems have found their place in the aseptic compounding of PN. They ensure precision in measurements and bar code scanners ensure correct product identification. Those with integrated systems for prescribing tools and labelling units have the added benefit of eliminating manual transcribing, and hence a reduction in associated errors. These systems have revolutionized workflow efficiency in aseptic units, with increased productivity and capacity. It is important we respect automation vulnerabilities. All systems should be validated and regularly audited to ensure patient safety. Human error cannot be completely eliminated. If an error in data entry occurs during the prescribing stage and is not highlighted in pharmacy, this could potentially be carried through the compounding and labelling stages, and if missed lead to the infusion of an incorrect formulation.

Standardization in PN provision has become accepted practice in many countries, especially for adult patients. Standardization can involve using an agreed selection of MCB or a selection of inhouse (local) compounded stock formulations. MCB are terminally sterilized, licensed products with shelf-life of up to 2 years. They can be stored at room temperature, and if no additions are made, can be dispensed directly from the hospital pharmacy, reducing workload in the aseptic unit. A reduction in available PN formulations may result in reduced frequency of laboratory monitoring due to less ability to change the PN formulation. It is important to note that the patient's nutritional/fluid requirements may not be met with standardized PN bags, and additional micronutrient/electrolyte/fluid infusions may be necessary for individual patients. Tailor-made stock formulations can be produced by inhouse or external compounding facilities, with a trained workforce and approved systems/processes. They will also require refrigerated storage, taking up considerable space and require temperature regulation during transportation to the clinical area for patient administration. Studies have demonstrated a reduction in medication errors through PN standardization, now recognized as being cost effective and time saving, without adverse effects.[37,38]

PARENTERAL NUTRITION ADMINISTRATION

A national evaluation of patient safety incidents in England and Wales,[18] was in agreement with an earlier US study[19] that recognized administration as the single most common origin of PN medication errors and for all reported degrees of harm in adults and children. Wrong infusion rate and improper dose/quantity were highlighted, although direct comparison of medication errors is difficult due to differences in reported categories. Inadvertently separately administrating ILE at the same rate as the nonlipid PN, and vice versa, in neonates and infants has been highlighted as a common incident type seen in case reports and observational studies.[23,39-41] Development of all-in-one MCB PN products for this age group could remove the need for separate ILE and nonlipid PN infusions.

Staff factors and equipment failure were highlighted as contributory factors in administration-related incidents by Mistry et al. in their evaluation of patient safety incidents.[20] Drug error reduction systems and "smart" infusion pumps have been introduced in healthcare to help reduce drug errors by using built-in drug libraries to impose dosing limits.[42] They aim to remove the element of human error when setting up infusion pumps. Studies have demonstrated a reduction in programming error rates but with the introduction of new error types, e.g., overriding pump warnings and outdated drug libraries.[42-46]

Extravasation is the accidental leakage of any liquid from a vein into the surrounding tissues when administering solutions such as medication or fluids, which can cause serious harm to the patient. Extravasation of PN is a safety consideration in both adult and pediatric patients. In a review of literature spanning 20 years, there were 19 reports of venous access accidents, of which 8 reports involved extravasation in patients, with incorrectly inserted venous access devices and inadequate confirmation of tip position.[18] Stringent venous access protocols that comply with international guidance for neonates may also reduce PN extravasation injuries.[47]

PARENTERAL NUTRITION MONITORING

Monitoring is a medication process stage that is key in all aspects of prescribing, compounding, and administration and has key implications for the provision of PN. There are many international guidelines for patient monitoring when PN is being delivered; and in the UK, the National Institute for and Health and Care Excellence (NICE) has produced a comprehensive monitoring list.[8] Environmental monitoring for microbial contamination within the aseptic unit and batch testing are methods employed to ensure all processes maintain sterility. Microbial contamination of PN though inadequate processes and/or monitoring has been shown to lead to fatal consequences in case reports around the world.[48-51] In the UK, it is recommended that additions to PN bags, including MCB, only occur in the pharmacy aseptic unit.[35]
- Clinical monitoring of the patient is key in ensuring safe delivery of PN and endorsement for continuation without any complications. This includes bedside patient monitoring such as temperature, heart rate, blood pressure, and fluid balance.

- Laboratory monitoring includes biochemical monitoring of serum urea, electrolytes, creatinine, liver function tests, and inflammatory markers such as C-reactive protein, and hematology monitoring of full blood count. Micronutrient monitoring is only recommended if indicated in longer-term patients, although this should not alleviate the need for full micronutrient provision. Inadequate biochemical monitoring has resulted in a case of hypophosphatemia in a patient at risk of refeeding syndrome.[52] An observational study has also demonstrated the association between failing to interrupt PN appropriately for blood sample collection and the incidence of spurious results.[53] As many as 87.5% of patients in this study underwent repeated blood sampling and 36.5% received unnecessary medical interventions such as administration of glucose and electrolytes, furosemide, insulin, and electrocardiogram tests.
- Implications of inadequate monitoring of venous access devices that result in extravasation of PN has already been discussed in the earlier section on administration.

The use of voluntary reporting methods from a local or national database to capture patient safety incidents presents a challenge, as investigators have minimal control over the data reported. Potential reporter bias in the form of missing data, underreporting, and subjectivity on applying scales for level of harm is accepted.[54] Nevertheless, incident reporting and auditing of practices/standards are vital in the healthcare setting to ensure safe provision of PN. This form of monitoring practices enables healthcare teams to recognize patterns in medication errors and implement systems to overcome further incidents from occurring, and to identify gaps in training and education of healthcare staff.

INCREASING PN SAFETY WITH A MULTIDISCIPLINARY NST

Nutrition support therapy is best performed as a collaborative effort among clinicians with specialized training and experience. In every clinical setting, safety is the responsibility of the prescriber, whether it be a physician, pharmacist, nurse, or dietitian, to recognize and report all PN-related medication errors, whether or not they reach the patient.[55] To improve patient nutrition status, clinical outcomes, and reduce costs associated with inappropriate management of patients, many healthcare facilities have implemented a NST in lieu of individual caregivers.[7] In the early days of PN, a NST that became common place in the USA, UK, and Taiwan in the 1990s[56] comprised a physician (usually a gastroenterologist) a pharmacist, and a specialist nurse, with dietitians playing a minor role. Over the years, the NST has become more multidisciplinary, also involving gastroenterologists with increasing responsibility taken by dietitians to assess nutrition status, determine the nutrition needs of patients, and in some countries, prescribe the nutrition regimen. This has sometimes meant less involvement from other clinicians and pharmacists; in particular, with advances in plastics and aseptic manufacturing technology, it is now possible to purchase a range of standard PN regimens in MCB, eliminating the need for in-house compounding. Consequently, some pharmacists have become "semidetached" from the NST, institutions in some countries have made NST redundant, and other countries have not adopted a team approach. A pilot survey of experts working in 10 countries on 5 continents, conducted by the international clinical nutrition section (ICNS) of the ASPEN, revealed several differences in nutrition therapy practices. Only 40%

of PN was prescribed by a full NST, 20% of institutions had no pharmacist reviewing PN orders and 50% had no quality management procedures in place.[57] In a recent meta-analysis that audited nine published studies on the benefits of NST between 2004 and 2019,[58] only one NST received a positive rating against a quality criteria checklist. The analysis revealed that inappropriate PN use varied from 4.3 to 18%, but overall a NST was associated with decreased incidence of inappropriate PN use.

CONCLUSION

A vast range of medication errors/patient safety incidents related to the provision of PN have been published for several decades. There is now sufficient published literature that harmful patient incidents are related to the inappropriate provision of PN in adults and children. We support the worldwide classification of PN as a high-risk medicine. Medication errors occur at all stages of the medication process, with incidents during the administration process being the most common. Mechanisms to reduce risk such as standardization, or the implementation of advanced computerized/automated technologies should be employed by all hospital pharmacies. The role of audit and incident reporting is a key learning tool to ensure safe practices. PN requires a multidisciplinary approach by trained healthcare professionals and prescribing managed by the NST that uses a shared conceptual framework to provide timely, cost-effective, safe, and appropriate nutrition therapy. Its main functions include full collaboration between all members to maximize patient therapeutic outcomes through provision and management of nutrition assessment, determination of micro/macronutrient needs, recommendations for appropriate EN/PN therapy. In all medication processes, the role of the hospital pharmacist in the NST is central to reducing risk associated with patient harm in PN provision. A unified team approach ultimately leads to cost-effective and safe nutrition therapy. A mixed-methods approach using a combination of quantitative and qualitative methods to provide greater insight into incidents should be adopted in future research to enhance understanding of contributory factors and to develop innovative procedures and interventions to further improve patient safety.

PARENTERAL NUTRITION SAFETY RECOMMENDATIONS

- Parenteral nutrition must be internationally classified as a high-risk medicine.
- Parenteral nutrition should be managed by a multidisciplinary NST that provides timely, cost-effective, and safe nutrition therapy.
- All hospitals should have local PN procedures that follow national and international standards and guidelines.
- Incident reporting and auditing of practices are vital to ensure safe provision of PN and for identifying gaps in training and education of healthcare staff.
- Compounding pharmacies should avoid PN preparation at the end of the working day.
- Standardization with MCB is cost/time effective and minimizes adverse effects.
- Stringent venous access protocols that comply with international guidance, especially for neonates, can reduce PN extravasation injuries.
- Minimize frequency of blood sampling and/or or other medical interventions.
- Standardization and computerized/automated technologies should be employed by all hospital pharmacies and incorporated into product specifications for PN.
- All compounding and administration systems should be validated and regularly audited to ensure patient safety.

REFERENCES

1. Barker LA, Gout BS, Crowe TC. Hospital malnutrition: prevalence, identification and impact on patients and the healthcare system. Int J Environ Res Public Health. 2011;8(2):514-27.
2. Jensen GL, Mirtallo J, Compher C, Forbes A, Grijalba RF, Hardy G, et al. Adult starvation and disease-related malnutrition: a proposal for etiology-based diagnosis in the clinical practice setting from the International Consensus Guideline Committee. JPEN J Parenter Enteral Nutr. 2010;34(2):156-9.
3. Tappenden KA, Quatrara B, Parkhurst ML, Malone AM, Fanjiang G, Ziegler TR. Critical role of nutrition in improving quality of care: an interdisciplinary call to action to address adult hospital malnutrition. JPEN J Parenter Enteral Nutr. 2013;37(4):482-97.
4. Agarwal E, Ferguson M, Banks M, Batterham M, Bauer J, Capra S, et al. Nutrition care practices in hospital wards: results from the Nutrition Care Day Survey 2010. Clin Nutr. 2012;31(6):995-1001.
5. British Association of Parenteral and Enteral Nutrition (BAPEN). (2011). The 'MUST' Explanatory Booklet: A Guide to the 'Malnutrition Universal Screening Tool' ('MUST') for Adults. [online] Available from: https://www.bapen.org.uk/pdfs/must/must-full.pdf. [Last accessed July, 2023].
6. Elia M. (2015). The cost of malnutrition in England and potential cost savings from nutritional interventions. In A Report from the Malnutrition Action Group of BAPEN and the National Institute for Health Research Southampton Biomedical Research Centre. [online] Available from: https://www.bapen.org.uk/pdfs/economic-report-full.pdf. [Last accessed July, 2023].
7. Cardenas D, Correia M, Hardy G, Gramlich L, Cederholm T, Van Ginkel-Res A, et al. The international declaration on the human right to nutritional care: A global commitment to recognize nutritional care as a human right. Clin Nutr. 2023;42(6):909-18.
8. National Institute for Health and Care Excellence. (2017). Nutrition support for adults: oral nutrition support, enteral tube feeding and parenteral nutrition. Clinical guidelines. [online] Available from: https://www.nice.org.uk/guidance/cg32. [Last accessed July, 2023].
9. World Health Organization. (2019). Medication Safety in High-risk Situations. Technical Report. [online] Available from: https://apps.who.int/iris/bitstream/handle/10665/325131/WHO-UHC-SDS-2019.10-eng.pdf?ua=1. [Last accessed July, 2023].
10. Institute for Safe Medication Practices. ISMP List of High-Alert Medications in Acute Care Settings [online] Available from: https://www.ismp.org/sites/default/files/attachments/2018-08/highAlert2018-Acute-Final.pdf2018. [Last accessed July, 2023].
11. Ayers P, Adams S, Boullata J, Gervasio J, Holcombe B, Kraft MD, et al. A.S.P.E.N. parenteral nutrition safety consensus recommendations. JPEN J Parenter Enteral Nutr. 2014;38(3):296-333.
12. Mirtallo JM. Consensus of parenteral nutrition safety issues and recommendations. JPEN J Parenter Enteral Nutr. 2012;36(2 Suppl):62S.
13. National Confidential Enquiry into Patient Outcome and Death (NCEPOD). (2010). A Mixed Bag. An enquiry into the care of hospital patients receiving parenteral nutrition. [online] Available from: https://www.ncepod.org.uk/2010report1/downloads/PN_report.pdf. [Last accessed July, 2023].
14. World Health Organization. Medication Errors. (2016). Technical Series on Safer Primary Care. [online] Available from: https://www.who.int/publications/i/item/9789241511643. [Last accessed July, 2023].
15. European Medicines Agency. (2015). Safer use of medicines by preventing medication errors 2015 [online] Available from: https://www.ema.europa.eu/en/news/safer-use-medicines-preventing-medication-errors [Last accessed July, 2023].
16. NHS England. (2023). Report a patient safety incident. [online] Available from: https://www.england.nhs.uk/patient-safety/report-patient-safety-incident/#:~:text=Patient%20safety%20incidents%20are%20any,action%20to%20keep%20patients%20safe [Last accessed July, 2023].

17. White R. Quality parenteral nutrition: an ideal mixed bag. Proc Nutr Soc. 2011;70(3):285-92.
18. Mistry P, Smith RH, Fox A. Patient safety incidents related to the use of parenteral nutrition in all patient groups: A systematic scoping review. Drug Saf. 2022;45(1):1-18.
19. Storey MA, Weber RJ, Besco K, Beatty S, Aizawa K, Mirtallo JM, et al. Evaluation of parenteral nutrition errors in an era of drug shortages. Nutr Clin Pract. 2016;31(2):211-7.
20. Mistry P, Fox A, Latter S. National evaluation of harm associated with patient safety incident reports related to the provision of parenteral nutrition to patients, using a national incident reporting system. Nutr Clin Pract. 2023.
21. Pittiruti M, Hamilton H, Biffi R, MacFie J, Pertkiewicz M; ESPEN. ESPEN Guidelines on Parenteral Nutrition: central venous catheters (access, care, diagnosis and therapy of complications). Clin Nutr. 2009;28(4):365-77.
22. Al Nemri AM, Ignacio LC, Al Zamil FA, Al Jarallah AS. Rare but fatal complication of umbilical venous catheterization. Congenit Heart Dis. 2006;1(4):180-3.
23. Sacks GS, Rough S, Kudsk KA. Frequency and severity of harm of medication errors related to the parenteral nutrition process in a large university teaching hospital. Pharmacother. 2009;29(8):966-74.
24. Ayers P, Foster J, Kanorwala A, Jenkins A, Raymer K, Byrd L, et al. Electronic health record and parenteral nutrition functionality: A gap analysis. Nutr Clin Pract. 2021;36(2):433-9.
25. Boullata JI, Guenter P, Mirtallo JM. A parenteral nutrition use survey with gap analysis. JPEN J Parenter Enteral Nutr. 2013;37(2):212-22.
26. Ahmed Z, Garfield S, Jani Y, Jheeta S, Franklin BD. Impact of electronic prescribing on patient safety in hospitals: Implications for the UK. Clinical Pharmacist. 2016;8.
27. NHS Improvement. Pharmacy Aseptic Services Review. Summary of Key Findings. [online] Available from: https://www.sps.nhs.uk/wp-content/uploads/2018/04/NHSI-Aseptic-Summary-and-Findings_280318.pdf2018 [Last accessed July, 2023].
28. Department of Health & Social Care. Transforming NHS Pharmacy Aseptic Services in England [online] Available from: https://assets.publishing.service.gov.uk/government/uploads/system/uploads/attachment_data/file/931195/aseptic-pharmacy.pdf2020 [Last accessed July, 2023].
29. The European Statements of Hospital Pharmacy. Eur J Hosp Pharm. 2014;21(5):256-8.
30. Ruktanonchai D, Lowe M, Norton SA, Garret T, Soghier L, Weiss E, et al. Zinc deficiency-associated dermatitis in infants during a nationwide shortage of injectable zinc - Washington, DC, and Houston, Texas, 2012-2013. MMWR Morb Mortal Wkly Rep. 2014;63(2):35-7.
31. Brown EW, McClellan NH, Minard G, Maish 3rd GO, Dickerson RN. Avoiding patient harm with parenteral nutrition during electrolyte shortages. Hosp Pharm. 2018;53(6):403-7.
32. Holcombe B, Mattox TW, Plogsted S. Drug Shortages: Effect on Parenteral Nutrition Therapy. Nutr Clin Pract. 2018;33(1):53-61.
33. ASHP guidelines on compounding sterile preparations. Am J Health Syst Pharm. 2014;71(2):145-66.
34. Boullata JI, Holcombe B, Sacks G, Gervasio J, Adams SC, Christensen M, et al. Standardized competencies for parenteral nutrition order review and parenteral nutrition preparation, including compounding. Nutr Clin Pract. 2016;31(4):548-55.
35. Beaney AM. Quality Assurance of Aseptic Preparation Services: Standards Handbook, 5th edition. London: Pharmaceutical Press; 2016.
36. Bateman R, Donyai P. Errors associated with the preparation of aseptic products in UK hospital pharmacies: lessons from the national aseptic error reporting scheme. Qual Safety Health Care. 2010;19(5):e29.
37. Berlana D, Almendral MA, Abad MR, Fernández Ana, Torralba A, Cervera-Peris M, et al. Cost, time, and error assessment during preparation of parenteral nutrition: multichamber bags versus hospital-compounded bags. JPEN J Parenter Enteral Nutr. 2019;43(4):557-65.
38. Poh BY, Benajmin S, Hayward TZ, 3rd. Standardized hospital compounded parenteral nutrition formulations do not guarantee safety. Am Surg. 2011;77(6):e109-11.
39. Bora KM, Hedge MW. Neonatal triglyceride levels after massive lipid bolus - Implications for lipid rescue. Clin Toxicol. 2009;47(7):760.

40. Cole C, Robertson S. Nine cases of unintentional rapid infusion of lipid emulsion in children: root cause analysis and changes to practice. Arch Dis Child. 2014;99:e3.
41. Hicks RW, Becker SC, Chuo J. A summary of NICU fat emulsion medication errors and nursing services: data from MEDMARX. Adv Neonatal Care. 2007;7(6):299-308.
42. Ohashi K, Dalleur O, Dykes PC, Bates DW. Benefits and risks of using smart pumps to reduce medication error rates: a systematic review. Drug Saf. 2014;37(12):1011-20.
43. Hsu KY, DeLaurentis P, Bitan Y, Degnan DD, Yih Y. Unintended patient safety risks due to wireless smart infusion pump library update delays. J Patient Saf. 2019;15(1):e8-e14.
44. Lyons I, Furniss D, Blandford A, Chumbley G, Iacovides I, Wei L. Errors and discrepancies in the administration of intravenous infusions: a mixed methods multihospital observational study. BMJ Qual Saf. 2018;27(11):892-901.
45. Melton KR, Timmons K, Walsh KE, Meinzen-Derr JK, Kirkendall E. Smart pumps improve medication safety but increase alert burden in neonatal care. BMC Med Inform Decis Mak. 2019;19(1):213.
46. Schnock KO, Dykes PC, Albert J, Ariosto D, Call R, Cameron C. The frequency of intravenous medication administration errors related to smart infusion pumps: a multihospital observational study. BMJ Qual Saf. 2017;26(2):131-40.
47. British Association of Perinatal Medicine. (2015). Use of central venous catheters in neonates (Revised 2018), A BAPM Framework for Practice [online] Available from: https://www.bapm.org/resources/10-use-of-central-venous-catheters-in-neonates-revised-2018. [Last accessed July, 2023].
48. Gehring S, Zepp F, Mildenberger E. Contamination of parenteral nutrition solution causes severe endotoxinemia/bacteremia in 11 children treated in a PICU/NICU. Pediatr Critical Care Med. 2011;12(3):A12.
49. Habsah H, Zeehaida M, Van Rostenberghe H, Noraida R, Wan Pauzi WI, Fatimah I, et al. An outbreak of Pantoea spp. in a neonatal intensive care unit secondary to contaminated parenteral nutrition. J Hosp Infect. 2005;61(3):213-8.
50. Staes C, Jacobs J, Mayer J, Allen J. Description of outbreaks of health-care-associated infections related to compounding pharmacies, 2000-12. Am J Health Syst Pharm. 2013;70(15):1301-12.
51. Tresoldi AT, Padoveze MC, Trabasso P, Veiga JF, Marba ST, von Nowakonski A, et al. Enterobacter cloacae sepsis outbreak in a newborn unit caused by contaminated total parenteral nutrition solution. Am J Infect Control. 2000;28(3):258-61.
52. Lin KK, Lee JJ, Chen HC. Severe refeeding hypophosphatemia in a CAPD patient: a case report. Renal Failure. 2006;28(6):515-7.
53. Fairholm L, Saqui O, Baun M, Yeung M, Fernandes G, Allard JP. Monitoring parenteral nutrition in hospitalized patients: issues related to spurious bloodwork. Nutr Clin Pract. 2011;26(6):700-7.
54. Williams SD, Ashcroft DM. Medication errors: how reliable are the severity ratings reported to the national reporting and learning system? Int J Qual Health Care. 2009;21(5):316-20.
55. Sacks GS. Safety surrounding parenteral nutrition systems. JPEN J Parenter Enteral Nutr. 2012;36(2 Suppl):20s-2s.
56. Allwood MC, Hardy G, Sizer T. Roles and functions of the pharmacist in the nutrition support team. Nutrition. 1996;12(1):63-4.
57. Pounds TI, Hardy G. Pharmacy services for safe parenteral nutrition. In: Babar Z-U-D, editor. Pharmacy Practice Research Case Studies, 1st edition. United States America: Elsevier; 2021.
58. Stidham MA, Douglas JW. Nutrition Support Team Oversight and Appropriateness of Parenteral Nutrition in Hospitalized Adults: A Systematic Review. JPEN J Parenter Enteral Nutr. 2020;44(8):1447-60.

CHAPTER 20

Nutrient–Drug: Interactions and Compatibility

T Mohan S Maharaj, Varalakshmi Diwakarla

INTRODUCTION

"Tell me what you eat and I shall tell you who you are."—The relationship between food health and pleasure summed up by Anthelme Brillat-Savarin, a French gastronome in 1825.[1]

Ancient wisdom has unequivocally emphasized nutrition-health-medication interactions. Ayurvedic texts describe several food–drug interactions.[2] Modern medicine is only recently beginning to understand the phenomenon and its implications.

The scope of drug–nutrient interactions (DNIs) is immense. Drug–drug interactions have been extensively studied and are routinely monitored by physicians and pharmacists in critically ill patients. There is sparse literature pertaining to the subject of DNIs. The reasons are multifactorial. These include poor scientific understanding, knowledge gaps, challenges in relevant study design, conduct, and standardization, lack of meaningful measurable endpoints such as biomarkers, and absence of regulatory requirements by authorities to name a few. The void is larger in critical care nutrition due to complex and dynamic pathophysiology, polypharmacy, comorbidities, interventions, and heterogeneity in disease and treatment response. Although we are beginning to understand the implications and application of available data, strategies, and practices to mitigate harm and better outcomes and safety in the intensive care patient population are grossly deficient. Further focused clinical research is required to fill existing knowledge gaps and provide evidence-based directions.

This chapter aims to provide the reader with an overview of current understanding and help the clinician identify, evaluate, and manage DNIs.

DEFINITION

A broad definition of a DNI is an interaction resulting from a physical, chemical, physiologic, or pathophysiologic relationship between a drug and a nutrient, multiple nutrients, food, or nutritional status.[3]

CLINICAL SIGNIFICANCE

An interaction is considered significant if it changes therapeutic drug response or compromises the nutritional status causing malnutrition. There may be an effect on disposition including absorption, distribution, and elimination of either drug or nutrient. The effect is defined as the physiological action of a drug or nutrient at the cellular or subcellular level.

RISK FACTORS

The most commonly identified risk factors are comorbid conditions requiring long-term medication, multiple medications, extremes of age, gastrointestinal (GI) failure, patients on continuous enteral nutrition support, and critical illness.

CLASSIFICATION

The most accepted classification is based on the cause or precipitating factor, the factor influenced by the interaction, and the potential effect or consequence.[3] There are five groups of interactions as depicted in **Table 1**.

MECHANISMS OF DRUG–NUTRIENT INTERACTIONS[3]

The interactions can be pharmaceutical, pharmacokinetic (PK) or pharmacodynamic. A working model as depicted in **Figure 1** by Choi et al.[5] incorporates all factors contributing to drug–nutrient interactions.

Pharmaceutical interactions involve physicochemical reactions that take place in the delivery device, e.g., a feeding tube, a central venous catheter (CVC), or the

TABLE 1: Classification of drug–nutrient interactions.[3]

Precipitating factor	Object of the interaction	Potential consequence
Nutritional status	Drug	Treatment failure or drug toxicity
Food or food component	Drug	Treatment failure or drug toxicity
Specific nutrients or other dietary Supplement ingredient	Drug	Treatment failure or drug toxicity
Drug	Nutritional status	Altered nutritional status
Drug	Specific nutrient	Altered nutrient status

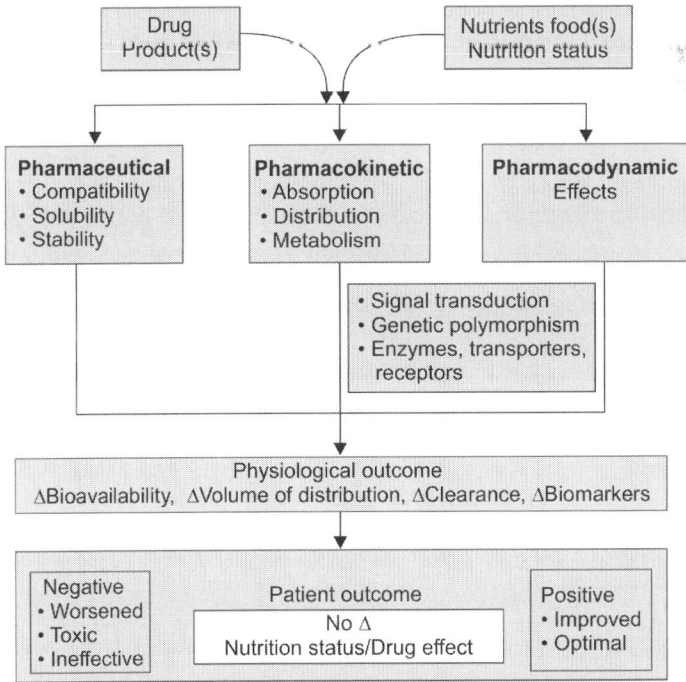

Fig. 1: Working model of drug–nutrient interactions.[6]

GI tract lumen. These include precipitation and chelation.

Pharmacodynamic interactions involve the clinical effect in the case of a drug and the physiologic effect in the case of a nutrient. These can be synergistic, additive, or antagonistic. Measurement is by drug response and nutritional status.

Pharmacokinetic interactions involve changes in bioavailability, the volume of distribution, and clearance. Enzymes and transporters needed for absorption, distribution, and elimination may be shared by drugs and nutrients resulting in potentially significant interactions. Transporters form the largest family of membrane proteins in humans, including members of solute carrier transporter and ATP-binding cassette transporter families. They play pivotal roles in the absorption, distribution, and excretion of xenobiotic and endogenous molecules.[4] Enzymes such as cytochrome P450 (CYP) are involved in phase 1 metabolism of xenobiotics and endogenous substances in the liver, cytochrome PA4 in enterocytes, which are a part of presystemic metabolism of drugs in the gut, and esterases, which inactivate prodrugs may mediate potential DNIs.[5]

Drug–nutrient interactions may be understood according to the site and mechanism of interactions as depicted in **Table 2**.

Another useful classification is the biopharmaceutical drug disposition classification.[7] This classification was formulated to evaluate *in vivo* performance of drugs based on *in vitro* permeability and solubility data and provided techniques for categorizing drugs based on solubility and permeability properties as well as dosage form dissolution, which when combined with physiological variables helps understand and evaluate DNIs **(Fig. 2)**.

EFFECT OF FOOD ON DRUGS

Concurrent administration of food and drugs changes the GI tract milieu. The rate and amount of drug absorption may be altered. It is important to understand that a change in the amount of absorption rather than rate leads to significant interactions. The Food and Drug Administration (FDA)-recommended test meal is designed to bring about extreme physiological disturbances in the GI tract to detect interactions. Many studies use modified test meals which should be borne in mind while interpreting results and making recommendations.

Individual dietary components may have specific effects. Dietary proteins and

TABLE 2: Location and mechanisms of drug–nutrient interactions.

Site of Interaction	Consequence	Mechanism of Interaction
In drug (or nutrient) delivery device or gastrointestinal lumen	Reduced bioavailability	Physiochemical reaction and inactivation
Gastrointestinal mucosa	Altered bioavailability	Altered transporter and/or enzyme function
Systemic circulation or tissues	Altered distribution/effect	Altered transporter, enzyme, or other physiologic function
Organs of excretion	Altered clearance	Antagonism, impairment, or modulation of elimination

Source: Chan LN. Drug-nutrient interaction in clinical nutrition. Curr Opin Clin Nutr Metab Care. 2002;5(3): 327-32.

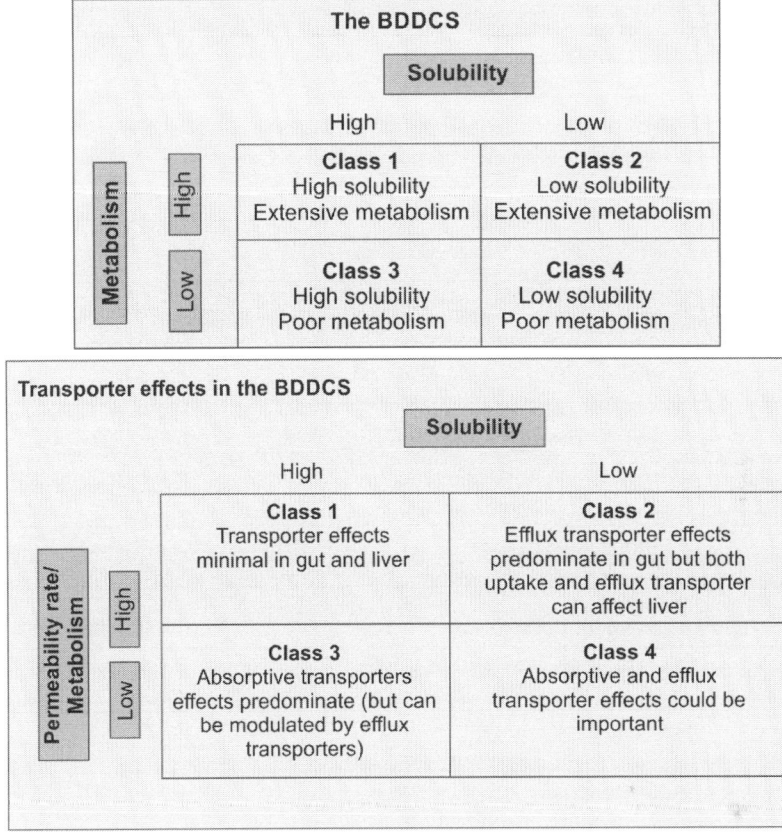

Fig. 2: The biopharmaceutical drug disposition classification system (BDDCS).

protein supplements increase drug metabolism through enzyme and transporter induction.

Cytochrome P450s play an important role in metabolism and clearance of most clinically utilized drugs and other xenobiotics. They are important in metabolism of endogenous compounds including fatty acids, sterols, steroids, and lipid-soluble vitamins. Soy protein isolates and soy significantly alter the expression and activity of CYP enzymes in a species, organ, and cell-type specific manner.[8]

Juices such as grapefruit interact with drugs depending on furanocoumarin and flavonoid content **(Table 3)**.[9] The common PK parameters affected are area under the concentration–time curve. The common potential interactions are depicted in **Table 4**.

Vitamins, Minerals, and Other Herbal Dietary Supplements

There is an ever increasing use of dietary supplements in general population and also in specific disease states. DNIs are being extensively studied in this population. Trials to establish clinically significant interactions are very challenging and therefore sparse. Supplements such as ginseng and echinacea can influence transporters and enzymes leading to drug interactions.

TABLE 3: Fruit juice–drug interactions.[9]

Fruit juice type	Examples of drugs	Suggested mechanism
Grapefruit	• CYP3A4 substrates • HMG-CoA reductase inhibitors (simvastatin, lovastatin) • Immunosuppressives (cyclosporine) • Antiarrhythmics (amiodarone) • Anticonvulsants (carbamazepine) • PDE5 inhibitor (sildenafil) • Antimalarial agent (artemether)	via CYP3A4, or/and P-gp
Orange	Bisphosphonates (alendronate)	Physicochemical interaction
	• Antihistamines (fexofenadine) • Beta-blocker (atenolol) • Anti-asthmatic agent (montelukast)	OATP transporters, or/and P-gp
Calcium-fortified orange juice	• Aluminum and iron supplements • Antibiotics (fluoroquinolones)	Physicochemical interaction
Seville orange	PDE5 inhibitor (sildenafil)	via CYP3A4
Pomegranate	PDE5 inhibitor (sildenafil)	via CYP3A4
Pomelo	PDE5 inhibitor (sildenafil)	Physicochemical interaction
	Immunosuppressives (cyclosporine)	P-gp
Apple	• Antihistamines (fexofenadine) • Beta-blocker (atenolol) • Anti-asthmatic agent (montelukast) • Antihypertensive agent (aliskiren) • Antihistamines (fexofenadine)	OATP transporters, or/and P-gp
Blueberry	TNF-α inhibitor (etanercept)	Beneficial interaction suggested to be due to anti-oxidant/anti-inflammatory properties of blueberries

(CYP3A4: cytochrome P450 3A4; HMG-CoA: β-hydroxy β-methylglutaryl-CoA; OATP: organic anion transporting polypeptides; PDE5: phosphodiesterase type 5; TNF-α: tumor necrosis factor alpha)

TABLE 4: Nutrient–drug interactions.

Vitamin/mineral supplement	Affected medication	Effect of interaction	Management of interaction
Vitamin A	Retinoids (isotretinoin and acitretin)	*Risk of toxicity:* Nausea, vomiting, dizziness, blurred vision, poor muscle coordination	Avoid concomitant use
Pyridoxine (Vitamin B)	• Levodopa • Phenytoin	• Decreased efficacy leading to Parkinsonian symptoms • Risk of seizure	• Recommend carbidopa/levodopa combination • Discontinue pyridoxine or increase phenytoin dose

Contd...

Contd...

Vitamin/mineral supplement	Affected medication	Effect of interaction	Management of interaction
Vitamin E	Warfarin	Risk of bleeding	Avoid doses >800 IU/day of vitamin E
Vitamin K	Warfarin	Decreased efficacy; risk of thromboembolism	Maintain consistent intake of vitamin K
Niacin	HMG-CoA reductase inhibitors	Risk of myopathy or rhabdomyolysis	Avoid self-treatment with niacin
Folic acid	Methotrexate	Prevents adverse events or toxicities from methotrexate	Recommend supplementation in patients taking methotrexate for rheumatoid arthritis or psoriasis
Calcium	• Fluoroquinolones and tetracyclines • Levothyroxine and bisphosphonates	• Decreased efficacy; risk of antibiotic failure • Decreased efficacy; risk of hypothyroidism	• Avoid concomitant calcium supplementation • Separate doses by at least 4 hours
Aluminum and magnesium	Fluoroquinolones, tetracyclines, bisphosphonates, and levothyroxine	Decreased efficacy of affected medication	Separate doses by at least 2 hours
Iron	• Fluoroquinolones, tetracyclines, digoxin, and levothyroxine • Methyldopa	• Decreased efficacy of affected medication • Worsening of hypertension	Separate doses by at least 2 hours. Avoid concomitant use
Potassium (including salt substitutes)	ACE Inhibitors, angiotensin receptor blockers, digoxin, indomethacin, prescription potassium supplements, and potassium-sparing diuretics	Hyperkalemia	Avoid concomitant supplementation without physician's supervision

(ACE: angiotensin-converting enzyme; HMG-CoA: β-hydroxy β-methylglutaryl-CoA)
Source: Sulli MM, Ezzo DC. Drug Interactions with vitamins and minerals. US Pharm. 2007;1:42-55.

Nutritional Status and Drug Interactions

Pharmacokinetic and pharmacodynamic data on drug disposition in malnutrition are not commonly found. Drug distribution and drug clearance are most affected and can potentially alter the clinical response.

Both fixed dose and body weight-based calculations of intravenous (IV) drug doses are unreliable in underweight and obese patients. Although lean body weight fares better than ideal body weight, such principles are not universally applicable. Several alternate body size descriptors which use mathematical calculations including height and weight similar to body surface area-based dosage calculations used in antineoplastic drug dosing are available but not backed by clinical studies. Humans have varied adipose tissue mass, muscle mass, and organ functions which may not correlate with height and weight. This creates a high probability of under- and overdosing which in turn cause treatment failure or toxicity. Higher treatment failure rates have been widely observed in obese patients treated with fixed-dose oral antibiotics and IV antibiotics as well.[10]

Forty kilograms is an arbitrary benchmark to differentiate pediatric from adult dosing recommendations. Population PK data is generated from observations across body weights 60 kilograms to 120 kilograms, in general. This may not be applicable to patients with higher weights. It may be practically impossible to get useful data from population studies for patients with extreme weights and extrapolation from available data may be imprecise.

Allometry is the study of the relationship of body size with shape, anatomy, physiology, and behavior. West, Brown, and Enquist in 1997 derived a hydrodynamic theory that states that metabolic rate scales as the $\frac{3}{4}$ power with body weight. Allometry-based dosage scales are available for many drugs.

Several calculations based on a combination of ideal body weight, adjusted body weight, and measured weight are available. Lean body weight using available formulas are proposed by Humes.[11]

Lean body weight derived from empirical data using bioelectrical impedance analysis is another technique. All the above calculations provide similar results. These empiric approaches mitigate the risk of overexposure and toxicity but do not account for the diversity of human body phenotypes that can alter tissue drug distribution and clearance.

Body phenotype identification is key to further dose refinement. Body mass index (BMI), waist–hip ratio, and waist circumference are crude and nonspecific measures. Body weight alone provides a one compartment framework. Two compartment frameworks comprise fat mass (FM) and fat-free mass (FFM). Equations have been developed to estimate this FFM using height and weight against measured FFM using hydrodensitrometry, air displacement plethysmography, and hydrometry. Dual-energy X-ray absorptiometry estimates of a third compartment (bone mineral content) that allows FFM to lean tissue mass extrapolation. Further assumption that adult total body water (TBW) is 73%, permits fractionation of the body in four compartments (FM, TBW, lean tissue mass, and bone mineral content) using multifrequency bioelectric impedance analysis.[12] Neutron activation analysis[13] is the most sophisticated technique that gives a breakup of the human body into six core elements. These methods are research tools and are not useful for everyday drug dosing considerations **(Table 5)**.

Parameter	Formula
Ideal body weight (IBW)	Males: 50 + [0.91 × (height in cm − 152.4)]
	Females: 45.5 + [0.91 × (height in cm − 152.4)]
Lean body weight (LBW)	Boer:
	Males: (0.407 × W) + (0.267 × H) − 19.2
	Females: (0.252 × W) + (0.473 × H) − 48.3
	W = body weight in kg, H = body height in cm
	Hume:
	Males: (0.32810 × W) + (0.33929 × H) − 29.5336
	Females: (0.29569 × W) + (0.41813 × H) − 43.2933
	W = body weight in kg, H = body height in cm
Adjusted body weight (AjBW)	IBW + 0.4 × (AjBW − IBW)

TABLE 5: Commonly used calculations for drug dose adjustment.

EFFECT OF DRUGS ON NUTRITION

Direct Effects

Drugs can influence food intake, digestion, absorption, and elimination. Intake may be impaired by dysgeusia, xerostomia, stomatitis, nausea, vomiting, diarrhea and physical characteristics such as bad odor or taste.

Indirect Effects

Drugs can impair ability to procure, process, and ingest food by causing gait disturbances, cognitive dysfunction, visual disturbances, and movement disorders.

Nutrient Metabolism

Macronutrient Metabolism

Weight gain, dyslipidemia, and hyperglycemia are documented metabolic adverse effects of antipsychotics whereas appetite suppressants cause weight loss.

Specific Nutrients

Similar to general macronutrients, effect of drugs on specific nutrients is multifactorial involving intake, digestion, absorption, and elimination. Development of overt classic nutrient deficiency due to an interaction is very rare. Carbamazepine decreases biotin absorption.[14] Antiepileptic drugs such as phenytoin, phenobarbital, and carbamazepine affect vitamin D metabolism and bone health.[15] Valproic acid causes carnitine deficiency causing impaired intermediary metabolism and subsequent hepatotoxicity. Simple supplementation of the deficient nutrient does not always mitigate problems. Further studies are needed to establish the role of prophylactic nutrient supplementation.

Drug–Nutrient Stability and Incompatibility

Parenteral Nutrition

Parenteral nutrition (PN) is administered to achieve set nutritional targets in special situations, which entail enteral nutrition unavailable or inadequate. It involves IV administration of carbohydrates as glucose, protein as amino acids, and fat as lipid emulsions along with electrolytes, vitamins, and micronutrients. Standard PN preparations are company manufactured, containing compartmentalized nutrients which are to be mixed prior to administration to optimize stability. Individualized pharmacy blended preparations are available in some centers. In general, standard preparations are found to be better.[16] Standard PN preparations are far from ideal. The common issues encountered being IV access, relatively lower concentrations of macronutrients, mixture stability, and compatibility issues with other nutrients and IV medications. PN infusions are incompatible with many IV medications. PN is, therefore, administered through a dedicated lumen through central venous access, except when short-term low osmolarity peripheral preparations suffice. Critically ill patients need multiple IV medications. PN should ideally be stopped with every medication and lines flushed before and after administration. This may lead to undernutrition and fluid overload in a fragile patient. Y-site connecters become necessary for administration of IV medication. Chemical degradation may not be very relevant because of low contact time but physical degradation.

Stability and Compatibility

A PN system or formulation is unstable if there is chemical, physical, or microbiological degradation or deterioration altering its pharmacological action or pharmaceutical characteristic. This includes potential loss of drug/PN component or altered properties leading to potential therapeutic failure, toxicity, or adverse events.[17] Factors affecting parenteral nutrition solutions are listed in **Table 6**.

A PN system is incompatible if on contact with another entity, such as drugs or excipients, there is physical and/or chemical degradation. Drug-parenteral nutrition solution interactions are listed in **Table 7**.

Assessing and establishing incompatibilities is challenging because of differences in PN formulations and IV medications in terms of concentration, excipients, additives such as vitamins and trace elements, container material, delivery systems and environmental factors such as storage temperature and exposure to light. It is imperative that incompatibilities become very significant in pediatric populations, especially neonates due to limited IV access and body size. Both precipitates and large oil droplets can potentially be dangerous upon infusion. Case reports of pulmonary emboli with fatal outcomes after the administration of total parenteral nutrition (TPN) containing calcium phosphate precipitates[18] and deaths of neonatal patients caused by an incompatibility between ceftriaxone and calcium-containing products[19] have contributed to safety guidelines. Animal studies have indicated that enlarged oil droplets can harm the lungs and liver because of emboli-like effects. Increased frequency of hypertriglyceridemia and impaired plasma clearance of lipids have been reported. Compatibility data hence becomes vital. Consensus regarding tests to check incompatibility or assessment criteria are lacking. The United States Pharmacopeia included droplet size requirements in 2007, stating that the mean droplet diameter (MDD) in lipid injectable emulsions should be <500 nm, measured by dynamic light scattering (DLS) or laser diffraction (LD), and that the volume-weighted percentage of fat with droplet diameter above 5 μm (PFAT5) measured by light obscuration (LO), should be ≤0.05%. These regulations are in general applicable to PN preparations also. Studies have shown that a combination of tests and technologies are required along with theoretical prediction are required to optimize compatibility testing.[20]

Assessment of precipitates is by visual examination with Tyndall light or other visual examination methods, turbidimetric measurements, colorimetric measurement, LO, DLS, microscopy, and pH-measurements. Parenteral emulsion stability may be investigated using visual observation with or without a centrifugation step, determination of zeta potential, measurement of dynamic surface tension, measurement of peroxide levels, and pH-measurements. Droplet size measurement techniques are microscopy, DLS, LD, flow cytometry, Coulter counter, and LO. Artificial intelligence tools using neural networks are under development to predict potential incompatibilities in the drug development phase.[21]

ENTERAL NUTRITION AND DRUGS

Most critically ill patients receive multiple drugs through enteral route after initial stabilization along with enteral nutrition. Interactions in this realm have not received needed attention. Various types of drug-enteral nutrition interactions are shown in **Table 8**.

IDENTIFICATION OF DRUG–NUTRIENT INTERACTIONS[6]

An informed scientific systematic approach will maximize prediction and recognition

CHAPTER 20 | Nutrient–Drug: Interactions and Compatibility

TABLE 6: Factors affecting parenteral nutrition solutions.[17]

Nutritive factors	Amino acids	• Higher concentrations improve emulsion stability and reduce Ca-P precipitation • Some acidic AAs cause creaming and cracking of the emulsion • Oxidizing agents like cysteine affect the bioavailability of easily oxidizable substances like ascorbic acid
	Glucose	• Concentrated glucose solutions cause disruption of the lipid phase • Maillard process may affect the bioavailability of AAs and may even produce toxic compounds • Lower glucose concentration potentially increases Ca-P precipitation
	Lipid	• Emulsifying agents, such as lecithin phospholipid, help maintaining stability of LEs is acronym for lipid emulsions • LEs in PNS are most stable at a pH of 8 • Composite lipid formulas are more stable compared to purely long-chain triglycerides formula
	Electrolytes	• Overall concentration individual cation burden, and electrolytes ratios have important effects on stability • High concentration of cations destabilizes lipid droplets • Ca-P precipitation is influenced by multiple factors. Low pH, calcium and phosphate concentrations prevent precipitation and maintain solubility
	Vitamins	• The least stable of all nutrients in PNS. Stability could be affected by photodegradation oxidation and interaction with storage material • Minimizing contact time, by adding vitamins to PNS immediately before use, may help to reduce stability and compatibility effects
	Trace elements	• Some trace elements may form insoluble salts • Copper can exacerbate degradation of vitamins • Positively charged trace elements may have a role in neutralizing the negative charge of the lipid emulsion and cause instability
Non-nutritive factors	pH	• Acidic pH values may jeopardize the integrity and stability of LEs, while alkaline pH favors the stability of the emulsion and maintains its uniformity • The Ca-P precipitation process depends on the pH of the medium, lower pH value maintains solubility
	Oxygen	• Components of PNS are subject to oxidative degradation in the presence of oxygen • Polyunsaturated fatty acids could be oxidized to harmful lipid hydroperoxides
	Light	• Light protection measures protect light sensitive compounds, such as photosensitive vitamins, from photo-oxidation • Exposure to daylight is more hazardous than artificial light due to the ultra-violet wave spectrum involved
	Temperature	• Standard refrigeration temperatures increase the storage life of PNS • Lipid peroxidation, and Ca-P precipitation may be accelerated by the increase of ambient temperature prior to and during the use of PNS
	Preparation and mixing order	Adding lipids firstly to the glucose compartment may increase lipid degradation due to high acidity of the dextrose solution before additional buffering compounds are added
	Co-infusion/ addition of drug	The addition, or concurrent administration of the IVM to PNS increases the risks of the stability and incompatibility problems
	Infusion sets, and containers	Infusion sets and containers also play a role in the stability of PNS in terms of light protection, oxygen barriers, and direct interactions

(AA: amino acid; Ca-P: calcium-phosphate precipitation; IVM: intravenous medication; LE: lipid emulsion; PNS: parenteral nutrition solutions)

TABLE 7: Drug-PNS with electrolytes interactions sourced from Drugs.com drug interaction checker.

Interaction	Drug class	Drug name	Adverse effect	Recommendation
Major	Potassium-sparing diuretics	• Amiloride • Spironolactone • triamterene	Hyperkalemia	
	Angiotensin Receptor blockers	• Azilsartan medoxomil • Candesartan • Eprosartan • Irbesartan • Losartan • Olmesartan • Telmisartan • Sparsentan • Valsartan	Hyperkalemia	*Caution:* Concurrent use with potassium salts, patients with renal impairment, diabetes, old age, severe or worsening heart failure, dehydration, or concomitant therapy with other agents that increase serum potassium such as nonsteroidal anti-inflammatory drugs, beta-blockers, cyclosporine, heparin, tacrolimus, and trimethoprim. Avoid combinations unless absolutely necessary and the benefits outweigh the potential risks
	Angiotensinogen-converting enzyme (ACE) inhibitors	• Benazepril • Captopril • Enalapril • Enalaprilat • Fosinopril • Lisinopril • Moexipril • Perindopril • Quinapril • Ramipril • Trandolapril	Hyperkalemia	*Caution:* If ACE inhibitors must be used concurrently with potassium salts, particularly in patients with renal impairment, diabetes, old age, severe or worsening heart failure, dehydration, or concomitant therapy with agents causing increase in serum potassium such as nonsteroidal anti-inflammatory drugs, beta-blockers, cyclosporine, heparin, tacrolimus, trimethoprim, and licorice
	• Aldosterone • Antagonists	• Eplerenone • Finerenone	Hyperkalemia	Contraindicated with potassium salts or potassium-sparing diuretics
	Antimicrobials	Ceftriaxone	Ceftriaxone – Calcium precipitates	• Contraindicated coadministration via a Y site in all patients • Contraindicated co-administration even at a different IV site within 48 hours of each other in neonates up to 28 days age

Contd...

Contd...

Interaction	Drug class	Drug name	Adverse effect	Recommendation
		Trimethoprim	Hyperkalemia	• Serum potassium, sodium levels and renal function need close monitoring when co administered with other potassium-sparing drugs or potassium salts, particularly in patients receiving high-dose or long-term trimethoprim treatment and in patients with renal impairment, diabetes, old age, severe or worsening heart failure, or dehydration. A dosage reduction of trimethoprim is recommended in renal dysfunction (50% reduction for CrCl between 15 and 30 mL/min)
Moderate				
	Renin–Angiotensin system inhibitors	Aliskiren	Hyperkalemia	Caution is advised if aliskiren is used in combination with potassium-sparing diuretics or potassium salts. Routine monitoring of electrolytes and renal function may be indicated, particularly in patients with renal impairment, diabetes, old age, worsening heart failure, or a risk for dehydration
	Nondepolarizing neuromuscular blocker (NMB)	• Atracurium • Cisatracurium • Mivacurium • Pancuronium • Rocuronium • Vecuronium	Magnesium salts enhance the effects of nondepolarizing NMBs	Close monitoring for excessive or prolonged neuromuscular blockade
	Calcium channel blockers (CCBs)	• Amlodipine • Clevidipine • Felodipine • Isradipine • Levamlodipine • Nicardipine • Nifedipine • Nimodipine • Nisoldipine • Bepridil • Diltiazem • Verapamil	Calcium in PNS may decrease the effectiveness of CCBs by saturating calcium channels	Monitor the effectiveness of CCB therapy during coadministration

Contd...

Contd...

Interaction	Drug class	Drug name	Adverse effect	Recommendation
	Radiopharmaceutical diagnostic agent	Indium oxyquinoline in-111	Decrease chemotaxis and cause false-negative results with Indium In-111-labeled leukocyte studies	Be aware of possible diagnostic interference
	Magnesium salts		Hypermagnesemia	Clinical and laboratory monitoring for signs of hypermagnesemia especially in elderly and patients with renal impairment

TABLE 8: Types of interactions between drugs and nutrients.

Type of interaction	Comments	Examples
Absorption	Interactions may occur between drugs and nutrients that are only orally administered or by enteral-feeding distribution systems. The oral bioavailability of the active drug increase or decrease because of these interactions	Tetracycline, alendronate, phenytoin, and levodopa display reduced absorption with food; grape juice reduces the absorption of carbamazepine
Postabsorption	Occurs after the drug molecule or the nutritional component reach the systemic circulation and may result in altered distribution within the various tissues, systemic metabolism, or penetration into a specific site	Foods rich in vitamin K (or its supplementation) alter the pharmacodynamics of warfarin
Elimination	Numerous pathways may be involved, such as antagonism, modulation, or decreased renal or enterohepatic transport	High-protein diets increase the elimination of propranolol; alkaline diets increase the excretion of barbiturates, diuretics, sulfonamides, acetylsalicylic acid, aminoglycosides, and penicillins and decrease the excretion

Source: Heldt T, Loss SH. Drug-nutrient interactions in the intensive care unit: literature review and current recommendations. Rev Bras Ter Intensiva. 2013;25(2):162-7. doi:10.5935/0103-507X.20130028.

of DNIs in clinical practice and optimize patient safety.

DRUG-NUTRITION INTERACTIONS IN THE ICU

A combination of comorbidities, polypharmacy, compromised organ function, and altered physiology due to disease and/or therapeutic interventions makes critically ill patients a high-risk population for DNIs. Studies in this area are very few and leave many knowledge gaps.

Challenges

Most critically ill patients are unable to eat normally. Enteral nutrition via nasogastric, orogastric, nasojejunal, gastrostomy, or jejunostomy routes is administered to provide nutrition. GI dysfunction because of nausea, vomiting, dysmotility, compartment syndrome, altered microbiome, and malabsorption is very common and contributes to worse outcomes. Withholding feeds before and after drug administration will lead to dangerous undernutrition and may not be practical. PN on the other hand can interact with drugs and alter drug efficacy. Extracorporeal therapies add more complexity. Establishing a drug–nutrition interaction as the cause for an event is a daunting task. **Tables 9 and 10** provides a framework for a systematic multilevel approach which may be helpful in identification of DNIs. Further evaluation and redressal is even more complex. Clinical pathways to this end are almost nonexistent in current practice. **Boxes 1 and 2** provide useful clinical pearls.

MANAGEMENT

Drug–nutrient interactions in general develop gradually except in the case of warfarin/Vitamin K and monoamine oxidase (MAO) inhibitors/tyramine. Most situations do not warrant urgent action. In critically ill patients with limited reserve and high severity of illness, there is a higher risk of harm. Drugs with a low therapeutic index may cause toxicity. Thus, urgent decisions to change therapeutic strategies may be warranted. The interventions may include an empirical administration of a nutrient in the event of suspected nutrient deficiency

TABLE 9: Identifying drug–nutrient interactions (DNIs) at multiple levels.[6]

Clinician	Institution	Patient
• Recognize DNIs systematically as part of a focused patient assessment • Understand underlying mechanisms of interactions and thereby predict DNIs and intervene appropriately • Understand drug disposition physiology • Access to information including drug product information, post-marketing observational studies, case reports	• Standardized hospital policy for patient assessment, patient care plans, medication chart review, safe medication administration, and patient monitoring and education • Abide by local regulation • Set up a team comprising physicians, pharmacists, dieticians, and nurses to coordinate care • Targeted monitoring for DNIs in high-risk patients or for high-risk medications • Integrated decision support systems	• Thorough nutrition history • Physical examination • Clues • Therapeutic outcome does not match expectation • Nutrition assessment to identify status and causation • Drug interaction probability scores to establish cause

TABLE 10: Drug interaction probability score by Horn and Hansten.[22]

The drug interaction probability scale (DIPS) is designed to assess the probability of a causal relationship between a potential drug interaction and an event. It is patterned after the Naranjo ADR probability scale (Clin Pharmacol Ther 1981;30:239-45).

Directions:
- Circle the appropriate answer for each question, and add up the total score.
- Object drug = Drug affected by the interaction.
- Precipitant drug = Drug that causes the interaction.
- Use the unknown (Unk) or not applicable (NA) category if (a) you do not have the information or (b) the question is not applicable (e.g., no dechallenge; dose not changed, etc.).

Contd...

Contd...

Questions	Yes	No	Unk or NA
1. Are there previous *credible* reports of this interaction in humans?	+1	−1	0
2. Is the observed interaction consistent with the known interactive properties of precipitant drug?	+1	−1	0
3. Is the observed interaction consistent with the known interactive properties of object drug?	+1	−1	0
4. Is the event consistent with the known or reasonable time course of the interaction (onset and/or offset)?	+1	−1	0
5. Did the interaction remit upon dechallenge of the *precipitant* drug with no change in the object drug? (if no dechallenge, use unknown or NA and skip question 6)	+1	−2	0
6. Did the interaction reappear when the precipitant drug was readministered in the presence of continued use of object drug?	+2	−1	0
7. Are there reasonable alternative causes for the event?[a]	−1	+1	0
8. Was the object drug detected in the blood or other fluids in concentrations consistent with the proposed interaction?	+1	0	0
9. Was the drug interaction confirmed by any objective evidence consistent with the effects on the object drug (other than drug concentrations from questions 8)?	+1	0	0
10. Was the interaction greater when the precipitant drug dose was increased or less when the precipitant drug dose was decreased?	+1	−1	0

[a]Consider clinical conditions, other interacting drugs, lack of adherence, risk factors (e.g., age, inappropriate doses of object drug). A NO answer presumes that enough information was presented so that one would expect any alternative causes to be mentioned. When in doubt, use unknown or NA designation.

Total score____   Highly probable: >8
　　　　　　　　 Probable: 5–8
　　　　　　　　 Possible: 2–4
　　　　　　　　 Doubtful: <2

BOX 1: Drug–nutrient interactions in enteral feeding in the intensive care unit (ICU).[23]

- *Knowledge of the type and location of the feeding tube:*
  - *Stomach:* Choice for drugs that act on this site, such as antacids and ketoconazole
  - *Duodenum:* Preferable route for drugs susceptible to gastric acidity (such as digoxin, carbamazepine, ciprofloxacin, and tetracycline)
- *Drugs that alter nutrients:*
  - *Diuretics:* Hyponatremia, hypernatremia, hypokalemia, and dehydration
  - *Steroids:* Changes in sodium, potassium, and glucose
  - *Angiotensin-converting enzyme inhibitors:* Hyperkalemia
  - *Amphotericin B:* Hypokalemia and hypomagnesemia
  - *Calcium supplements:* Hypophosphatemia
- *Nutrients that affect drugs:*
  - *Phenytoin:* Requires interruption of the diet for 1–2 hours
  - *Quinolones:* Reduced serum levels when administered with food
  - *Itraconazole:* Increased absorption with nutrients
    Warfarin: Decreased anticoagulation with vitamin K
  - *Alendronate:* Decreased absorption with food

BOX 2: Precautions for drug administration through feeding tubes.[23]
- Determine the type, caliber, and location of the distal end of the tube
- Administer liquid medication whenever possible
- Choose a gastric tube over a duodenal tube whenever possible
- Avoid crushing drug capsules or programmed/extended release—drug formulations
- Administer each drug separately
- Administer the entire programmed dose
- Do not mix drugs with nutrients
- Nutrition deficit should be addressed by using nutrient dense feeds
- Dilute viscous or hyperosmolar solutions with 60–90 mL water
- Rinse the tube with 30 mL water before and after drug administration
- Participate in continuous training

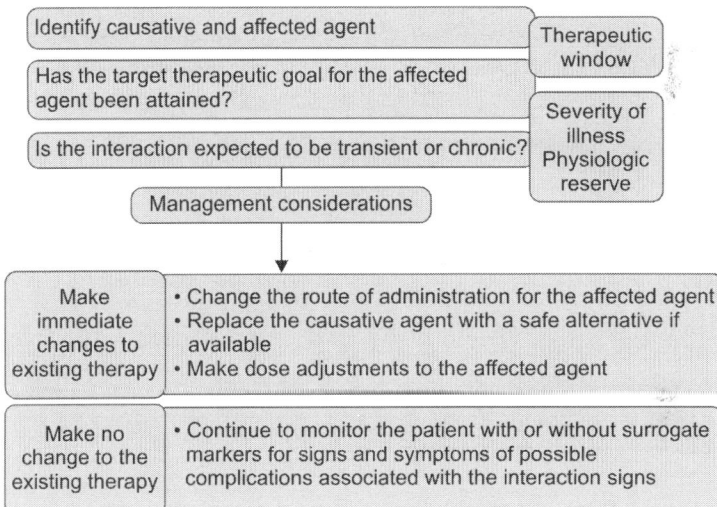

Flowchart 1: Approach to management of drug–nutrition interactions.[24]

or withholding a drug in a suspected case of drug toxicity due to a DNI or using alternate regimens or routes of administration. A practical approach is depicted in **Flowchart 1**.

FUTURE

We need more research in the field targeting the following areas:[24]
- Developing a common language and concept in the understanding, evaluation, and management of DNIs
- Understanding the mechanisms of DNIs
- Population- and gene-based research to compare incidence and risk factors of specific DNIs
- Outcomes research that addresses the short-term and long-term clinical significance and economic impact of specific DNIs.

CONCLUSION

Drug nutrition interactions are common and significant. Recognition, evaluation, and management strategies lack robust evidence. Clinicians should be aware of possible DNIs based on case reports, and postmarketing studies. Understanding basic PK and pharmacodynamic concepts, extrapolation from *in vitro* studies, and good clinical judgement will help manage patients safely.

REFERENCES

1. Drees BM, Barthel B. We are what we eat. Mo Med. 2022;119(5):479-80.
2. Sarkar PK, Chaudhari S, Chattopadhyay A. Concept of interactions between consumable substances in Ayurveda with special reference to foods and drugs. Drug Metabol Drug Interact. 2013;28(3):147-52.
3. Santos CA, Boullata JI. An approach to evaluating drug-nutrient interactions. Pharmacotherapy. 2005;25(12):1789-800.
4. Liang Y, Li S, Chen L. The physiological role of drug transporters. Protein Cell. 2015;6(5):334-50.
5. Choi JH, Ko CM. Food and Drug Interactions. J Lifestyle Med. 2017;7(1):1-9.
6. Boullata JI, Hudson LM. Drug-nutrient interactions: a broad view with implications for practice. J Acad Nutr Diet. 2012;112(4):506-17.
7. Amidon GL, Lennernäs H, Shah VP, Crison JR. A theoretical basis for a biopharmaceutic drug classification: The correlation of in vitro drug product dissolution and in vivo bioavailability. Pharm Res. 1995;12(3):413-20.
8. Ronis MJ. Effects of soy containing diet and isoflavones on cytochrome P450 enzyme expression and activity. Drug Metab Rev. 2016;48(3):331-41.
9. Petric Z, Žuntar I, Putnik P, Bursać Kovačević D. Food-drug interactions with fruit juices. Foods. 2020;10(1):33.
10. Barber KE, Loper JT, Morrison AR, Stover KR, Wagner JL Impact of obesity on ceftriaxone efficacy. Diseases. 2020;8:27.
11. Hume R. Prediction of lean body mass from height and weight. J Clin Pathol. 1966;18(4):38991.
12. Pai MP. Antimicrobial dosing in specific populations and novel clinical methodologies: Obesity. Clin Pharmacol Ther. 2021;109(4):942-51.
13. Kehayias JJ, Valtueña S. Neutron activation analysis determination of body composition. Curr Opin Clin Nutr Metab Care. 1999;2:453-63.
14. Mock DM, Dyken ME. Biotin catabolism is accelerated in adults receiving long-term therapy with anticonvulsants. Neurology. 1997;49(5):1444-7.
15. Siniscalchi A, De Arro G, Michniewicz A, Gallelli L. Conventional and new antiepileptic drugs on vitamin d and BONE HEALTH: What we know to date? Curr Clin Pharmacol. 2016;11(1):69-70.
16. Alfonso JE, Berlana D, Ukleja A, Boullata J. Clinical, ergonomic, and economic outcomes with multichamber bags compared with (hospital) pharmacy compounded bags and multibottle systems: a systematic literature review. JPEN J Parenter Enteral Nutr. 2017;41(7):1162-77.
17. Farhan M, McCallion N, Bennett J, Cram A, O'Brien F. Stability and compatibility of parenteral nutrition solutions; a review of influencing factors. Eur J Pharm Biopharm. 2023;187:87-95.
18. Hill SE, Heldman LS, Goo EDH, Whippo PE, Perkinson JC. Fatal microvascular pulmonary emboli from precipitation of a total nutrient admixture solution. JPEN J Parenter Enteral Nutr. 1996;20:81-7.
19. Bradley JS, Wassel RT, Lee L, Nambiar S. Intravenous ceftriaxone and calcium in the neonate: assessing the risk for cardiopulmonary adverse events. Paediatrics. 2009;123:e609-13.
20. Staven V, Wang S, Grønlie I, Tho I. Development and evaluation of a test program for Y-site compatibility testing of total parenteral nutrition and intravenous drugs. Nutrition J. 2016;15(1).
21. Patel S, Patel M, Kulkarni M, Patel MS. DE-INTERACT: A machine-learning-based predictive tool for the drug-excipient interaction study during product development—Validation through paracetamol and vanillin as a case study. Int J Pharm. 2023;637(122839):378-5173.
22. Horn JR, Hansten PD, Chan LN. Proposal for a new tool to evaluate drug interaction cases. Ann Pharmacother. 2007;41(4):674-80.
23. Heldt T, Loss SH. Drug-nutrient interactions in the intensive care unit: literature review and current recommendations. Rev Bras Ter Intensiva. 2013;25(2):162-7.
24. Chan LN. Drug-nutrient interactions. JPEN J Parenteral Enteral Nutr. 2013;37(4):450-9.

CHAPTER 21: Fluid and Electrolytes in Critical Illness

Bharat Jagiasi, Priya Sonavdekar

INTRAVENOUS FLUIDS

■ INTRODUCTION

Total body water content accounts for approximately 60% of total body weight (TBW) in young male adult and about 50% in young adult female. Total body fluid is divided further into intracellular and extracellular fluids (ECFs). Intracellular fluid (ICF) accounts for two-thirds of TBW and ECF for one-third of TBW. ECF comprises interstitial compartment and intravascular compartment (plasma) **(Fig. 1)**. The small narrow spaces between tissues and organs are called the interstitial compartment, filled with fluid. When excessive fluid starts accumulating in interstitial space edema starts developing. The main component of the intravascular compartment is blood. The average volume of blood in humans is approximately 70–75 mL/kg.

■ FLUIDS

Fluids are by far the most commonly administered intravenous (IV) treatment in inpatient care.

Crystalloids

Crystalloids are mainly made up of water and electrolytes, which can cross a semipermeable cell membrane, and it is the most common choice of IV fluid used for resuscitation worldwide. There are three types of crystalloids, given according to their tonicity, the ability to make water move into or out of a cell by osmosis **(Flowchart 1)**.

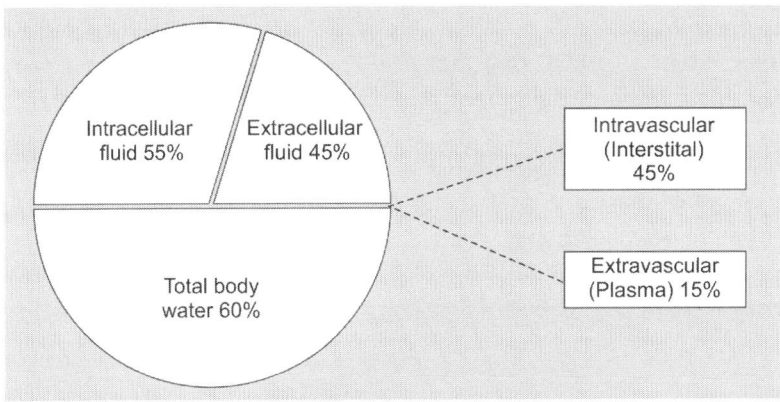

Fig. 1: Distribution of total body water.

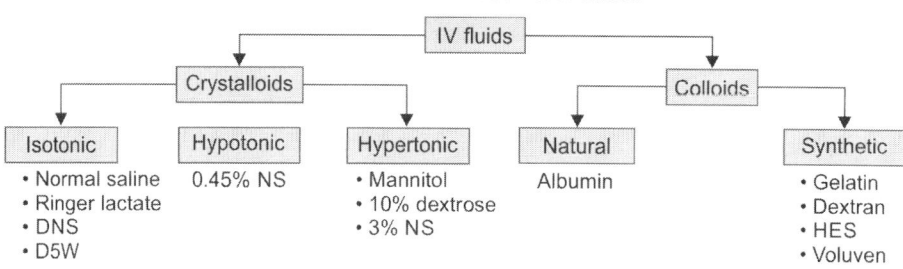

Flowchart 1: Classification of IV fluids.

(DNS: dextrose normal saline; D5W: dextrose 5% in water; HES: hydroxyethyl starch; IV: intravenous; NS: normal saline)

Tonicity is solute concentration relative to another solution on the opposite side of a cell membrane.

The osmolarity of a solution is determined by the amount of solute dissolved in a solvent.

A solution with few particles has a low osmolarity, while a solution with a high number of particles has a high osmolarity. Water moves through the semipermeable membranes of the body from low-to-high osmolarity to create a balance of water and solutes. Osmotic pressure determines water distribution among the different fluid compartments, particularly between the ECF and ICF.

The three types of crystalloids are:
1. *Hypotonic:* When the ECF has fewer solutes (osmolarity) than the fluid in the cells, water will move from extracellular space into the cells.
2. *Hypertonic:* When the ECF has more solutes (osmolarity) than within the cells, water flows out of the cells.
3. *Isotonic:* Both the extracellular and ICFs have the same osmolarity, so there is no water movement between them.

0.9% Normal Saline

Composition: Na-154, Cl-154
Type: Isotonic
Distribution: It mainly stays in ECF.

Indications

- Intravascular resuscitation like state of hypovolemic shock
- Metabolic alkalosis in cases of vomiting and diarrhea
- Hypovolemic natremia
- Diabetic ketoacidosis (DKA), hypercalcemia, and fluid challenge
- Brain injury

Contraindications/Drawbacks

It has a high concentration of chloride, hence causing hyperchloremia.

It has to be cautiously used and/or avoided in case of renal disease as it can cause acute tubular damage, which can decrease output and cause acute kidney injury (AKI).

Since it stays entirely in extravascular—it increases volume, so best avoided in congestive heart failure (CHF) and cirrhosis.

Dextrose Normal Saline

Composition: 0.9% saline 5% dextrose
Distribution: ECF
Type: Isotonic

Indications

- Fluid deficit with calorie
- Can be given in cases of vomiting and diarrhea.
- Fluid compatible with blood transfusion.

Contraindications/Drawbacks

- Can cause hyperglycemia, if given in large volumes leading to osmotic diuresis.
- Avoided in patients with diabetes.
- Cautious use in patients with anasarca.

Ringer Lactate

Type: Isotonic

Distribution: Stays in ECF; expand the intravascular volume, so it helps in case of severe hypovolemia. Composition is most physiologically similar to plasma. Hence, large volumes can be administered.

Indications

- Fluid losses due to burns and trauma
- Gastrointestinal (GI) losses due to diarrhea
- Acute blood loss in case of surgical patients.

Contraindications/Drawbacks

- Metabolites in the liver hence cannot be given to a patient with chronic liver disease as lactate is converted to bicarbonate in the liver.
- Avoided in patients with lactic acidosis.
- Cannot be given along blood products as Ca binds with citrate leading to reduced anticoagulant activity.
- Cannot be given in case of metabolic alkalosis as it has bicarbonate and can worsen the condition.

3% Normal Saline

Composition:

One litre of fluid contains: Sodium 154.0 mEq chloride 154.0 mEq.

Type: Hypertonic

Distribution: It has high osmolarity and tonicity; hence, osmotic pressure gradient draws water out of intracellular space, increasing ECF.

Indications

- Patient with cerebral edema
- Severe hyponatremia

Contraindications/Drawbacks

- Requires constant monitoring for potential complications. Serum Na to monitor at regular intervals.
- Requires a definite volume to be administered with an actual infusion rate over a definite period.
- Have to be administered with the central line as it causes phlebitis in the peripheral line.

25% Dextrose

Composition: 100 mL of 25% dextrose contains 25 g of glucose.

Type: Hypertonic

Indications

- Used for correction of hypoglycemia or hyperglycemic coma
- For hyperkalemia.

Contraindications/Drawbacks

- In case of traumatic brain injury as it may cause cerebral edema due to its nature of distribution in ECF.
- Avoided in diabetic patients unless hypoglycemic coma.

Balanced and Nonbalanced Crystalloids (Table 1)

Generally, two broad categories of crystalloid preparations are available for IV use in the intensive care unit (ICU). These categories are physiologically buffered (balanced) preparations containing electrolytes and buffers in concentrations that approximate those found in normal human plasma.

TABLE 1: Comparison between balanced and unbalanced crystalloids with human plasma.

	Sodium (Na)	Potassium (K)	Chloride (Cl)	Calcium (Ca)	Magnesium (Mg)	Lactate	Acetate	Gluconate	Osmolarity
Normal saline (0.9%)	154	–	154	–	–	–	–	–	308
Ringer's lactate	130	4	109	1.5	–	28	–	–	276
Plamsalyte	140	5	98	–	3	–	27	23	293
Plasma	136–145	3.5–4.5	98–106	4.4–5.2	1.6–2.4	Bicarbonate 21–30			280–300

The other category is neither buffered nor balanced, and it does not contain physiological concentrations of electrolytes.

Plasmalyte

Plasmalyte is balanced IV fluid with sodium and chloride concentrations and other electrolytes identical to human plasma. The osmolality is the same as that of the plasma with the buffering effect.

Plasmalyte has no acidifying effect, has a better buffering effect (sodium bicarbonate) and is, therefore, more effective than isotonic saline in countering metabolic acidosis in diabetic ketosis and trauma. In acute/chronic kidney disease, plasmalyte administration caused less deviation of the electrolyte balance than both isotonic saline and Ringer's lactate, as it does not cause hyperchloremia and acidosis since the composition of plasmalyte is more similar to the ECF than any other crystalloid. Although plasmalyte is the best choice for IV, there is no benefit concerning clinical outcomes relative to other unbalanced fluids.

Plasmalyte is used on the same indications as the buffered Ringer's solutions. This fluid might also be considered in trauma patients and children because it is isotonic.

The clinical trial (SMART trial) was conducted in a cluster-randomized, multiple-crossover trial in five intensive care units at an academic center where balanced crystalloids and saline are used for IV fluid administration in critically ill adults. A study suggested that using balanced crystalloids for IV fluid administration resulted in a lower rate of the composite outcome of death from any cause, new renal-replacement therapy (RRT), or persistent renal dysfunction than using saline.

TABLE 2: Characteristic of colloids per 100 mL infusion.

Type of fluid	Effective plasma volume expansion	Duration of expansion
5% albumin	70–130 mL	16 hours
25% albumin	400–500 mL	16 hours
6% hetastarch	100–130 mL	24 hours
Dextran 40	100–150 mL	6 hours

Colloids (Table 2)

Colloids are IV fluids that contain high molecular weight microscopic substances suspended in crystalloid solutions. Colloids can remain in the intravascular space longer than crystalloids due to macromolecules in solution, which create more significant osmotic pressure in the circulation. Because of their high molecular weight, colloidal substances penetrate the healthy semipermeable endothelial barrier only slowly. While crystalloid electrolyte solutions distribute evenly to intravascular and extravascular spaces, colloids expand intravascular. This effect is partially lost with inflammation-altered vascular permeability.

The primary function of colloids is to use as second-line treatment for volume resuscitation. Theoretically, the colloid volume required to maintain the same intravascular filling is up to three times smaller than that of crystalloids. However, this advantage is lost when inflammatory conditions like sepsis damage the endothelial glycocalyx.

Colloids can be divided into two groups: (1) "Semi-synthetic" hydroxyethyl starch (HES), gelatin and dextran solutions and "natural" (human albumin solution). (2) Semi-synthetic colloids were preferred because they were cheaper and more readily available than their natural counterparts.

Albumin[1]

It is a physiological plasma protein. It maintains oncotic pressure. human serum albumin is commercially available in 5% (50 g/L) and 25% (250 g/L).

Distribution: plasma volume expansion occurs due to interstitial fluid shifts from the extravascular to the intravascular compartment, expanding roughly the same as the volume infused. Oncotic pressure lasts 12–18 hours.

Indications

- Plasma volume expansion in cases of acute hypovolemic shock, burns, and severe acute albumin loss.
- Correction of hypoproteinemia—in cases of liver disease, malnutrition, diuretic resistant nephrotic syndrome, and septic shock.
- Exchange fluid in therapeutic plasmapheresis in certain neurological diseases or cancers, in large volume ascites paracentesis to replace removed plasma.

Contraindications

- Contraindicated in severe anemia or congestive cardiac failure, acute respiratory distress syndrome causes pulmonary edema, traumatic brain injury increases chances of 30-day mortality due to an increase in vasogenic edema and disruption in the blood-brain barrier.
- Albumin is considered a relatively safe, although more expensive, alternative for volume resuscitation of ICU patients with semi-synthetic colloids.

The SAFE study conducted on 6,997 patients who required volume resuscitation in ICU was randomized into two groups where one group received 4% albumin and other received 0.9% normal saline (NS) and found no difference in mortality, stay of ICU or days of mechanical ventilation or RRT. The Albumin Italian Outcome Sepsis (ALBIOS) study showed that albumin did not improve 28- and 90-day survival. However, post-hoc analysis found a reduction in 90-day mortality for the albumin group in patients with septic shock. Surviving sepsis guidelines for the management of sepsis and septic shock 2021 suggest using albumin, which cannot tolerate a large number of crystalloids, as a second line of resuscitation.

Gelatin Polymer (Haemaccel)[2]

It is a colloidal plasma substitute which contains a polymer of degraded gelatin 35 g with electrolytes such as Na, K, Cl, and Ca.

- *Type:* Semi-synthetic colloids
- *Distribution:* Because of its lower molecular weight colloid osmotic effect of gelatins lasts longer than other colloids.

- *Indication:* For rapid expansion of volume intraoperative or to reduce the total volume of fluid replacement, it expands volume by 50% of infused volume.
- For priming heart-lung machine.
- *Contradiction/complication:* The use of gelatin is found to be associated with an increase in anaphylaxis (urticaria and bronchospasm) and AKI and mortality.

Dextran

- *Type:* Semi-synthetic colloids
  Dextran is a mixture of glucose polymers of variable sizes, derived from bacteria. *Leuconostoc mesenteroides*, commercially available in two forms dextran 40 and dextran 70.
- *Distribution:* It effectively expands intravascular volume, but it is not a substitute for blood or plasma as it lacks clotting factors and oxygen carrying properties.

Indication

They are approved for vascular surgery because of their rheological properties, decreasing blood viscosity and potentially improving microvascular flow, especially after grafting.

Rapid expansion of plasma volume in case of surgeries; cautiously to be used in patients with pulmonary edema or chronic heart failure and chronic liver disease.

Contraindication/Complication

- As dextrans are associated with renal failure, avoid in case of oligoanuria, allergic reactions (urticaria) and changes in viscoelastic measurements and fibrinolysis, producing increased coagulopathy, these solutions should not be used for volume resuscitation.
- Should be given cautiously in patients receiving heparin as it tends to increase the anticoagulation effect.
- Contains Ca hence it should be avoided along with blood transfusion.
- Given its cost and no substantial benefit over crystalloids, its use should be discouraged in perioperative and severely dehydrated patients.

Hydroxyethyl Starch and Voluven (Tetrastarch)

Commercially available as 6% hetastarch. It is a synthetic colloid available as a 6% solution in isotonic saline.

Distribution: Plasma volume expanders like albumin and dextran but found to be more potent than 5% serum albumin. It has higher colloidal osmotic pressure than 5% albumin, causing more significant plasma volume expansion (30%) and lasts up to 24 hours. It is cheaper than 5% albumin.

Indications

It is safer and effective plasma expander; and can be used to correct hypovolemia.

Contraindications

- Increase in serum amylase during and 3–5 days after discontinuation of transfusion
- Allergic reactions can occur.
- Not to be used in congestive cardiac failure, impaired renal failure, or acute pancreatitis

Based on randomized trials of HES versus crystalloids done on patients with sepsis, HES solutions should not be used in patients with septic shock.

In 2012, the CHEST trial also reported that HES 130/0.4 in saline (Voluven) was associated with more negative outcomes than isotonic saline in 7,000 patients treated for different diagnoses in the intensive care setting. There was no difference in mortality, but serum creatinine rose more in the HES group.

Fluid Therapy

Fluid therapy is widely used for restoring fluids and electrolytes, as a drug carrier and for nutrition. It shows immediate response due to direct infusion in the intravascular compartment and correction of severe fluid and electrolyte disturbances. It affects the cardiovascular, renal, GI, and immune systems. Fluid administration should, therefore, always be accompanied by careful consideration of the risk/benefit ratio. Apart from the need to constantly assess fluid responsiveness, it is also essential to periodically reconsider the type of fluid being administered. Every specific disease requires a particular fluid therapy.

Fluids may expand the intravascular compartment, improving cardiac output (CO) and end-organ perfusion. However, hypo- and hypervolemia have been associated with several unfavorable outcomes, including AKI, respiratory complications, increased lengths of stays, admission costs, and 30-day mortality rates. Hence, ROSE concept was established.

Three primary indications for IV fluid administration are resuscitation, replacement, and maintenance. Resuscitation fluids are used to correct an intravascular volume deficit or acute hypovolemia; replacement solutions are prescribed to correct existing or developing deficits that cannot be compensated by oral intake alone; maintenance solutions are indicated in hemodynamically stable patients that are not able/allowed to drink water in order to cover their daily requirements of water and electrolytes.

The ROSE concept and the four phases of fluid therapy: Resuscitation (R), Optimization (O), Stabilization (S), and Evacuation (E) have been shown in **Figure 2**.

Step 1: Resuscitation—in the resuscitation phase, when a patient presents with hemodynamic shock, the aim of the treatment is resuscitation and correction of shock with the achievement of an adequate perfusion pressure by giving rapid fluid bolus along with vasopressor if required. In the initial phase, we aim for positive fluid balance.

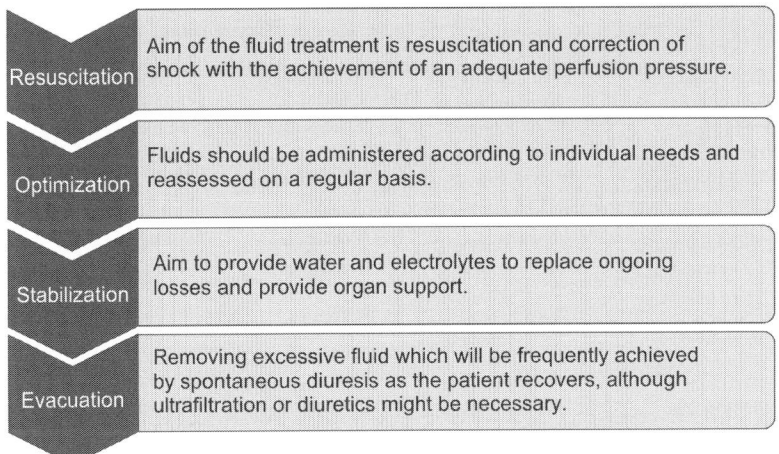

Fig. 2: Steps in ROSE concept. Intravenous fluid therapy in the perioperative and critical care setting: Executive summary of the International Fluid Academy.[3]

Step 2: Optimization—in this phase, the patient is no longer hypovolemic but is hemodynamically unstable. We aim to optimize and maintain adequate tissue perfusion and oxygenation to prevent and limit organ damage. Hence, few things are essential to keep in mind before administrating fluid, such as type of fluid—decide the type of fluid crystalloid (balanced/unbalanced), (isotonic/hyper-/hypotonic), rate of fluid—calculate the total amount of fluid you want to give, objective—to maintain hemodynamic stability, limits—to avoid increased central venous pressure or EVLI (extravascular lung water index).

We can insert arterial and central lines to get the exact status of patients' hemodynamics along with echocardiography, X-ray imaging and arterial blood gas (ABG).

Step 3: Stabilization—in this phase, fluid management aims to ensure water and electrolytes to replace ongoing losses and provide organ support. We try to maintain a neutral balance to avoid fluid overload, which may cause congestive cardiac failure or pulmonary edema, may increase in mechanical ventilator days or increase in ICU length of stay.

Step 4: Evacuation/De-escalation—in this stage, we try to maintain a negative balance in case of fluid overload with late goal-directed fluid removal (LGFR) to remove the excessive fluid. We stopped fluid if no longer needed and achieved spontaneous diuresis or hemodialysis if required as the patient recovers. Therapeutic goals should consider the patient's primary pathology, underlying life goals, preferences regarding aggressive medical therapy and response to treatment. Like other medical therapies, fluid therapy should be tailored to the individual patient's needs.

HYPOKALEMIA

Hypokalemia is generally defined as a serum potassium level of <3.5 mEq/L (3.5 mmol/L). Moderate hypokalemia is a serum level of 2.5–3.0 mEq/L, and severe hypokalemia is <2.5 mEq/L.

Causes

- *Osmotic diuresis:* Mannitol and hyperglycemia can cause osmotic diuresis.
- Increased GI losses (nasogastric suction, vomiting, and diarrhea)
- Hypomagnesemia
- Antifungal agents (amphotericin B, azoles, and echinocandins)
- Verapamil (with overdose)
- *Renal tubular disorders:* Types I and II renal tubular acidosis
- Cushing syndrome (causes kidneys to excrete K^+)
- Too much water intake
- Inadequate consumption of K^+

Symptoms

- Lethargy
- Cardiac arrhythmia—ST depression, shallow T wave, and U wave.
- Respiratory muscle weakness
- Hypokalemia periodic paralysis or leg cramps
- Tachycardia
- Low blood pressure.

Laboratory Parameters

- Evaluate serum potassium
- Check glucose levels in patients with known or suspected diabetes mellitus, if a persistent loss despite the sufficient correction, then look for other reasons.
- Serum renin, aldosterone, and cortisol
- Pituitary imaging to evaluate for Cushing syndrome

- Evaluation for a renal workup to look for a renal tubular disorder
- Thyroid function studies in patients with tachycardia.

Management

- Watch other electrolytes like magnesium (will also decrease. It is hard to get K^+ to increase if magnesium is low); watch glucose, sodium, and calcium all go hand-in-hand and play a role in cell transport.
- Administer oral supplements for potassium with doctor's order: Usually for levels 2.5–3.5 given with food can cause GI upset.
- IV potassium for levels <2.5 (*never ever give potassium* via IV push or by IM or subcutaneous routes).
- Do not increase the rate. It has to be given slowly; patients who are to receive >40–60 mEq/h should be on a cardiac monitor and monitored for ECG changes.
- IV K^+ correction causes phlebitis or infiltrations if given via peripheral lines; always needs central access if frequent correction is needed or K < 2.5.
- Do not give diuretics—LASIX or thiazides (waste more potassium) if a patient is normotensive; on the contrary, if a patient is hypertensive or in congestive cardiac failure K sparing diuretics may be considered.
- Watch heart rhythm and regular laboratory monitoring of serum K after giving correction.

■ HYPERKALEMIA

Hyperkalemia is defined as a serum potassium concentration greater than approximately 5.0–5.5 mEq/L in adults. Levels higher than 7 mEq/L can lead to significant hemodynamic and fatal cardiac consequences; levels exceeding 8.5 mEq/L qualify as severe hyperkalemia.

Causes

- Excessive K intake
- Intake of potassium-sparing drugs like spironolactone
- Tissue damage leading to cellular movement of K from intracellular to extracellular in conditions such as insulin deficiency, burns, rhabdomyolysis, hemolysis, and tumor lysis syndrome.
- Renal failure leading to impaired renal excretion of potassium
- Adrenal insufficiency.

Signs and Symptoms

- Frank muscle paralysis
- Dyspnea, respiratory failure due to muscle weakness
- Palpitations
- Nausea or vomiting
- Decrease in urine output
- Paresthesia
- *ECG:* Tall, peaked T waves with a narrow base, best seen in precordial leads, shortened QT interval, and prolonged PR interval.

Laboratory Parameters

- Check serum potassium
- *Arterial or venous blood gas:* If acidosis is suspected.

If persistent hyperkalemia in spite of taking anti-K measures, then look for other causes:

- *Serum uric acid and phosphorus tests:* For tumor lysis syndrome
- *Serum creatinine phosphokinase (CPK), urine myoglobin test:* For crush injury or rhabdomyolysis
- *Serum cortisol and aldosterone levels:* To check for mineralocorticoid deficiency when other causes are eliminated.

Management

- Stop ongoing IV potassium and hold all PO potassium supplements, if any.

- May consider loop diuretics/thiazides such as lasix or hydrochlorothiazide but should be avoided in volume-depleted states.
- Administer a hypertonic solution of glucose and regular insulin to pull the potassium into the cell (10 U of regular insulin in 25% dextrose 100 mL), also called GI drip.
- Potassium binders include cation exchange resins such as K-BIND.
- Correct severe metabolic acidosis with sodium bicarbonate, three ampules in 5% dextrose/sterile water until bicarbonate normalizes.
- Consider β-adrenergic agonist therapy, e.g., nebulized albuterol given by nasal inhalation over 15 minutes.
- Prepare chronic kidney/renal disease (CKD) patients ready for dialysis. Most renal patients get dialysis regularly and will have high potassium.
- Watch heart rhythm and regular laboratory monitoring of serum K after taking anti-K measures.

HYPONATREMIA

- Normal sodium levels are from 135 to 145 mEq/L.
- Hyponatremia is defined as serum sodium concentration <135 mEq/L with mild hyponatremia from 130 to 120, moderate hyponatremia from 120 to 110, and severe hyponatremia below 110 mEq/L.

Causes

Depending on the volume status:
- If hypovolemic, there is a possibility of intake of diuretics, loss of fluids from the body in case of severe vomiting and diarrhea.
- If hypervolemic, increased intake of fluids, congestive cardiac failure, or decompensated cirrhosis (called dilutional hyponatremia).
- If euvolemic, SIADH high levels of the antidiuretic hormone (ADH) are produced, causing your body to retain water instead of excreting it normally in your urine.

Symptoms

- *In mild cases:* Nausea, vomiting, and headache.
- *In moderate cases:* Confusion, altered mental status, drowsiness, restlessness, and irritability.
- *In severe hyponatremia:* Seizures, or coma.

Approach to Hyponatremia (Flowchart 2)[4]

- *Rate of correction:*
  - 0.5–1 mEq/L/h or a total of 8–10 mEq/L in 24 hours
  - When the process is acute (duration of <2 days) or when severe neurological dysfunction is present, correction of the serum (Na^+) can be 1–2 mEq/L per hour until symptoms improve, then slowed to no more than 0.5 mEq/L per hour.
- Correct at a rate no >12 mEq/L/day
- Overly rapid correction can precipitate central pontine myelinolysis (CPM).
- Consider adding tolvaptan 15 mg per oral qid; titer dose according to sodium levels if resistant to initial measures.
- Monitor serum sodium levels 6 hourly.

HYPERNATREMIA

Hypernatremia is categorized as serum sodium concentration <145 mEq/L.

Mild (146–149 mEq/L), moderate (150–169 mEq/L), and severe (≥170 mEq/L).

CHAPTER 21 | Fluid and Electrolytes in Critical Illness

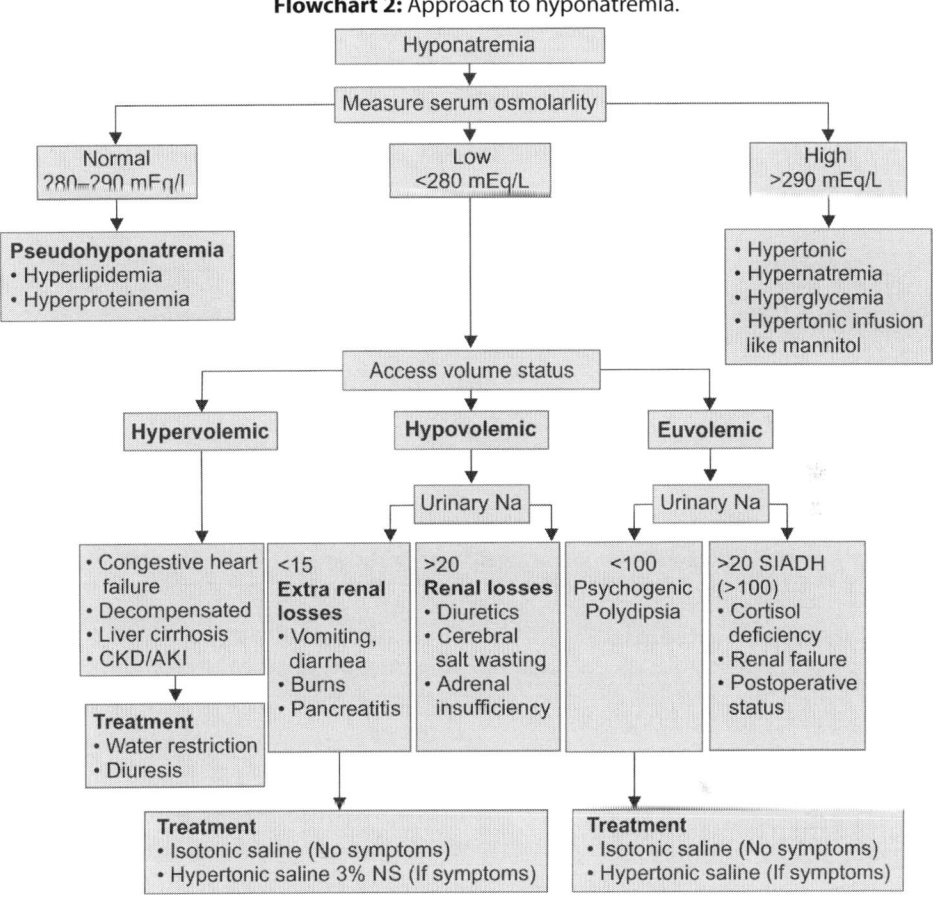

Flowchart 2: Approach to hyponatremia.

(AKI: acute kidney injury; CKD: chronic kidney disease; SIADH: syndrome of inappropriate antidiuretic hormone secretion)

Causes

- Depending on volume status if hypervolemic, increased Na intake like saline solutions or sodium bicarbonate administration.
- If hypovolemic, extrarenal losses, diarrhea, vomiting, fistulas, decreased free water intake. Renal losses such as osmotic diuresis if the patient is receiving IV mannitol or IV diuretics.
- If euvolemic, like extrarenal losses like insensible free water loss from the skin if a patient has a fever or respiratory system, e.g., in ICU where patients are mechanically ventilated, losses can be ≥500 mL/day. In state of euvolemia, increased urinary sodium indicates SIADH, cortisol deficiency, postoperative status or renal failure.

Symptoms

- *Central nervous system symptoms:* Cognitive dysfunction, confusion, abnormal speech, irritability, and seizures.
- In case of dehydration—tachycardia and oliguria.

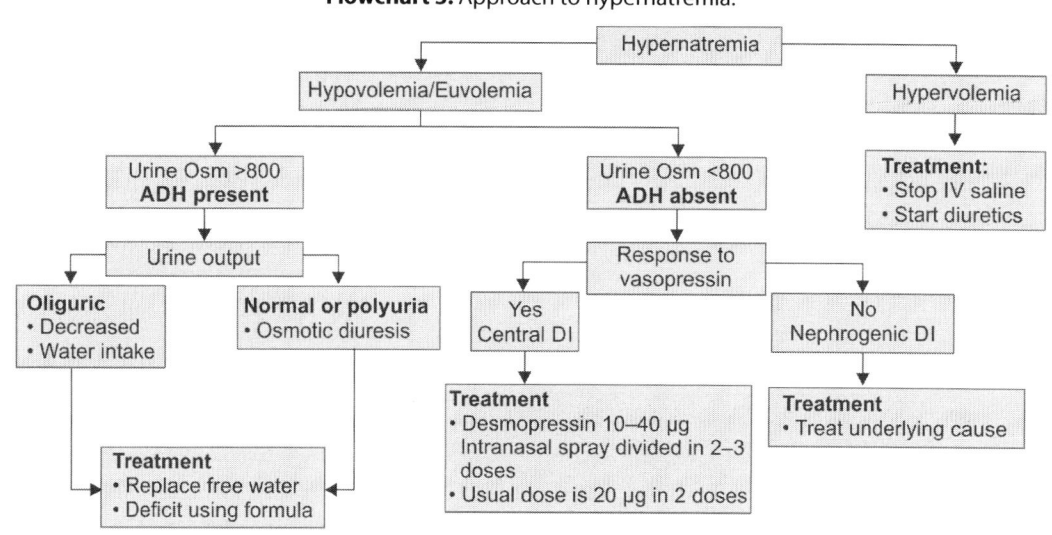

Flowchart 3: Approach to hypernatremia.

(ADH: antidiuretic hormone; DI: diabetes insipidus; IV: intravenous)

Approach to Hypernatremia (Flowchart 3)

Formula to calculate free water deficit:

Free water deficit = Body weight (kg) × Percentage of total body water (TBW) × [(Serum Na/140) − 1]

- Rate of free water infusion should depend on the total volume required to replace in case of hypovolemia and targeted Na to be achieved.
- Rate of correction of Na should be targeted by 8–10 mEq/L in 24 hours. Correct at a rate no >12 mEq/L/day.
- If the patient can tolerate per oral, then administer free water per oral
- Monitor serum sodium levels 6 hourly.
- Excessive/rapid correction can cause fluid shifts, which result in water entering the cells, leading to cerebral edema and fatal brain herniation.

HYPERPHOSPHATEMIA

Hyperphosphatemia is defined as a serum level above 4.5 mg/dL, but it is usually clinically significant only when levels are >5 mg/dL.

Causes

- *Decreased excretion:* Renal failure
- *Increased intake/absorption:* Phosphate supplements, enema/laxatives.
- *Transcellular shift:* Rhabdomyolysis, tumor lysis syndrome, metabolic acidosis, hemolysis, and insulin deficiency.

Clinical Features

- Hyperphosphatemia causes hypocalcemia by precipitating calcium out of the blood and decreasing vitamin D production.
- It is this secondary hypocalcemia that can cause muscle cramping, tetany, and seizures. Chronic hyperphosphatemia can also lead to metastatic calcifications in joints, tissues, and arteries.

Management

- Dietary restriction alone may suffice for the control of hyperphosphatemia in persons with normal renal insufficiency.

Hyperphosphatemia usually resolves in 6-12 hours in patients with normal renal function.
- In patients with mild renal function, phosphate excretion can be increased by saline infusion coupled with loop diuretics.
- In patients with hyperphosphatemia with renal failure, hemodialysis should be considered early in the management.
- When chronic, use phosphate binders like calcium carbonate.

HYPOPHOSPHATEMIA

Hypophosphatemia is defined as mild (2-2.5 mg/dL), moderate (1-2 mg/dL), or severe (<1 mg/dL).

Causes

- *Increased excretion:* Extrarenal—diarrhea and vomiting. Renal losses: Vitamin D deficiency, diuretics, volume expansion, and hyperparathyroidism.
- *Decreased intake:* Dietary deficiency, anorexia, chronic alcoholism, malabsorption, and antacids.
- *Transcellular shift:* Refeeding syndrome, DKA, and hypomagnesemia.

Clinical Features

- Mild-to-moderate hypophosphatemia is usually asymptomatic, but significant clinical manifestations can occur with severe hypophosphatemia.
- Severe hypophosphatemia can be manifested as seizures, arrhythmias, cardiomyopathy, and insulin resistance.
- The ED patients most likely to have hypophosphatemia are those malnourished with alcohol withdrawal or sepsis and patients with DKA or alcohol ketoacidosis in whom reintroduction of insulin and glucose causes phosphate uptake into cells.

Management

- Because hypophosphatemia is often coupled with hypokalemia, patients with hypophosphatemia also require potassium repletion.
- IV preparations are available as sodium phosphate (Na_2PO_4 and $NaPO_4$) or potassium phosphate (K_2PO_4 and KPO_4), and the rate of infusion and choice of initial dosage should be based on the severity of hypophosphatemia and presence of symptom.
- If oral is not tolerated, then,
    In case of severe 0.6 mmol/kg IV over 6 hours, watch for hypotension; if any, discontinue the infusion.
    In the case of moderate 0.4 mmol/kg IV over 6 hours.
- Oral phosphorous, 250-500 mg twice daily, can be given to stable or asymptomatic patients weekly.
- Treat vitamin D deficiency, if any.

HYPOCALCEMIA

Hypocalcemia is defined as a total serum calcium concentration <8.4 mg/dL in the presence of normal plasma protein concentrations or as a serum ionized calcium concentration (<1.17 mmol/L).

Causes

- Always check vitamin D and parathyroid hormone (PTH) levels.
- If vitamin D is low—low dietary intake, and liver disease.
- If vitamin D is normal—hypoalbuminemia in cirrhosis, nephrosis, malnutrition, burns, chronic illness, sepsis, acute pancreatitis, and hypomagnesemia.
- Hyperphosphatemia
- *Parathyroid hormone-related:* Surgery like thyroidectomy and pseudohypoparathyroidism.

Symptoms

- *Muscular:* Weakness, fatigue, spasms, and cramps
- *Neurologic:* Tetany, Chvostek sign, digital paresthesia, impaired memory, confusion, hallucinations, dementia, seizures, and extrapyramidal disorders.
- *Dermatologic*: Hyperpigmentation, coarse, brittle hair, dry, and scaly skin
- *Cardiovascular:* Heart failure, ventricular arrhythmias, torsade de pointes, and vasoconstriction
- *Skeletal:* Osteodystrophy, rickets, and osteomalacia.

Management

- *IV calcium gluconate:* If hypocalcemia is severe and the patient is experiencing muscle cramps or spasms (tetany), a bolus of 1 ampule of calcium gluconate in 20 mL NS can be given over 20 minutes, followed by a slow IV of 10 calcium gluconate ampules in 500 mL of NS can be given over 10-12 hours. Monitor calcium levels 6 hourly/12 hourly. ECG changes should be monitored.
- *Oral calcium supplement:* Calcium pills or supplements 1-2 g of elemental Ca TID may be used to restore your calcium to normal levels.
- *Vitamin D supplement:* People with chronic hypocalcemia should take a vitamin D supplement and calcium pills so that their bodies can properly absorb the calcium. It can add 0.25-4 µg calcitriol.
- *Synthetic form of PTH:* If you have hypoparathyroidism causing hypocalcemia, intake of PTH.
- Monitor serum calcium, ionized calcium, magnesium, and phosphorus levels.

HYPERCALCEMIA

Hypercalcemia is diagnosed by a serum calcium concentration >10.4 mg/dL or ionized serum calcium >5.2 mg/dL.

Causes

- Always check vitamin D and PTH levels.
- *If vitamin D is high:* Sarcoidosis, exogenous vitamin D like in dialysis patients, and acromegaly.
- *If vitamin D is normal:* In decreased Ca excretion such as volume depletion, milk-alkali syndrome, or bone reabsorption in conditions like Paget's disease, any malignancy or metastasis, hyperthyroidism, and calcitriol overdose.
- Parathyroid hormone-related—primary hyperparathyroidism.

Symptoms

- Neurological: Muscle weakness, fatigue, headache, mental instability, lethargy, confusion, psychotic behavior, stupor, and coma.
- Gastrointestinal: Abdominal pain, constipation, nausea, vomiting, and peptic ulcer.
- Renal: Nephrolithiasis, nephrocalcinosis, and renal failure.
- Cardiovascular: Arrhythmias, bradycardia, short QT interval, AV block, bundle branch block, and arrest (rare).
- Skeletal: Bone pain and arthralgia.

Management

General guidelines:
- Correct volume depletion with IV fluids; if ECG changes, then begin rapid-acting therapy; if chronic underlying disease, consider bisphosphonates as it has a delayed effect and lasts longest (2-4 weeks).

- *Hydration:* IV fluids 2–4 L over 24 hours. maintain rate to achieve a urine output of 100–150 mL/h.
- *Inhibition of bone resorption:*
  - Calcitonin: 4–8 IU IM or subcutaneously in 12 hours
  - Bisphosphonates: Zoledronate—4 mg over 15 minutes IV
- Low calcium diet
- Dialysis, if required
- Treat the underlying disease.

HYPOMAGNESEMIA

Hypomagnesemia is diagnosed if serum magnesium <1.5 mEq/L.

Causes

- *Reduced intake:* Starvation and malabsorption.
- *Extrarenal loss:* Diarrhea, vomiting, and prolonged GI drainage.
- *Renal loss:* Osmotic diuresis and chronic alcoholism.
- *Others:* Amphotericin B, pancreatitis, and burns.

Symptoms

Insomnia, tachycardia, confusion, increased deep tissue reflex, and convulsion.

Management

- *Mild cases:* Oral elemental Mg supplements.
- *In severe cases:* IV magnesium sulfate 1 AMP to give slowly in 100 mL NS over 30 minutes to decrease the chance of cardiac arrest. It can be repeated twice a day for 2–3 days depending upon serum magnesium levels. In the case of chronic conditions, the continuous infusion should be considered.
- Continuous magnesium sulfate is also given in case of preeclampsia to prevent seizures.
- The dose has to be decreased in case of renal insufficiency.

HYPERMAGNESEMIA

Hypermagnesemia is diagnosed if serum magnesium >5 mEq/L.

Causes

- Excessive magnesium intake
- Renal insufficiency
- Laxatives overuse
- Over aggressive IV magnesium administration
- Tumor lysis syndrome
- DKA

Symptoms

Flushing, lethargy, muscle weakness, and decreased deep tissue reflex.

Management

- Stop IV administration
- IV calcium gluconate over 10–15 minutes slowly
- Diuretics along with IV fluids
- Avoiding laxatives containing magnesium
- Decrease dietary intake of magnesium.

CONCLUSION

Fluids and electrolytes are the cornerstone of critical care, serving as fundamental therapies and interventions. A comprehensive understanding of their role is essential, as they are routinely employed in patient management. Mastery of these crucial elements ensures the delivery of optimal care in critical settings.

REFERENCES

1. Ghosh S. Handbook of Intravenous Fluids; 1st edition; 2022.
2. Pandya S. Practical Guidelines on Fluid Therapy, 2nd edition; 2020.
3. Malbrain MLNG, Langer T, Annane D, Gattinoni L, Elbers P, Hahn RG, et al. Intravenous fluid therapy in the perioperative and critical care setting: Executive summary of the International Fluid Academy (IFA). Ann Intensive Care. 2020;10(1):64.
4. Kollef M, Isakow W. Washington Manual of Critical Care; 2nd edition; 2012.

SECTION 5

Nutrition in Specific Situations

22. **Nutrition in Medical ICU Patients**
    Chitra Mehta, Yatin Mehta
23. **Nutrition in Pediatric ICUs**
    Anshu Joshi
24. **Nutritional Therapy in the Perioperative Period**
    Robert Martindale, Sarah Warren, Malissa Warren
25. **Nutrition in Cardiac and Cardiothoracic Intensive Care**
    Shweta Suri Kandpal
26. **Clinical Nutrition in Oncology**
    Vanessa Fuchs-Tarlovsky
27. **Nutrition in Severe Acute Pancreatitis**
    Deekshu Kapoor, Adarsh Chaudhary
28. **Nutrition in Short Bowel Syndrome and Enterocutaneous Fistulas**
    Gil Hardy, Chen Liu, Emma Ludlow, Ian Bissett
29. **Nutrition in Critically Ill Patients with Renal Failure**
    Penmetsa Vijay Varma, Rajasekara Chakravarthi, Mahesh Kota
30. **Nutrition in Critically Ill Patients with Respiratory Failure**
    Dhruva Chaudhry, Vineela Surapaneni
31. **Nutrition in the Critical Patient with Obesity**
    Anna Ferreira, Idiberto José, Zotarelli Filho, Durval Ribas Filho
32. **Nutrition in Critically Ill Patients with Liver Dysfunction and Failure**
    Keerti Brar, Rahul Harne, Sweta J Patel
33. **Nutrition in Major Trauma and Burns**
    Khusrav Bajan, Shradha K Bajan
34. **Nutrition in Neurology and Neurosurgical Patients**
    Barkha Bindu, Amit Goyal, Indu Kapoor, Hemanshu Prabhakar
35. **Nutrition in Solid Organ Transplantation and Immunocompromised Patients**
    Pooja Tyagi, Sweta J Patel, Jagadeesh KN
36. **Nutritional Support in a Critically Ill Parturient**
    Sunil T Pandya, Nishanth Aasuri

CHAPTER 22

Nutrition in Medical ICU Patients

Chitra Mehta, Yatin Mehta

INTRODUCTION

Due to advancement in medical technology and improved patient care there has been threefold increased survival of critically ill patients. This, however, has led to another serious issue of having a huge patient population with prolonged functional impairment associated with poor quality of life and frequent healthcare visits. Malnutrition has been found to contribute significantly toward this, and nutritional management forms an important pillar of multimodal interventions used for taking care of these intensive care unit (ICU) survivors.[1]

Nutritional care plan must start from the day of admission to ICU. It is essential to meet patients' energy requirement during the ICU stay as well as in post-ICU discharge phase to avoid proteolysis related muscle loss. Many ICU patients, postrecovery, have been found to progress to a chronic state of protein catabolism and persistent inflammation called as persistent inflammatory catabolic syndrome (PICS). This is associated with poor quality of life even after 12 months of discharge secondary to substantial muscle loss and sarcopenia.[1,2]

Malnutrition is defined as the state where there is deficiency of either total calorie count or protein, resulting in reduced body cell mass and organ dysfunction. It may occur secondary to either reduced absorption from the intestine, inadequate oral intake, or increased requirement by the body. During ICU stay protein breakdown has been reported to increase from 12 to 16 g of nitrogen/day to about 30 g of nitrogen/day, in some patients. This contributes toward huge muscle loss these patients develop. Malnutrition is quite common, easily overlooked, and missed in patients especially those who are critically sick. This contributes toward their prolonged ICU and prolonged hospital stay, increased complication, and mortality.[1-3]

ASSESSMENT OF NUTRITIONAL STATUS

It is a must to identify ICU patients who are at high nutritional risk. Malnutrition has been reported to exist in about 60% of patients even in developed countries like UK. The American Society for Parenteral and Enteral Nutrition (ASPEN) and the European Society of Parenteral and Enteral Nutrition (ESPEN) guidelines recommend tools like nutritional Risk Screening 2002 (NRS-2002), and NUTRIC scores to ascertain the nutrition risk in critically ill patients. Patients with NRS-2002 ≤3, or NUTRIC score ≤5 are not at nutritional risk, and do not need to be given any specialized nutrition therapy during the first week of ICU stay at least.[4,5]

Next step is assessment of nutritional status of ICU patients. Anthropometric measurements like skin-fold thickness and mid-arm circumference have not been found to be accurate in this subset of patients. Biochemical tests have their own set of limitations like albumin is known to fluctuate and fall rapidly as acute phase reactant. Hemoglobin levels may also be not helpful in the setting off ongoing hemorrhage or hemolysis. Other biochemical markers such as transferrin, lymphocyte count, and prealbumin may be influenced by various factors like patient's hydration status. Body mass index (BMI) is an important predictor of mortality but fails to depict acute changes in nutritional status. Low body mass can also be assessed with the help of ultrasonography or computed tomography.

Subjective global assessment (SGA) has been found to be a reliable assessment tool, and can help in inferring outcomes in ICU patients. It incorporates targeted history and physical examination of the patients. It has also been found to be reproducible as well.

Nutritional assessment is an important but lengthy process. As per the Indian nutritional guidelines for critically sick patients, it is desirable to maintain 1:25 nutritionist to critically ill patient ratio for the purpose.[6,7]

ENERGY REQUIREMENTS ESTIMATION

Nutritional management in ICU must be very precise in order to prevent both overfeeding and underfeeding. Underfeeding has been found to be associated with prolonged mechanical ventilation, prolonged hospital stay, and poor outcome. Overfeeding may lead to elevated levels of glucose, urea, deranged liver function tests, hypercapnia, and refeeding syndrome which again contribute to prolonged hospital stay and poor outcomes.

Using conventional predictive equations like Harris-Benedict equation is not suitable as it is too long and time consuming. Inaccuracies have been reported to be as high as 60% with these equations.

Harris-Benedict Equation

For male basal metabolic rate (BMR) = 13.75 × weight (kg) + 5 × height (cm) − 6.78 × age (years) + 66

For female BMR = 9.56 × weight (kg) + 1.85 × height (cm) − 4.68 × age (years) + 65

Drawbacks with Harris-Benedict equation led physicians to use indirect calorimetry which is currently the reference standard to assess basal metabolic rate and caloric requirement in critically ill patients. This is currently recommended by both ASPEN and ESPEN guidelines. Limited availability of its monitors however restricts its use in ICU.[3,4,5,7]

MACRONUTRIENTS

As per Indian guidelines, the protein requirement in ICU is about 1.2–2 g/kg bodyweight/day, and caloric requirement is in the range of 25–30 kcal/kg bodyweight/day. However, patients who are severely hypercatabolic like polytrauma and burns patients, may benefit from 120:1, or 100:1 ratio of kilocalorie: nitrogen. A balanced administration of carbohydrates and lipids is recommended. The optimal ratio for these is however not known. Toronto formula is recommended for caloric requirement calculation in patients with acute burns.

Electrolyte status should be closely monitored to timely identify any significant decrease in the levels of phosphorus, potassium, or magnesium. In such a situation of hypoelectrolytemia, the caloric intake should be reduced by 50% for next few days along with electrolyte correction.

Essential fatty acids requirement remains unexplored and unanswered. Unsaturated fats in excess amounts have been associated with increased incidence of immunosuppression and lung injury. It has been advised to keep glucose/lipid ratio on the lower side. In addition, ASPEN guidelines recommend lipid levels <1.5 g/kg/day in the parenteral formulation being administered in these patients. It helps keeping insulin resistance and hyperglycemia in check. Glutamine is not routinely recommended except in burns and trauma patients by majority of guidelines.[4,5]

As per current guidelines, enteral feeding should be commenced early during ICU stay as it is associated with reduced infection rate. The expected caloric target should be achieved over 3 days to avoid overfeeding and its complications. This is based on the concept of hypocaloric nutrition for the 1st week of ICU stay as recommended by ESPEN guidelines. Isocaloric enteral nutrition (EN) can be commenced after that. If somehow the enteral nutrition is not able to meet caloric goals, parenteral nutrition (PN) can be used to supplement remaining caloric balance between day 3 and 7 of ICU admission. ASPEN guidelines strongly recommend maximization of all efforts to initiate EN before switching to PN. ESPEN and ASPEN guidelines further recommend early restoration of physical activity in critically sick patients to counter the muscle breakdown and protein loss.[4,5,7,8]

MICRONUTRIENTS

This is often an overlooked aspect of nutritional therapy in ICU. Critically sick patients are predisposed to developing acute and chronic micronutrient (MN) deficiency such as vitamins, zinc, and trace elements. Vitamin A losses in urine have been found to occur in patients with sepsis. Selenium, copper, and zinc losses occur via exudates in burns patients. Selenium and zinc are lost in trauma patients through their drains. Selenium is regarded as one of the most important MNs.

Vitamins are organic compounds, usually acting as cofactors for metabolic pathway enzymes. Trace elements are structurally integral part of enzymes, and are also involved in electron transfer. Thus, ingestion of MNs is essential for immunity, normal metabolism, and antioxidant defense. The body stores of MNs deplete after 1 week. Trace elements in commercial feeds are usually sufficient to cover only for needs of healthy people receiving 1,500 kcal/day. So, there is a growing consensus of using early intravenous delivery of MNs during first 7 days of EN like in those receiving PN. It is about 100–200 mg of thiamine, 1 vial of multivitamins, and 1 vial of trace elements. Few trials have shown benefit of using four to five times higher doses of MNs in patients on PN.

As per ESPEN 2019 guidelines, antioxidants like vitamin C should be used only if there is evidence of deficiency. Vitamin D should be given in high doses (5,00,000 IU) in the first week of ICU admission if the patient is showing its deficiency.[4-7]

Daily requirements of electrolytes, trace elements, and vitamins are elicited in **Table 1**.

ROUTE OF NUTRITION

All major guidelines recommend using EN over PN unless there is a contraindication to the former. EN is considered to be more physiologic, maintains structural and functional integrity of the gut and associated microbiota, reduces peptic ulceration, minimizes mucosal atrophy, and reduces bacterial translocation from the intestine. Early EN has been advocated even in patients with acute pancreatitis.

TABLE 1: Daily requirements.

Electrolytes (mmol/kg/d)		Vitamins		
Sodium	1.0–2.0	*Fat soluble*		
Potassium	0.7–1.0	Vitamin A	Retinol	3,300 IU
Calcium	0.1	Vitamin D		200 IU
Magnesium	0.1	Vitamin E		10 IU
Chloride	1.0–2.0	Vitamin K		2–4 mg/wk
Phosphate	0.4	Vitamin C		100 mg
Trace elements (micrograms)		*Water soluble*		
Zinc	2,500–4,000	Vitamin B_1	Thiamine	3 mg
Selenium	30–60	Vitamin B_2	Riboflavin	3.6 mg
Copper	500–1,500	Vitamin B_3	Niacin	40 mg
Chromium	10–15	Vitamin B_5	Pantothenic acid	15 mg
Magnesium	150–800	Vitamin B_6	Pyridoxine	4 mg
		Vitamin B_7	Biotin	60 µg
		Vitamin B_9	Folic acid	0.4 mg
		Vitamin B_{12}	Cyanocobalamin	5 mg

Patients who are drowsy, or not able to take adequate oral caloric intake may receive EN either through nasogastric tube, nasojejunal route, or percutaneous endoscopic gastrostomy tube. Ryle's tube can be inserted nasally in most of the patients. Patients on ventilation can have an orally placed tube in order to reduce the incidence of sinusitis. Nasal route is contraindicated in patients with base of skull fracture or epistaxis.

Postpyloric feeding with nasojejunal placement is recommended who are at risk of aspiration, or have a feeding intolerance and gastroparesis despite using prokinetic agents.

Small bowel ileus is less frequent as compared to gastric ileus and is usually less prolonged.

Scientific formula feeding is preferred to blenderized diet for the risk of bacterial contamination and inconsistent nutrition content. Closed system ready to hang formula feeds should be used whenever possible. Large volume feeds put the patient at risk of aspiration so continuous feeding with the help of pump or gravity bags should be used.[4,5,7]

GASTRIC FEEDING INTOLERANCE

To prevent underfeeding and aspiration it is very essential to regularly monitor the patient for feeding intolerance. Gastric residual volume (GRV) monitoring should be done at 6-to-8-hour interval. As per ASPEN guidelines GRV of >500 mL is used to define feeding intolerance. As per Indian guidelines this can be between 300 and 500 mL of GRV. Patients who are intolerant of feeds should be shifted to continuous mode of feeding, and prokinetic agents like metoclopramide (10 mg IV TDS) or erythromycin (250 mg IV TDS) should be added.[4,5,7]

TYPES OF FEEDS

As discussed previously blenderized hospital prepared feeds should be avoided because of unpredictable levels of micronutrients and macronutrients, high osmolality, and viscosity leading to increase incidence of tube blockages. As per recommendation, standard polymeric formula feed should be initiated. Polymeric preparations contain intact protein, carbohydrates, and fats which need to be digested before getting absorbed. These also contain of electrolytes, vitamins, trace elements, and fiber. These are usually lactose free.[4,5,7]

Elemental Preparation

These formula feeds contain macronutrients in predigested form like protein as peptides or amino acids, carbohydrates as mono- or disaccharides and fats as medium chain triglycerides (MCT). These are usually preferred in patients who have malabsorption syndrome pancreatic insufficiency or persistent diarrhea.[4,5,7]

Immune Enhancing Enteral Nutrition

These may be used in acute respiratory distress syndrome (ARDS) patients and polytrauma patients. Routine use is not recommended. Glutamine should not be used in patients with multiorgan failure, or in severe sepsis.

Disease-specific Feeding

- In hepatic failure patients, a whole protein formula should be used. Energy intake should be targeted at 35–40 kcal/kg bodyweight/day. And protein intake should be 1.2–1.5 g/kg bodyweight/day. Hepatic specific formula feeds have not been found to be associated with any additional benefit, and therefore are not recommended.
- In patients with acute kidney injury protein intake should not be restricted. Daily protein recommended is 1.2–1.7 g/kg bodyweight/day. If there is significant dyselectrolytemia, a nephrospecific designed formula feed having low phosphate and potassium may be considered.
- In patients with respiratory failure, routine use of disease-specific low carbohydrate and high fat formula feed is not recommended.[4,5,7]

Energy Dense Formulae

These are not routinely recommended as these may cause delay in gastric emptying, diarrhea, hyperglycemia, decreased water, and protein administration. This may, however, be tried if patient is not able to tolerate full volume isocaloric nutrition, or if fluid restriction needs to be done.[8]

High Protein Formula

These are recently being used to meet the protein and nonprotein caloric targets so as to minimize the risk of overfeeding related to nonprotein calories. Whey protein formulae are being used for this purpose. It sounds most logical to use this in the late or recovery face of critical illness. This, however, needs to be investigated in future.[8]

PARENTERAL NUTRITION

Absolute indication for PN is persistent gastrointestinal failure. It can be given either to supplement EN, i.e., partial parental nutrition (PPN), or as a sole source of nutrition. It is recommended, however, after a week of failure of EN to meet metabolic demands of the patient despite using prokinetic agents or using nasojejunal route of feeding.[4,5,7]

COMPLICATIONS OF NUTRITION THERAPY

Ogilvie Syndrome and Bowel Ischemia

Hemodynamically, unstable patients requiring more than two vasopressors may develop these complications in face of receiving full EN due to mesenteric ischemia. To prevent this low-dose EN is recommended in first 2 days of ICU admission in patients who are receiving small or moderate doses of vasopressors. EN should be delayed in patients who are on higher dosages of vasopressors.[7,8]

Refeeding Syndrome

It is a lethal metabolic response to full feeding in patients who are malnourished, or have been having variable length of starvation before being admitted to ICU. This condition becomes evident during the first few days of nutritional support. It may present in the form of respiratory failure, muscle weakness, seizures, cardiac failure, and death.

It occurs due to electrolyte shifts that occur during the transition from a catabolic state using fat and protein as energy sources to the natural state of using carbohydrates as the main source of energy. Using glucose as a substrate leads to elevated circulating insulin levels resulting in depletion of thiamine levels, and plasma electrolyte levels due to intracellular shift of electrolytes. At risk, patients should be identified and must receive liberal doses of thiamine and other B vitamins intravenously for the first 3 days of feeding. EN should be introduced gradually giving only 500 kcal/day, or 25% of the estimated caloric target on day 1, which may then be progressed to 100% over next 4 days. All critically sick patients should actually be considered at risk of developing refeeding syndrome. Regular monitoring of serum phosphate levels for initial few days is recommended.[6,8]

Overfeeding

Many patients inadvertently end up being overfed which is as deleterious as underfeeding. It results in hyperglycemia, uremia, cholestasis, hyperlipidemia, hypercapnia, and fluid overload. It is more common with PN. PN, in addition to above, also predisposes patients to develop hepatobiliary diseases like acalculous cholecystitis.

Diarrhea

Enteral feeding is the main culprit for causing diarrhea in ICU. Diarrhea is defined as passage of three or more loose stools, or more frequent stools than is normal for the person. Such patients may benefit with peptide-based formula feeds or mixed fiber containing formula feeds. It is important to rule out *Clostridium difficile* infection before this. Probiotics may prove to be helpful in some patients, though their routine use cannot be recommended.[6-8]

NUTRITION DURING RECOVERY FROM CRITICAL ILLNESS

Many patients recovering from mechanical ventilatory support may face the issue of postextubation dysphagia. This compromises their ability to take desired caloric diet. Active deglutition rehabilitation should be an important part of nutritional support in these patients.[1,7,8]

NUTRITIONAL INTAKE POST-ICU

After an ICU stay, patients who have lost a lot of strength and muscle mass should receive more calories and protein for a long time. We need to take into account whether patients who leave the hospital after an ICU stay will be able to take oral calories and protein to heal well at home.

ROLE OF ANABOLIC/ANTICATABOLIC AGENTS

The HP-ONS trial and another recent trial indicated the possible role of anabolic and catabolic therapies, such as propranolol, oxandrolone, and other drugs intended to increase lean muscle mass, in enabling meaningful recovery of quality of life.[1]

CONCLUSION

Medical nutrition plays an important role in management of critically ill patients in medical ICU. This, however, needs to be done in a systematic approach by ICU professionals. Early EN should be emphasized upon, and PN should be instituted in case there is failure to achieve full EN despite best efforts. Regular monitoring of electrolytes cannot be overstressed upon. Nutritional management should continue right through the critical phase to recovery and rehabilitative phase of illnesses.

REFERENCES

1. Van Zanten ARH, De Waele E, Wischmeyer PE. Nutrition therapy and critical illness: practical guidance for the ICU, post-ICU, and long-term convalescence phases. Crit Care. 2019;23:368.
2. De Jonghe B, Bastuji-Garin S, Durand MC, Malissin I, Rodrigues P, Cerf C, et al. Respiratory weakness is associated with limb weakness and delayed weaning in critical illness. Crit Care Med. 2007;35:2007-15.
3. Singer P. Preserving the quality of life: nutrition in the ICU. Crit Care. 2019;23(Suppl 1):139.
4. Singer P, Blaser AR, Berger MM, Alhazzani W, Calder PC, Casaer MP, et al. ESPEN guideline on clinical nutrition in the intensive care unit. Clin Nutr. 2019;38(1):48-79.
5. Compher C, Bingham AL, McCall M, Patel J, Rice TW, Braunschweig C, et al. Guidelines for the provision of nutrition support therapy in the adult critically ill patient: The American Society for Parenteral and Enteral Nutrition. JPEN J Parenter Enteral Nutr. 2022;46(1):12-41.
6. Wellesley H, Frenchay Hospital, Bristol, UK. Nutrition in ICU. [online] Available from: https://www.coursehero.com/file/118709304/60-englishpdf. [Last accessed June, 2023].
7. Mehta Y, Sunavala JD, Zirpe K, Tyagi N, Garg S, Sinha S, et al. Practice Guidelines for Nutrition in Critically Ill Patients: A Relook for Indian Scenario. Indian J Crit Care Med. 2018;22(4):263-73.
8. Preiser JC, Arabi YM, Berger MM, Casaer M, McClave S, Montejo-González JC, et al. A guide to enteral nutrition in intensive care units: 10 expert tips for the daily practice. Crit Care. 2021;25:424.

CHAPTER 23

Nutrition in Pediatric ICUs

Anshu Joshi

INTRODUCTION

Malnutrition is a key challenge in the pediatric intensive care settings/units (PICU) and is associated with poor outcomes clinically. Critically ill patients/children are always at high risk of getting malnourished and worsening nutritional status (NS). Many children may be undernourished at the time of PICU admission. Early identification of pediatric undernutrition leads to adequate and effective nutritional interventions resulting in better clinical outcomes.

UNDERNUTRITION IN PEDIATRIC CRITICAL ILLNESS

Stress Response: Metabolism Changes

Altered metabolism in critical conditions leads to metabolic, neuroendocrine, and immunologic changes. There is higher protein catabolism, increase in hepatic protein synthesis, insulin resistance, consequent hyperglycemia, and increased lipolysis.

Pediatric critical illness can be characterized in three phases: (1) acute, (2) stable, and (3) recovery phase. The early acute phase manifests with severe catabolic changes. It is an adaptation to provide free amino acids (AAs) and calories to vital tissues while triggering catabolic pathophysiology. Protein loss is high and results in loss of lean body mass (LBM). Various signaling pathways trigger proteolysis by the ubiquitin-proteasome complex (UPS) and autophagy. Forkhead box protein O (FOXO) and UPS are the most important ones. Inflammatory cytokines amplify the body protein catabolism.

Acute phase is followed by phase of stabilization and some metabolic responses remain similar. In the recovery phase begins with anabolism and protein synthesis. Patients can also progress to recovery or chronic critical illness (CCI). Patients may show multiple phenotypes. There can be persistent inflammation with/without immunosuppression. The sustained inflammation continues catabolism with loss of LBM causing deterioration in muscle function and worsening of NS.

NUTRITIONAL STATUS ASSESSMENT

All critically ill children should undergo nutritional assessment within 48 hours of PICU admission. This helps identify preexisting undernutrition and also to understand worsening of nutrition status during PICU stay.

The NS assessment can be performed with various parameters such as anthropometry, physical examination, and biochemical assessment such as serum proteins and inflammatory markers. NS assessment should include static and dynamic NS indices before and during PICU stay. It helps integration of malnutrition etiology/consequences with clinical management.

ANTHROPOMETRY

Weight, height/length, mid-upper arm circumference (MUAC), and head circumference (in children <36 months) are important parameters. Z-scores for body mass index (BMI)-for-age (BMIz) or weight-for-length z-scores (WLz) in children <2 years, or weight-for-age z-scores (WAz) are important calculations for reference.

Growth faltering (failure to thrive) is a dynamic approach that allows to assess growth progress according to WHO cut-off points.

Underlying chronic diseases correlate with the risk for malnutrition and faltering growth at PICU admission.

Laboratory Parameters

Though controversial, serum biomarkers help in diagnosing or monitoring undernutrition. However, they have low specificity and reflect the presence of underlying inflammation and hypermetabolism. C-reactive protein (CRP), serum albumin, and prealbumin are commonly used. Not many studies show their predictive value on NS.

Nutritional Status Deterioration

Weight loss or a decline of NS indicators during PICU stay indicates NS deterioration. Illness severity and length of PICU stay account for NS deterioration. Underlying inflammation, oxidative stress and underfeeding in are contributory. Acquired undernutrition and muscle loss often leads to weaning failure and post-PICU weakness.

Muscle Mass Wasting

Muscle protein loss with negative nitrogen balance is high in PICU patients. Early and rapid muscle loss in ventilated children is common. Early identification of muscle wasting is very important. It becomes challenging to evaluate muscle loss in critically ill children. Current methods available have various limitations in PICU. Skinfold thickness, MUAC, and bioelectrical impedance analysis (BIA) are affected by hydration and may not be very reliable. It is impractical to perform computerized tomography (CT) or magnetic resonance imaging (MRI) at bedside. Ultrasound is noninvasive and available at the bedside, may be promising tool to evaluate muscle mass in critically ill children. Quadriceps femoris is most measured.

METABOLIC ALTERATIONS IN THE PICU CHILD

There is hypercatabolism causing release of increased amounts of glucose, AAs, and fatty acids. There are changes in energy expenditure (EE). Inflammatory cytokines like interleukin (IL)-1β, IL-6, IL-12, IL-18, tumor necrosis factor alpha (TNF-α), and interferon gamma (IFN-γ) mediate metabolic changes; hormonal responses with growth hormone (GH), thyroid-stimulating hormone (TSH), and insulin growth factor binding proteins (IGFBPs). Increased gluconeogenesis, fatty and carbohydrate oxidation with LBM loss is seen.

Cytokine cascade initiates metabolic response to tissue injury. Proinflammatory interleukins [IL-1β, TNF-α, IL-18, IL-12, IL-17, INF-γ, and granulocyte-macrophage colony-stimulating factor (GM-CSF)] participate in cellular activation, tissue destruction, and necrosis. Anti-inflammatory interleukins [IL-10, IL-13, IL-1ra, and transforming growth factor beta (TGF-β)] cause dampening and reversing of the inflammation.

The stress responses results in alterations at the hypothalamic-anterior pituitary axes resulting in increased cortisol, GH, T_3, and rT_3 secretion. Sympathetic nervous system increases catecholamine secretion. Increased resistance to the actions of the GH at the peripheral tissues is also seen. Due to disrupted peripheral conversion of T_4, severe stress causes decline of circulating levels of T_3 with increase in rT_3 to preserve energy.

Cortisol levels increase in acute phase. Cortisol suppresses immune and inflammatory reactions because of cytokines activity or other inflammatory mediators. Stress hypercortisolism causes increased calorie generation by increasing carbohydrate, fat, and protein catabolism and suppressing inflammation. It also increases vasopressor response to catecholamines. However, it also causes impaired wound healing and myopathy.

MACRONUTRIENT METABOLISM IN PICU CONDITIONS

Carbohydrate and Lipid Metabolism

Stress-induced hyperglycemia is a consequence of increased gluconeogenesis and insulin resistance. Proinflammatory cytokines also prevent insulin to be secretion by activating α-adrenergic receptors. Increased catecholamines result in elevated glucagon levels causing gluconeogenesis despite elevated insulin levels. Muscle catabolism releases alanine which enhances gluconeogenesis. Hepatic insulin resistance is mediated by glucagon, epinephrine, and cortisol. Peripheral insulin resistance is mediated by cytokines and hormones. Peripheral insulin resistance continues even after recovery, especially in pediatric patients.

Hypertriglyceridemia caused due to stress response is troublesome because of the existing endothelial dysfunction and hyperinflammation. Parenteral lipid infusions cause worsening of hypertriglyceridemia.

Protein Metabolism

In healthy conditions, there is a balance between protein intake, turnover, and loss for maintaining LBM, sustaining protein homeostasis, and LBM growth. Prealbumin has shorter half-life and is better to evaluate the response of plasma protein pool to dietary intake of proteins, in comparison to albumin, which has a longer half-life.

Starvation, immobility in PICU and inflammation result in protein and LBM loss. Organ dysfunctions can prolong inflammation and catabolism. This causes chronic cumulative nitrogen deficit. Proteins breakdown for providing substrate for calorie generation and body protein metabolism. This is not reversed by provision of dietary proteins because it is regulated by stress hormones, neural mediators, and cytokines. On the other hand, inflammation also causes increased protein synthesis, especially in the liver and immune cells. AA released from breakdown of body protein stores are preferentially used for gluconeogenesis, oxidation, and synthesis of acute phase reactants.

Protein synthesis in muscles decreases and protein catabolism increases vis-à-vis increased whole body protein synthesis. Preferential protein degradation over protein synthesis in skeletal muscles leads to LBM loss. This also causes growth failure in children.

This catabolic response may not respond anabolically to exogenous nutritional intervention in comparison to simple starvation. Stress response, induced insulin resistance, high cortisol, and high levels of cytokines reduce the response to dietary protein intake. Injury and inflammation reduce anabolic response to nutrients.

Adequate calories of energy are required for utilization of the dietary protein since nitrogen utilization is adversely affected by caloric deficits. Protein synthesis increases when dietary proteins are supplied with adequate calories. Children require uninterrupted supply of energy generating substrates and proteins for maintaining adequate growth.

ENERGY EXPENDITURE IN CRITICALLY ILL CHILDREN

Adequate energy intake improves clinical outcomes. The determination of energy requirement in PICU is challenging. Adequate nutrition recommendations should avoid both underfeeding and overfeeding. Energy requirements are based on the specific phase of critical illness. Various factors such as medicines for sedation, muscle relaxants, ventilation, and high body temperature affect energy requirements. Resting energy expenditure (REE) is important and is usually measured with indirect calorimetry (IC). If not feasible, then REE may be calculated using standard predictive equations as per latest guidelines recommendations.

Indirect Calorimetry in PICU

To plan guide nutritional support and determine total energy requirements, American Society for Parenteral and Enteral Nutrition (ASPEN) recommends measuring REE, with the help of indirect calorimeter, once the acute phase is over.

Criteria Proposed by the ASPEN to Identify Patients for REE Measurement by IC in PICU

- Underweight (BMI <5th percentile for age), at risk of overweight (BMI >85th percentile for age) or overweight (BMI >95th percentile for age)
- Children with >10% weight gain or loss during ICU stay
- Failure to consistently meet prescribed caloric goals
- Failure to wean or need to escalate respiratory support
- Need for muscle relaxants for >7 days
- Neurologic trauma (traumatic, hypoxic and/or ischemic) with evidence of dysautonomia
- Oncologic diagnoses (including children with stem cell or bone marrow transplant)
- Children with thermal injury
- Children requiring mechanical ventilator support for >7 days
- Children suspected to be severely hypermetabolic (status epilepticus, hyperthermia, systemic inflammatory response syndrome, dysautonomic storms, etc.) or hypometabolic (hypothermia, hypothyroidism, pentobarbital, or midazolam coma, etc.)
- Any patient with ICU length of stay (LOS) >4 weeks may benefit from IC to assess adequacy of nutrient intake.
- If REE measurement with IC is not feasible then predictive equations as per latest guidelines recommendations can be used to estimate REE.

NUTRITION INTERVENTION

Enteral nutrition (EN) should be initiated early in all eligible PICU children, unless contraindicated. Institutional EN guidelines should be in place regarding the patient eligibility for EN, timing to initiate EN, and stepwise rate of increase in calorie and proteins as well as for detecting and managing intolerance.

Suitability of EN with regard to the clinical diagnosis in PICU patients and patients receiving vasopressors should be evaluated on individual patient basis.

Delay in nutrition initiation, feeding intolerance, and consequent interruptions, and long fasting periods are common barriers in achieving nutrition adequacy. Hence, efforts should be undertaken to minimize the interruptions.

Nutrient delivery via the enteral route should be done stepwise in children tolerating EN. In such cases, commencement of parenteral nutrition (PN) should be delayed. Initiation time of supplemental PN for insufficient EN is not well established. The threshold and initiation timing of PN should be decided on case basis. Supplemental PN can be deferred for 1 week after PICU admission in patients with normal baseline nutritional state and low risk of nutritional deterioration. However, it can be initiated in the first week in PICU children who are severely malnourished or at risk of NS worsening and/or did not receive any EN during the first week of PICU admission.

Even small amounts of nutrient delivered via enteral route are beneficial for overall gastrointestinal health, mucosal integrity, and motility. Early initiation of EN (within 24–48 hours of admission) and achievement of up to two-thirds of the nutrient adequacy goals in the first week improves patient clinical outcomes.

Energy intake should not exceed resting EE in the early and acute phase of illness in PICU. Energy intake should match for energy debt, physical activity, rehabilitation, and growth after acute phase of critical illness is over. Cumulative energy deficits during the first week may be associated with poor outcomes. Timely achievement of nutrition adequacy goals and matching the same with energy balance prevents cumulative caloric deficit or excesses. Energy requirements can be increased by approximately 1.3 times REE in the stable phase to enable catch-up growth. This can be further increased in the recovery phase.

Parenteral Glucose Intake

The amount of glucose to be provided by PN should be decided by:
- Energy intake requirements and the risks associated with overfeeding
- Phase of illness
- Total macronutrient intake by both enteral and parenteral routes
- Glucose intake apart from nutrition, e.g., with medication

Existing latest ESPEN guidelines can be followed while deciding the daily dosage parenteral glucose intake in children according to body weight and phase of illness.

Lipid Intake

Intravenous lipid emulsions (ILE) are integral component of PN intervention. They can be used exclusively or given complementary to EN intervention. Parenteral lipid intake should not be >3 g/kg/day in children. In preterm infants, newborns, and older children who are on short-term PN, composite ILEs provide more balanced nutrition than pure soybean oil (SO) ILEs. For PN lasting longer than a few days, composite ILEs with or without fish oil (FO) should be preferred. In infants and children, 20% ILEs is preferable. Carnitine supplementation can be considered in those receiving PN for >4 weeks on an individual basis. In patients receiving ILEs and cases with a marked risk for hyperlipidemia, liver function markers and triglyceride concentrations should be monitored regularly. Plasma triglyceride concentrations during infusion >3 mmol/L (265 mg/dL) in infants or >4.5 mmol/L (400 mg/dL) in older children may warrant daily intake reduction of ILEs.

Protein/Amino-acid Intake

Minimum daily enteral protein intake of 1.5 g/kg avoids negative nitrogen balance. Higher protein intake to prevents cumulative negative protein balance. In PICU patients, daily optimal protein intake required may be higher to attain a positive protein balance. Negative protein is associated with poor outcomes.

A minimum amino acid intake of 1.0 g/kg/day should be administered in stable infants and children to avoid negative balance. In stable children aged 3–12 years, an amino acid intake of 1.0–2.0 g/kg/day is adequate. An amino acid intake of at least 1.0 with a maximum of 2.0 g/kg/day in stable adolescents is considered adequate. Additional supplementation of glutamine is not permitted in infants and children up to the age of 2 years.

CONCLUSION

Adequate and timely nutrition intervention during PICU stay is important to meet patient's basal metabolic needs, support substrate metabolism in response to stress and illness, and prevent the excess LBM loss. Nutrition care in PICU helps offset the burden of stress. Rational dietary intervention, either EN or PN should be individualized to the patient, the phase of illness, and existing NS. EN is associated with improved clinical outcomes and decreased LOS. Objective criteria for monitoring feeding intolerance should be followed. Further large-scale studies are warranted to study the impact of nutrition in specific phases of critical illness. Optimal approaches need to be determined for objective assessment, prescription, and delivery of nutrition care in PICU population.

SUGGESTED READING

1. Eveleens RD, Verbruggen SCAT, Joosten KFM. The role of parenteral nutrition in paediatric critical care, and its consequences on recovery. Pediatr Med. 2020;3:24.
2. Irving SY, Albert BD, Mehta NM, Srinivasan V. Strategies to optimize enteral feeding and nutrition in the critically ill child: a narrative review. Pediatr Med. 2022;5:9.
3. Joosten K, Embleton N, Yan W, Senterre T; ESPGHAN/ESPEN/ESPR/CSPEN working group on pediatric parenteral nutrition. ESPGHAN/ESPEN/ESPR/CSPEN guidelines on pediatric parenteral nutrition: Energy. Clin Nutr. 2018;37(6 Pt B):2309-14.
4. Lapillonne A, Fidler Mis N, Goulet O, van den Akker CHP, Wu J, Koletzko B, et al. ESPGHAN/ESPEN/ESPR/CSPEN guidelines on pediatric parenteral nutrition: Lipids. Clin Nutr. 2018;37(6 Pt B):2324-36.
5. Mesotten D, Joosten K, van Kempen A, Verbruggen S; ESPGHAN/ESPEN/ESPR/CSPEN working group on pediatric parenteral nutrition. ESPGHAN/ESPEN/ESPR/CSPEN guidelines on pediatric parenteral nutrition: Carbohydrates. Clin Nutr. 2018;37(6 Pt B): 2337-43.
6. Moreno YMF, Ventura JC, de Almeida Oliveira LD, Silveira TT, Hauschild DB. Undernutrition in critically ill children. Pediatr Med. 2020;3:22.
7. Orellana RA, Coss-Bu JA. Metabolic alterations in the critically ill child: a narrative review. Pediatr Med. 2021;4:8.
8. van Goudoever JB, Carnielli V, Darmaun D, Sainz de Pipaon M; ESPGHAN/ESPEN/ESPR/CSPEN working group on pediatric parenteral nutrition. ESPGHAN/ESPEN/ESPR/CSPEN guidelines on pediatric parenteral nutrition: Amino acids. Clin Nutr. 2018;37(6 Pt B):2315-23.
9. Veldscholte K, Joosten K, Jotterand Chaparro C. Energy expenditure in critically ill children. Pediatr Med. 2020;3:18.

CHAPTER 24

Nutritional Therapy in the Perioperative Period

Robert Martindale, Sarah Warren, Malissa Warren

INTRODUCTION

As with any patient admitted to an intensive care unit (ICU), the surgical patient exhibits variable catabolic stresses that may be associated with significant increase in morbidity and mortality. Optimal nutritional support is fundamental to minimize the adverse outcomes. Historically, the primary challenge in providing high-quality surgical nutrition has been the lack of robust and high-quality evidence with very few adequately powered randomized trials to guide practice. However, in recent years, numerous high-quality, evidence-based studies have been conducted, making for new challenges of sorting through the rapidly expanding literature in order to determine who will benefit from nutrition intervention.[1,2]

Widespread variation exists among surgeons regarding the use of enteral nutrition (EN), parenteral nutrition (PN), and supplemental parenteral nutrition (SPN). Fortunately, high-quality sources for perioperative nutrition management exist, including guidelines and detailed synthesis and analysis of the existing literature. These include the joint 2016 American Society of Parenteral and Enteral Nutrition (ASPEN)/Society of Critical Care Medicine (SCCM) nutrition guidelines, the European Society Parenteral and Enteral Nutrition (ESPEN) practical guidelines for nutrition in surgery, and the Critical Care Nutrition, an academic research organization (website: https://criticalcarenutrition.com).[3-5] The Critical Care Nutrition site includes the reviews of surgical nutrition evidence and current nutrition studies, feeding guides, calculators, protocols, slide presentations, and educational materials intended for clinicians. These resources may provide an excellent starting point for a clinician or a team interested in learning more or initiating surgical nutrition protocols. Recent data demonstrate significantly improved patient outcomes when nutrition support protocols incorporate best practices and are appropriately tailored to the patient.[6] Some of the primary benefits of nutrition support protocols include decreased local and systemic infections, attenuation of systemic inflammation, and improved metabolic/physiologic profiles. It is important to note that benefits observed with early nutritional therapy in the ICU setting do not appear directly correlated with the dose (both volume and caloric) of delivered nutrition. Recent studies indicate that excessive or overly aggressive nutrition intervention for the purpose of achieving estimated energy demands can nullify positive physiologic effects of more temperate nutrition therapy and lead to unnecessary morbidity.[7] For this reason, surgical nutrition protocols should be routinely updated based on evolving evidence. Nutritional therapy in the perioperative period should serve as a proactive therapeutic strategy to ameliorate or attenuate the metabolic stress of surgery, modulate the immune response, and maintain gastrointestinal integrity and physiology rather than an aggressive approach to meet metabolic needs as quickly as possible.

NUTRITION ASSESSMENT

Determining whether a patient will benefit from nutritional therapy requires thorough understanding of the patient's present nutrition status and anticipated extent of catabolic injury as the result of surgical intervention. To evaluate a patient for surgery, a comprehensive evaluation of objective and subjective data is required. Routine nutrition screening should be performed on all patients prior to major surgery. Several screening tools or risk calculations have been proposed such as NUTRIC (Nutrition Risk in Critically Ill) score, Nutrition Risk Screening 2002 (NRS-2002), subjective global assessment (SGA), and mini nutritional assessment, which are reviewed in other chapters of this text. The use of screening and risk assessment is variable and not standardized, though select tools have been validated in the literature in surgical populations.[8] Nutrition screening helps to identify patients at risk for malnutrition and who require more comprehensive assessment and likely nutrition intervention. Nutrition assessment of the surgical patient consists of detailed medical and surgical history, nutritional intake and weight trends, laboratory data, and evaluation of body composition through nutrition focused physical exam (NFPE) that may also include mid-arm circumference, hand grip strength, and ultrasound or computed tomography (CT) and measurement of muscle quantity and quality. The use of cross-sectional imaging via CT is shown to be the best predictor of outcome for most surgical procedures.[9]

Other functional tools or measures of daily activities such as gait speed, sit to stand, and timed stair tests are common in preoperative assessment and may be helpful to identify those patients at highest risk for functional decline in the postoperative period.[10] Lastly, visceral protein levels, albumin, and prealbumin are frequently and inaccurately considered in nutrition screening and assessment as markers of nutrition status. It is critical to understand that the production of visceral proteins is reduced during the times of stress irrespective of the patients' nutritional status and should be considered as indicators of inflammation or metabolic status rather than determinant of how nutritionally replete the patient may be.[11]

PREHABILITATION FOR THE SURGICAL PATIENT

Achieving optimal surgical outcomes following major surgery is inherently challenging. Patients often present for surgery deconditioned and malnourished with or without sarcopenia (loss of muscle mass and decline in function).[12] The concept of preparing the patient for major surgery or prehabilitation is nothing new. Level one data supporting the concept is widely published across surgical specialties, including visceral cancer surgery, orthopedics, neurosurgery, and many other elective surgery procedures. The features of prehabilitation programs typically include smoking cessation, weight loss if obese, glycemic control, and a "healthy diet" for weeks to months prior to surgery. Recommendations for the "healthy diet" focus on complex carbohydrates and whole foods such as fruits, vegetables, and whole grains that are rich in dietary fiber and vitamins and minerals. Increased protein intake, 1.2-2 g/kg, spread throughout the day for at least 1-4 weeks prior to surgery is also recommended. Then, immune-enhancing nutrition supplementation is encouraged for 5 days prior to surgery. Immune-enhancing nutrition is typically defined as a formula containing at least two or more nutrients, including omega-3 fatty acids [docosahexaenoic acid (DHA) and eicosapentaenoic acid (EPA)], arginine, and nucleotides.[13] In addition to nutrition management, prehabilitation programs usually include a resistance exercise program that is individualized to the patient. Psychosocial and stress reduction strategies are also important components for surgery preparation. Prehabilitation programs have consistently shown significant benefit, especially in the patients with neoplastic disease and/or frailty.[14]

INITIATING NUTRITION THERAPY IN THE POSTOPERATIVE SETTING

The two most common areas of contention and debate surrounding nutrition in the surgical patient are: (1) the optimal timing for starting supplemental nutrition and (2) the benefits or disadvantages of EN versus PN. Although there is no universal agreement for when to initiate nutritional therapy in surgical patients, there is consensus to start enteral feedings early for optimal effects on the gut, defined as within 24-48 hours of surgical insult. Several major studies consistently demonstrated that early enteral feedings confer benefits by reducing infections and organ failure, decreasing length of stay, and potentially reducing mortality rates, when compared to delayed initiation of enteral feeding or the use of PN. Interestingly, recent research has shown that these benefits of early EN appear to be relatively independent to the actual nutritional dose (calories delivered)

but are likely related to the non-nutritional benefits, such as minimizing adverse changes in gut permeability, curtailing immuno-suppression, and positively impacting the gut microbiome.[15]

Clinicians must consider the preexisting nutritional status of the surgical patient to determine the route and timing of nutrition after surgery. If no evidence of significant malnutrition or elevated nutrition risk exists at the time of surgery, then PN should be considered if unable to feed enterally 5-7 days after surgery. For malnourished patients, PN should be initiated earlier if enteral is contraindicated or not tolerated, for example, as soon as the patient is hemodynamically stable in the postoperative setting, within 24-48 hours. Though evidence supports early EN in postoperative setting regardless of nutrition status, the timing of initiation remains controversial. Many surgeons still follow dogma that "normal" bowel sounds or passing of flatus and/or stool is required before starting EN. However, current literature and consensus guidelines suggest that the return of bowel function (i.e., bowel sounds, flatus, and bowel movement) is not necessary for initiation of EN.[16] Early tolerance to small amounts of EN is universally accepted, but a significant number of critically ill surgical patients, 30-70%, can have gastrointestinal dysfunction related to a variety of factors.[4]

Several factors have been found to improve the delivery of EN and are recommended for all surgical patients requiring supportive nutrition therapy. These include: (1) the initiation of EN at a slow rate (10-20 cc/h) and then slow advancement to the calculated "goal" rate, (2) the use of higher thresholds of gastric residual volumes (>500), and (3) the postpyloric feeding if there are persistent high gastric residuals/emesis/

distension or in patients who are at high risk for aspiration. The optimal method to ensure maximized use of adequate nutritional support is having all the above included in a local protocol or algorithm using best practice and evidence-based guidelines.[3,4] However, despite the mentioned recommendation and overwhelming literature supporting nutrition therapy in surgical patients, suboptimal caloric delivery is unfortunately more the rule than the exception in the postoperative setting following major surgery. This is primarily due to interruption of feedings for procedures, imaging studies, and elevated gastric residuals or other signs of feeding intolerance. EN administration is often delayed or interrupted in the critically ill surgical patient requiring vasopressors; however, the surgical and critical care literature supports early delivery of EN in patients who are not on escalating doses or are stable on low doses of vasopressors.[17] Patients who are hemodynamically unstable, requiring an escalation of vasopressors or requiring multiple high-dose vasopressor agents, are unlikely to tolerate EN. In this setting, providing aggressive EN increases risk for bowel-related complications, such as ischemia, dilation with perforation, or anastomotic breakdown. For patients who have undergone gastrointestinal surgery and are critically ill, it is important that collaborative decisions for early feeding are reached among the multidisciplinary team caring for the patient.

Enteral versus Parenteral Nutrition

The debate over the indications, benefits, and risks of enteral versus parenteral delivery of nutritional therapy continues to be a focus of scientific investigation. Although the enteral route is proven optimal when tolerated, it may have significant limitations and unwanted side effects in many critically ill and surgical patients. Several recent, large, randomized controlled trials have challenged the dogma that EN is superior to PN in critically ill patients.[18,19]

Currently, there remains general support for the superiority of EN over PN among patients who are able to receive and tolerate enteral feeding. However, the pendulum is swinging to a more balanced perspective with greater acceptance of PN or SPN as a viable option in the critically ill and surgical patient unable to receive adequate EN.[18,20] In addition, a 2022 meta-analysis of studies demonstrated no difference in mortality when comparing EN versus PN, but there was a decrease in infectious complications and length of stay associated with EN.[18]

The maintenance of the gut mucosal integrity is the other proposed advantage of EN over PN therapy. Enteral nutrients support the luminal microbiome and prevent the conversion of a healthy microbiome to a pathobiome due to overgrowth of pathogens and loss of normal colonic flora as can occur with disuse of the gut during PN therapy. In addition to gut disuse, the other adverse effects of PN include vascular access complications (infection and thrombosis), cholestasis and hepatocellular damage, glucose, and electrolyte disturbances. If PN is used in the surgical patient, some of these adverse effects are addressed by modifying the PN formulation and utilizing second generation intravenous lipid emulsions (ILE).

Estimating Caloric Requirements and Selecting the Optimal Dose

Although determining the optimal dose of PN or EN to deliver in the perioperative period for the surgical critically ill patient may seem relatively straightforward, calorie and protein requirements remain poorly understood, widely debated, and highly complex. The traditional teaching on this subject has almost exclusively focused on estimating the "caloric needs" of the surgical patient. Much less consideration has been given to estimate their physiologic and metabolic readiness and the patient's ability to tolerate and/or utilize the macronutrient load. It is critical to understand that perioperative surgical critical illness-induced catabolism is entirely different from simple protein/calorie malnutrition (or "starvation"). Major surgery and surgical complications can lead to significant inflammatory response, insulin resistance, and disruption and dysfunction of the patient's intrinsic macronutrient processing capacity. As a result, nutritional supplementation is not just a matter of supplying adequate calories and nutritional substrates. Early aggressive feeding regimens in the immediate postoperative and critically ill patient, particularly high-calorie feeding during peak periods of inflammation, may have a paradoxical effect of inducing cellular, tissue, and organ injury, without providing any substantive nutritional benefit.[21] The concept of staged introduction of calories and protein substrates is now supported by numerous lines of evidence detailing the ultimate fate of supplied nutrients and the potential adverse effects of overfeeding in the surgical and medical hyperdynamic patients.[7] To estimate caloric and energy needs, the three main methods that are utilized in the majority of surgical ICUs are: (1) indirect calorimetry, (2) predictive equations, and (3) simplified weight-based calculation. There is a paucity of level 1 evidence examining the optimal method for estimating caloric needs; however, no conclusion on a standardized method has been determined.

It is also important to understand that the surgical patient's energy and macronutrient requirements are not static and have significant and variable changes depending on the degree of inflammation, underlying metabolism and physiology, and metabolic response to the delivered nutrition. Therefore, the nutrition assessment and calculation of nutrient goals should be reevaluated and adjusted frequently to accurately account for the dynamic nature of surgical metabolic response and stage of disease.

Finally, there has been keen interest, which has driven recent re-evaluation of primary nutrient sources (lipid, protein, and carbohydrates) and the numerous other potential supplements as well as varying ratios and combinations of these components. A complete review of nutrient makeup for the surgical perioperative description of this topic is beyond the scope of this short chapter, but several key summary points are as follows:

- Carbohydrates, proteins, and fats/lipids are the backbone nutritional components, and there appears to be no evidence for very low or very high protein or carbohydrate/fat ratio strategies.
- Soybean ILE have proinflammatory effects and have been associated with adverse outcomes in surgical patients. A second-generation ILE using a mixed lipid solution (olive oil, medium chain triglycerides, fish oil, and less soybean oil) has numerous metabolic advantages for patients in the perioperative period.[22,23]
- "Immune-enhancing" formulas have shown significant benefit in select surgical populations in both the preoperative and perioperative periods.[24] These formulations generally contain fish oils and arginine with added nucleotides.

- Glutamine supplementation by parenteral or enteral routes should not be routinely used in surgical or critically ill patients, and particularly in patients with shock or multiple organ failure.

TROPHIC FEEDING, HYPOCALORIC FEEDING, AND PERMISSIVE UNDERFEEDING

As noted previously in this chapter, multiple studies have suggested that many of the benefits of nutrition in the surgical patient are not dependent on the overall amount of delivered energy and macronutrients or the aggressiveness of achieving 100% of the target or goal calories.[25] There is growing level one data to support the potential adverse effects of delivering excessive protein and/or caloric content, including volume overload, hyperglycemia, mitochondrial dysfunction, metabolic stress, renal injury, immunosuppression (primarily from soy-based lipids), and increased respiratory expenditures.[26,27] This has led to significant debate for correct targets and timing to reach total calories and protein delivery in the surgical patient, particularly in the early acute phase of illness. In these patients, we must balance the need for nutritional delivery to provide critical organ metabolic substrate, and when possible, enteral support to attempt to maintain a "normal" microbiome and prevent conversion to a pathobiome.[28]

Recent interest and evidence, including several level-1 randomized clinical trials, evaluate various levels of "permissive underfeeding" strategies. These studies include the EDEN, PermiT (Permissive Underfeeding versus Target Enteral Feeding in Adult Critically ill Patients), INTACT, CALORIES, EPaNIC (Early Parenteral Nutrition Completing Enteral Nutrition in Adult Critically Ill Patients), NUTRIREA-2, NUTRIREA-3, and the Swiss SPN trial. These studies suggest that it is best to generally provide a significantly lower volume of initial feeding that is slowly increased in the postoperative setting (5-7 days) based on the patient's response and illness acuity.[6]

TRAUMA/BURNS

The trauma patients comprise a significant proportion of surgical patients needing nutrition and metabolic support. These patients commonly present with a level of complexity that often makes early nutrition delivery challenging. In fact, the hyperdynamic and catabolic metabolism is compounded by a variety of other factors, such as tissue trauma, immobility, insulin resistance, and quasi-starvation. Like all critically ill patients, starting nutrition early within the first 24-48 hours after resuscitation has been found to improve outcomes. As discussed earlier, clinicians should consider lower energy and protein provision during the initial phases or trauma management with a plan to ramp up to goals over the first 5-7 days that range in the region of 20-35 kcal/kg/day. The amount of protein delivered at a level is approximately 2 g/kg/day.[29]

Traumatic brain injury (TBI) is a widely discussed subset of patients. Trauma patients with TBIs have greatly improved outcomes with early feeding.[30] As with other surgical patients, enteral is the preferred method of nutrient delivery. Another subset of trauma patients in which the route of nutrition delivery is commonly misguided is patients with an open abdomen. Contrary to popular belief, the open abdomen patient can and should be started on early nutrition with the caveat that no bowel injury is present and that bowel continuity has been restored. In addition, protein losses can be high due to significant exudate volume that is emitted from an open abdomen, 10–20 g protein per liter of abdominal fluid lost. The protein provision should account for additional protein lost in abdominal fluid. Early conservative enteral feeding has been shown to decrease anastomotic leaks and decrease mortality.[31] Burn injury patients with a large surface area burn have also been found to require a significant amount of micro- and macronutrients secondary to the metabolic demands that result from burn injury. The additional resources are available from the global associations and the ASPEN/SCCM nutrition guidelines.[32]

EVOLVING NOVEL STRATEGIES FOR THE SURGICAL CRITICAL CARE PATIENT

The surgical critically ill population is a prime target for new and evolving metabolic support regimens as major surgery and/or traumatic injury can induce a cascade of metabolic changes that lead to rapid and significant inflammatory response and lean body tissue loss.[33] Attempting to modulate the inflammatory response has been widely variable in response. One consistent agent which has proven benefit is the fish oils, EPA and DHA. The benefit of fish oils is noted not only in preventing excessive inflammation initially, but also enhancing inflammation resolution. The discovery of lipid mediators, specialized pro-resolving mediators (SPMs), derived from essential fatty acids, EPA, and DHA, has revolutionized the concept of inflammation resolution at several metabolic levels.[34]

Microbiome management is another novel surgical strategy that promises to be critical in enhancing surgical outcomes (**Fig. 1**). Healthcare providers should consider the "microbiome" as an organ just as the liver, gastrointestinal tract, heart, and kidney are considered organs. Understanding the role of the gut microbiota in the surgical patient before, during, and after

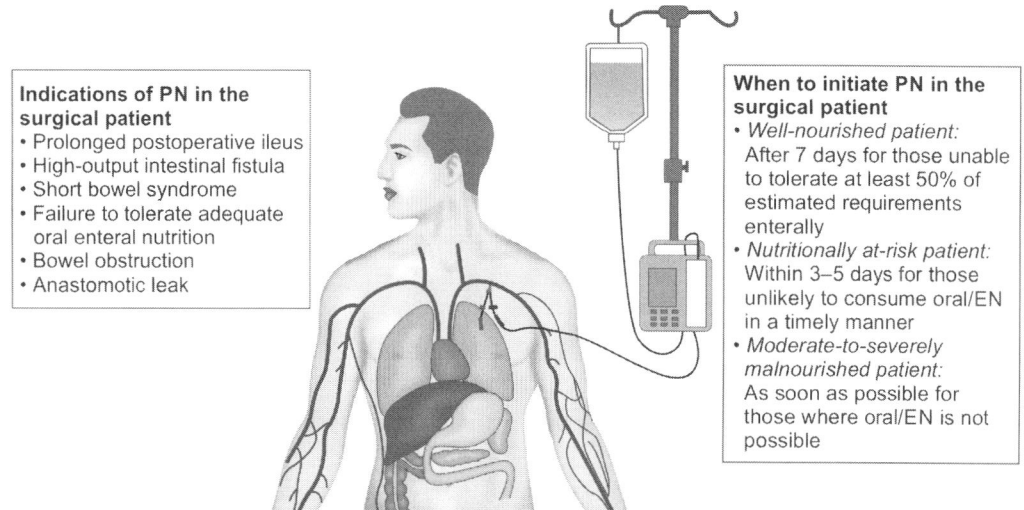

Fig. 1: Criteria for PN. (EN: enteral nutrition; PN: parenteral nutrition)

the insult of surgery will likely guide our methods to restore and promote its function more effectively. When the microbiome is optimally supported, it is presumed it will function in the postoperative setting to keep the host safe and healthy by preventing the conversion of a normal microbiome to a pathobiome.[33] In addition to early enteral feeding discussed throughout this chapter, the other examples of microbiota-targeted strategies may include using complex nutrition formulas, pre- and probiotics, fecal microbiota transplants, personalized gut bacteria profiles, or a combination of these methods. However, defining the microbiome in the perioperative setting and determining the method to optimally support it remains to be clarified.[35]

CONCLUSION

Nutritional support or therapy in the surgical population requires close attention to details. Prehabilitation and the global success of enhanced recovery after surgery (ERAS) programs have clearly revolutionized perioperative surgical metabolic therapy. The detailed approach to nutrition therapy in the surgical patient has shown beneficial in long- and short-term outcomes in multiple prospective randomized trials. In the postoperative setting, the choice of the best timing, route of nutrient delivery, dose, composition, and the need for supplementation will vary and is clearly dependent on the metabolic and catabolic stress anticipated during and after surgery. Simplistic policies that take a universal approach and attempt to provide full caloric support regardless of the patient's status and disease severity will often result in overfeeding and will have no benefit (or even harm) to the patient. EN remains the preferred route of feeding, when possible, although PN is no longer considered to have the risk once reported in older studies and should be utilized in the appropriate patient. The horizon is bright for surgical nutrition as many high-quality randomized trials are underway and the science is rapidly expanding to include cellular and mitochondrial metabolism as well as the microbiome and its crucial role in surgical metabolism.

REFERENCES

1. Williams DGA, Molinger J, Wischmeyer PE. The Malnourished Surgery Patient. Curr Opin Anaesthesiol. 2019;32(3):405-11.
2. Gillis C, Wischmeyer PE. Preoperative Nutrition and the Elective Surgical Patient: Why, How, and What? Anaesthesia. 2019;74: 27-35.
3. McClave SA, Martindale RG, Vanek VW, McCarthy M, Roberts P, Taylor B, et al. Guidelines for the Provision and Assessment of Nutrition Support Therapy in the Adult Critically Ill Patient: Society of Critical Care Medicine (SCCM) and American Society for Parenteral and Enteral Nutrition (ASPEN). JPEN J Parenter Enteral Nutr. 2016;40(2):159-211.
4. Weimann A, Braga M, Carli F, Higashiguchi T, Hübner M, Klek S, et al. ESPEN Practical Guideline: Clinical Nutrition in Surgery. Clin Nutr. 2021;40(7):4745-61.
5. Critical Care Nutrition. The Sustain CSX Randomized Clinical Trial. [online] Available from: www.criticalcarenutrition.com/ [Last accessed August, 2023].
6. Yeh DD, Martin M, Sakran JV, Meier K, Mendoza A, Grant AA, et al. Advances in Nutrition for the Surgical Patient. Curr Probl Surg. 2019;56(8):343-98.
7. van Zanten AR, De Waele E, Wischmeyer PE. Nutrition Therapy and Critical Illness: Practical Guidance for the ICU, Post-ICU, and Long-Term Convalescence Phases. Crit Care. 2019;23(1):368.
8. House M, Gwaltney C. Malnutrition Screening and Diagnosis Tools: Implications for Practice. Nutr Clin Pract. 2021;37(1):12-22.

9. Yang TR, Luo K, Deng X, Xu L, Wang RR, Ji P. Effect of Sarcopenia in Predicting Postoperative Mortality in Emergency Laparotomy: A Systematic Review and Meta-analysis. World J Emerg Surg. 2022; 17(1):36.
10. Russell MK. Functional Assessment of Nutrition Status. Nutr Clin Pract. 2015;30(2): 211-8.
11. Evans DC, Corkins MR, Malone A, Miller S, Mogensen KM, Guenter P, et al. The Use of Visceral Proteins as Nutrition Markers: An ASPEN Position Paper. Nutr Clin Pract. 2021;36(1):22-8.
12. Sayer AA, Alfonso C-J. Sarcopenia Definition, Diagnosis, and Treatment: Consensus is Growing. Age Ageing. 2022;51(10): afac220.
13. Shen J, Dai S, Li Z, Dai W, Hong J, Huang J, et al. Effect of Enteral Immunonutrition in Patients Undergoing Surgery for Gastrointestinal Cancer: An Updated Systematic Review and Meta-analysis. Front Nutr. 2022;9:941975.
14. Molenaar CJL, Minnella EM, Coca-Martinez M, ten Cate DWG, Regis M, Awasthi R, et al. Effect of Multimodal Prehabilitation on Reducing Postoperative Complications and Enhancing Functional Capacity Following Colorectal Cancer Surgery. JAMA Surg. 2023;158(6):572-81.
15. McClave SA, Lowen CC, Martindale RG. The 2016 ESPEN Arvid Wretlind Lecture: The Gut in Stress. Clin Nutr. 2018;37(1):19-36.
16. Caddell KA, Martindale R, McClave SA, Miller K. Can the Intestinal Dysmotility of Critical Illness be Differentiated from Postoperative Ileus? Current Gastroenterology Reports. 2011;13(4):358-67.
17. Wischmeyer PE. Enteral Nutrition can be given to Patients on Vasopressors. Crit Care Med. 2020;48(1):122-5.
18. Reignier J, Boisrame-Helms J, Brisard L, Lascarrou JB, Ait Hssain A, Anguel N, et al. Enteral versus parenteral early nutrition in ventilated adults with shock: A randomised, controlled, multicentre, open-label, parallel-group study (NUTRIREA-2). Lancet. 2018;391(10116):133-43.
19. Patel JJ, Rice TW, Mundi MS, Stoppe C, McClave SA. Nutrition Dose in the Early Acute Phase of Critical Illness: Finding the Sweet Spot and Heeding the Lessons from the NUTRIREA Trials. JPEN J Parenter Enteral Nutr. 2023;47(7):859-65.
20. Gao X, Liu Y, Zhang L, Zhou D, Tian F, Gao T, et al. Effect of Early vs. Late Supplemental Parenteral Nutrition in Patients Undergoing Abdominal Surgery. JAMA Surg. 2022; 157(5):384.
21. Merker M, Felder M, Gueissaz L, Bolliger R, Tribolet P, Kägi-Braun N, et al. Association of Baseline Inflammation with Effectiveness of Nutritional Support among Patients with Disease-Related Malnutrition: A Secondary Analysis of a Randomized Clinical Trial. JAMA Netw Open. 2020;3(3):e200663.
22. Martindale RG, Berlana D, Boullata JI, Cai W, Calder PC, Deshpande GH, et al. Summary of Proceedings and Expert Consensus Statements from the International Summit 'Lipids in Parenteral Nutrition.' JPEN J Parenter Enteral Nutr. 2020;44(Suppl 1): S7-20.
23. Calder PC, Waitzberg DL, Klek S, Martindale RG. Lipids in Parenteral Nutrition: Biological Aspects. JPEN J Parenter Enteral Nutr. 2020;44(Suppl 1):S21-7.
24. Adiamah A, Skořepa P, Weimann A, Lobo DN. The Impact of Preoperative Immune Modulating Nutrition on Outcomes in Patients Undergoing Surgery for Gastrointestinal Cancer: A Systematic Review and Meta-analysis. Annals of Surg. 2019; 270(2):247-56.
25. Patel JJ, Martindale RG, McClave SA. Controversies Surrounding Critical Care Nutrition: An Appraisal of Permissive Underfeeding, Protein, and Outcomes. JPEN J Parenter Enteral Nutr. 2017:014860711772190.
26. Hermans AJ, Laarhuis BI, Kouw IWK, van Zanten ARH. Current Insights in ICU Nutrition: Tailored Nutrition. Curr Opin Crit Care. 2023;29(2):101-7.
27. Moonen HP, van Zanten AR. Mitochondrial Dysfunction in Critical Illness during Acute Metabolic Stress and Convalescence. Curr Opin Crit Care. 2020;26(4):346-54.

28. Trone K, Rahman S, Green CH, Venegas C, Martindale R, Stroud A. Synbiotics and Surgery: Can Prebiotics and Probiotics Affect Inflammatory Surgical Outcomes? Curr Nutr Rep. 2023;12(2):238-46.
29. Heyland DK, Weijs PJ, Coss-Bu JA, Taylor B, Kristof AS, O'Keefe GE, et al. Protein Delivery in the Intensive Care Unit: Optimal or Suboptimal? Nutr Clin Pract. 2017;32(suppl 1):58S-71S.
30. Jeong H, Kim JH, Choo YH, Kim M, Lee S, Ha EJ, et al. Nutrition Therapy for Patients with Traumatic Brain Injury: A Narrative Review. Korean J Neurotrauma. 2023;19(2):177.
31. Goh EL, Chidambaram S, Segaran E, Garnelo Rey V, Khan MA. A Meta-analysis of the Outcomes Following Enteral vs Parenteral Nutrition in the Open Abdomen in Trauma Patients. J Crit Care. 2020;56:42-8.
32. Koyro KI, Bingoel AS, Bucher F, Vogt PM. Burn Guidelines—an International Comparison. Eur Burn J. 2021;2(3):125-39.
33. Martindale RG. Novel Nutrition Strategies to Enhance Recovery after Surgery. JPEN J Parenter Enteral Nutr. 2023;47(4):476-81.
34. Chiang N, Serhan CN. Specialized Pro-Resolving Mediator Network: An Update on Production and Actions. Essays Biochem. 2020;64(3):443-62.
35. Zheng Z, Hu Y, Tang J, Xu W, Zhu W, Zhang W. The Implication of Gut Microbiota in Recovery from Gastrointestinal Surgery. Front Cell Infect Microbiol. 2023;13:1110787.

CHAPTER 25

Nutrition in Cardiac and Cardiothoracic Intensive Care

Shweta Suri Kandpal

DISEASE BURDEN

Cardiovascular diseases (CVD) like ischemic heart disease (IHD) and cerebrovascular diseases like stroke account for 17.7 million deaths and are the leading cause. In accordance with the World Health Organization, India accounts for one-fifth of these deaths worldwide, especially in younger population. The results of Global Burden of Disease study state age-standardized CVD death rate of 272 per 100,000 population in India, which is much higher than that of global average of 235.[1]

India has a high burden of acute coronary syndrome and ST-elevation myocardial infarction (MI). Also, on one hand, hypertensive heart disease is a leading pathology in India, associated with 261,694 deaths in 2013 (an increase of 138% in comparison with 1990). On the other hand, rheumatic heart disease (RHD) in India continues to remain in large proportions, accounting for about 1.5–2 per 1,000 individuals.[2] Indians are usually affected earlier than the western population by almost a decade.

Cardiovascular morbidity and mortality data from hospitals does not represent the overall CVD burden. In 2016, 28.1% of total deaths and 14.1% of total disability-adjusted life years (DALYs) compared with 15.2% and 6.9%, respectively in 1990 were attributed to CVDs. Among the states, the rates of CVD were highest in states of Kerala, Punjab, and Tamil Nadu. The highest prevalence of raised cholesterol levels and blood pressure was also seen in these states.[2]

Significantly higher (about thrice) prevalence of coronary artery disease (CAD) is seen in migrant Asian Indians than the native population of the US. The likelihood of hospitalization for complications of CAD is two to four times higher in Indians as compared to other ethnic groups. Their admission rates are also five to ten times higher, especially for patients younger than 40 years. The occurrence of CAD in Indians residing in India is 21.4% for diabetics and 11% for nondiabetics.

At present in India, chronic diseases contribute to an estimated 53% of deaths and 44% of DALYs lost. CVD and diabetes are highly prevalent in urban areas. Hypertension and dyslipidemia, although common, are inadequately detected and treated.[3]

RISK FACTORS

The four main risk factors, which showed consistently significant associations across all South Asian countries in both sexes were:
1. Current and former smoking
2. High $ApoB_{100}$/Apo-I ratio
3. *History of hypertension:* Almost 30% of adult Indians are found to be hypertensive, of which 34% are in urban areas and 28% are in rural areas.[4]
4. *History of diabetes:* Diabetes mellitus prevalence has grown exponentially in the

urban areas of India, it has nearly doubled over last 20 years, from 9 to 17%. On the other hand, in rural areas, it has jumped from 2 to 9%.[5]

Certain dietary habits have also been implicated with higher risk of CVD. As opposed to the notion that Indians are predominantly vegetarian, and thus their consumption of fruits and vegetables would be sufficient, the rate of consumption is found to be low in India.

According to a study by P Joshi et al., the rates of consumption of fruits and vegetables were surprisingly lower in South Asian group compared with controls from other areas, despite vegetarianism being common among Indians. Consumption of green leafy vegetables and fruits is associated with lower risk of coronary heart disease (CHD). Also lower risk is seen with a greater number of servings consumed (P for trend <0.001).[6]

The National Family Health Survey-3 (NFHS-3) that covered a large national population of 156,316 individuals in India also reported 50% of the population agreed to having been consuming zero or only 1 serving of fruit in a week.

A large portion of total fat in the Indian diet comprises partially hydrogenated vegetable oils with high trans fat content. This oil is consumed especially in urban adult slum dwellers belonging to lower socioeconomic strata (SES) common in urban adult slum dwellers.[7,8]

Research has proved the direct connection of transfatty acids with CVDs, breast cancer, shortening of pregnancy period, risks of preeclampsia, disorders of nervous system and vision in infants, colon cancer, diabetes, obesity, and allergy.[5]

SPECTRUM OF DISEASE

The spectrum of the CVDs ranges from dyslipidemia, hypertension, IHD to valvular heart disease to cardiomyopathies to heart failure (HF).

The most common causes of HF are RHD and CAD. RHD burdens 0.25–0.3 million 20% get HF with a 3% annual mortality. CAD burdens 29.8 million 30-day HF rate of 5%. Hypertension 25–40% in urban, 10–15% in rural with total of 118.2 million 5–10% get HF.[9]

NUTRITION CONSIDERATIONS

The inflammatory process of atherosclerosis contributes to major incidence and mortality of CVD.

Inflammatory processes involve the accumulation of lipids and lipid-laden macrophages in the subendothelial area of the arterial wall.[10,11]

The main mediators of CAD development are C-reactive protein (CRP), interleukin (IL)-1, IL-6, IL-8, IL-1β, IL-18, monocyte chemoattractant protein (MCP)-1, and tumor necrosis factor (TNF)-α. The expression of these proinflammatory mediators may possibly correlate with disease severity.[12,13] Nutrition has shown to modify oxidative stress and systemic inflammation. A lack of physical activity and a high energy intake are associated with proinflammatory cytokines secretion.

Current evidence suggests that healthy dietary patterns have common patterns like:

- An increased consumption of fiber, antioxidants, vitamins, minerals, polyphenols, monounsaturated, and polyunsaturated fatty acids [monounsaturated fatty acid (MUFA) and polyunsaturated fatty acid (PUFA), respectively]
- Decreased salt, refined sugar, saturated, and trans fats intake
- Consumption of carbohydrates of low glycemic index.

Thus, this implies a high intake of fruits, vegetables, legumes, fish and seafood, nuts, seeds, whole grains, vegetable oils [mainly, extra virgin olive oil (EVOO)], and dairy foods together with a low intake of pastries, soft drinks, and red and processed meat.

Diets such as the Mediterranean and DASH (Dietary Approaches to Stop Hypertension) dietary interventions are extensively analyzed for effects on CV outcome. Both these dietary patterns have shown to downregulate low-grade inflammation and thereby allowing better control of body weight, which in turn also improve other risk factors, and are correlated with lower incidence of CVD. In comparison with the conventional low-fat, high-carbohydrate DASH diet, a modified DASH diet higher in vegetable fats and lower in carbohydrates—i.e., more similar to a Mediterranean diet—produces larger cardiometabolic benefits.[14,15]

Interestingly, MeDiet seems to modulate the expression of proatherogenic genes as *cyclooxygenase-2 (COX-2), MCP-1,* and *low-density lipoprotein (LDL) receptor-related protein* (LRP1), reducing plasmatic levels of plaque stability and rupture-related molecules as matrix metallopeptidase 9 (MMP-9), IL-10, IL-13, or IL-18.[16,17]

Corley et al. studied 792 participants aged 70 years from the Lothian Birth Cohort 1936 for the association between biomarkers of systemic inflammation (CRP and fibrinogen) and specific single foods (fruits and vegetables). A 168-item food frequency questionnaire (FFQ) was used to measure the dietary intake. They concluded that a higher fresh fruit intake was associated with lower CRP levels (≤3 mg/L) ($\beta = 0.100$, 95% CI 0.82, 0.99). However, there was no statistically significant association between vegetables and CRP. Similar pattern ($p < 0.05$) was seen between fibrinogen levels and fruit intake ($\beta = 0.083$) or combined fruits and vegetables intake ($\beta = 0.084$).[18]

The HELENA cross-sectional study was carried out to show that a healthy diet might reduce adiposity and systemic inflammation, also concluded that fruits and nuts had a negative relation with IL-4 (all subjects, $p<0.05$; both) and TNF-α (only girls, $p=0.036$).[19]

Multiple meta-analyses have shown the anti-inflammatory effects of olive oil (OO) rich diets. Improvements in inflammatory status, oxidative stress, and endothelial dysfunction has been seen with the bioactive components of EVOO, that is also the key food of the MeDiet.

Schwingshackl et al. conducted a meta-analysis in 30 randomized controlled trials (RCTs) (3,106 participants and daily consumption of 1 mg and 50 mg OO). They found a statistically significant decrease in CRP (–0.64 mg/L, $p < 0.0001$, n = 15 trials) and IL-6 (–0.29 mg/L, $p < 0.04$, n = 7 trials) as compared to the controls. Subjects with highest OO intake (0.6%, $p < 0.002$) also demonstrated significant increase in the flow-mediated dilatation (FMD) value.[20,21]

Numerous studies from the PREDIMED study and other studies related to the MeDiet have concluded that EVOO added to MeDiet causes decrease in levels of N-terminal pro-brain natriuretic peptide (NT-proBNP) I has also shown to decrease the progression of intima media thickness (IMT) in people with elevated baseline IMT. There has been an improved systolic and diastolic BP in both hypertensive and nonhypertensive patients, and also a decreased expression and concentration of circulating inflammatory biomarkers that are related to atherosclerosis were noted.[22,23]

Multiple large prospective cohort studies have shown reduced CVD morbidity and mortality with the consumption of nuts, especially peanuts and walnuts.[24,25]

An umbrella review of meta-analysis suggested that individuals consuming the highest amounts of dietary fiber intake can significantly reduce their incidence and mortality from CVD. Mechanistically, these beneficial effects may be due to dietary fiber actions on reducing total serum and low-density lipoprotein cholesterol concentrations between 9.3–14.7 mg/dL and 10.8–13.5 mg/dL, respectively.[26] These findings lend support to the hypothesis that a high-fiber diet is associated with lower plasma levels of IL-6 and TNF-α-R2.[27]

Protective effect of micronutrients is implicated via three ways:
1. Attenuating endothelial cells damage
2. Enhancing the production of nitric oxide (NO)
3. Impeding oxidation of LDL cholesterol (LDL-c).

Proinflammatory biomarkers have been associated with higher CVD risk in case of deficiency of dietary antioxidants, such as Zn, Se, and vitamins C and E. Zinc deficiency plays a role in inflammation, mainly elevating inflammatory response as well as damage to host tissue. Zinc is involved in the modulation of the proinflammatory response by targeting nuclear factor kappa B (NF-κB), a transcription factor that is the master regulator of proinflammatory responses. It is also involved in controlling oxidative stress and regulating inflammatory cytokines.[28]

Results of a meta-analysis indicated that magnesium supplementation reduces CRP levels among individuals with inflammation (CRP levels >3 mg/dL). This finding suggests that magnesium supplements may have a beneficial role as an adjuvant for the management of low-grade chronic systemic inflammation.[29]

A number of bioactive compounds such as omega-3 fatty acids, lycopene, or polyphenols, present in the diet tend to reduce levels of LDL-c, improving inflammatory and oxidative stress biomarkers and thus have beneficial effects on atherosclerosis development.[30]

Potential anti-atherogenic effects have been demonstrated by PUFAs, as Omega-3 fatty acid (Ω-3 PUFA), α-linolenic acid (ALA), eicosapentaenoic acid (EPA), and docosahexaenoic acid (DHA). These improve the lipid and lipoprotein profile, oxidation, thrombosis, endothelial function, BP, plaque stability, CV mortality, platelet aggregation, modulating concentration or expression of proinflammatory markers (adhesion molecules, cytokines, etc.), and immune cells and thereby decrease the risk of CVDs.[31,32]

Lycopene is a lipophilic and an unsaturated carotenoid. It is present in red-colored fruits and vegetables, such as papaya, watermelons, tomatoes, etc. Multiple epidemiological observational and interventional studies have demonstrated that lycopene might have the potential to decrease the atherosclerotic risk, especially in initial stages of atherosclerosis, thus, preventing endothelial dysfunction (NO bioavailability and blood flow) and LDL oxidation. Lycopene might also improve the metabolic profile by affecting cholesterol synthesis and BP, by reducing arterial stiffness. It may also modulate the expression of proinflammatory markers and platelet aggregation.[33-35]

Another study suggested a 6–15% reduction of LDL-c with a daily dose of 2–3 g of plant sterols or phytosterols. Similar reductions were also noted by Demonty et al. in their meta-analysis. They observed an 8.8% reduction in LDL-c after administering a daily dose of 2.15 g of phytosterols.

As a matter of fact, plant sterols have been proposed as a complement of statins treatment in order to decrease the risk of CVD. Although more research is needed as available data is inconsistent.[36-38]

The most abundant dietary antioxidants present in most plant-origin foods and beverages are polyphenols. They have multiple beneficial effects in the prevention of CVD. The important food sources of polyphenols are fruit and vegetables, red wine, black and green tea, coffee, EVOO, and chocolate, and also nuts, seeds, herbs, and spices.

Numerous scientific papers have suggested that the mechanism of the beneficial effects of polyphenols may be by delaying progression of atherosclerosis through several ways:

- Modulation of signaling and transcription pathways, such as NF-κβ
- Antioxidant systems
- Inhibition of leukocyte migration and infiltration inside plaque
- decreased adhesion molecules levels
- Impeding the encoding of proinflammatory cytokines
- Decreased BP due to the enhanced NO production
- Enhancing lipid metabolism, coagulation activity, and endothelial function

The dietary consumption of polyphenols was shown to be inversely associated with cardio- and cerebrovascular diseases due to the anti-inflammatory and antiatherogenic properties of polyphenols, such as inhibition of peroxyl radical-induced DNA strand breakage, inhibition of platelet aggregation and of the expression of adhesion molecules to the endothelium, and protection of LDL from oxidative damage.[39-41]

CARDIAC CACHEXIA

Cachexia, that is caused by congestive heart failure (CHF), is called cardiac cachexia. This leads to increased morbidity and mortality. It is known to worsen skeletal muscle degradation. Cardiac cachexia by definition is the loss of edema-free muscle mass with or without affecting fat tissue. The primary cause is loss of balance between protein synthesis and degradation. It may also occur due to intestinal malabsorption. This loss of balance may be the result of altered endocrine mediators such as insulin, insulin-like growth factor 1, leptin, ghrelin, melanocortin, growth hormone and neuropeptide Y.[42]

According to the 2008 criteria, cardiac cachexia is characterized by: A loss of 5% of body weight during the last 12 months, without edema + a body mass index of <20 kg/m^{2+} the presence of at least three of the following clinical findings:

- Decreased muscular strength
- Anorexia
- Low body mass free of fat
- Fatigue
- Elevated reactive C-protein and IL-6
- Hypoalbuminemia <3.2 g/dL
- Hemoglobin <12 g/dL (anemia)

Cachexia is a nutritional syndrome because nutrients such as protein and calories are required to reverse it, and anorectic components participate in it.[43,44]

The degree of progression of cachexia is strongly linked to deficiency in the concentration of vitamin D. Other micronutrient deficiencies are also shown to influence the progression of HF. Thus, this unintentional cachexia is associated with poor survival in HF patients.[45]

Cachexia causes deficiencies in micronutrients and trace elements such as calcium, magnesium, zinc, iron, thiamine, vitamins E and K, and folate. Vitamin E along with omega-3 fatty acids have shown to improve survival. It has also been demonstrated that supplementation with vitamin C leads to an improvement of various quality of life aspects. Selective deficiency of selenium, calcium, and thiamine have also been linked to HF syndrome. Nutrients such as vitamins C and E and beta-carotene, are antioxidants and thus, they may have a protective effect on the vasculature.[46,47]

Cachexia is related to malnutrition. Except for cancer cachexia, all other causes of cachexia respond to judicious nutritional support. Cachexia must be treated cautiously to avoid overfeeding syndrome that may lead to serious complications or death.[48]

Enteral nutrition (EN) should always be preferred over parenteral feeding. If parenteral nutrition (PN) becomes mandatory and unavoidable, the general guidelines should be followed: 35 kcal/kg of body weight/day, 1.2 g of protein/kg/day, and a 70:30 glucose:lipid ratio for the nonprotein energy.[49]

Patients with CHF, whether cachectic or not, should restrict their daily sodium intake to about 2 g. Foods rich in salt such as cheese, sausages, crisps, tinned soup and vegetables, ham, bacon, tinned meat, and tinned or smoked fish should therefore be avoided. Long periods of fasting are mostly harmful. The cachectic patients should be advised to eat small, frequent meals. Fluid overload should be avoided, and in patients with severe symptoms or those requiring high doses of diuretics, fluid restriction (1.5–2.0 L/day) should be advised. It is suggested that multiple micronutrient supplementation is beneficial for cachectic patients, and it should contain antioxidant supplements and B-group vitamins.[50,51]

Vitamin D also has antihypertensive effects and improves endothelial function, and therefore, it may reduce the predictors of HF if it is timely administered. Vitamin D also serves as an anti-inflammatory agent and suppresses serum concentrations of parathormone, that is associated with impaired heart function. Calcium supplementation may result in a slight improvement in hemodynamic parameters, thus, it may be useful for the treatment of HF.[52-54]

Coenzyme Q_{10} has also proven to have positive effects.[55]

Food that negatively influence inflammatory processes can be recommended, such as fish oil supplements, olives, walnuts, flaxseed oil, any fruits or vegetables, garlic, ginger, turmeric, sunflower seeds, eggs, herring, or nuts.[56]

The therapeutic concepts comprise interventions with appetite stimulants, anabolic steroids, and growth hormone.

Appetite stimulants such as megestrol acetate and medroxyprogesterone acetate have been suggested to stimulate appetite and weight gain. The optimal dose of megestrol appears to be 800 mg daily with doses ranging from 160 to 1,600 mg daily.[57]

■ CARDIAC SURGERY

Nutrition support is widely being identified and accepted as a clinically pertinent aspect of the intensive care treatment of cardiac surgery patients.

Patients undergoing cardiac surgery experience a systemic inflammatory response that attributes to acute and persistent organ injury. With a growing older population undergoing complex cardiosurgical procedures, the incidence of comorbidities and malnutrition rises. The nutritional status and adequate nutrition therapy are important factors associated with the outcome of patients.

Iatrogenic malnutrition is mainly due to delayed initiation of nutrition support after cardiac surgery. It is also attributed by an inadequate supplementation of protein and energy. The European Society for Clinical Nutrition and Metabolism (ESPEN) as well as the American Society for Clinical Nutrition and Metabolism (ASPEN) recommend the initiation of EN within 24 hours after surgery and a supplementation of 25–30 kcal and 1.5–2.5 g of protein/day and kilogram ideal body weight for critically ill patients.[59,60]

The primary role of postoperative nutrition support is to maintain nutritional status and energy requirements in the catabolic period after surgery. Although evidence suggests that early oral and/or enteral food intake is possible, it diminishes the risk of infectious complications and favors shorter hospital stays, yet an interruption of nutritional intake is usually observed after surgery. Early nutrition is thus, encouraged by international nutrition societies to enhance recovery after surgery **(Box 1)**. The function of the gastrointestinal (GI) tract is an important factor for initiation of EN after abdominal surgery; however, as recommended by the revised ASPEN guidelines, the key determinant for initiation of nutrition in cardiac surgery patients is hemodynamic stability.[61,62]

In case of hemodynamic instability, EN is considered to be contraindicated as it may negatively affect gut integrity during a state of severe circulatory compromise in patients requiring high levels of vasopressor support, resulting in: (1) alteration of splanchnic perfusion and (2) an increased risk of GI complications, such as bowel ischemia. Also, there are pertinent practical obstacles such as the multiple interruptions of enteral feeding, pyloric dysfunction, and intestinal atony, which are frequently seen in patients after major surgical procedures.

Existing guidelines recommend the initiation of PN in all critically ill patients within 3–7 days after admission if EN is contraindicated or cannot be tolerated in patients with low nutrition risk and within 24 hours in patients with high nutrition risk.[59,60]

Parenteral nutrition assures attaining energy and protein targets and avoids the potential complications of EN. Concerns regarding PN are the potential risk of overfeeding with hyperglycemia, elevated liver enzymes, and increased rate of bloodstream infections.

Growing interest is seen with intravenous fish oil (FO)-based lipid emulsions (LEs) as part of the PN support. FO is rich in ω-3-PUFAs, such as EPA and DHA, which exhibit anti-inflammatory and immunomodulatory effects. Evidence received from small phase II trials on FO-containing emulsions in cardiac surgery have demonstrated that preoperative FO infusion is a promising strategy to alter the biological and clinical response to cardiac surgery with the use of cardiopulmonary bypass (CPB).[63-65]

The ESPEN Expert Group currently supports the use of olive oil and FO in nutrition support in surgical and nonsurgical ICU patients although it recommends further research to provide stronger evidence.[66]

In view of the insufficient evidence, recent guidelines state that routine supplementation with glutamine cannot be recommended

---

BOX 1: Nutrition support: Benefits in cardiac surgery.

To summarize, nutrition support enhances the recovery of patients in following ways:[58]
- Maintenance of metabolism
- Inhibition of catabolism
- Maintenance of gut-integrity
- Decreased postoperative complications
- Enhanced wound healing
- Maintaining adequate hydration and euglycemia

due to the unproved clinical benefits in cardiac surgery patients and even a risk of harm, which has been demonstrated in critically ill patients.

Selenium is a trace element that is necessary for body's multiple regulatory and metabolic functions, especially during stress. An observational study demonstrated that majority of patients undergoing cardiac surgery had a significant selenium deficiency prior to CPB, which was further aggravated with rising CPB time, associated with an insufficient capacity to withstand the stress of surgery.

Scanty data is available regarding vitamin supplementation in cardiac surgery patients. However, thiamine and vitamins D and C are the most commonly implicated and have been studied in several trials. Thiamine, the essential cofactor for pyruvate dehydrogenase function, is responsible for adequate aerobic metabolism.[67]

Sufficient nutrition support and intervention have shown to attenuate metabolic response to stress and favorably modulate immune responses. Nutritional support in critically ill patients prevents further metabolic deterioration and loss of lean body mass. Decrease in length of hospital stay, morbidity rate, and improvement in patient outcomes have highlighted the importance of nutrition support in the critically ill patients. Practice guidelines relevant for cardiac ICU are highlighted in **Table 1**.[68]

TABLE 1: Recommended practice guidelines.[68]

S. No.	Recommendation	Level of evidence
1.	All the critically ill patients should undergo nutrition assessment, on admission.	A I
2.	Observation of signs of malnutrition (e.g., cachexia, edema, muscle atrophy, BMI <20 kg/m²) is critical.	A I
3.	Enteral nutrition (EN) should be started early, preferably within first 24–48 hours	A I
4.	In case, the nutrition requirement is not met adequately with EN even after 7 days of ICU admission, then usage of parenteral nutrition (PN) may be considered.	A I
5.	Nutritional support should be considered as of therapeutic benefits and not just supportive or adjunctive.	A I
6.	Electrolytes should be strictly monitored in the patient on nutrition therapy.	B V
7.	Assessment of drug–nutrient interaction to be done on daily basis.	B V
8.	Tube feeding to be considered if even 50–60% of nutrition targets are not met adequately within 72 hours of oral nutrition support.	C
9.	Clinical monitoring of gut functioning should be started early when the patient is HD stable.	C
10.	Once the patient has been fluid resuscitated and stabilized on declining doses of <2 vasopressors, EN may be started cautiously at low rates.	A I
11.	Enteral nutrition should be administered within 24–48 hours, once the patient is stable with vasopressors.	A I
12.	In persistent shock, early EN should be avoided.	A I
13.	Feeding should be tailored as per the patient's requirement and level of tolerance.	C
14.	Protein requirement for most critically ill patients is in range of 1.2–2.0 g/kg body weight/day	A I
15.	Calories should be in range of 25–30 kcal/kg body weight/day for most critically ill patients.	A I
16.	EN should be considered over PN.	A I

Contd...

Contd...

S. No.	Recommendation	Level of evidence
17.	Combination of EN and PN should not be routinely recommended, except for specific indications.	A II
18.	Nasogastric (NG) route should be the first choice of enteral feeding. Jejunal route can be used if required.	A I
19.	Continuous formula feeding with pumps or gravity bags can be preferably done via fine-bore (8F–12F) tubes.	A I
20.	Scientific formula feed should be preferred over blenderized feeds to minimize feed contamination.	B III
21.	Whenever feasible, closed system ready-to-hang formula feeds should be preferred.	B III
22.	Blenderized formulae are more likely to have bacterial contamination than other hospital-prepared diets.	B IV
23.	Hygienic methods of feed preparation, storage, and handling of both formula feeds and blenderized feeds are necessary.	B III
24.	Gastric residual volume (GRV) should be measured by syringe aspiration and not by suction pump.	A II
25.	Gastric residual volume of <300 mL can be refed if it is not blood stained.	B V
26.	Holding EN for GRVs <500 mL in the absence of other signs of intolerance should be avoided.	A I
27.	However, GRV cutoff range of 300–500 mL can be considered, in Indian ICUs.	C
28.	In case of high GRVs, efforts should be made to continue feeding with reduced volumes.	C
29.	Prokinetic agents such as metoclopramide and erythromycin can be recommended in patients with intolerance and risk of aspiration.	A I
30.	Nurses should be trained for monitoring tolerance.	C
31.	EN should not be interrupted in the event of diarrhea.	A I
32.	Feeds can be continued while evaluating the etiology of diarrhea.	A I
33.	Use of a soluble fiber-containing formula or small peptide semielemental formula in divided doses over 24 hours may benefit to patients with persistent diarrhea (after exclusion of hyperosmolar agent intake and *Clostridium difficile* infection).	A I
34.	Routine use of probiotics across the general population of ICU patients is not recommended. Probiotics should be used only for selected medical and surgical patient populations, for which RCTs have documented safety and outcome benefit.	A I
35.	Preexisting micronutrients deficiency should be evaluated/assessed.	B V
36.	Patients on formula feeds may not require additional micronutrients, vitamins, and trace elements, if they are on complete and balanced formula feeds.	A I
37.	Micronutrients can be supplemented in patients on blenderized feeds and those on PN.	C
38.	Immune-modulating nutrients should not be used routinely.	A I
39.	In ICU patients with very severe illness and not tolerating >700 mL enteral formulae per day, immune nutrients should not be used.	A I
40.	Immune-modulating nutrients could be considered for patients with TBI and perioperative patients in the surgical ICU.	A I
41.	Glutamine is not recommended in critically ill patients with multiple organ failure.	B V

(BMI: body mass index; HD: hemodynamic; ICU: intensive care unit; RCTs: randomized controlled trials; TBI: traumatic brain injury)

MONITORING

To obtain high-quality nutrition care, nutritional practices should be documented from the very first step, i.e., with diagnosis and then with assessment, intervention, and monitoring.[68]

- Documentation of body weight and its review on weekly basis is recommended. (A II)
- Documentation of the below mentioned is also recommended (C):
  - Screening and assessment tools used along with their scores and the weekly review scores
  - Nutritional diagnosis
  - Nutrition care plan on daily basis
  - Infectious complications and stool frequency on daily basis.

CONCLUSION

Nutrition is now targeted to be of therapeutic importance in improving patient outcomes. Early, optimum, and adequate nutrition is implicated in improving overall prognosis of the patients. It has also shown to reduce the length of stay. EN is preferable in majority of cases. Scientific nutrition intervention is very important to achieve better clinical outcomes.

REFERENCES

1. Prabhakaran D, Jeemon P, Roy A. Cardiovascular diseases in India: Current epidemiology and future directions. Circulation. 2016;133:1605-20.
2. Kumar AS, Sinha N. Editorial cardiovascular disease in India: A 360 degree overview. Med J Armed Forces India. 2020;76:1-3.
3. Srinath RK, Shah B, Varghese C, Ramadoss A. Responding to the threat of chronic diseases in India. Lancet. 2005;366:1744-9.
4. Anchala R, Kannuri NK, Pant H, Khan H, Franco OH, Di Angelantonio E, et al. Hypertension in India: a systematic review and meta-analysis of prevalence, awareness, and control of hypertension. J Hypertens. 2014;32:1170-7.
5. Gupta R, Guptha S, Sharma KK, Gupta A, Deedwania P. Regional variations in cardiovascular risk factors in India: India heart watch. World J Cardiol. 2012;4:112-20.
6. Joshi P, Islam S, Pais P, Reddy S, Dorairaj P, Kazmi K, et al. Risk factors for early myocardial infarction in South Asians compared with individuals in other countries. JAMA. 2007;297:286-94.
7. Dhaka V, Gulia N, Ahlawat KS, Khatkar BS. Trans fats-sources, health risks and alternative approach – a review. J Food Sci Technol. 2011;48:534-41.
8. Misra A, Sharma R, Pandey RM, Khanna N. Adverse profile of dietary nutrients, anthropometry and lipids in urban slum dwellers of northern India. Eur J Clin Nutr. 2001;55:727-34.
9. Chaturvedi V, Parakh N, Seth S, Bhargava B, Ramakrishnan S, Roy A, et al. Heart Failure in India: The INDUS (INDia Ukieri Study) Study. J Pract Cardiovasc Sci. 2016;2(1):28-35.
10. Lu H, Daugherty A. Recent highlights of ATVB atherosclerosis. Arterioescler Thromb Vasc Biol. 2015;35:485-91.
11. Micha R, Peñalvo JL, Cudhea F, Imamura F, Rehm CD, Mozaffarian D. Association between dietary factors and mortality from heart disease, stroke, and type 2 diabetes in the United States. JAMA. 2017;317:912-24.
12. Ozawa M, Shipley M, Kivimaki M, Singh-Manoux A, Brunner EJ. Dietary pattern, inflammation, and cognitive decline: The Whitehall II prospective cohort study. Clin Nutr. 2017;36:506-12.
13. Atkins JL, Whincup PH, Morris RW, Lennon LT, Papacosta O, Wannamethee SG. Dietary patterns and the risk of CVD and all-cause mortality in older British men. Br J Nutr. 2016;116:1246-55.
14. Mozaffarian D. Dietary and policy priorities for cardiovascular disease, diabetes, and obesity: A comprehensive review. Circulation. 2016;133:187-225.

15. Silveira BKS, Oliveira TMS, Andrade PA, Hermsdorff HHM, Rosa COB, Franceschini SDCC. Dietary pattern and macronutrients profile on the variation of inflammatory biomarkers: Scientific Update. Cardiol Res Pract. 2018;2018:4762575.
16. Llorente-Cortés V, Estruch R, Mena MP, Ros E, González MA, Fitó M, et al. Effect of Mediterranean diet on the expression of pro-atherogenic genes in a population at high cardiovascular risk. Atherosclerosis. 2010; 208:442-50.
17. Casas R, Sacanella E, Urpí-Sardà M, Chiva-Blanch G, Ros E, Martínez-González MA, et al. The effects of the mediterranean diet on biomarkers of vascular wall inflammation and plaque vulnerability in subjects with high risk for cardiovascular disease. A randomized trial. PLoS ONE. 2014;9:e100084.
18. Corley J, Kyle JA, Starr JM, McNeill G, Deary IJ. Dietary factors and biomarkers of systemic inflammation in older people: The Lothian Birth Cohort 1936. Br J Nutr. 2015;114:1088-98.
19. Arouca A, Michels N, Moreno LA, González-Gil EM, Marcos A, Gómez S, et al. Associations between a Mediterranean diet pattern and inflammatory biomarkers in European adolescents. Eur J Nutr. 2018;57:1747-60.
20. Wongwarawipat T, Papageorgiou N, Bertsias D, Siasos G, Tousoulis D. Olive Oil-related Anti-inflammatory effects on atherosclerosis: Potential clinical implications. Endocr Metab Immune Disord Drug Targets. 2018;18:51-62.
21. Schwingshackl L, Christoph M, Hoffmann G. Effects of olive oil on markers of inflammation and endothelial function-A systematic review and meta-analysis. Nutrients. 2015;7:7651-75.
22. Fitó M, Estruch R, Salas-Salvadó J, Martínez-Gonzalez MA, Arós F, Vila J, et al. Effect of the Mediterranean diet on heart failure biomarkers: A randomized sample from the PREDIMED trial. Eur J Heart Fail. 2014;16:543-50.
23. Sala-Vila A, Romero-Mamani ES, Gilabert R, Núñez I, De La Torre R, Corella D, et al. Changes in ultrasound-assessed carotid intima-media thickness and plaque with a Mediterranean diet: A substudy of the PREDIMED trial. Arterioscler Thromb Vasc Biol. 2014;34:439-45.
24. Guasch-Ferré M, Liu X, Malik VS, Sun Q, Willett WC, Manson JE, et al. Nut consumption and risk of cardiovascular disease. J Am Coll Cardiol. 2017;70:2519-32.
25. Aune D, Keum N, Giovannucci E, Fadnes LT, Boffetta P, Greenwood DC, et al. Nut consumption and risk of cardiovascular disease, total cancer, all-cause and cause-specific mortality: A systematic review and dose-response meta-analysis of prospective studies. BMC Med. 2016;14:207.
26. McRae MP. Dietary fiber is beneficial for the prevention of cardiovascular disease: An umbrella review of Meta-analyses. J Chiropr Med. 2017;16:289-99.
27. Ma Y, Hébert JR, Li W, Bertone-Johnson ER, Olendzki B, Pagoto SL, et al. Association between dietary fiber and markers of systemic inflammation in the Women's Health Initiative Observational Study. Nutrition. 2008;24:941-9.
28. Gammoh NZ, Rink L. Zinc in Infection and Inflammation. Nutrients. 2017;9:624.
29. Simental-Mendia LE, Sahebkar A, Rodriguez-Moran M, Zambrano-Galvan G, Guerrero-Romero F. Effect of magnesium supplementation on plasma C-reactive protein concentrations: A systematic review and meta-analysis of randomized controlled trials. Curr Pharm Des. 2017;23:4678-86.
30. Casas R, Castro-Barquero S, Estruch R, Sacanella E. Nutrition and cardiovascular health. Int J Mol Sci. 2018;19:3988.
31. Massaro M, Scoditti E, Carluccio MA, DeCaterina R. Nutraceuticals and prevention of atherosclerosis: Focus on omega-3 polyunsaturated fatty acids and Mediterranean diet polyphenols. Cardiovasc Ther. 2010;28:e13-9.
32. Hamer M, Steptoe A. Influence of specific nutrients on progression of atherosclerosis, vascular function, haemostasis and inflammation in coronary heart disease patients: A systematic review. Br J Nutr. 2006;95:849-59.
33. Kaliora AC, Dedoussis GV. Natural antioxidant compounds in risk factors for CVD. Pharmacol Res. 2007;56:99-109.

34. Valderas-Martinez P, Chiva-Blanch G, Casas R, Arranz S, Martínez-Huélamo M, Urpi-Sarda M, et al. Tomato sauce enriched with olive oil exerts greater effects on cardiovascular disease risk factors than raw tomato and tomato sauce: A randomized trial. Nutrients. 2016;8:170.
35. Mozos I, Stoian D, Caraba A, Malainer C, Horbańczuk JO, Atanasov AG. Lycopene and vascular health. Front Pharmacol. 2018;9:521.
36. Ras RT, Geleijnse JM, Trautwein EA. LDL-cholesterol-lowering effect of plantsterols and stanols across different dose ranges: A meta-analysis of randomised controlled studies. Br J Nutr. 2014;112:214-9.
37. Cabra CE, Simas-Torres Klein MR. Phytosterols in the treatment of hypercholesterolemia and prevention of cardiovascular diseases. Arq Bras Cardiol. 2017;109:475-82.
38. Demonty I, Ras RT, van der Knaap HC, Duchateau GS, Meijer L, Zock PL, et al. Continuous dose-response relationship of the LDL-cholesterol-lowering effect of phytosterol intake. J Nutr. 2009;139:271-84.
39. Tressera-Rimbau A, Arranz S, Eder M, Vallverdú-Queralt A. Dietary polyphenols in the prevention of stroke. Oxid Med Cell Longev. 2017;2017:7467962.
40. González-Gallego J, García-Mediavilla MV, Sánchez-Campos S, Tuñón MJ. Fruit polyphenols immunity and inflammation. Br J Nutr. 2010;104:S15-27.
41. Bahramsoltani R, Ebrahimi F, Farzaei MH, Baratpourmoghaddam A, Ahmadi P, Rostamiasrabadi P, et al. Dietary polyphenols for atherosclerosis: A comprehensive review and future perspectives. Crit Rev Food Sci Nutr. 2019;59(1):114-32.
42. Soto ME, Pérez-Torres I, Rubio-Ruiz ME, Manzano-Pech L, Guarner-Lans V. Interconnection between cardiac cachexia and heart failure—protective role of cardiac obesity. Cells. 2022;11(6):1039.
43. Evans WJ, Morley JE, Argiles J, Bales C, Baracos V, Guttridge D, et al. Cachexia: A new definition. Clin Nutr. 2008;27:793-9.
44. Bowen TS, Schuler G, Adams V. Skeletal muscle wasting in cachexia and sarcopenia: Molecular pathophysiology and impact of exercise training. J Cachexia Sarcopenia Muscle. 2015;6:197-207.
45. Krim SR, Campbell P, Lavie CJ, Ventura H. Micronutrients in chronic heart failure. Curr Heart Fail Rep. 2013;10:46-53.
46. Mochamat, Cuhls H, Marinova M, Kaasa S, Stieber C, Conrad R, et al. A systematic review on the role of vitamins, minerals, proteins, and other supplements for the treatment of cachexia in cancer: A European Palliative Care Research Centre cachexia project. J Cachexia Sarcopenia Muscle. 2017;8:25-39.
47. Cleland Witte KK, Clark AL, Cleland JG. Chronic heart failure and micronutrients. J Am Coll Cardiol. 2001;37:1765-74.
48. Palesty JA, Dudrick SJ. Cachexia, malnutrition, the refeeding syndrome, and lessons from Goldilocks. Surg Clin N Am. 2011;91:653-73.
49. Mustafa I, Leverve X. Metabolic and nutritional disorders in cardiac cachexia. Nutrition. 2001;17:756-60.
50. Gibbs CR, Jackson G, Lip GY. ABC of heart failure. Non-drug management. BMJ. 2000;320:366-9.
51. Witte KK, Nikitin NP, Parker AC, von Haehling S, Volk HD, Anker SD, et al. The effect of micronutrient supplementation on quality-of-life and left ventricular function in elderly patients with chronic heart failure. Eur Heart J. 2005;26:2238-44.
52. Pfeifer M, Begerow B, Minne HW, Nachtigall D, Hansen C. Effects of a short-term vitamin D(3) and calcium supplementation on blood pressure and parathyroid hormone levels in elderly women. J Clin Endocrinol Metab. 2001;86:1633-7.
53. Sugden JA, Davies JI, Witham MD, Morris AD, Struthers AD. Vitamin D improves endothelial function in patients with type 2 diabetes mellitus and low vitamin D levels. Diab Med. 2008;25:320-5.
54. Schleithoff SS, Zittermann A, Tenderich G, Berthold HK, Stehle P, Koerfer R. Vitamin D supplementation improves cytokine profiles in patients with congestive heart failure: A double-blind, randomized, placebo-controlled trial. Am J Clin Nutr. 2006;83:754-9.

55. Berman M, Erman A, Ben-Gal T, Dvir D, Georghiou GP, Stamler A, et al. Coenzyme Q10 in patients with end-stage heart failure awaiting cardiac transplantation: A randomized, placebo-controlled study. Clin Cardiol. 2004;27:295-9.
56. Azhar G, Wei JY. Nutrition and cardiac cachexia. Curr Opin Nutr Metab Care. 2006;9:18-23.
57. von Haehling S, Doehner W, Anker SD. Nutrition, metabolism, and the complex pathophysiology of cachexia in chronic heart failure. Cardiovasc Res. 2007;73(2):298-309.
58. Hill A, Nesterova E, Lomivorotov V, Efremov S, Efremov S, Goetzenich A, Benstoem C, et al. Current evidence about nutrition support in cardiac surgery patients—What do we know? Nutrients. 2018;10(5):597.
59. Weimann A, Braga M, Carli F, Higashiguchi T, Hubner M, Klek S, et al. ESPEN guideline: Clinical nutrition in surgery. Clin Nutr. 2017;36(3):623-50.
60. McClave SA, Taylor BE, Martindale RG, Warren MM, Johnson DR, Braunschweig C, et al. Guidelines for the provision and assessment of nutrition support therapy in the adult critically ill patient: Society of critical care medicine (SCCM) and American society for parenteral and enteral nutrition (ASPEN). JPEN J Parenter Enteral Nutr. 2016;40(2):159-211.
61. ASPEN Board of Directors and the Clinical Guidelines Task Force Guidelines for the use of parenteral and enteral nutrition in adult and pediatric patients. JPEN J Parenter Enter Nutr. 2002;26:1SA-138SA.
62. Andersen HK, Lewis SJ, Thomas S. Early enteral nutrition within 24h of colorectal surgery versus later commencement of feeding for postoperative complications. Cochrane Database Syst. Rev. 2006:CD004080.
63. Heidt MC, Vician M, Stracke SKH, Stadlbauer T, Grebe MT, Boening A, et al. Beneficial effects of intravenously administered N-3 fatty acids for the prevention of atrial fibrillation after coronary artery bypass surgery: A prospective randomized study. Thorac Cardiovasc Surg. 2009;57:276-80.
64. Berger MM, Delodder F, Liaudet L, Tozzi P, Schlaepfer J, Chiolero RL, et al. Three short perioperative infusions of N-3 PUFAs reduce systemic inflammation induced by cardiopulmonary bypass surgery: A randomized controlled trial. Am J Clin Nutr. 2013;97:246-54.
65. Metcalf RG, James MJ, Gibson RA, Edwards JR, Stubberfield J, Stuklis R, et al. Effects of fish-oil supplementation on myocardial fatty acids in humans. Am J Clin Nutr. 2007;85:1222-8.
66. Calder PC, Adolph M, Deutz NE, Grau T, Innes JK, Klek S, et al. Lipids in the intensive care unit: Recommendations from the ESPEN expert group. Clin Nutr. 2018;37:1-18.
67. Benstoem C, Goetzenich A, Kraemer S, Borosch S, Manzanares W, Hardy G, et al. Selenium and its supplementation in cardiovascular disease–what do we know? Nutrients. 2015;7:3094-118.
68. Mehta Y, Sunavala JD, Zirpe K, Tyagi N, Garg S, Sinha S, et al. Practice guidelines for nutrition in critically ill patients: A relook for Indian scenario. Indian J Crit Care Med. 2018;22(4):263-73.

CHAPTER 26

Clinical Nutrition in Oncology

Vanessa Fuchs-Tarlovsky

INTRODUCTION

Cancer is one of the leading causes of mortality worldwide; its incidence and prevalence have increased in recent years. Due to its pathophysiological characteristics, nutrition has important implications in developing the disease and maintaining the oncologic patient.

The oncological patient may also be affected by the type of antineoplastic treatment and its associated effects, so other alterations related to decreased intake and muscle depletion, as well as anorexia, may occur.

Malnutrition is a frequent problem in cancer patients, occurring in 40-80% of cases; its frequency varies according to the location, clinical stage of the disease, and treatment implemented. It is associated with increased morbidity and mortality and is the cause of death in up to 20% of patients.[1]

Malnutrition is prevalent in 15-20% of patients at the time of cancer diagnosis and up to 90% during treatment. In clinical practice worldwide, there is underdiagnosis and undermanagement of malnutrition. Because of this, timely counseling and management are essential, as it is known that a good nutritional status contributes to recovery, response to treatment, and quality of life, and, in some cases, works as an adjuvant in antineoplastic treatment.

This chapter reviews the fundamental concepts for cancer patient's diagnosis and nutritional management.

NUTRITIONAL ALTERATIONS IN CANCER

Cachexia

Cachexia is a frequent complication in the oncologic patient; it is defined according to the international consensus (IC) of 2011 as a "multifactorial syndrome characterized by a decrease in skeletal muscle (with or without loss of fat mass), which cannot be completely reversed by conventional nutritional support and generates a progressive functional failure".[2] Its etiology is multicausal, although it is mainly associated with decreased intake and metabolic changes resulting from cancer.[3]

PATHOPHYSIOLOGY OF CANCER CACHEXIA

There is no specific cause for the development of cachexia syndrome, but its main causative factor is the exacerbation of the immune response and increased production of proinflammatory cytokines due to neoplastic activity.[4]

In solid tumors, tumor growth demands more significant energy expenditure and hyperactivation of the immune system. In the first phase, there is a negative energy and protein balance due to increased energy demands and caloric deficiency in intake. At the metabolic level, there are digestive alterations, hormonal responses related to the underlying disease, increased proteolysis, lipolysis, and inflammatory mediators such as tumor-necrosis factor-α (TNF-α) and interleukins that induce anorexia—the decrease in energy intake results in a hypermetabolic catabolic state with increased glucagon, cortisol, and catecholamines. In addition, the production of anabolic mediators such as growth hormone, insulin-like growth factor-1 (IGF-1), testosterone, and ghrelin is reduced.[4,5] It presents clinically as a decreased bodyweight with muscle and fat loss.

Inflammation is fundamental in developing cachexia and affects various tissues including skeletal muscle, fat, brain, and liver. The central proinflammatory cytokines are TNF-α, interferon-gamma (IFN-γ), and interleukin-1, 6, and 8 (IL-1, IL-6, and IL-8).[6] The effects of proinflammatory cytokines on macronutrient metabolism are presented **(Table 1)**.

The IC classifies cachexia into three stages: (1) Precachexia, (2) cachexia, and (3) refractory cachexia. It is crucial to consider that not all patients go through each stage and that the onset of clinical signs may occur before there is significant weight loss **(Fig. 1)**.[2]

For the diagnosis of cachexia, the following characteristics are considered: Weight loss >5% or body mass index (BMI) <20 kg/m^2 accompanied by a weight reduction of 2% or the presence of sarcopenia (appendicular skeletal mass index in the male sex <7.26 kg/m^2; female <5.45 kg/m^2) and loss of at least 2% of the weight. In refractory cachexia, in addition to weight loss, the presence of signs of disease progression and response to antineoplastic treatment are taken into consideration, which in these patients is little or null, they also present low physical performance score (WHO 3-4), and their life expectancy is <3 months.[2]

TABLE 1: Cytokine effects on protein and lipid metabolism in cancer cachexia.

	Protein	*Carbohydrate*	*Lipid*
TNF-α	• Increased muscle proteolysis • Increased protein oxidation • Increased hepatic protein synthesis	• Increased glycogenolysis • Decreased glycogen synthesis • Increased glucogenesis • Increased glucose clearance • Increased lactate production	• Decreased lipogenesis • Decreased LPL in fat tissue
IL-1	Increased hepatic protein synthesis	• Increased gluconeogenesis • Increased glucose clearance	• Increased lipolysis • Decreased LPL synthesis • Increased fatty acid synthesis
IL-6	Increased hepatic protein synthesis		• Increased lipolysis • Increased fatty acid synthesis
IFN-γ			• Decreased lipogenesis • Increased lipolysis • Decreased LPL activity

(IFN-γ: interferon-gamma; IL: interleukin; LPL: lipoprotein lipase; TNF: tumor-necrosis factor)
Source: Obtained from Fuchs-Tarlovsky V, Isenring E. Nutrition therapy in patients with cancer and immunodeficiency. In: Creci G (Ed). Nutrition in the critically ill patient. United States: CRC Press; 2013.

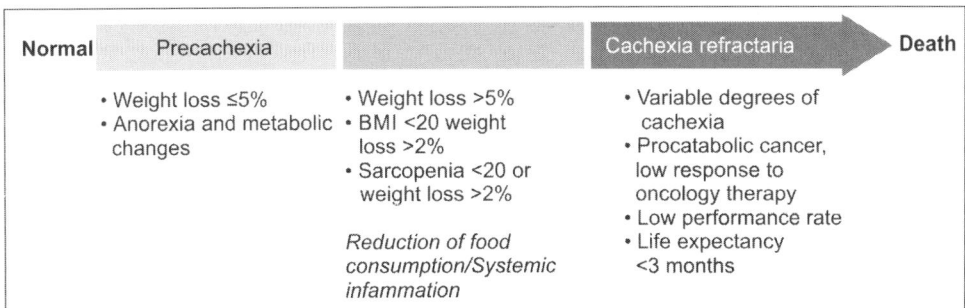

Fig. 1: Stages of cachexia. (BMI: body mass index)
Source: Adapted from Fearon K, Strasser F, Anker SD, Bosaeus I, Bruera E, Fainsinger RL, et al. Definition and classification of cancer cachexia: an international consensus. Lancet Oncol. 2011;12(5):489-95.

The severity of the disease can be classified according to the degree of weight loss in combination with the depletion of energy reserves and body protein mass. However, progression varies according to the type of cancer, stage of disease, presence of systemic inflammation, low food intake, or poor response to antineoplastic therapy.

So far, the only validated screening test for cachexia staging is the *Cancer Cachexia Score* (CASCO). This scale assesses five components: (1) Weight loss and composition, (2) inflammation/metabolic disturbances/immunosuppression, (3) physical performance, (4) anorexia, and (5) quality of life. The score ranges from 0 to 100 and is classified as follows: No cachexia (<14), mild (15-28), moderate (29-46), and severe (47-100).[7]

The initial design of the test in 2011 contemplated the state of precachexia and corresponded to a score of PPC = 0 and IMDI + CV DF + AN + CV > 35; however, in the validation of the difficulty in 2017, there is no mention of the validity of this cut-off point. The authors of the test propose a brief version of the screening. However, both tests are little used in practice due to the number of items it evaluates; the most used classification is the one proposed by the IC.[7]

Sarcopenia

The operational definition of sarcopenia in the latest update of the European Working Group on Sarcopenia in Older People (EWGSOP2) defines it as a progressive and generalized alteration of skeletal muscle associated with increased adverse effects including falls, fractures, physical disability, and mortality.[8] The term has been coined primarily in the older adult population; however, because of its phenotypic characteristics, it has been transpolated to other areas where such a condition may coexist with other disorders, such as cancer. The definition is still a matter of discussion among experts, and they currently need to be a global consensus for its diagnosis. The European Society for Clinical Nutrition and Metabolism (ESPEN) adheres to the definition provided by EWGSOP, adapting it to the nutritional context of the geriatric or nongeriatric adult patient.[9,10]

Sarcopenia has been divided into categories by cause: Primary sarcopenia is an age-related pathology preceded by a state of frailty; secondary sarcopenia is associated with other pathophysiological mechanisms related to a disease state, physical activity, or nutritional status.[9] By its time of evolution:

Acute when it has <6 months of development and chronic when it is ≥6 months. A state known as sarcopenic obesity, a condition of reduced body mass accompanied by excess adiposity, has also been categorized.[8,9]

European Working Group on Sarcopenia in Older People describes the possible coexistence of malnutrition and sarcopenia resulting from decreased intake, poor nutrient bioavailability, or high-energy requirements, such as cancer and cachexia.[8]

Probable sarcopenia is one in which decreased muscle strength is present; frank sarcopenia is confirmed by decreased muscle in quantity and quality tests, while severe sarcopenia, in addition to the above criteria, is accompanied by poor physical performance **(Table 2)**.

The tests to evaluate each diagnostic criterion for sarcopenia are listed in **Table 3** with their respective cut-off points.

Severe sarcopenia alone increases the risk of death; in the case of the elderly, it can amount to 76% of death when present with slowed walking speed.[11] In cancer patients, the prevalence is 20–70% depending on the

TABLE 2: Operational definition of sarcopenia according to EWGSOP2.

Criteria	Definition	Diagnosis
1. Low muscle strength	Probable sarcopenia	Criterion 1
2. Low quantity or quality of muscle	Confirmed diagnosis	Criterion 2
3. Low physical performance	Severe sarcopenia	Criteria 1, 2, and 3

(EWGSOP2: European Working Group on Sarcopenia in Older People 2018)
Source: Adapted from Cruz-Jentoft AJ, Bahat G, Bauer J, Boirie Y, Bruyère O, Cederholm T, et al. Sarcopenia: revised European consensus on definition and diagnosis. Age Ageing. 2019;48(1):16-31.

TABLE 3: Validated diagnostic tests for assessing the diagnostic criteria for sarcopenia.

Criteria	Tests	Cut-off points Female	Cut-off points Male
Muscle strength	• Tensile strength *(Grip strength)* • Chair stand test *(Chair stand test)*	<16 kg >15 s for five elevations	<27 kg
Muscle mass/ skeletal muscle quality	• MAE evaluated by DXA muscle mass assessment (MMAS) • SMM predicted by BIA (SMM) • Cross-sectional area of the lumbar muscle by CT and MRI • Muscle quality of half or whole body assessed by biopsy, CT, and MRI	<15 kg	<20 kg
Physical performance	• Gait speed • *Short physical performance battery (SPPB)* test • *Time-up-and-go* dynamic functional balance test *(Time-up-and-go test)* TUG • 400 m hike or long-distance walk	≤0.8 m/s ≥8 points in the test ≥20 s Fails to complete or takes ≥6 minutes to complete the test	

(ASM: appendicular skeletal mass; BIA: bioimpedance analysis; CT: computed tomography; DXA: dual-energy X-ray absorptiometry; MRI: magnetic resonance imaging; MSM: musculoskeletal stress markers)
Source: Adapted from Cruz-Jentoft AJ, Bahat G, Bauer J, Boirie Y, Bruyère O, Cederholm T, et al. Sarcopenia: revised European consensus on definition and diagnosis. Age Ageing. 2019;48(1):16-31.

type of tumor. It is more frequent in women (56%). In de novo diagnoses, the prevalence is 14–16%, and treatment with chemotherapy increases the majority, which increases the risk of toxicity by these drugs.[12-14]

Anorexia

Anorexia in cancer is defined as nonvolitional loss of appetite, also known as secondary anorexia.[15] In the oncologic patient, it is a crucial component in the pathogenesis of cachexia and sarcopenia, but it can occur independently. There are different causes of anorexia; among them there is the release of proinflammatory cytokines, lactate, and parathyroid hormone-related peptide, tumors that cause dysphagia or alterations of intestinal function; tumors that alter nutrients; tumors that cause hypoxia, a peripheral increase of tryptophan and accumulation of serotonin and changes in the peripheral release of hormones that influence feeding. It results from central and peripheral alterations, the hypothalamic mechanisms that control feeding under normal conditions. At the cerebral level, the presence of neuroinflammation alters the satiety-mediating neurons (proopiomelanocortin-producing neurons) and the prophagic neurons [neuropeptide Y (NPY)].[15]

It is an independent adverse prognostic factor in cancer and is associated with other symptoms **(Table 4)**, which the medical and nutritional assessment can identify. Anorexia can be reversed by adequate dietary support.

Assessment of Nutritional Status

To evaluate the nutritional status of the oncologic patient, validated screening tools have been designed in different languages. Early and properly performed screening ensures timely care and the possibility of patient recovery.

In European countries, there is evidence of underdiagnosis of malnutrition during the first hospitalization for cancer and subsequent hospitalizations; in countries such as Italy, the average time between the first nutritional prescription and the patient's death is 3.5 months.[16]

It is known that oncology patients present a high risk of malnutrition because of the tumor or treatment. The most used nutritional screening is the patient-generated subjective global assessment (PG-SGA) can be used as a nutrition screening, assessment, or measure to estimate the patient outcome.[17] However, because it has to be performed by a healthcare professional, it is often used

TABLE 4: Symptoms associated with anorexia.

	Symptoms associated with anorexia	Test
Anorexia	• Decreased appetite • Early satiety • Changes in the sense of taste • Changes in smell • Depression • Dysphagia • Painful swallowing	• Visual analog pain scale questionnaire • Evaluation of portion size • Evaluation of taste and smell perception thresholds • Psychiatric scales • Endoscopic evaluation of swallowing • Pain scales

Source: Laviano A, Koverech A, Seelaender M. Assessing pathophysiology of cancer anorexia. Curr Opin Clin Nutr Metabol Care. 2017;20(5):340-5.

as part of a much more comprehensive nutritional assessment. This is based on a combination of known prognostic indicators of weight loss and functional status, as well as clinical aspects of dietary intake and its impairments (including symptoms of nutritional impact), which allow the identification of malnutrition and assessment of nutritional status.

It is recommended that patients should be assessed during the planning or initiation of antineoplastic therapy and reassessed periodically (weekly or every clinic visit).

In 2019, the Expert Group of the Malnutrition Initiative [Global Leadership Initiative on Malnutrition (GLIM)], its acronym in English, released the criteria for the diagnosis of malnutrition, which considers body composition in its various forms of assessment as one of the diagnostic criteria. The tool includes two phases, the first is a risk screening tool, and the second is the malnutrition diagnosis and grading of malnutrition. For that purpose it uses both etiological and phenotypical criteria.[18]

Despite its recent publication and the incipiency of validations in different countries, the first studies in cancer patients have shown that the GLIM criteria have a predictive value for mortality at 6 months in oncology patients similar to the PG-SGA.[19]

As part of the assessment of nutritional status, an individualized evaluation consisting of anthropometric and biochemical data, clinical signs and symptoms, and dietary aspects should be considered in addition to the measurement of nutritional risk.[20]

Several factors must be taken into account to determine an adequate nutritional diagnosis; among them:[13]

- Food intolerance or rejection
- Changes in snack patterns
- Prescription and over-the-counter drugs, herbal preparations, and complementary or alternative medicine products
- Factors affecting food availability
- Energy and protein intake
- Changes in food and fluid intake
- Adequacy and appropriateness of nutrient intake or administration
- Current daily consumption by enteral, parenteral, and other means of feeding
- Changes in type, texture, or temperature of foods and liquids
- Use of medical/food supplements

Anthropometric Evaluation

It is advisable to assess the following anthropometric measurements in the adult oncology patient:[21]

- Height
- Current weight
- Weight history
- Usual weight
- Recent weight change (in the last 6 months)
- Percentage of usual weight
- Body mass index
- Electrical bioimpedance (to assess body composition, including body water), if available.

Any unintentional weight loss of >10% of their usual weight in the adult patient is momentous.

Assessing the previous factors is necessary for a correct nutritional diagnosis and an adequate nutritional support plan. It is essential to measure and record body weight regularly, as it is not always obvious when someone is losing weight as an effect of volume gain or water retention and disease-related changes in the body, e.g., ascites, which could mask a loss of lean body mass weight and changes in composition.

Body mass index has limitations if taken as the sole measure of nutritional status. Malnutrition may be overlooked in patients within the "healthy" or "overweight" range for BMI, despite significant weight loss.[14]

Monitoring food intake, biochemical indicators, body weight, and composition is essential to assess patient outcomes.[15]

Evaluation and Interpretation of Biochemical Data

Biochemical indicators to be considered include:[11]

- *Serum proteins:* Albumin and prealbumin.
- Renal function from blood urea nitrogen (BUN), creatinine, and blood glucose.
- *Hematological data:* Hemoglobin, hematocrit, ferritin, platelet count, mean corpuscular volume, among others.
- Plasma concentrations of serum electrolytes
- Leukocyte and total neutrophil counts
- C-reactive protein to determine chronic inflammation

It is worth mentioning that several of these indicators will be affected by both the disease and its treatment. Albumin is a very sensitive indicator to inflammation since the higher the CRP, the lower the albumin concentrations, even when measured twice on the same day; when there is a surgical procedure involved that implies inflammation, albumin concentrations will be lower, so it cannot be taken as the only data to evaluate nutritional status.[7] The concentration of albumin, a thyroxine transporter protein with a short half-life (2-3 days), is the most helpful indicator since it is less altered by inflammation.

Hematological data may vary due to the frequent transfusions these patients receive and the ability of tumors to form new blood vessels that increase the demand for iron and other nutrients. The white formula can vary significantly due to antineoplastic treatments, which produce secondary damage to these elements.

It is worth mentioning that the patient's hydration status must be considered before the interpretation of laboratory tests. If the patient is dehydrated, the figures cannot be viewed until rehydrated.

Clinical Indicators

Signs and symptoms develop due to a deficiency or excess of some nutrients and the various symptoms caused by cancer and antineoplastic treatments. They are clinical indicators that extend throughout the course of the disease and that, to a lesser or greater extent, may denote an inadequate nutritional status.[15]

As mentioned above, the metabolic changes developed by certain types of cancer are closely linked to cachexia, characterized by the loss of lean and body fat mass. A patient is likely to mask the loss of muscle mass if they have excess adipose tissue before developing cancer, so it is essential to have the necessary skills to diagnose a state of cachexia during the patient's physical evaluation.

The complete physical evaluation should include observation for signs of edema, ascites, temporal lobe atrophy, and muscle atrophy.

Similarly, it should be evaluated if there are or have been gastrointestinal (GI) symptoms such as those mentioned throughout the chapter, as well as an assessment of the oral cavity that includes dentition and the functional capacity of the patient to carry out chewing and swallowing correctly. Subclinical signs denoting the presence of any GI symptoms of interest, such as vomiting, can be evaluated using the oral cavity.[13]

Dietary Indicators

Intake analysis and assessment of dietary habits provide information about patients' energy and other nutrient intake. Comparing standard input with recommendations will possibly highlight the likelihood of inadequate intake and thus identify risk situations. It is worth mentioning that in many oncology patients, there are changes in food taste (dysgeusia), which further affects proper nutrition.

The instruments available and recommended to carry out the dietary evaluation are:[8]
- Food consumption frequency questionnaires
- 24-hour reminder
- Usual diet
- Food diary

Because of the complex relationships between dietary habits and the tools already mentioned, others have been developed, such as the *alternative healthy eating index* and *the dietary quality index*.[16] These tools enhance the ability to understand these phenomena, although they also increase costs to such an extent that they cannot be used routinely in clinical practice. Likewise, self-administered methods have been described, such as the *eating assessment table*, which has advantages over existing conventional methods and is affordable enough for clinical practice.[17]

Functional Evaluation

In addition to the tools mentioned above, which assess nutritional status, diet quality and quantity, and other prognostic indicators, questionnaires, and scales have been developed that have proven effective in the cancer patient assessment process.

The *activities of daily living questionnaire* (ADLQ)[18] assess routine activities such as eating, bathing, dressing, continence, etc., that the general population performs daily without assistance. It is imperative to determine the functional capacity with which the patient performs each activity to predict what type of assistance they will require throughout the evolution of their disease.

Another of these tools is the "Karnofsky Scale", a subjective assessment that aims to determine cancer patients' general well-being. This tool is handy since the history of the disease process can be analyzed through periodic evaluations and comparisons. These scores range from 100 to 0, where 100 indicates good health and 0 is equivalent to death.[19]

Validated scales for measuring the quality of life can help to measure treatment success since one of the most critical goals in oncology is to preserve as much of the patient's quality of life as possible. This is where nutritional status plays a vital role.

Calculation of Requirements

Providing the cancer patient with sufficient nutritional intake is essential to maintain or prevent weight loss associated with the disease or antineoplastic treatment.

Indirect calorimetry (IC) remains the gold standard for calculating the energy requirement of cancer patients. However, an indirect calorimeter is only sometimes available in clinical practice, so there is some basis for performing the calculation necessary to develop a dietary plan.

The following guidelines are a guide for calculating the energy requirements of oncology patients:[21]
- *Patients with normal metabolism:* 25–30 kcal/kg/day
- *In hypermetabolism or for weight gain:* 30–35 kcal/kg/day

- *Patients with obesity:* 21–25 kcal/kg/day (when weight maintenance is the goal, requirements may be increased if nutritional status deteriorates).

It is essential to mention that the requirements may exceed 35 kcal/kg/day when the patient requires it, either to maintain or increase the weight or simply because of the etiology of the type of cancer.

Similarly, the provision of adequate protein, both in quality and quantity, is essential to prevent or reduce a negative nitrogen balance and to meet the patient's need to synthesize protein:

- *Nonstressed patients:* 1–1.5 g/kg/day
- *Patients with hypermetabolism or protein losses:* 1.5–2.5 g/kg/day

Using the usual or ideal weight is recommended to make these calculations. Still, if the patient's weight is well below their average weight, it is recommended to start with the current weight and gradually increase it until reaching the calculation based on their usual weight.

On the other hand, it should be considered that cancer patients, especially those undergoing chemotherapy or radiotherapy, usually present in a state of dehydration due to inadequate fluid intake caused by diarrhea, xerostomia, mucositis, dysgeusia, dysphagia, and odynophagia.[22] Patients with these alterations should be monitored for signs or symptoms of dehydration, such as dark and concentrated urine, decreased urination, dry mouth, acute weight loss, and fatigue.

The recommended fluid intake in cancer patients is 30–35 mL/kg/day. It should be considered that the consumption can be higher, especially in case of diarrhea, vomiting, or fistulas.[22]

It is also essential to ensure that serum electrolyte concentrations are within the normal range since, due to tumor activity, the effects of proinflammatory cytokines, infectious processes, poor digestion, and malabsorption, deficiencies that may compromise the patient's hydroelectrolyte and hemodynamic stability are recurrent.

TYPES OF CANCER WITH MAJOR NUTRITIONAL IMPLICATIONS

The presence of cachexia and accelerated and involuntary weight loss represents the most frequent secondary diagnosis in cancer patients. However, some types of cancer compromise to a greater extent the nutritional status of patients, which is due to the impossibility they have to cover their energy-protein requirements as a consequence of the location and type of the tumor, as well as the stage at which the disease is diagnosed, and the side effects of the oncological treatments used.

Head and Neck Cancer

Head and neck cancer (H&N) affects the nutritional status due to the location and histological lineage of the tumor. In these cases, the area of the cancer is associated with swallowing disorders, thus directly affecting food consumption.

The treatment of patients with advanced clinical stage H&N cancer consists of the concomitant administration of radiotherapy (60–65 Gy) and chemotherapy (platinum and 5-fluorouracil), together of before surgery instead of adjuvant and neoadjuvant. Radiotherapy is applied in daily sessions for 7 weeks (35 days), and chemotherapy in cycles every 21 days for 5 days until completing three cycles.[23]

Metabolic stress caused by surgery for H&N cancer is associated with hypermetabolism and protein loss. Side effects, such as diarrhea, vomiting, nausea, dysphagia, odynophagia, xerostomia, hypogeusia or ageusia, and mucositis, depend on the size of the resection and result in decreased food intake, which in turn can lead to malnutrition.

Likewise, all the previously mentioned symptoms and frequent weight loss in these patients affect their quality of life, resulting in additional anxiety and depression.

In a Dutch study,[24] the authors demonstrated that patients with H&N cancer who are malnourished have an increased risk of complications, as there is a close relationship between malnutrition and specific immunological indicators that is important for establishing a prognosis.

Lung Cancer

Lung cancer is usually asymptomatic, so this disease is diagnosed when it is in its advanced stages. Less than 15% of cases appear as localized cancers at the time of diagnosis, and only about 20% of patients present to the specialist with cancer, making them candidates for curative treatment.

Among the factors that are considered carcinogenic in this type of cancer, tobacco consumption is number one, followed by other sources of nicotine; then come environmental factors, such as radon, pollution, and asbestos, while those considered nonenvironmental include socioeconomic factors, gender, race, and ethnicity of origin, genetic factors, etc.[1]

The nutritional status of lung cancer patients is affected by a wide variety of factors, including:
- Adequacy of nutrient intake
- Weight loss
- Presence of symptoms related to antineoplastic treatment
- Cachexia

Like most cancers, patients with this specific disease have disease-specific symptoms such as mucositis, dysgeusia, dysphagia, nausea/vomiting, early satiety, malabsorption, and depression.

Lung cancer represents a high energy expenditure due to the tumor or the disease since it compromises a primary function of the organism, such as respiration. Since it is in the lung, the risk of patients presenting pleural effusion is much higher. With parenteral nutritional support, the supply of nutrients and all the liquids administered to the patient must be restricted.[25]

Recently, symptoms have been described that have implications for the nutritional status of patients with lung and GI tract cancer; these include loss of appetite, early satiety, and changes in food taste.

■ DIGESTIVE SYSTEM CANCER
Esophageal Cancer

Between 50 and 80% of patients with esophageal cancer are diagnosed with poor nutritional condition. This situation is due to dysphagia, a persistent symptom in patients with this disease. Poor dietary status potentially increases the risk of developing postoperative complications, resulting in increased recovery time after surgery and decreased quality of life for patients.[26]

The most frequent and characteristic symptoms of esophageal cancer patients are mucositis, odynophagia, and dysphagia.[11] More than 90% of patients with esophageal cancer develop dysphagia, making this a significant complication in this population. Therefore, the most frequent histopathological strain, which is very aggressive, makes them a considerable population for evaluation and nutritional treatment.

Gastric Cancer

Surgical treatment of this type of cancer involves partial or total stomach resection, which undoubtedly alters its function as a reservoir. This will lead the patient to present, in the case of partial or complete resection, early satiety and deficient absorption of vitamin B_{12}. After a gastrectomy, the characteristic of the stomach to "store" food is affected to the point of being able to cause involuntary regurgitations; likewise, the capacity or volume of the organ decreases.[27]

If the esophageal sphincter needs to be removed during surgery, it has been observed that patients present reflux in 80% of the cases. Likewise, suppose the procedure includes an alteration of the pyloric function. In that case, biliary reflux can reach causing significant damage since, unlike reflux caused by gastric acids, this is not controllable with medications. Since it cannot be neutralized using drugs, it can affect the squamous epithelium of the esophagus.

On the other hand, when the parietal cells found in the proximal part of the stomach are resected, a loss of intrinsic factor occurs, which results in malabsorption of vitamin B_{12}, which, in turn, can cause the patient to develop megaloblastic anemia.

Another critical problem to be treated is *dumping* syndrome, which causes intolerance to simple sugars due to high osmolar load; for this reason, the diet in these patients should be deficient in sugars and divided into fifths, sixths, or more times a day in small portions.[27]

Hepatic Cancer or Hepatocarcinoma

Liver cancer is relevant because it is the mortality and the fifth most frequent cancer worldwide. The treatment par excellence of this disease is the total resection of the tumor, as long as it is feasible to perform the surgery. This usually implies the elimination of a significant portion of the cirrhotic liver, functionally compromised.

The nutritional implications of this type of cancer are centered on managing the patient's nutritional status since it can be a determining factor for adequate postoperative recovery.[16] In the first instance, it is recognized that a good dietary status represents a lower risk for the patient to present complications of the surgical treatment. In addition, the implementation of nutritional support either by enteral or parenteral route, preoperatively and postoperatively, can contribute to the survival of the hepatocyte and promote a regenerative response of the remaining hepatic segments.

Pancreatic Cancer

At present, pancreatic cancer is one of the most aggressive cancers. Nutritionally speaking, it is cancer with the highest incidence of cachexia, as about 80% of patients diagnosed with pancreatic cancer present with some cachexia during the course of the disease.[28] So much so that up to one-third die from cachexia-related complications of developing immobility and severe impairment of respiratory muscles resulting in cardiopulmonary failure and impaired immunity.

Cachexia, in this population, is closely related to a decrease in essential human functions, which reduces the quality of life, the response rate to chemotherapy and radiotherapy, and, therefore, survival.

A key component in developing cachexia and one of the important nutritional implications in this patient population is hypercatabolism resulting from tumor metabolism, systemic inflammation, and other effects mediated by the tumor itself.

On the other hand, decreased food intake can promote and maintain weight loss associated with cancer. Mechanical digestive disturbances may produce a loss of appetite. Patients with pancreatic cancer suffer from pronounced pain, fatigue, nausea, dysphagia, gastroparesis, duodenal stenosis, pancreatic insufficiency, malabsorption, constipation, and difficulty in managing glycemia.[28]

It is important to emphasize that the symptoms mentioned above are a direct consequence of tumor invasion, which can lead to obstruction of the pancreatic duct or the GI tract, particularly the second portion of the duodenum, causing deficiency of lipids, amino acids, and inorganic nutrients such as calcium, magnesium, and iron.

Likewise, patients with pancreatic cancer experience symptoms characteristic of antineoplastic treatment. Treatment usually consists of surgery, if it is feasible to perform this procedure, and adjuvant chemotherapy; if it is not possible to complete the surgical procedure, and if the prognosis is good in the short term, treatment is carried out with the application of chemotherapies with which it is hoped to reduce the size of the tumor and thus avoid complications such as those mentioned in the previous section.

If the surgical procedure is performed, which in this case is a pancreatoduodenectomy (better known as *Whipple*), in which the objective is the resection of the pancreatic head mass, the patient may present worsening of the pancreatic insufficiency and a more significant decrease in oral intake.

Additionally, tumor-derived factors contribute to metabolic abnormalities in this type of cancer. Two of the most studied are *lipid mobilizing factor* (LMF) and *proteolysis inducing factor* (PIF), which implications are most important for nutritional status, the most important being the development and progression of cachexia.[5,28]

Therefore, it is of utmost importance to provide the pancreatic cancer patient with the best possible multidisciplinary support and to counteract the secondary causes of anorexia, which include pain, nausea, pancreatic insufficiency, and constipation. Treatment is based on oncologic therapy that best controls the tumor, nutritional support, and pharmacological treatment for pain and symptom control.[23]

Colon and Rectal or Colorectal Cancer

Colon and rectal cancer currently rank third in incidence and fourth in mortality worldwide.[1] It is essential to evaluate the nutritional implications of this type of cancer, given the high rate of malnutrition to which the treatment can lead the patient and other factors that determine this alteration, such as the location, type, and stage of the tumor.

Most patients who undergo surgical treatment already present a previous state of malnutrition, so it is also essential to emphasize adequate preoperative nutritional support since it has been shown that a good nutritional status contributes to better postoperative recovery and reduces the risk of developing infectious complications.[29]

This type of cancer treatment is inclined to surgical intervention whenever feasible. It is aimed at the resection of the tumor if it is localized and sometimes includes the resection of certain portions of the cancer site.[29] The colon is responsible for reabsorbing fluids and electrolytes, so sectioning the terminal portion of the ileum and colon can significantly affect the body's water-electrolyte balance. If the peristalsis function is affected or anatomical anomalies are present due to surgical treatment, abnormal growth of colonic bacteria can occur, which can cause metabolic acidosis and malabsorption of both energy substrates and inorganic nutrients.

The use of antineoplastic treatments, such as adjuvant chemotherapy or radiotherapy, implies the symptoms mentioned above typical of these therapies, namely: Nausea, vomiting, fatigue, and dysgeusia, among others, which, as has been observed throughout this section, compromise the patient's nutritional status and even quality of life.[11]

It should be emphasized that the evaluation of the nutritional status and nutritional support, if necessary, of all patients who undergo surgery are a determining factor in postoperative recovery and contribute to the maintenance of the cancer patient's immune system.

As part of the follow-up and evaluation of patients with lung, pancreatic, head and neck, and GI cancers, or those who are at high risk of malnutrition or who have had significant unintentional weight loss (>10% in the last 6 months), nutritional impact symptoms, markers of inflammation and other signs of weight loss that may indicate cachexia or precachexia should be monitored and evaluated and followed up as necessary to intervene nutritionally at the right time and in the right way.

Hematologic Cancer

Although hematologic cancer does not usually cause cachexia and the risk of malnutrition observed in most studies is lower than in solid tumors, nutritional monitoring of this patient population is of utmost importance.

It has been observed that the resting enery expenditure (REE) of once-hematologic patients does not vary considerably compared to healthy patients.[24-26] However, it is 9.8% (178.2 kcal) higher than in non-oncologic patients. It is accompanied by a reduction in fat-free mass (FFM) obtained by electrical bioimpedance after the first cycle of chemotherapy.[27]

The expected effects of chemotherapeutic treatment in patients with hematologic cancer are decreased food intake and a worsening nutritional status. After the first month of treatment, there is evidence of a 23% reduction in caloric intake. Likewise, the quality of the diet in terms of diversity and micronutrients is affected by the side effects of chemotherapy. There is insufficient evidence on the impact of the nutritional deterioration in hematologic patients. According to a report on patients over 15 years of age in Malaysia, malnutrition is a 19.4% prevalence after the first cycle of chemotherapy in leukemias.[28]

As a result of the treatment, the patient's acceptance of the diet is reduced, and GI disorders occur in up to 72% of patients, where the most common symptom is nausea (59%).[29]

Diet acceptance in hematological patients is significantly reduced during chemotherapy, and GI disorders occur in up to 72% of patients, where the most common symptom is nausea (59%).[29]

ADJUVANT MEDICAL-NUTRITIONAL THERAPY IN ANTINEOPLASTIC TREATMENT

It is essential to consider the different implications that the different types of antineoplastic treatments can have on the nutritional aspect to prevent the development of side effects that compromise the adequate dietary status of the patient.

A nutritional intervention accompanied by nutritional support therapy is a proactive way to improve the nutritional status of cancer patients undergoing oncologic treatment. The goal of providing nutritional support to cancer patients is to minimize or prevent the weight loss that accompanies the disease, as well as to decrease nitrogen loss and specific nutrient deficiencies.

Radiotherapy

This can affect healthy cells close to the radiation field, leading to several side effects for the patient. Whether these side effects arise will depend on the radiation dose and the duration and site at which it is applied.[24] Additionally, these effects may be aggravated by implementing adjuvant therapies such as chemotherapy. Medical literature reports that the most significant weight loss in patients receiving radiation therapy occurs between the 4th and 8th week of treatment.

If radiation therapy is delivered to any part of the digestive system, adverse effects that compromise nutritional status are likely to develop.

Chemotherapy

Chemotherapy treatments are cytotoxic drugs that stop the growth of cancer cells, either by apoptosis or by preventing cell differentiation and proliferation. This therapy aims to attack rapidly replicating cells, including those in the bone marrow and GI tract; therefore, chemotherapy has adverse effects that impair the nutritional status of the cancer patient.[30]

Chemotherapeutic agents are classified according to their mechanism of action and can be administered intravenously or orally. Due to their elimination or metabolism pathways, specific chemotherapeutic agents have more toxic effects on the kidneys and liver. As these therapies are systemic treatments, they affect the whole body.

Due to the potential for damage to the epithelium and mucosa of the GI tract, antineoplastic therapies may cause nausea, vomiting, diarrhea or constipation, mucositis, stomatitis and esophagitis, early satiety, altered gastric motility and taste sensation, immunosuppression, and infections.[11]

Continued nutritional intervention throughout cancer diagnosis and treatment can prevent or decrease complications and the severity of side effects.

Surgery

Depending on the surgery site, nutritional status and function may be affected. For example, oropharyngeal surgery can lead to chewing and swallowing difficulties. Gastrectomy can cause early satiety, malabsorption, vitamin D and B_{12} deficiencies, hypoglycemia, and *dumping* syndrome. Intestinal resections can lead to maldigestion and malabsorption of energy substrates and inorganic nutrients, as well as fluids and electrolytes.

Realistic and achievable goals for nutritional support include minimizing the effects of energy and substrate starvation, preventing specific nutrient deficiencies, and supporting the acute inflammatory response until the hypermetabolic answer resolves and healing occurs. Sufficient energy intake should be achieved to meet patients' energy needs.

Immunotherapy

Also called *biological therapy* or *biotherapy* takes advantage of the patient's immune system to fight cancer. It uses substances synthesized by the body or formulated in laboratories to boost the patient's immune system and restore the body's natural antibodies against cancer.

Immunotherapy can cause various symptoms, such as fever, nausea, vomiting, anorexia, and asthenia, which also affect dietary intake.[11] These uncontrolled symptoms can lead to weight loss and malnutrition, delay treatment or recovery and promote complications from an infection.

Diet Therapy in the Cancer Patient

Nutritional support is integral to managing cachexia and includes providing dietary advice, oral nutritional supplements, and enteral and parenteral feeding if required.

Ideally, cancer patients and those receiving antineoplastic treatment should preferably meet their nutritional needs orally, which is physiologically superior and should be maintained as long as possible.

Modified textures, energy added with supplements in the form of powders or liquids and soft solids, and spacing of meal time are essential management tips to help the patient to carry and complete their antineoplastic treatment while minimally compromising nutritional status.

Some achievable goals for nutritional support include:[7] Minimization of the effects of starvation in terms of energy and other substrates, since using n-3 fatty acids as part of the treatment, has shown significant benefits on the stimulation of hunger and an increase in muscle mass when protein is provided in sufficient quantities.

PREVENTION OF SPECIFIC NUTRIENT DEFICIENCIES

Nutritional Support to Control the Acute Inflammatory Response

It is essential to consider that there is usually a negative energy balance resulting from a decreased energy intake caused by anorexia or hypophagia and an increased energy expenditure in absolute value that is not adapted to the conditions of semination. The increase in energy expenditure is usually mild but varies depending on the type of cancer and the clinical stage or degree of progression (usually 100–300 kcal/day). However, if this is not compensated by increased energy and protein intake, it can cause a loss of body fat (0.5–1 kg) and preferably muscle mass (1–2.3 kg/month).[7,25]

Regarding diet, carbohydrates remain the primary energy source in hypermetabolic patients and should comprise approximately 50–60% of nonprotein energy.[25]

Protein requirements are markedly increased in oncologic patients. The high rate of catabolism is refractory to protein, but protein synthesis is sensitive to amino-acid infusions, making a nitrogen balance possible if parenteral nutritional support is warranted; otherwise, the protein source should come from the oral route of the highest possible quality.

The recommended non-protein energy to nitrogen ratio is generally 150:1. Still, patients under enormous amounts of stress, such as the oncologic patient, require a lower percentage, as low as 100:1.[11] Fluids and electrolytes should be provided to maintain adequate diuresis and average serum electrolyte concentration.

The priorities in the care of the cancer patient determine the timing of when nutritional support should be implemented.[15]

Enteral Nutritional Support

The consensus indicates that it should be preferred as a feeding route if the bowel is functional. The use of enteral feeding should be considered when the patient cannot meet their energy requirements orally and, in those cases, where the benefit of receiving metabolic support outweighs the risks.[26]

Therefore, the enteral route is preferred for providing nutritional support to the cancer patient. This route has several advantages over parenteral feeding: easy administration, good tolerance, promotes mucosal growth and development, stimulates the immune system, helps to maintain the barrier function of the GI tract, and involves much lower costs.

Nasoenteral tube feeding is the most appropriate access route to administer enteral feeding. It is also widely used because it can be placed into the stomach, duodenum, or jejunum. This route should be used only when enteral feeding is required for a short period (<4 weeks). Ostomies (gastrostomy and jejunostomy) are indicated when the patient requires enteral feeding for over 30 days or when there is any nasal obstruction.

The limitations of enteral feeding are the risk of broncho-aspiration and its contraindication in patients with ileus or intestinal obstruction. In an article published by Kirby et al., the authors discuss the advantages and changes in the nutritional management of critically ill patients, patients with GI disease, or selected cancers. According to the authors, mechanical obstruction is the only contraindication to enteral feeding.

Parenteral Nutritional Support

Parenteral feeding should be reserved for those patients who cannot tolerate nutritional intake by mouth or along the GI tract or who cannot meet the necessary daily requirements of energy, carbohydrates, lipids, or proteins. This is the case of patients with uncontrolled diarrhea, intense mucositis, or some advanced peritoneal neoplasms that do not allow peristalsis or nutrient absorption.

The findings of different published studies show that the timely implementation of nutritional support, i.e., before presenting marked signs or symptoms of cachexia, has a more significant positive effect than in those patients who were provided with this support in later stages.[15]

Home Nutritional Support

Home nutritional support, both enteral and parenteral, is becoming increasingly common. Implementing nutritional support outside a clinical setting requires special care to avoid contamination risks. The personnel who provide this support, or the patient, should be instructed in the techniques and measures necessary to carry out the nutritional support in the best possible way.

In the case of enteral feeding, and if the case requires it, the patient or caregiver should be taught how the formula should be prepared and under what sanitary conditions. It has been shown that carrying out these practices gives the patient a certain feeling of independence and makes them focus on the positive aspects.

In the case of parenteral feeding, this requires much more technical expertise. Home parenteral nutrition support is appropriate for patients with a safe home environment and a team with the necessary skills to provide this service. In this case, it requires adequate equipment at home, such as infusion pumps. That parenteral nutrition is delivered daily or every third day if the formula and conditions allow, as well as adequate care of the route it is administered, to avoid infections that prevent further parenteral support.

Recent evidence shows that this type of nutritional support increases the quality of life and preserves the nutritional status of cancer patients, even when provided as palliative treatment.

Palliative Care

Palliative care should be carried out with great care. It is not aimed at improving the patient's nutritional status or curing the disease but rather at minimizing conditions that cause the patient to suffer, such as pain, and providing as much comfort as possible. Such care is provided when there is little or no chance of a cure, and further treatment is no longer feasible.

The aggressiveness or content of palliative nutritional support depends on the prognosis of the disease and the wishes of the patient and family members. The patient should be provided with adequate hydration and the minimum requirements; likewise, the contribution of these two components should be communicated and accepted by the treating medical team, the patient, and their family members.

Nutrients with Pharmacological Actions in Cancer

The use of antioxidants added to medical nutrition therapy in cancer patients continues to be controversial. A recent study found that the addition of antioxidants in specific doses during cancer treatment maintains hemoglobin concentrations and results in a better quality of life in a group of women with cervical cancer undergoing cancer therapy with cisplatin and concomitant radiotherapy.

However, nutrition management guidelines for head and neck cancer patients recommend that antioxidants should not be taken during medical oncology treatment due to possible tumor protection. Therefore, further studies and clinical judgment by the healthcare professional are needed before making routine recommendations regarding antioxidants.

Eicosapentaenoic Acid

If suboptimal symptoms or inadequate food intakes have been treated, and the oncology patient continues to suffer from weight loss and a low BMI, as stated in the new Academy of Nutrition and Dietetics (AND) guidelines, dietary supplements with high doses of eicosapentaenoic acid (EPA) may be considered as an adjunct to a nutritional intervention (2 g/day is recommended).[22]

The research indicates as a strong and imperative recommendation the use of food supplements containing fish oil (current consumption of 0.26–0.60 g EPA per day) and medical-food supplements that also include it (current consumption of 1.1–2.2 g EPA per day), as it turns out to have a significant effect on the preservation or improvement of weight and muscle mass, as well as on the increase of appetite in patients with cachectic cancers.

Glutamine

As dictated by the 2014 AND cancer guidelines, there are currently limited studies in head and neck patients and transplanted patients with progenitor cells who received glutamine that has not established the effectiveness of L-alanyl-L-glutamine in the treatment or prevention of oral mucositis.

When parenteral feeding is required in patients undergoing hematopoietic cell transplantation, the experienced and knowledgeable health professional may recommend using parenteral glutamine in doses ranging from 0.2 to 0.5 g/kg daily.

The most recent studies indicate that parenteral glutamine should be initiated in the early stages of treatment. Parenteral glutamine is associated with improved nitrogen balance and decreased morbidity. However, a decrease in hospital stay was only seen when allogeneic and autologous transplantation data were combined.

What is it expected of a doctor to know about nutrition in oncology?

It is expected that an oncologist has elementary knowledge about nutrition as well as an interest in tracking nutritional risk and preventing malnutrition as an additional complication in oncology patients, as well as to refer it to a nutritionist in case the patient needs special attention or if the tumor that the patient has will produce cachexia.

They must consider that an early multimodal approach can improve cancer patients' treatment tolerance and quality of life. We must assume that the first nutritional approach should be counseling on food properties and, in a critical case, using nutrition supplements. If necessary, nutritional support should be used on time.[30]

CONCLUSION

The treatment of oncologic patients requires interdisciplinary work to improve their conditions during cancer treatment and their quality of life and minimize the side effects of the treatment. The evaluation of nutritional status should be performed from the time of diagnosis of the patient because the dietary implications of the disease may have occurred before diagnosis; detecting the risk of malnutrition should be part of the initial comprehensive management of the oncology patient.

Once a nutritional deficiency is established, it is essential to structure a treatment plan. In acute stages, it should consist of intensive individualized nutritional support according to the most current recommendations for this type of patient; given the symptomatology of the cancer patient, any feeding mode and route can be used, sometimes a mixed course should be used to supply the patient's energy requirements (e.g., enteral feeding in conjunction with supplementary parenteral feeding).

The follow-up of these patients should be constant and based on the symptoms that appear in order not to reduce the nutritional intake at any time. A patient whose disease becomes chronic requires follow-up feeding strategies. If this is achieved, the patient will have a greater chance of cure, survival, and improved quality of life, which are essential goals in oncology.

REFERENCES

1. Paval DR, Patton R, McDonald J, Skipworth RJE, Gallagher IJ, Laird BJ. A systematic review examining the relationship between cytokines and cachexia in incurable cancer. J Cachexia Sarcopenia Muscle. 2022;13(2):824-38.
2. Fearon K, Strasser F, Anker SD, Bosaeus I, Bruera E, Fainsinger RL, et al. Definition and classification of cancer cachexia: An international consensus. Lancet Oncol [Internet]. 2011;12:489-95.
3. Raff S, Rome I, Baracos VE, Fearon K, Strasser F, Anker SD, et al. Definition and classification of cancer cachexia: an international consensus. Lancet Oncol. 2011;12:489-95.
4. Baker Rogers J, Minteer JF. Cachexia. StatPearls. 2020.
5. Serpe R, Demurtas L, Puzzoni M, Madeddu C, Scartozzi M. Cancer cachexia assessment: new tools for oncologists. Recent Prog Med. 2016;107:515-24.
6. Peixoto da Silva S, Santos JMO, Costa e Silva MP, Gil da Costa RM, Medeiros R. Cancer cachexia and its pathophysiology: links with sarcopenia, anorexia and asthenia. J Cachexia Sarcopenia Muscle. 2020;11:619-35.
7. Argilés JM, Betancourt A, Guàrdia-Olmos J, Peró-Cebollero M, López-Soriano FJ, Madeddu C, et al. Validation of the CAchexia SCOre (CASCO). Staging cancer patients:

The use of miniCASCO as a simplified tool. Front Physiol. 2017;8:92.
8. Cruz-Jentoft AJ, Bahat G, Bauer J, Boirie Y, Bruyère O, Cederholm T, et al. Sarcopenia: revised European consensus on definition and diagnosis. Age Ageing. 2019;48:16-31.
9. Cederholm T, Barazzoni R, Austin P, Ballmer P, Biolo G, Bischoff SC, et al. ESPEN guidelines on definitions and terminology of clinical nutrition. Clin Nutr. 2017;36:49-64.
10. Cruz-Jentoft AJ, Sayer AA. Sarcopenia. Lancet. 2019;393(10191):2636-46.
11. Bachettini NP, Bielemann RM, Barbosa-Silva TG, Menezes AMB, Tomasi E, Gonzalez MC. Sarcopenia as a mortality predictor in community-dwelling older adults: a comparison of the diagnostic criteria of the European Working Group on Sarcopenia in Older People. Eur J Clin Nutr. 2020;74:573-80.
12. Ryan AM, Power DG, Daly L, Cushen SJ, Ní Bhuachalla È, Prado CM. Cancer-associated malnutrition, cachexia and sarcopenia: the skeleton in the hospital closet 40 years later. Proceed Nutr Soc. 2016;75:199-211.
13. Davis MP, Panikkar R. Sarcopenia associated with chemotherapy and targeted agents for cancer therapy. Ann Palliat Med. 2019;8:86-101.
14. Oflazoglu U, Alacacioglu A, Varol U, Kucukzeybek Y, Salman T, Taskaynatan H, et al. Prevalence and related factors of sarcopenia in newly diagnosed cancer patients. Support Care Cancer. 2020;28:837-43.
15. Laviano A, Koverech A, Seelaender M. Assessing pathophysiology of cancer anorexia. Curr Opin Clin Nutr Metabol Care. 2017;20:340-5.
16. Caccialanza R, Goldwasser F, Marschal O, Ottery F, Schiefke I, Tilleul P, et al. Unmet needs in clinical nutrition in oncology: a multinational analysis of real-world evidence. Ther Adv Med Oncol. 2020;12:1758835919899852.
17. Gómez-Candela C, Canales Albendea MA, Palma Milla S, de Paz Arias R, Díaz Gómez J, Rodríguez-Durán D, et al. Intervención nutricional en el paciente oncohematológico. Nutr Hosp. 2012;27:669-80.
18. Cederholm T, Jensen GL, Correia MITD, Gonzalez MC, Fukushima R, Higashiguchi T, et al. GLIM criteria for the diagnosis of malnutrition—A consensus report from the global clinical nutrition community. Clin Nutr. 2019;38:1-9.
19. Contreras-Bolívar V, Sánchez-Torralvo FJ, Ruiz-Vico M, González-Almendros I, Barrios M, Padín S, et al. GLIM Criteria Using Hand Grip Strength Adequately Predict Six-Month Mortality in Cancer Inpatients. Nutrients. 2019;11:2043.
20. Suverza A, Haua K. El ABCD de la evaluación del estado de nutrición. México: McGraw Hill; 2010. p. 349.
21. Neamat-Allah J, Wald D, Hüsing A, Teucher B, Wendt A, Delorme S, et al. Validation of anthropometric indices of adiposity against whole-body magnetic resonance imaging—a study within the German European Prospective Investigation into Cancer and Nutrition (EPIC) cohorts. PLoS One. 2014;9:e91586.
22. Arends J, Bachmann P, Baracos V, Barthelemy N, Bertz H, Bozzetti F, et al. ESPEN guidelines on nutrition in cancer patients. Clin Nutr [Internet]. 2017;36:11-48.
23. Poulia KA, Sarantis P, Antoniadou D, Koustas E, Papadimitropoulou A, Papavassiliou AG, et al. Pancreatic cancer and cachexia—Metabolic mechanisms and novel insights. Vol. 12, Nutrients. 2020;12(6):1543.
24. Ting CS, Wen WW, Bahari L, Sriram RK. Comparison of Measured Resting Energy Expenditure between Cancer Patients and Non-Cancer Controls. Asian J Diab. 2019;23-8.
25. Gómez-Candela C, Serrano Labajos R, García-Vazquez N, Valero Pérez M, Morato Martínez M, Santurino Fontecha C, et al. Proceso completo de implantación de un sistema de cribado de riesgo nutricional en el hospital universitario La Paz de Madrid. Nutr Hosp. 2013;28:2165-74.

26. Khor SM, Mohd Baidi B. Assessing the resting energy expenditure of cancer patients in the penang general hospital. Malays J Nutr. 2011;17:43-53.
27. Galati PC, Chiarello PG, Simões BP. Variation of resting energy expenditure after the first chemotherapy cycle in acute leukemia patients. Nutr Cancer. 2016;68:86-93.
28. Malihi Z, Kandiah M, Chan YM, Esfandbod M, Vakili M, Hosseinzadeh M, et al. The effect of dietary intake changes on nutritional status in acute leukaemia patients after first induction chemotherapy. Eur J Cancer Care (Engl). 2015;24:542-52.
29. Marx W, Kiss N, McCarthy AL, McKavanagh D, Isenring L. Chemotherapy-Induced Nausea and Vomiting: A Narrative Review to Inform Dietetics Practice. J Acad Nutr Diet. 2016;116:819-27.
30. Barreira JV. The Role of Nutrition in Cancer Patients. Nutr Cancer. 2021;73(11-12):2849-50.

CHAPTER 27

Nutrition in Severe Acute Pancreatitis

Deeksha Kapoor, Adarsh Chaudhary

INTRODUCTION

Acute pancreatitis (AP) is an inflammatory process of the pancreas characterized by autodigestion of the gland, activation of pancreatic enzymes, and an inflammatory cascade.[1] It is reported as one of the most common gastrointestinal (GI) diseases requiring admission to the hospital.[2] The incidence of acute pancreatitis worldwide is estimated to be 33.74 cases per 100,000 person-years.[3] Though the exact data on the prevalence of acute pancreatitis in India is lacking, the incidence is suspected to have increased in the last few years.[4] The diagnosis of AP is established when any two of the three parameters are present: typical upper abdominal pain with possible radiation to the back, elevated serum lipase or amylase levels to more than three times the upper limit of normal and characteristic findings of AP on abdominal imaging.[5] The clinical course of AP is highly variable, ranging from mild self-limiting disease to fulminant disease with multiorgan failure and high infection rates.[5] The modified Atlanta and the Determinant based classification systems are used to classify the disease and define the severity grades.[6,7] Patients with severe acute pancreatitis (SAP) have a higher incidence of infected pancreatic necrosis and a higher mortality rate.[2]

The medical management of AP typically discusses the importance of fluid therapy, adequate analgesia, the role of antibiotics, etc. The initial management in AP targets decreasing the systemic inflammatory response, pain control, and nutritional management. The traditional management of AP propagated the concept of "pancreas rest" with the premise that feeding the patient would stimulate the pancreas and increase the extent of inflammation. Eventually, evidence emerged that starvation had deleterious effects on intestinal barrier function[8] and the paradigm shifted from gut resting to gut arousing in AP.

This chapter discusses the importance and the main concepts of nutritional management in AP. The topic will be addressed in the following subheadings:

- How does the gut barrier get affected in AP?
- Why nutritional management is important?
- Nutritional assessment is important in which patients with AP?
- Which is better—parenteral nutrition or enteral nutrition?
- How to feed the patient—oral versus nasogastric versus nasojejunal versus. surgical jejunostomy?
- What to feed the patient—role of immuno-nutrition, the role of probiotics?
- Nutrition and feeding in special situations—intra-abdominal hypertension, abdominal compartment syndrome, and open abdomen.
- Nutrition in hemodynamically unstable patients.

HOW DOES THE GUT BARRIER GET AFFECTED IN ACUTE PANCREATITIS?

- At the initiation of AP, reflex splanchnic vasoconstriction occurs to preserve the blood flow to vital organs, resulting in tissue hypoxia and ischemic injury followed by reperfusion injury once the patient is resuscitated with fluids. This contributes to and worsens the ongoing inflammatory response.[9,10]
- Under normal circumstances, the intestinal epithelial barrier produces immunoglobulin A which is the first line of defense. In AP, the surge of inflammatory mediators causes increased capillary leakage, and the tight junctions are unable to maintain the gut barrier. This compromise in the gut barrier causes bacterial translocation and the release of toxins into the portal venous system and mesenteric lymph.[11] The gut mucosa is responsible for producing over two thirds of the antibody load in the body. Injury to the mucosa leads to not just decreased immunity but increased systemic events and increased susceptibility to microbiological infections.[12]
- This loss of epithelial barrier and bacterial translocation are postulated to contribute to secondary infection, infected pancreatic necrosis, and multiorgan failure as studies reveal that microorganisms responsible for infected necrosis are often enteric in origin.[13]
- The mucosal epithelium of the gut maintains two important roles in the healthy state—effective barrier against luminal bacteria and absorption of nutrients. Both these functions are disrupted in the setting of AP.[14]
- With the progression of pain and severity in AP, the patient stops eating, causing a decrease in the number of immunoglobulin A (IgA)-producing cells, further increasing the possibility of organ failure.
- The cytokine storm tumor necrosis factor-alpha [(TNF-α), interleukin (IL)-1, IL-6], the increase in the levels of stress hormones, cortisol, catecholamines and glucagon and the inability to eat worsen the nutritional status of the patient, creating a negative nitrogen balance of up to 20–40 mg/day. This state of nutritional compromise and increased resting energy expenditure further worsens the inflammation creating a vicious cycle. Therefore, poor tolerance to enteral nutrition presents a difficult challenge for the treating physicians and warrants a discussion on determining the timing, type, composition, and route of feeding.

WHY IS NUTRITIONAL MANAGEMENT IMPORTANT IN AP?

- The metabolic changes and their impact on nutrition in AP have been discussed in the previous section. Proper nutritional management helps in circumventing the catabolic state of AP and mitigating the systemic inflammatory response.
- Nutritional management has two important benefits—physiological benefits and outcome benefits. The physiological benefits of nutritional management in AP include preservation of the gut barrier integrity, prevention of bacterial overgrowth and translocation, maintenance of intestinal motility and IgA production, and an increase in splanchnic blood flow.[15] Important disease-related outcomes have been found to improve with enteral feeding in patients with AP. Enteral feeding has been shown to decrease mortality in AP and is probably one of the few interventions that have been shown

to have a mortality benefit in the management of AP.[16] The benefits extend to decreased rates of multiorgan failure and decreased length of hospital stay.[17]
- The historic concept of "nil by mouth" in AP has undergone a paradigm shift into gut-arousing and oral/enteral feeding and early enteral nutrition is now considered an imperative part of managing AP.
- Enteral nutrition is probably the only intervention in AP which has been consistently found to be effective in preventing negative clinical outcomes in terms of mortality, multiorgan failure and infectious complications.[18]

NUTRITIONAL ASSESSMENT IS IMPORTANT IN WHICH PATIENT?

- Acute pancreatitis is a severely catabolic state, and it is imperative to identify the nutritional risk. While patients who have mild-to-moderate disease are likely to experience recovery within 1–2 weeks, patients with severe AP run a more turbulent course.
- All patients with predicted severe AP are considered to be at nutritional risk.[19]
- Patients with mild-to-moderate AP should be screened using the Nutritional Risk Screening (NRS) 2002. Preexisting malnutrition is estimated to exist in about 30% of patients, while the elderly and chronic alcoholics are considered to be at nutritional risk.[20]

WHICH IS BETTER—PARENTERAL OR ENTERAL NUTRITION?

- The use of total parenteral nutrition (TPN) used to be the standard practice for the nutritional management of severe AP with the premise that it would avoid stimulation of the pancreas and provide nutrition in the meantime. However, TPN has many associated disadvantages such as septic complications, metabolic and electrolyte abnormalities, and associated costs. On the other hand, the use of enteral nutrition has the benefit of maintaining gut integrity and mucosal function. This strongly favors the early initiation of enteral nutrition over nil by mouth and TPN. Other advantages associated with early enteral feeding include its simplicity and low cost. However, chances of tube migration and ileus are potential issues that can reduce its use in clinical practice. A large body of evidence suggests that enteral feeding can be started as soon as it can be tolerated by the patient.
- A meta-analysis published by Al-Omran et al. in 2010 looked at data from 348 patients across eight randomized trials and reported decreased rates of mortality (RR = 0.50, 95% CI 0.28–0.91), multi-organ failure (RR = 0.55, 95% CI 0.37–0.91), infections and need for surgical intervention. The incidence of local complications and length of hospital stay was also found to be lower. When only patients with predicted severe AP were studied, the subgroup analysis revealed a decrease in mortality by 80% and a decrease in the rate of multiorgan failure by 55% in patients who received enteral nutrition.[21] Subsequently, multiple pooled analyses were published substantiating the benefit of enteral nutrition over parenteral nutrition.
- In 2017, Yao et al. investigated if enteral nutrition was beneficial in critically ill patients with severe AP. Data from five randomized controlled trials (RCTs), of 348 patients were analyzed which revelated a decrease in overall mortality (RR = 0.36, 95% CI 0.20–0.65) and a

decrease in the rate of multiorgan failure (RR = 0.39, 95% CI 0.21–0.73), substantiating clinical benefits even in critically ill patients.[22] Another study by Li et al. reported similar results.[23] Enteral nutrition was associated with lower rates of surgical interventions (27.4% vs. 69.4%, OR: 0.17, 95% CI: 0.05–0.62), and shorter length of hospital stay.[23]

- Though parenteral nutrition is not preferred over enteral nutrition, it finds its use when patients are not able to tolerate enteral nutrition, or as additional support when nutritional requirements are not being met. In certain complicated situations like bowel obstruction, ischemia or abdominal compartment syndrome, when enteral nutrition is contraindicated, parental nutrition is used.[24,25]

HOW TO FEED THE PATIENT—ORAL VERSUS NASOGASTRIC VERSUS NASOJEJUNAL VERSUS SURGICAL JEJUNOSTOMY?

- It is recommended that patients with mild AP be started with an oral diet as soon as clinically tolerable, and a low-fat soft diet can be initiated without the need for gradual escalation.[26,27] However, patients with severe AP may not be able to tolerate an oral diet early in the course of their disease, in which case enteral nutrition via nasogastric or nasojejunal access may be initiated.
- If early enteral nutrition or delayed oral feeding was better in patients with predicted severe AP, was studied in the Phython Trial, which was a superiority multicenter trial of 205 patients. Patients were divided into two groups—those who started on early (<24 hours) enteral nutrition and those who were encouraged to take the diet orally after 72 hours or on demand. No difference in the rate of mortality or infectious complications was found between the two groups, but on-demand initiation of feeding prevented the insertion of a tube in about 70% of patients.[28] A subsequent prospective study suggested that the best time to initiate enteral nutrition was the third day after hospital admission, the risk reduction to secondary infection was maintained while improving tolerance.[29]
- Once it is established that enteral nutrition is required, the route—nasogastric vs. nasojejunal access needs to be decided. Traditionally, nasojejunal route has been advocated as it has the theoretical advantage of bypassing the pancreas and avoiding stimulation of an inflamed gland. It has been found in some animal models of AP, that cholecystokinin-induced pancreatic secretion is reduced in patients with AP.[30,31] In that case, the benefit of delivering feed beyond the pylorus is minimal. Nasogastric vs. nasojejunal routes of feeding have been compared in three RCTs, and no difference was found in complication rates, mortality or feeding tolerance, abdominal pain, or diarrhea.[32-36] Nasogastric tubes are easier to place, do not require an endoscopic or fluoroscopic approach for placement, and are cheaper and more convenient to use. Nevertheless, nasojejunal tubes find use in patients with delayed gastric emptying or gastric outlet obstruction because of pancreatic head edema, pseudocyst or phlegmon formation.[36]
- Patients undergoing surgical necrosectomy, who have gastric outlet obstruction or delayed gastric emptying and are expected to require nutritional support for prolonged durations benefit from

a surgically placed tube jejunostomy. A surgically placed jejunostomy tube tends to be more durable, with less likelihood of dislodgement and abates repeated endoscopic or fluoroscopic repositioning of the tube.

WHAT TO FEED THE PATIENT? WHAT IS THE ROLE OF A SEMIELEMENTAL DIET, IMMUNO-NUTRITION, AND PROBIOTICS?

- The importance and benefits of enteral nutrition are well established. The next pertinent question is about the best possible formulation of feeds—semi-elemental versus polymeric, and the benefit of probiotics or of immuno-nutrition. It was theorized that the use of predigested or elemental compounds would act as "pancreas rest" as such a formulation would not require pancreatic enzymes for digestion and absorption. Feeding tolerance and clinical outcomes such as mortality and infectious complications are important to understand.
- *Polymeric versus semielemental diet:* Elemental or semielemental diet comprises medium and long-chain triglycerides, amino or oligopeptides, and maltodextrins over complex compounds. While polymeric diets consist of nonhydrolyzed proteins, long-chain triglycerides, maltodextrins and oligo-fructosaccharides. It was postulated that a semielemental diet would be better tolerated and more beneficial than a polymeric diet in patients with AP.[37] Most initial studies evaluating the benefit of enteral nutrition had used a semielemental diet while recent studies have used a polymeric diet.
- A small RCT of 30 patients revealed that both formulations were safe and tolerated, but the use of a semielemental diet was associated with some clinical benefits of reduced hospital stay and maintenance of weight.[38] However, a meta-analysis by Petrov et al., published in 2009 analyzed data from 1,070 patients from 20 trials and concluded that the use of a polymeric diet was not associated with an increased incidence of feeding intolerance, death or infectious complications in patients with AP. No significant difference was found even when only patients with severe AP were analyzed. The study also reported that there were no significant clinical benefits of using probiotics or immunonutrition.[39]
- Semielemental formulations may still find their use in patients of severe AP who have malabsorption or are in the initial phase of the disease. The use of elemental formulations may be associated with an increased incidence of diarrhea because of the high osmolar load.[40] A meta-analysis of data from 13 RCTs compared fiber-rich versus fiber-free formulations and reported a reduction in the incidence of diarrhea in the former.[41]
- *Immunonutrition:* Immune-enhancing compounds include glutamine, arginine, and omega-3 fatty acids. The most important and most studied compound among these is glutamine which is a nonessential amino acid in plasma and is known to have a positive effect on immune function in a variety of disorders.[42] Inadequate production of endogenous glutamine may result in glutamine depletion which may be associated with poor outcomes in patients with a critical illness.[43-45] Treatment with glutamine in patients with AP is expected to improve serum albumin levels, decrease the levels of C-reactive protein

and decrease infectious complications. The meta-analysis published by Petrov et al. in 2009 analyzed the data of 50 patients of severe AP comparing immuno-enhanced formulations versus no immunoenhancement.[39] The addition of immune compounds was not associated with improved rates of mortality, infectious complications, or feeding tolerance. Another meta-analysis published in 2015, reported benefits in mortality and length of hospital stay with the use of glutamine, but when a post hoc analysis was performed only of patients with severe AP, there was no significant reduction in mortality.[46] Though multiple meta-analyses have demonstrated the benefit of glutamine in terms of clinical outcomes, the studies are hugely criticized for being heterogeneous and having small sample sizes.[47,48] Moreover, the analysis may be affected by multiple confounding factors like drainage, debridement, and surgery. However, subgroup analysis has suggested a benefit in clinical outcomes in patients receiving total parenteral nutrition.[48] In fact, the current European Society for Clinical Nutrition and Metabolism (ESPEN) guidelines on nutrition in AP suggest that there is no routine role of immunonutrition in patients with severe AP, but glutamine at the rate of 0.20 g/kg/day may be supplemented in patients in whom enteral nutrition is either not possible or is contraindicated.[24]

- *Probiotics:* The effect of probiotic prophylaxis in patients with predicted severe AP was tested in the PROPATRIA trial which was a multicenter randomized, double-blinded, placebo-controlled trial and reported an increased incidence of intestinal ischemia and death.[49] A meta-analysis of six RCTs also did not reveal any statistically significant difference in the rate of mortality or length of hospital stay.[50] Probiotics, therefore, cannot be recommended in patients with AP.[24]

NUTRITION IN SPECIAL CONDITIONS—RAISED INTRA-ABDOMINAL PRESSURE OR ABDOMINAL COMPARTMENT SYNDROME

- It is a matter of debate whether patients developing complications of severe AP, such as intra-abdominal hypertension, abdominal compartment syndrome, or patients with an open abdomen should be fed enterally or not. Patients with severe AP who develop intra-abdominal hypertension or abdominal compartment syndrome are at a higher risk of mortality, from 30% to over 65%. It is logical to assume that enteral feeds in such patients tend to increase intra-abdominal pressures.[51,52] However, evidence from a small, randomized trial of 60 patients with predicted severe AP, revealed that feeding enterally did not increase intra-abdominal pressure, in fact, may help prevent intra-abdominal hypertension in patients with intra-abdominal pressure (IAP) <15 mm Hg and reduce disease severity.[53] But in patients with IAP >15 mm Hg, enteral nutrition was associated with a higher frequency of diarrhea.
- The latest guidelines on nutrition in AP from the European Society for Clinical Nutrition and Metabolism recommend that patients with IAP <15 mm Hg, shall be initiated on enteral nutrition while continuously monitoring the clinical condition and IAP for the patient.[24]
- In patients with IAP >15 mm Hg, enteral nutrition via nasojejunal access be tried.

- A slow feed, at 20 mL/h may be introduced and increased as per tolerance. If the patients do not tolerate feed or IAP rises, enteral nutrition is discontinued and parenteral nutrition is initiated.[24]
- Patients with abdominal compartment syndrome or IAP >20 mm Hg are better managed with parenteral nutrition.
- An open abdomen is a highly catabolic state with a nitrogen loss of almost 2 g/L of abdominal fluid output. Small amounts of enteral feeds are initiated in patients who have undergone a laparostomy, with supplemental or total parenteral nutrition. Feeds can be increased as per tolerance and are associated with higher fascial closure rates, decreased mortality, and infectious complications.[24]
- *Severe AP needing interventions:* In cases of severe AP, when interventions in the form of endoscopic or percutaneous drainage or endoscopic or surgical necrosectomy are needed, enteral or oral nutrition has been found to be safe. Feeds can be restarted within the first 24 hours of the procedure if the patient remains otherwise stable.[24]

HEMODYNAMICALLY UNSTABLE PATIENTS

- Any disturbance of intestinal epithelial hemostasis leads to an inflammatory response, and dysfunction of the gut mucosal barrier and is a driver of sepsis and multiorgan failure. Rapid changes occur in intestinal permeability and changes in the gut microbiome which is called dysbiosis.[54-56] Recent studies demonstrate that even if 20% of nutrition is established via the enteral route, it can help prevent dysbiosis, preserve innate immunity, and abate the loss of the gut mucosal barrier.[56]
- There exist valid concerns about enteral feeding in patients critically ill and on vasopressors, with response to the development of mesenteric ischemia and nonocclusive bowel necrosis. Patients who have increasing vasopressor requirements have increased serum lactates, increased intestinal fatty acid binding concentration, and 28-day mortality.[57] However, data from many studies on patients in cardiogenic shock receiving enteral nutrition demonstrate that enteral nutrition increased cardiac index, and splanchnic blood flow and preserves the absorptive capacity of the gut during vasopressor delivery.[58]
- Vasopressors may have a differential impact on the gut flow. Patients on epinephrine may have lower splanchnic blood flow, lower splanchnic oxygen, higher levels of lactates and lower gastric pH.[59] There is evidence to suggest that vasopressin may also be associated with gastric and enteric hypoperfusion in patients with septic shock.[60] Phenylephrine, on the other hand, increases splanchnic blood flow, with no significant difference in small bowel perfusion with norepinephrine. Concerns about feeding patients on vasopressors is real. In such patients, bowel ischemia and nonocclusive bowel necrosis occur at a rate of 0.3–8.5% and are associated with a mortality of 46–100%.[60] Patients may also have impaired GI mucosal perfusion without overt signs of shock. Literature also suggests that nonocclusive bowel necrosis is seen more frequently in patients receiving postpyloric small bowel feeding than those on gastric-delivered nutrition.[60] This goes to suggest that postpyloric feeds may be avoided in patients in shock until more evidence is available.

- Substantial recent evidence has expressed the safety and benefit of enteral nutrition on clinical outcomes in critically ill patients on vasopressors. A retrospective study of about 1,200 patients, needing vasopressors and mechanical ventilation within 2 days of admission, showed that when enteral nutrition was started early (<48 hours), was associated with a significant decrease in mortality. Even trophic feeds (<600 kcal/day, or 20 mL/h) were found to be associated with a decreased time on the mechanical ventilator and shorter stay.[61] Data also suggests that patients on norepinephrine <12.5 µg/min, phenylephrine use and exclusion or stoppage of dopamine and vasopressin, and tolerated enteral nutrition better.[62]
- The relevance of delivering enteral nutrition to patients who are critically ill and on vasopressors depends on the agent in use, the dose of vasopressors, certain markers, and feeding strategies.[64] Enteral nutrition is more compatible with norepinephrine, phenylephrine > epinephrine > and vasopressin. If the dose of norepinephrine (or equivalent doses) is <0.1 µg/kg/day, enteral nutrition can be safely instituted, maintain caution if the dose is increasing. Enteral nutrition is better avoided if the dose is >0.5 µg/kg/min.[63] During nutrition, it is prudent to monitor lactate levels, fluid requirements, any ongoing bleeding, etc. It is better to start with trophic gastric feeds and advance slowly as per tolerance. The feed should be tapered or stopped if the gastric residue increases, the patient develops abdominal distension, any new-onset abdominal pain, unexplained elevation in lactate levels and/or intra-abdominal hypertension of abdominal compartment syndrome.[64]

CONCLUSION

- The gut barrier function is significantly affected in SAP and is said to contribute to secondary infection, infected pancreatic necrosis and multiorgan failure.
- All patients with SAP should be considered at nutritional risk and patients with mild to moderate AP should be screened using the Nutritional Risk Screening 2002.
- Nutritional management in SAP is extremely important, as it preserves gut barrier function, prevents bacterial overgrowth and maintains intestinal motility and IgA production. It is also associated with decreased rates of multiorgan failure and mortality.
- The use of enteral nutrition, over parenteral nutrition has been proven beneficial and an oral diet can be attempted in patients with SAP, usually by the third day.
- The use of nasojejunal tubes has no specific advantage except in patients with gastric outlet obstruction because of pancreatic head edema, pseudocyst or phlegmon formation.
- The benefit of immunonutrition in patients with SAP is ambiguous. There is no role for the routine use of glutamine but is recommended in patients of SAP in whom enteral nutrition is either not possible or is contraindicated.
- In patients with raised intra-abdominal hypertension, enteral nutrition can be initiated if the inter-abdominal pressure is <15 mm Hg, while continuously monitoring the patient's clinical status and IAP.

REFERENCES

1. Sakorafas GH, Tsiotou AG. Etiology and pathogenesis of acute pancreatitis: current concepts. J Clin Gastroenterol. 2000;30(4): 343-56.

2. Boxhoorn L, Voermans RP, Bouwense SA, Bruno MJ, Verdonk RC, Boermeester MA, et al. Acute pancreatitis. Lancet. 2020; 396(10252):726-34.
3. Xiao AY, Tan MLY, Wu LM, Asrani VM, Windsor JA, Yadav D, et al. Global incidence and mortality of pancreatic diseases: a systematic review, meta-analysis, and meta-regression of population-based cohort studies. Lancet Gastroenterol Hepatol. 2016;1(1):45-55.
4. Krishna SG, Kamboj AK, Hart PA, Hinton A, Conwell DL. The Changing Epidemiology of Acute Pancreatitis Hospitalizations: A Decade of Trends and the Impact of Chronic Pancreatitis. Pancreas. 2017;46(4):482-8.
5. Lankisch PG, Apte M, Banks PA. Acute pancreatitis. Lancet. 2015;386(9988):85-96.
6. Banks PA, Bollen TL, Dervenis C, Gooszen HG, Johnson CD, Sarr MG, et al. Classification of acute pancreatitis—2012: revision of the Atlanta classification and definitions by international consensus. Gut. 2013;62(1):102-11.
7. Dellinger EP, Forsmark CE, Layer P, Lévy P, Maraví-Poma E, Petrov MS, et al. Determinant-based classification of acute pancreatitis severity: an international multidisciplinary consultation. Ann Surg. 2012;256(6):875-80.
8. Ralls MW, Demehri FR, Feng Y, Woods Ignatoski KM, Teitelbaum DH. Enteral nutrient deprivation in patients leads to a loss of intestinal epithelial barrier function. Surgery. 2015;157(4):732-42.
9. Oldenburg WA, Lau LL, Rodenberg TJ, Edmonds HJ, Burger CD. Acute mesenteric ischemia: a clinical review. Arch Intern Med. 2004;164(10):1054.
10. Li XY, He C, Zhu Y, Lu NH. Role of gut microbiota on intestinal barrier function in acute pancreatitis. World J Gastroenterol. 2020;26(18):2187-93.
11. Fanous MYZ, Phillips AJ, Windsor JA. Mesenteric lymph: The bridge to future management of critical illness. JOP. 2007;8(4):374-99.
12. Lenz A, Franklin GA, Cheadle WG. Systemic inflammation after trauma. Injury. 2007;38(12):1336-45.
13. Liu H, Li W, Wang X, Li J, Yu W. Early gut mucosal dysfunction in patients with acute pancreatitis. Pancreas. 2008;36(2):192-6.
14. Barash M, Patel JJ. Gut luminal and clinical benefits of early enteral nutrition in shock. Curr Surg Rep. 2019;7(10):21.
15. van Dijk SM, Hallensleben NDL, van Santvoort HC, Fockens P, van Goor H, Bruno MJ, et al. Acute pancreatitis: Recent advances through randomised trials. Gut. 2017;66(11):2024-32.
16. Lee PJ, Papachristou GI. New insights into acute pancreatitis. Nat Rev Gastroenterol Hepatol. 2019;16(8):479-96.
17. Hegazi RA, DeWitt T. Enteral nutrition and immune modulation of acute pancreatitis. World J Gastroenterol. 2014;20(43):16101-5.
18. Petrov MS. Enteral nutrition and the risk of mortality and infectious complications in patients with severe acute pancreatitis: a meta-analysis of randomized trials. Arch Surg. 2008;143(11):1111.
19. Roberts KM, Nahikian-Nelms M, Ukleja A, Lara LF. Nutritional aspects of acute pancreatitis. Gastroenterol Clin North Am. 2018;47(1):77-94.
20. Kondrup J. Nutritional risk screening (NRS 2002): a new method based on an analysis of controlled clinical trials. Clinical Nutrition. 2003;22(3):321-36.
21. Al-Omran M, AlBalawi ZH, Tashkandi MF, Al-Ansary LA. Enteral versus parenteral nutrition for acute pancreatitis. Cochrane Upper GI and Pancreatic Diseases Group, ed. Cochrane Database Syst Rev.
22. Yao H, He C, Deng L, Liao G. Enteral versus parenteral nutrition in critically ill patients with severe pancreatitis: a meta-analysis. Eur J Clin Nutr. 2018;72(1):66-8.
23. Li W, Liu J, Zhao S, Li J. Safety and efficacy of total parenteral nutrition versus total enteral nutrition for patients with severe acute pancreatitis: a meta-analysis. J Int Med Res. 2018;46(9):3948-58.

24. Arvanitakis M, Ockenga J, Bezmarevic M, Gianotti L, Krznaric Z, Lobo DN, et al. ESPEN guideline on clinical nutrition in acute and chronic pancreatitis. Clin Nutr. 2020;39(3):612-31.
25. Smit M, Buddingh KT, Bosma B, Nieuwenhuijs VB, Hofker HS, Zijlstra JG. Abdominal compartment syndrome and intra-abdominal ischemia in patients with severe acute pancreatitis. World J Surg. 2016;40(6):1454-61.
26. Li J, Xue GJ, Liu YL, Javed MA, Zhao X-L, Wan M-H, et al. Early oral refeeding wisdom in patients with mild acute pancreatitis. Pancreas. 2013;42(1):88-91.
27. Lariño-Noia J, Lindkvist B, Iglesias-García J, Seijo-Ríos S, Iglesias-Canle J, Domínguez-Muñoz JE. Early and/or immediately full caloric diet versus standard refeeding in mild acute pancreatitis: a randomized open-label trial. Pancreatology. 2014;14(3):167-73.
28. Bakker OJ, van Brunschot S, van Santvoort HC, Besselink MG, Bollen TL, Boermeester MA, et al. Early versus on-demand nasoenteric tube feeding in acute pancreatitis. N Engl J Med. 2014;371(21):1983-93.
29. Jin M, Zhang H, Lu B, Li Y, Wu D, Qian J, et al. The optimal timing of enteral nutrition and its effect on the prognosis of acute pancreatitis: a propensity score matched cohort study. Pancreatology. 2017;17(5):651-7.
30. Niederau C, Niederau M, Lüthen R, Strohmeyer G, Ferrell LD, Grendell JH. Pancreatic exocrine secretion in acute experimental pancreatitis. Gastroenterology. 1990;99(4):1120-7.
31. Czakó L, Yamamoto M, Otsuki M. Exocrine pancreatic function in rats after acute pancreatitis. Pancreas. 1997;15(1):83-90.
32. Nally DM, Kelly EG, Clarke M, Ridgway P. Nasogastric nutrition is efficacious in severe acute pancreatitis: a systematic review and meta-analysis. Br J Nutr. 2014;112(11):1769-78.
33. Singh N, Sharma B, Sharma M, Sachdev V, Bhardwaj P, Mani K, et al. Evaluation of early enteral feeding through nasogastric and nasojejunal tube in severe acute pancreatitis: a noninferiority randomized controlled trial. Pancreas. 2012;41(1):153-9.
34. Eatock FC, Chong P, Menezes N, Murray L, McKay CJ, Carter CR, et al. A randomized study of early nasogastric versus nasojejunal feeding in severe acute pancreatitis. Am J Gastroenterol. 2005;100(2):432-9.
35. Kumar A, Singh N, Prakash S, Saraya A, Joshi YK. Early enteral nutrition in severe acute pancreatitis: a prospective randomized controlled trial comparing nasojejunal and nasogastric routes. J Clin Gastroenterol. 2006;40(5):431-4.
36. Petrov MS, Correia MITD, Windsor JA. Nasogastric tube feeding in predicted severe acute pancreatitis: a systematic review of the literature to determine safety and tolerance. JOP. 2008;9(4):440-8.
37. Silk DBA. Formulation of enteral diets. Nutrition. 1999;15(7-8):626-32.
38. Tiengou LE, Gloro R, Pouzoulet J, Bouhier K, Read M-H, Arnaud-Battandier F, et al. Semi-elemental formula or polymeric formula: is there a better choice for enteral nutrition in acute pancreatitis? Randomized Comparative Study. J Parenter Enteral Nutr. 2006;30(1):1-5.
39. Petrov MS, Loveday BPT, Pylypchuk RD, McIlroy K, Phillips ARJ, Windsor JA. Systematic review and meta-analysis of enteral nutrition formulations in acute pancreatitis. Br J Surg. 2009;96(11):1243-52.
40. Whelan K. Enteral-tube-feeding diarrhoea: manipulating the colonic microbiota with probiotics and prebiotics: BAPEN Symposium 2 on 'Pre- and probiotics.' Proc Nutr Soc. 2007;66(3):299-306.
41. Elia M, Engfer MB, Green CJ, Silk DBA. Systematic review and meta-analysis: the clinical and physiological effects of fibre-containing enteral formulae: Systematic review and meta-analysis: Effects of fibre-containing enteral formulae. Aliment Pharmacol Ther. 2007;27(2):120-45.

42. Şahin H, Mercanlıgil SM, Inanç N, Ok E. Effects of glutamine-enriched total parenteral nutrition on acute pancreatitis. Eur J Clin Nutr. 2007;61(12):1429-34.
43. Foitzik T, Stufler M, Hotz HG, Klinnert J, Wagner J, Warshaw AL, et al. Glutamine stabilizes intestinal permeability and reduces pancreatic infection in acute experimental pancreatitis. J Gastrointest Surg. 1997;1(1):40-7.
44. Foitzik T, Kruschewski M, Kroesen AJ, Hotz HG, Eibl G, Buhr HJ. Does glutamine reduce bacterial translocation? Int J Colorectal Dis. 1999;14(3):143-9.
45. de Beaux AC, O'Riordain MG, Ross JA, Jodozi L, Carter DC, Fearon KCH. Glutamine-supplemented total parenteral nutrition reduces blood mononuclear cell interleukin-8 release in severe acute pancreatitis. Nutrition. 1998;14(3):261-5.
46. Jeurnink SM, Nijs MM, Prins HAB, Greving JP, Siersema PD. Antioxidants as a treatment for acute pancreatitis: A meta-analysis. Pancreatology. 2015;15(3):203-8.
47. Asrani V, Chang WK, Dong Z, Hardy G, Windsor JA, Petrov MS. Glutamine supplementation in acute pancreatitis: a meta-analysis of randomized controlled trials. Pancreatology. 2013;13(5):468-74.
48. Yong L, Lu QP, Liu SH, Fan H. Efficacy of glutamine-enriched nutrition support for patients with severe acute pancreatitis: a meta-analysis. J Parenter Enteral Nutr. 2016;40(1):83-94.
49. Besselink MG, Van Santvoort HC, Buskens E, Boermeester MA, van Goor H, Timmerman HM, et al. Probiotic prophylaxis in predicted severe acute pancreatitis: a randomised, double-blind, placebo-controlled trial. Lancet. 2008;371(9613):651-9.
50. Gou S, Yang Z, Liu T, Wu H, Wang C. Use of probiotics in the treatment of severe acute pancreatitis: a systematic review and meta-analysis of randomized controlled trials. Crit Care. 2014;18(2):R57.
51. Marvin RG, McKinley BA, McQuiggan M, Cocanour CS, Moore FA. Nonocclusive bowel necrosis occurring in critically ill trauma patients receiving enteral nutrition manifests no reliable clinical signs for early detection. Am J Surg. 2000;179(1):7-12.
52. Burlew CC, Moore EE, Cuschieri J, Jurkovich GJ, Codner P, Nirula R, et al. Who should we feed? A Western Trauma Association multi-institutional study of enteral nutrition in the open abdomen after injury. J Trauma Acute Care Surg. 2012;73(6):1380-8.
53. Sun JK, Li WQ, Ke L, Tong ZH, Ni HB, Li G, et al. Early enteral nutrition prevents intra-abdominal hypertension and reduces the severity of severe acute pancreatitis compared with delayed enteral nutrition: a prospective pilot study. World J Surg. 2013;37(9):2053-60.
54. Clark JA, Coopersmith CM. Intestinal crosstalk: a new paradigm for understanding the gut as the "motor" of critical illness. Shock. 2007;28(4):384-93.
55. Wischmeyer PE, McDonald D, Knight R. Role of the microbiome, probiotics, and 'dysbiosis therapy' in critical illness. Curr Opin Crit Care. 2016;22(4):347-53.
56. Krezalek MA, Yeh A, Alverdy JC, Morowitz M. Influence of nutrition therapy on the intestinal microbiome. Curr Opin Clin Nutr Metab Care. 2017;20(2):131-7.
57. Piton G, Cypriani B, Regnard J, Patry C, Puyraveau M, Capellier G. Catecholamine use is associated with enterocyte damage in critically ill patients. Shock. 2015;43(5):437-42.
58. Revelly JP, Tappy L, Berger MM, Gersbach P, Cayeux C, Chioléro R. Early metabolic and splanchnic responses to enteral nutrition in postoperative cardiac surgery patients with circulatory compromise. Intensive Care Med. 2001;27(3):540-7.
59. Nygren A, Thorén A, Ricksten SE. Vasopressors and intestinal mucosal perfusion after cardiac surgery: norepinephrine vs. phenylephrine: Crit Care Med. 2006;34(3):722-9.
60. Bruns BR, Kozar RA. Feeding the postoperative patient on vasopressor support: feeding and pressor support. Nutr Clin Pract. 2016;31(1):14-7.

61. Patel JJ, Kozeniecki M, Biesboer A, Peppard W, Ray AS, Thomas S, et al. Early trophic enteral nutrition is associated with improved outcomes in mechanically ventilated patients with septic shock: a retrospective review. J Intensive Care Med. 2016;31(7):471-7.
62. Mancl EE, Muzevich KM. Tolerability and safety of enteral nutrition in critically ill patients receiving intravenous vasopressor therapy. J Parenter Enteral Nutr. 2013;37(5):641-51.
63. Reignier J, Boisramé-Helms J, Brisard L, Lascarrou JB, Hssain AA, Anguel N, et al. Enteral versus parenteral early nutrition in ventilated adults with shock: a randomised, controlled, multicentre, open-label, parallel-group study (NUTRIREA-2). Lancet. 2018;391(10116):133-43.
64. Wischmeyer PE. Enteral nutrition can be given to patients on vasopressors. Crit Care Med. 2020;48(1):122-5.

CHAPTER 28

Nutrition in Short Bowel Syndrome and Enterocutaneous Fistulas

Gil Hardy, Chen Liu, Emma Ludlow, Ian Bissett

INTRODUCTION

An enterocutaneous fistula (ECF) is an abnormal connection between the small intestine and the abdominal skin surface. A double-barreled enterostomy (stoma) or temporary double enterostomy (DES) is a surgical procedure used either when an immediate joining of the intestine should be avoided or to divert intestinal contents (chyme) away from a downstream surgical anastomosis/join to allow time for the join to heal, especially if the surgery was performed in high-risk circumstances such as acute peritonitis.[1] Enteroatmospheric fistulas (EAF) are intestinal fistulas in which the small bowel is completely exposed through the abdominal wall. EAF are typically left open for many months, during which time chyme has usually been discarded. EAF patients often initially present with sepsis requiring immediate and careful control of an underlying infection comprising broad-spectrum antibiotics, percutaneous drainage, or surgery before reaching a stable clinical state.[2]

Short bowel syndrome (SBS) occurs subsequent to greatly reduced functional surface area of the small intestine. The syndrome is characterized by intestinal failure (IF); the inability of the gut to absorb sufficient macronutrients, micronutrients, or fluid. Prolonged diversion of intestinal contents from the distal small bowel and colon can also cause atrophy, leading to an increased risk of prolonged postoperative ileus following stoma reversal or fistula closure and impaired distal bowel function. Patients with DES or EAF of the small bowel frequently have high intestinal fluid losses, which often result in serious complications.[3-5] These include fluid and electrolyte disturbances such as dehydration, renal impairment, metabolic acidosis, hypokalemia, hyponatremia and hypomagnesaemia, which often culminate in prolonged hospital stays or recurrent readmissions.[6-9]

Other common sequelae include calcium and other electrolyte disturbances, micronutrient deficiencies such as zinc, iron, vitamin B_{12}, and fat-soluble vitamins. The associated malabsorption of carbohydrates, lactose, and protein, and development of metabolic acidosis, gastric acid hypersecretion, steatorrhea, diarrhea, and dehydration commonly lead to malnutrition in the form of weight loss, hypoalbuminemia and anemia.[6] Cumulatively, these sequelae result in IF.

NUTRITIONAL MANAGEMENT OF INTESTINAL FAILURE

Comprehensive nutritional management is key to achieving an optimal outcome and has traditionally involved three phases: the acute phase when parenteral nutrition (PN) and replacement of excess fluid and electrolyte losses are the focus of care, followed by the adaptation phase, when the intestine adapts to the changes, and finally the maintenance phase, when longer term stability is reached.[10] Recommendations for prescribing PN vary depending on the presence or absence of the ileocecal valve, jejunum, and functional colon. Patients with residual small bowel length of 100 cm or less usually require PN. The PN regimen should be high in lipid energy, protein, carbohydrates, and micronutrients. Although early PN can be lifesaving, treatment goals should focus on early transition to enteral nutrition (EN) and eventually oral food.

Parenteral nutrition mitigates the risks associated with IF, but such therapy is not curative and merely compensates for fluid and nutritional losses without improving bowel function. In addition, PN is accompanied by risks (described in more detail in Chapter 19) such as catheter-related complications (e.g., thrombosis and infection), gut dysfunction (e.g., microbiome dysbiosis or inflammation), hepatobiliary dysfunction [e.g., derangement of liver function tests (LFTs) or cholestasis] and metabolic complications such as hyperglycemia. Moreover, inpatient management of IF patients is expensive, with one cohort study estimating the daily cost per patient up to GBP 1102[11] and for long-term hospitalization estimated at USD 150,000 per annum.[12]

The incidence of IF in patients with enterostomies is underestimated. Many may develop Type 2 IF due to SBS, requiring PN, sometimes at home home parenteral nutrition (HPN) until they have recovered enough for surgical re-establishment of intestinal continuity, typically 6–12 months after primary surgery.[1,13] Patients may need to be nil by mouth and are at high risk of dehydration and disease-related malnutrition (DRM) due to high fluid losses and intestinal malabsorption. Dehydration occurs in up to 20% of patients with enterostomies and is the cause of 40% of readmissions,[14] with a high relative risk of acute renal failure.[15] High output stoma (HOS) is defined as producing losses greater than 1.5 L/day but may involve losses of several liters daily resulting in marked water and electrolyte deficiencies.[16] While transient HOS is not uncommon in the early postoperative period, if this continues for several days, a cause should be sought. A short bowel (<200 cm jejunum remaining) is the most common reason, but partial small bowel obstruction, intra-abdominal sepsis and *Clostridium difficile* infection should be considered, and appropriate investigations performed.[17] A stenosis at or near to the stoma is common and may be detected by visual and digital examination of the stoma. HOS accompanied by low albumin, raised C-reactive protein (CRP), elevated neutrophil count, and intestinal ileus may indicate intra-abdominal infection, which is usually identified by abdominal CT scan. Other causes include administration of prokinetic drugs (e.g., metoclopramide) or premature withdrawal of opioids or steroids.

As the sodium concentration of small bowel stomal fluid is high (approximately 100 mmol/L), intravenous rehydration with a balanced crystalloid solution is frequently necessary. Common intravenous solutions used include plasmalyte 148 and 0.9% saline and should be accompanied by restricted oral intake, whilst monitoring weight and fluid balance charts. Hypotonic fluids (e.g., water or tea) should be restricted to <0.5 L/24 hours as these cause a net efflux of sodium into the bowel lumen that is then lost through the stoma. In contrast, hypertonic fluid such as an elemental diet will cause a net flow of fluid out of the bowel lumen (together with sodium) reducing (inducing) water, sodium, and magnesium depletion. Oral rehydration solutions that facilitate glucose absorption and/or sodium and magnesium supplementation are useful but correcting sodium depletion alone may be adequate.[16]

FISTULOCLYSIS AND CHYME REINFUSION THERAPY IN ADULTS

Fistuloclysis, involving infusion of EN, bile or chyme through the distal fistula, represents an alternative to the management of gastrointestinal surgery patients until surgical reconnection enables a return to use of the entire remaining gastrointestinal tract.[18-22] Bile reinfusion (BR) in combination with PN and/or EN in 20 postoperative patients improved nutritional status and allowed better control of fluid and electrolyte balances. BR-enabled optimal utilization of the remaining absorptive capacity for EN leading to early discharge home for 18/20 patients.[23]

Chyme is a semifluid mass of partially digested food, saliva, gastric juice, biliopancreatic and intestinal secretions, whereby food is transformed into absorbable nutrients by enzymatic digestion and under the influence of bile salts. When all of the nutrients have been absorbed from chyme, the remaining indigestible or nonabsorbable waste is eliminated as stool. Chyme reinfusion therapy (CRT) establishes an extracorporeal circulation of chyme between the collection stoma bag and the downstream small intestine and is one of several distal feeding or fistuloclysis techniques all of which are recommended by the American Society for Parenteral and Enteral Nutrition (ASPEN)[24] and the European Society for Clinical Nutrition and Metabolism (ESPEN)[25] for restoration of digestive function. One cohort study of DES and EAF patients, with outputs exceeding 1,000 mL/day, found a reduction in the volume of intestinal losses by >90% when CRT was optimally implemented.[26] Normalization of electrolyte abnormalities, reduced need for intravenous fluids, and significant improvements in creatinine clearance have also been reported. This may be due to restoration of the ileal break, causing inhibition of gastric emptying and reduction in gastric secretions, thus slowing gut motility which allows for increased absorption and reduced outputs.

Chyme reinfusion therapy also leads to improvement in a range of nutritional biomarkers.[26,27] These include significant increases in serum albumin, net nitrogen absorption (89% increase), net fat absorption (91% increase), body mass index (BMI), and plasma citrulline concentration (a biomarker of intestinal function which parallels enterocyte mass).[26] In clinical practice, this may manifest as earlier cessation of PN with avoidance of the PN-associated risks detailed above. Layec et al. found that all 37 patients admitted to hospital with EAF were weaned from their PN in a median of 3 days (interquartile range: 0–14) of CRT initiation.[28] Reduced dependence on PN appears long-lasting, with no patients requiring PN after a median follow-up period of 25 months.

The impact of CRT on recovery of bowel function following DES reversal or EAF repair has been less well investigated but two publications have produced promising results. A retrospective study of 117 Crohn disease patients (33 with CRT and 84 without) assessed the impact of CRT on rates of postoperative ileus and postoperative diarrhea (defined as three or more loose or liquid stools per day).[29] They found a significant reduction in the incidence of postoperative ileus within the CRT group

(11.5% vs. 42.3%, $p = 0.012$). However, the reduction in the rate of postoperative diarrhea was not significant following propensity-score matching (7.7% vs. 23.1%, $p = 0.191$). The second retrospective cohort study found that CRT was an independent significant protective factor against postoperative complications, recurrent fistula and ileus in 159 EAF patients who underwent definitive surgical repair (multivariate odds ratios of 0.161, 0.382, and 0.209, respectively).[30]

CLINICAL BENEFITS OF CHYME REINFUSION THERAPY IN NEONATES AND PEDIATRICS

Chyme reinfusion therapy is a recognized refeeding technique for premature infants with SBS[33-37] and is associated with improvements in numerous nutritional biomarkers and shorter duration of PN. About 60% of pediatric patients and neonates in a neonatal intensive care unit (NICU) were able to be weaned[12] completely off PN. Positive weight gain has been observed, with fewer incidences of stomal prolapse in CRT patients (0% vs. 100% in those not undergoing CRT). This was thought to be due to improved nutritional status, likely resulting in increased tissue tensile strength.[38] Normalization of liver function derangements, serum electrolytes, and fluid balance are also observed. Specifically, improvements were seen in alkaline phosphatase (ALP), gamma-glutamyl transferase (GGT), and serum bilirubin levels, with one study showing a statistically significant reduction in the mean peak bilirubin level after CRT (155 vs. 275 µmol/L; $p <0.001$) and improvements in serum hematocrit (37.8% vs. 29.7%; $p = 0.0227$), and hemoglobin levels (12.2 vs. 9.65 g/dL; $p = 0.0282$).[34-38]

Chyme reinfusion therapy also results in rehabilitation and maturation of the distal bowel following DES reversal surgery. In particular, a reduction in the size discrepancy between the proximal and distal intestine has been seen which was statistically significant in one study (25% vs. 53%; $p = 0.034$).[39-41] This is ascribed to the trophic effect of CRT that facilitates an easier DES reversal operation with a significant reduction in the rates of postoperative anastomotic leakage (3% vs. 20%; $p = 0.029$).[35] CRT also significantly increased distal ileum villus length, crypt width and depth.[42]

LIMITATIONS OF CHYME REINFUSION TECHNOLOGY

A combination of factors has contributed to CRT failing to gain widespread popularity. Manual collection of proximal DES or EAF output into a stoma bag, followed by refrigeration, sieving to remove large food particles then, after processing, manually reinfusing chyme can be very demanding and resource intensive. Input and expertise from specialist stomal nurses as well as multidisciplinary team members can be time consuming and poorly tolerated by staff and patients, who find manual handling of chyme to be smelly and disgusting.

Chyme reinfusion therapy has been associated with some adverse events (AEs) in both adults and neonates, particularly when initiated after the distal gut has been defunctioned for a prolonged period of time. Spasmodic abdominal discomfort and pain, mild constipation and diarrhea, nausea and vomiting have been reported. AEs in neonatal and pediatric populations are also most commonly gastrointestinal, with mild diarrhea and prolapse of the distal DES limb, most likely resulting from bolus rather than continuous reinfusion. Leakage, backflow, or loss of intestinal contents causing peristomal skin irritation, amplified by the increased challenges of fitting stoma appliances have limited use of CRT, especially in the neonatal population. Infrequent more serious AEs have included intestinal perforation with recurrent hemorrhage around the distal EAF site, necessitating multiple blood transfusions.[31]

Reinfusion of cooled chyme can affect patient tolerability but may be attributable to an excessively rapid rate. Additionally, significant modification to the patient's diet further reduced patient tolerability. Nevertheless, <5% of one cohort prematurely stopped CRT[1] when required to only consume pureed meals. Tube blockage, tube dislodgement, and even tube migration into the distal stoma or EAF limb have until recently, been technical challenges associated with CRT. Collectively, these limitations associated with earlier CRT methodologies have slowed progress and technological advancements.

Financial costs associated with CRT may limit its use in lower-income healthcare settings. However, discussion of costs should take into account the economic burden of the alternative management options which likely involves prolonged, expensive inpatient PN, and protracted use of stoma appliances.[32]

TECHNOLOGICAL INNOVATIONS IN CHYME REINFUSION THERAPY

A novel, purpose-built closed system has been developed through a collaboration between surgical and bioengineering teams in New Zealand (NZ) to overcome many of the described limitations to encourage routine use of CRT. The Insides® System (The Insides Company, Auckland, NZ) consists of three components: (1) A hand-held, portable, battery-operated and rechargeable driver unit, (2) a compact impeller pump that is placed within a standard stoma appliance, and (3) an intestinal feeding tube that is inserted into the distal stoma or fistula limb and connected to the pump inside the stoma appliance. To activate the pump, the driver unit is held adjacent, but external, to the stoma appliance. Magnetic coupling between the driver and the impeller pump allows activation and subsequent intermittent bolus CRT without physical contact with chyme. The driver has five speed settings to facilitate patient control of the infusion rate based on the DES or EAF output viscosity and individual comfort **(Fig. 1)**.

The tube carries the following key features: (1) A plastic guidewire that allows easy insertion into the distal DES limb, (2) the remaining portion of the tube, external to the stoma, that can be cut to fit an individual patient's stoma appliance, (3) a 90° retention sleeve to create a low profile to reduce device protrusion, and (4) a biconcave half-balloon tip that allows adequate tube retention below the abdominal fascia without placing excessive pressure on the bowel wall as depicted in **Figure 2**. The feeding tube is replaced every 28 days by a healthcare professional for the duration of therapy and the impeller device is changed by the carer or patient every 3 days.

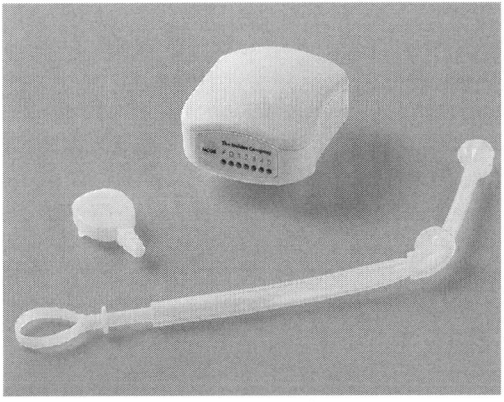

Fig. 1: The Insides® System.

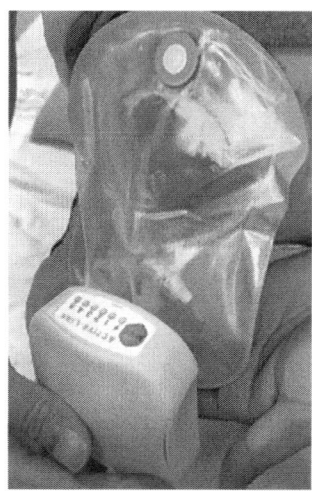

Fig. 2: Chyme reinfusion front facing.

The first feasibility clinical study in 10 patients with either a small bowel stoma, an ECF, or an EAF was captured over 740 patient-days of device use.[41] Clinical benefits included cessation of PN in four out of five patients (80%), median weight gain of 2.6 kg, and improvement in LFTs over the reinfusion period with only one out of seven patients (14%) developing postoperative ileus following ileostomy reversal. Patients were able to be fully mobile and independent whilst undergoing CRT, thereby leading to high usability of the system amongst patients. Staff acceptability was also high, with 11/12 nursing staff reporting very low levels of disgust associated with device use. There were no serious device-related AEs or microbiological complications. Microbiology safety studies of the stoma contents were conducted in parallel with device development and demonstrated no growth of pathogenic bacterial species within the chyme despite 8 hours of continuous testing.

In a subsequent clinical study involving 19 adult ileostomy patients using The Insides System and 549 patient-days of device use, CRT patients experienced the following clinical benefits: 11 patients exhibiting a reduction in net stoma losses per day, with a median reduction of 452 mL. Five of the nine patients (56%) using loperamide at baseline ceased or reduced their dosages. Fourteen patients underwent ileostomy reversal with a median length of post-operative stay of 3.5 days (range: 1–28) and a 21% rate of prolonged postoperative ileus.[42]

CHYME REINFUSION THERAPY TECHNOLOGICAL INNOVATIONS IN NEONATAL AND PEDIATRIC POPULATIONS

Following the successful design and implementation of a dedicated adult CRT system, innovation has since focused on improved systems for pediatric cohorts, and critically ill neonates suffering from necrotizing enterocolitis (NEC). Preliminary data with a novel system for pediatric CRT (The Insides® Neo) has been obtained from five neonatal IF patients with a median age 110 days and weight 1.8 kg. They experienced an average of 0.6% weight gain, improvement in electrolyte profiles, creatinine and LFTs. One baby showed a 91% reduction in alanine transaminase (ALT) and return to the reference range from 335 to 29 U/L with CRT over 2 months. Nurses and medical staff emphasize that The Insides® Neo System facilitates a more streamlined chyme refeeding process, resulting in more available nursing hours to provide better patient care and education. Parents report that this new system is easy to use and helps their babies grow prior to surgery.[43]

CONCLUSIONS AND FUTURE RESEARCH DIRECTIONS

Preoperative stimulation of the distal small or large bowel prior to stoma reversal or fistula repair via CRT is a promising therapy for minimizing the high rates of morbidity associated with DES or EAF of the small bowel in both adult and pediatric patients. The novel closed CRT systems, developed in NZ, have significantly advanced the field of CRT. Clinical studies have shown benefits associated with The Insides® System include reduction of fluid losses, improved nutrition status whilst weaning earlier from PN, and cessation or reduction of antidiarrheal medication use. The system overcomes many of the earlier challenges when undertaking CRT manually, now allowing most patients to remain fully independent and mobile during its use. CRT advancements have the potential to become the standard of nutrition care in pediatric NEC patients and adult IF patients with high output DES or EAF of the small bowel, as well as for loop ileostomates in the community. If better postoperative outcomes with CRT are confirmed in larger multicenter randomized trials, this will further aid the goal of optimum nutrition, achieving earlier discharge from hospital, facilitate home management of therapy with potentially improved quality of life.

REFERENCES

1. Picot D, Layec S, Seynhaeve E, Dussaulx L, Trivin F, Carsin-Mahe M, et al. Chyme reinfusion in intestinal failure related to temporary double enterostomies and enteroatmospheric fistulas. Nutrients. 2020;12(5):1376-91.
2. Bhama AR. Evaluation and management of enterocutaneous fistula. Dis Colon Rectum. 2019;62(8):906-10.
3. Martinez JL, Luque-de-Leon E, Mier J, Blanco-Benavides R, Robledo F. Systematic management of postoperative enterocutaneous fistulas: factors related to outcomes. World J Surg. 2008;32(3):436-43;discussion 444.
4. Gutierrez IM, Kang KH, Jaksic T. Neonatal short bowel syndrome. Semin Fetal Neonatal Med. 2011;16(3):157-63.
5. Bafford AC, Irani JL. Management and complications of stomas. Surg Clin North Am. 2013;93(1):145-66.
6. Dudrick SJ, Panait L. Metabolic consequences of patients with gastrointestinal fistulas. Eur J Trauma Emerg Surg. 2011;37(3):215-25.
7. Hayden DM, Pinzon MC, Francescatti AB, Edquist SC, Malczewski MR, Jolley JM, et al. Hospital readmission for fluid and electrolyte abnormalities following ileostomy construction: preventable or unpredictable? J Gastrointest Surg. 2013;17(2):298-303.
8. Justiniano CF, Temple LK, Swanger AA, Xu Z, Speranza JR, Cellini C, et al. Readmissions with dehydration after ileostomy creation: rethinking risk factors. Dis Colon Rectum. 2017;61(11):1297-305.
9. Assaf D, Hazzan D, Ben-Yaacov A, Laks S, Zippel D, Segev L, et al. Predisposing factors for high output stoma in patients with a diverting loop ileostomy after colorectal surgeries. Ann Coloproctol. 2021;39:3-7.
10. Couper C, Doriot A, Siddiqui MTR, Steiger E. Nutrition management of the high-output fistulae. Nutr Clin Pract. 2021;36(2):282-96.
11. Saunders J, Parsons C, King A, Stroud M, Smith T. The financial cost of managing patients with type 2 intestinal failure; experience from a regional centre. e-SPEN Journal. 2013;8(3):e80-5.
12. Bhat S, Cameron NR, Sharma P, Bissett IP, O'Grady G. Chyme recycling in the management of small bowel double enterostomy in pediatric and neonatal populations: A systematic review. Clin Nutr ESPEN. 2020;37:1-8.
13. Liu MY, Tang HC, Yang HL, Chang SJ. Is jejunostomy output nutrient or waste in short bowel syndrome? Experience from six cases. Asia Pac J Clin Nutr. 2016;25(2):430-5.
14. Messaris E, Sehgal R, Deiling S, Koltun WA, Stewart D, McKenna K, et al. Dehydration is the most common indication for readmission after diverting ileostomy creation. Dis Colon Rectum. 2012;55:175-80.

15. Jafari MD, Halabi WJ, Jafari F, Nguyen VQ, Stamos MJ, Carmichael JC, et al. Morbidity of diverting ileostomy for rectal cancer: Analysis of the American College of Surgeons National Surgical Quality Improvement Program. Ann Surg. 2013;79:1034.
16. Nightingale JMD. How to manage a high-output stoma. Frontline Gastroenterol. 2021;13(2):140-151.
17. Seifarth C, Augustin LN, Lehmann KS, Stroux A, Lauscher JC, Kreis ME, et al. Assessment of risk factors for the occurrence of a high-output ileostomy. Front Surg. 2021;8:642288.
18. Kwun H. Re-feeding of chymus into a high-output jejunostomy: a nursing care study. World Council Enterostomal Ther J. 1999;19:20-1.
19. Bhat S, Sharma P, Cameron NR, Bissett IP, O'Grady G. Chyme reinfusion for small bowel double enterostomies and enteroatmospheric fistulas in adult patients: A systematic review. Nutr Clin Pract. 2020;35(2):254-64.
20. Ribeiro-junior MA, Yeh DD, Augosto S. The role of fistuloclysis in the treatment of patients with enteroatmospheric fistulas. Arq Bras Cir Dig. 2021;34(2):e1605.
21. Blaauw R, Du Toit A, Boutall A. Opinions of South African dietitians on fistuloclysis as a treatment option for intestinal failure patients. South Afr J Clin Nutr. 2018;31(2):6-11.
22. Du Toit A. Nutritional management of a complicated surgical patient by means of fistuloclysis. South Afr J Clin Nutr. 2014;27(4):230-6.
23. Chada R, Madhulika J, Yadav V, et al. Nutritional adequacy during bile reinfusion in post-surgical patients. NCP. 2023 in press.
24. Kumpf VJ, de Aguilar-Nascimento JE, Diaz-Pizarro Graf JI, Hall AM, McKeever L, Steiger E, et al. ASPEN-FELANPE guidelines: Nutrition support of adult patients with enterocutaneous fistula. JPEN J Parenter Enteral Nutr. 2017;41(1):104-12.
25. Cuerda C, Pironi L, Arends J, Bozzetti F, Gillanders L, Jeppesen PB, et al. ESPEN practical guideline: Clinical nutrition in chronic intestinal failure. Clin Nutr. 2021;40(9):5196-220.
26. Picot D, Garin L, Trivin F, Kossovsky MP, Darmaun D, Thibault R. Plasma citrulline is a marker of absorptive small bowel length in patients with transient enterostomy and acute intestinal failure. Clin Nutr. 2010;29(2):235-42.
27. Picot D, Layec S, Dussaulx L, Trivin F, Thibault R. Chyme reinfusion in patients with intestinal failure due to temporary double enterostomy: A 15-year prospective cohort in a referral centre. Clin Nutr. 2017;36(2):593-600.
28. Layec S, Seynhaeve E, Trivin F, Carsin-Mahé M, Dussaulx L, Picot D. Management of entero-atmospheric fistulas by chyme reinfusion: A retrospective study. Clin Nutr. 2020;39:3695-702.
29. Duan M, Cao L, Gao L, Gong J, Li Y, Zhu W. Chyme reinfusion is associated with lower rate of postoperative ileus in Crohn's disease patients after stoma closure. Dig Dis Sci. 2020;65(1):243-9.
30. Tian W, Zhao R, Xu X, Zhao Y, Luo S, Tao S, et al. Chyme reinfusion reducing the postoperative complications after definitive surgery for small intestinal enteroatmospheric fistula: A cohort study. Front Nutr. 2020;9:708534.
31. Haddock CA, Stanger JD, Albersheim SG, Albersheim SG, Casey LM, Butterworth SA. Mucous fistula refeeding in neonates with enterostomies. J Pediatr Surg. 2015;50(5):779-82.
32. Al-Harbi K, Walton JM, Gardner V, Fitzgerald PG. Mucous fistula refeeding in neonates with short bowel syndrome. J Pediatr Surg. 1999;34(7):1100-3.
33. Wong KK, Lan LC, Lin SC, Chan AWA, Tam PKH. Mucous fistula refeeding in premature neonates with enterostomies. J Pediatr Gastroenterol Nutr. 2004;39(1):43-5.
34. Gause CD, Hayashi M, Haney C, Rhee D, Karim O, Weir BW, et al. Mucous fistula refeeding decreases parenteral nutrition exposure in postsurgical premature neonates J Pediatr Surg. 2016;51(11):1759-65.

35. Lau EC, Fung AC, Wong KK, Tam PK. Beneficial effects of mucous fistula refeeding in necrotizing enterocolitis neonates with enterostomies. J Pediatr Surg. 2016;51(12):1914-6.
36. Inoue S, Odaka A, Muta Y, Beck Y, Sobajima H, Tamura M, et al. Recycling small intestinal contents from proximal ileostomy in low-birth-weight infants with small bowel perforation. J Pediatr Gastroenterol Nutr. 2017;64(1):e16-8.
37. Drenckpohl D, Vegunta R, Knaub L, Holterman M, Wang H, Macwan K, et al. Reinfusion of succus entericus into the mucous fistula decreases dependence on parenteral nutrition in neonates. Infant Child Adolesc Nutr. 2012;4(3):168-74.
38. Elliott T, Walton JM. Safety of mucous fistula refeeding in neonates with functional short bowel syndrome: A retrospective review. J Pediatr Surg. 2019;54(5):989-92.
39. Gardner VA, Walton JM, Chessell L. A case study utilizing an enteral refeeding technique in a premature infant with short bowel syndrome. Adv Neonatal Care. 2003;3(6):258-68.
40. Tanaka A, Nakayama-Imaohji H, Shimono R, Suzuki M, Fujii T, Kubo H, et al. Nutritional benefit of recycling of bowel content in an infant with short bowel syndrome. J Pediatr Gastroenterol Nutr. 2017;65(3):e75-6.
41. Sharma P, Davidson R, Davidson J, Keane C, Liu C, Ritchie SR, et al. Novel chyme reinfusion device for gastrointestinal fistulas and stomas: feasibility study. Br J Surg. 2020;107(9):1199-210.
42. Liu C, Bhat S, Bissett I, O'Grady G. A review of chyme reinfusion: new tech solutions for age old problems. Journal of the Royal Society of New Zealand. 2022. DOI: 10.1080/03036758.2022.2117832.
43. Harrington. T, Ludlow E, Hardy G, et al. Can chyme reinfusion therapy (CRT) improve intestinal failure associated liver disease (IFALD) in adults and children? Clin Nutr. 2023.

CHAPTER 29

Nutrition in Critically Ill Patients with Renal Failure

Penmetsa Vijay Varma, Rajasekara Chakravarthi, Mahesh Kota

INTRODUCTION

Acute kidney injury (AKI) is a frequent complication of critical illness with the incidence ranging from 20 to 50% of intensive care unit (ICU) patients.[1] It is a proinflammatory condition which affects the metabolism of all macronutrients. Severe malnutrition, as defined by the subjective global assessment (SGA), can be observed in ~40% of patients with AKI in the ICU and is a major prognostic factor.[2] Severe malnutrition severely impairs patient's outcome, whether defined in terms of length of hospital stay, increased risk of complications (sepsis, bleeding, arrhythmia, respiratory failure, etc.), or increased in-hospital mortality.

Metabolic abnormalities associated with AKI/acute kidney disease (AKD)[3] are:
- Protein catabolism
- Alteration of metabolism of specific amino acids [several nonessential amino acids (e.g., tyrosine) become conditionally essential, and there are alterations in the intra- and extracellular amino acid pools]
- Hyperglycemia caused by both peripheral insulin resistance and the activation of hepatic gluconeogenesis
- Reduction of lipolysis and impaired fat clearance resulting in hypertriglyceridemia
- Depletion of antioxidant systems
- Induction of a proinflammatory state
- Immunodeficiency.

NUTRITIONAL ASSESSMENT

Who should be screened for malnutrition?
Any hospitalized patient with AKI/AKD, especially those staying for >48 hours in the ICU, should be screened for malnutrition **(Table 1)**. Few existing screening tools have been evaluated in this population; however, none of these have been validated. They include:
- Malnutrition universal screening tool (MUST) score—low sensitivity in these patients
- The Nutritional Risk Screening (NRS) 2002 tool—identifies patients considered malnourished by SGA and predicts worse clinical outcomes
- Recently, a new renal inpatient nutritional screening tool (renal iNUT) was specifically developed for hospitalized patients with AKI/AKD showing a good sensitivity, specificity, and positive predictive value against the SGA.[4]

A general nutritional assessment should include patient history, report of unintentional weight loss or decrease in physical performance before hospital or ICU admission, physical examination, general assessment of body composition, muscle mass, and strength.

How to assess lean body mass, muscle mass, and function?
Body composition assessment should be preferred to anthropometry measurements

TABLE 1: Nutritional markers used in acute kidney injury (AKI) and their limitations.

Markers	Limitations
Body weight and BMI	• Poor nutritional assessment tools • Cannot take into account the frequent presence of fluid overload • Cannot distinguish fat from muscle stores • May miss sarcopenic obesity.
Nutritional scores (SGA)	• More studied in CKD population than in AKI group • Difficult to apply in ICU setting
Serum albumin	• Negative phase reactant • Levels should not be interpreted alone
Anthropometry (skinfold, triceps, arm circumference, etc.)	Affected by edema
Energy expenditure	Prediction formulas are not constantly accurate in critically ill patients (they are generally based on body weight)
Protein catabolic rate or protein equivalent of nitrogen emergence	Measurements require calculations based on urea kinetics during RRT + collection of dialysates

(AKI: acute kidney injury; BMI: body mass index; CKD: chronic kidney disease; ICU: intensive care unit; RRT: renal replacement therapy; SGA: subjective global assessment)

when diagnosing and monitoring malnutrition in hospitalized patients with AKI/AKD.

While dual-energy X-ray absorptiometry (DEXA), computed tomography (CT) scan at the level of third lumbar vertebra (CT), and magnetic resonance imaging (MRI) are considered the reference standard techniques for the assessment of skeletal muscle mass and body composition, however, they cannot be used routinely for nutritional status assessment in ICU or more in general in-hospitalized patients.[5] As a potential alternative method, the use of ultrasound for the assessment of muscle mass has been recently investigated in hospitalized patients with AKI.

NORMAL ENERGY EXPENDITURE

The human body combusts organic fuels (lipids, carbohydrates, and proteins) in combination with oxygen and produces heat, kcal, and waste. The energy yield differs from 9.1 kcal/g for lipids, 4 kcal/g for protein, and 3.75 kcal/g for glucose.

Normal nutritional requirements [daily energy expenditure (EE)] can be measured/calculated by the following methods:

- *Indirect calorimetry (IC):* The gold standard for measuring individual caloric needs is represented by IC, a noninvasive method allowing resting energy expenditure (REE) assessment based on oxygen consumption and carbon dioxide production measurements in the exhaled air.[6] Unfortunately, IC measurements are not widely used in daily hospital routine.
- *Prediction equations:* Basal energy expenditure (BEE) kcal/24 hours

    Men = 66 + (13.7 × weight in kg) + (5.0 × height in cm) – (6.7 × age in years)

    Women = 655 + (9.6 × weight in kg) + (1.8 × height in cm) – (4.7 × age in years)

    Resting energy expenditure = 1.2 × BEE

    Energy expenditure in critical illness—EE should always be measured, or calculated, and then corrected depending on the concomitant condition; in most cases, it does not exceed 1.3 × BEE, though it may reach 1.5 – 1.7 × BEE in some cases.

- *Weight based formulae:* In practice, we use simplified computations – 25–35 kcal/kg ideal body weight (BW) depending on activity and stress. In AKI, the reference BW used is the preadmission dry weight for normal and overweight patients. For obese patients, the ideal BW to reach a BMI = 25 kg/m² should be considered.
- *Definitions and terminologies:*
  - Actual BW is the weight measured during hospitalization.
  - Ideal BW is the weight related to the height to obtain a body mass index (BMI) of 23 kg/m².
  - Adjusted BW is usually used in obese and is calculated as (actual BW – ideal BW) × 0.33 + ideal BW.

Equations and formulations aiming at REE estimation are largely inadequate, thus carrying the risk of clinically significant under- and overfeeding depending on the BW used for calculations. While published prediction equations and weight-based formulae provide valid estimates of energy requirements at the population level, both methods are subject to significant bias and imprecision when applied to individual patients.

If calorimetry is not available, using VO_2 (oxygen consumption) from pulmonary arterial catheter or VCO_2 (carbon dioxide production) derived from the ventilator will give a better evaluation on EE than predictive equations.

Which patients should receive nutritional treatment?
Medical nutrition therapy should be provided to any patient with AKI/AKD, AKI on chronic kidney disease (CKD) who stays in the ICU for >48 hours.

Route and timing of feeding: In line with the European Society for Clinical Nutrition and Metabolism (ESPEN)[7] and the European Society of Intensive Care Medicine (ESICM)[8] guidelines, oral nutrition should be started as early as possible while considering the risk of complications (e.g., aspiration). If oral intake is not possible or is not sufficient to meet at least 70% of daily requirements, early enteral nutrition (EN) (within 48 hours) at a low and progressive rate should be performed/initiated rather than delaying EN. EN is the most physiologic route of feeding in comparison to parenteral nutrition (PN), and in general has been linked to lower infection rates, shorter ICU, and hospital stay.

When is PN indicated?
In case of contraindications to oral and EN, PN should be implemented within 3–7 days. Early and progressive PN can be provided instead of no nutrition in case of contraindications for EN in severely malnourished patients.

CALORIE REQUIREMENTS

In critically ill patients, actual EE should not be the target during the first 72 hours. Because in the early phase of critical illness, there is an endogenous energy production of 500–1,400 kcal/day, early full feeding adding up to this amount may cause overfeeding.[7] Hence, hypocaloric nutrition (not exceeding 70% of EE) should be administered in the early phase of acute illness. After day 3, caloric delivery can be increased up to 80–100% of measured EE. To avoid overfeeding, early full EN and PN shall not be used in critically ill patients but shall be prescribed within 3–7 days. Usually calorie requirements are achieved 70% from carbohydrates and 30% from fats.

In patients undergoing renal replacement therapy (RRT), the total energy provision by additional calories given in the form of citrate (1 mmol provides 0.59 kcal), lactate (1 mmol provides 0.32 kcal), and glucose from dialysis/hemofiltration solutions should be included in the calculations to determine the total daily energy provision to avoid overfeeding.

PROTEIN REQUIREMENTS

Protein requirements are mainly determined by baseline illness; however, prolonged RRT can exert a negative influence on protein balance.

The following protein intakes are recommended by the latest ESPEN guidelines:[7]

Hospitalized patient with AKI, AKI on CKD:
- *Without acute/critical illness:* 0.8–1.0 g/kg BW/day
- *With acute/critical illness, not on RRT:* Start with 1 g/kg BW/day, and gradually increase up to 1.3 g/kg BW/day if tolerated
- *With acute/critical illness on conventional intermittent kidney replacement therapy (KRT):* 1.3–1.5 g/kg/day
- *With acute/critical illness on continuous renal replacement therapy (CRRT) or prolonged intermittent renal replacement therapy (PIRRT):* 1.5 g/kg/day up to 1.7 g/kg/day.

Kidney replacement therapies as CRRT or PIRRT such as sustained low-efficiency dialysis (SLED) have become the treatment modality of choice in critically ill patients with AKI. These modalities of intensive RRT, due to their prolonged schedules and the type of membranes used, can exert a negative influence on protein balance by inducing amino acid and peptide/protein losses (up to 15–20 g/day and 5–10 g/day, respectively). Besides, since amino acids are low molecular weight substances with a sieving coefficient near 1.0, many amino acids such as cysteine, arginine, alanine, and glutamine can be readily filtered from the blood into effluent.

It is important to note that protein prescription shall not be reduced in order to avoid or delay RRT start in critically ill patients with AKI, AKI on CKD, or CKD with kidney failure (KF).

A medical conservative approach consisting of moderately restricted protein regimens may be considered only in the case of metabolically stable patients with AKI or CKD without any catabolic condition/critical illness and not undergoing RRT.

MICRONUTRIENT REQUIREMENT

Because of increased requirements during AKI and critical illness and large effluent losses during RRT, trace elements and water soluble vitamins should be monitored and supplemented. Increased attention should be given to selenium, zinc, copper, vitamin C, folate, and thiamine.

ELECTROLYTES REQUIREMENTS

Electrolytes abnormalities are common in patients with AKI, AKI on CKD receiving RRT, and shall be closely monitored.

Common laboratory abnormalities include hypophosphatemia, hypokalemia, and hypomagnesemia. Dialysis solutions containing potassium, phosphate, and magnesium should be used to prevent electrolyte disorders during RRT.

CONCLUSION

The presence of KF in critically ill patients identifies a highly heterogeneous group of subjects with widely varying nutrient needs and intakes. Since they are at high risk of malnutrition, nutritional status should be thoroughly assessed and interventions should be tailored taking into account the catabolic state and need for RRT. Nutrition in AKI is an under-researched area and well-designed randomized controlled trials (RCTs) are the urgent need of the hour.

REFERENCES

1. Case J, Khan S, Khalid R, Khan A. Epidemiology of acute kidney injury in the intensive care unit. Crit Care Res Pract. 2013;2013:479730.
2. Mehta H. Why is acute kidney injury more demanding in terms of nutritional support? J Renal Nutr Metab. 2019;5:28-31.
3. Fiaccadori E, Regolisti G, Maggiore U. Specialized nutritional support interventions in critically ill patients on renal replacement therapy. Curr Opin Clin Nutr Metab Care. 2013;16:217-24.
4. Jackson HS, McLoughlin HL, VidalDiez A, Banerjee D. A new renal inpatient nutrition screening tool (Renal iN): a multicenter validation study. Clin Nutr. 2018;30:2297303.
5. Buckinx F, Landi F, Cesari M, Fielding RA, Visser M, Engelke K, et al. Pitfalls in the measurement of muscle mass: a need for a reference standard. J Cachexia Sarcopenia Muscle. 2018;9:269-7.
6. Oshima T, Berger MM, De Waele E, Guttormsen AB, Heidegger CP, Hiesmayr M, et al. Indirect calorimetry in nutritional therapy. A position paper by the ICALIC study group. Clin Nutr. 2017;36:651-62.
7. Fiaccadori E, Sabatino A, Barazzoni R, Carrero JJ, Cupisti A, De Waele E, et al. ESPEN guideline on clinical nutrition in hospitalized patients with acute or chronic kidney disease. Clin Nutr. 2021;(4):1644-68.
8. Reintam Blaser A, Starkopf J, Alhazzani W, Berger MM, Casaer MP, Deane AM, et al. Early enteral nutrition in critically ill patients: ESICM clinical practice guidelines. Intensive Care Med. 2017;43:380-98.

CHAPTER 30

Nutrition in Critically Ill Patients with Respiratory Failure

Dhruva Chaudhry, Vineela Surapaneni

INTRODUCTION

Acute respiratory failure (ARF) is a life-threatening condition where patients experience inadequate gas exchange due to lung injury, compromised lung function, or increased metabolic demands. It is characterized by hypoxemia, hypercapnia, or both, and is associated with a high mortality rate.[1] Nutritional therapy plays a crucial role in the management of patients with ARF, as malnutrition and undernutrition can exacerbate the clinical outcomes of these patients.[2]

This chapter will discuss the importance of nutritional therapy in patients with ARF, the specific nutritional requirements of these patients, and various nutritional strategies to improve patient outcomes.

IMPORTANCE OF NUTRITIONAL THERAPY IN ARF PATIENTS

In patients with ARF, the physiological stress response to critical illness leads to increased metabolic demands and catabolism resulting in the rapid depletion of energy and protein stores.[3] This condition referred to as acute illness-related malnutrition has been associated with poor clinical outcomes including increased infection rates, prolonged mechanical ventilation, longer hospital stays, and higher mortality.[4] Consequently, timely and adequate nutritional therapy is essential to mitigate these adverse effects and improve patient outcomes.

NUTRITIONAL REQUIREMENTS IN ARF PATIENTS

Energy Requirements

The energy requirements of critically ill patients with ARF depend on several factors including age, weight, gender, and underlying medical conditions. It is crucial to accurately estimate the patients' energy expenditure to avoid under- or overfeeding, both of which have been associated with poor outcomes.[5]

Indirect calorimetry is the gold standard for measuring energy expenditure in critically ill patients.[6] However, if this method is not available, predictive equations such as the Harris–Benedict equation or the Penn State equation can be used, although their accuracy in critically ill patients is limited.[3]

Protein Requirements

Protein requirements in critically ill patients with ARF are higher than in healthy individuals due to the increased protein breakdown associated with the stress response to critical illness. Current guidelines recommend providing 1.2–2.0 g of protein per kilogram of body weight per day to optimize protein balance and promote anabolism.[7] This protein intake should be adjusted based on individual patient characteristics and clinical course.

Micronutrient Requirements

Micronutrients such as vitamins and minerals play a vital role in various metabolic and immune functions. Deficiencies in micronutrients can impair immune response, delay wound healing, and increase the risk of infections in critically ill patients.[8] Therefore, supplementation of vitamins and trace elements including vitamin C, vitamin D, zinc, selenium, and copper is recommended in patients with ARF.[7]

NUTRITIONAL STRATEGIES IN ARF PATIENTS

Enteral Nutrition

Enteral nutrition (EN) is the preferred method of providing nutritional support to critically ill patients with ARF, as it preserves gut function, reduces bacterial translocation, and is associated with a lower risk of complications compared to parenteral nutrition (PN).[9] EN should be initiated within 24-48 hours of admission to the intensive care unit (ICU) or the onset of ARF provided there are no contraindications.[7]

To minimize the risk of aspiration and ventilator-associated pneumonia, it is recommended to use a postpyloric feeding tube in patients with ARF who require mechanical ventilation.[9] Additionally, the use of prokinetic agents such as metoclopramide or erythromycin can improve gastric emptying and promote the tolerance of enteral feeding.[3]

Parenteral Nutrition

Parenteral nutrition is an alternative method of providing nutritional support in critically ill patients with ARF who cannot tolerate or have contraindications to EN. PN should be considered after 7-10 days of failed attempts to achieve adequate EN or in patients with severe gastrointestinal dysfunction.[7] However, PN is associated with a higher risk of complications such as infections, metabolic disturbances, and liver dysfunction compared to EN.[10]

Immunonutrition

Immunonutrition refers to the supplementation of specific nutrients with immunomodulatory properties such as omega-3 fatty acids, glutamine, and arginine to enhance the immune response and reduce inflammation in critically ill patients.[11] While some studies have shown beneficial effects of immunonutrition in critically ill patients, the evidence for its routine use in ARF patients remains inconclusive and further research is needed to determine its efficacy and safety.[3]

MONITORING AND ADJUSTING NUTRITIONAL THERAPY

Close monitoring of the nutritional status and clinical course of patients with ARF is essential to ensure optimal nutritional therapy. Parameters to monitor include body weight, serum proteins (albumin and prealbumin), electrolytes, blood glucose, and nitrogen balance.[7] Adjustments to nutritional therapy should be made based on the patients' clinical response, tolerance, and nutritional goals.

NUTRITIONAL CHALLENGES IN SPECIFIC ARF POPULATIONS

Obesity

Obesity presents unique challenges in managing the nutritional needs of patients with ARF. Obese patients are at higher risk of complications including prolonged mechanical ventilation and difficulty in

TABLE 1: Calculation of ideal body weight.
Males: 50 kg + (Height in inches − 60) × 2.3
Females: 45.5 kg + (Height in inches − 60) × 2.3

weaning from ventilatory support.[12] Accurate estimation of energy requirements is essential to prevent overfeeding and its associated complications such as hyperglycemia, hepatic steatosis, and increased carbon dioxide production.[7] The use of ideal body weight **(Table 1)** and indirect calorimetry can help provide a more accurate estimation of energy expenditure in obese patients.[6]

Protein requirements in obese patients with ARF should be based on ideal body weight to avoid overfeeding and promote anabolism.[7] Supplementation of specific micronutrients such as vitamin D and thiamine may be necessary, as deficiencies in these nutrients are more prevalent in obese individuals.[8]

Acute Respiratory Distress Syndrome

Acute respiratory distress syndrome (ARDS) is a severe form of ARF characterized by diffuse alveolar damage, increased pulmonary vascular permeability, and non-cardiogenic pulmonary edema leading to severe hypoxemia and decreased lung compliance.[1] Nutritional therapy in ARDS patients should focus on providing adequate energy and protein to support lung repair and prevent muscle wasting. However, overfeeding should be avoided, as it may exacerbate lung injury and impair weaning from mechanical ventilation.[5]

Enteral nutrition should be initiated within 24–48 hours of ARDS diagnosis, and the use of a high-protein as well as low-carbohydrate enteral formula has been suggested to reduce carbon dioxide production and improve respiratory function.[3] The use of omega-3 fatty acids and antioxidants such as vitamin C and E may have beneficial effects on lung function and inflammation in ARDS patients, but further research is needed to confirm these findings.[11]

Chronic Obstructive Pulmonary Disease

Chronic obstructive pulmonary disease (COPD) is a common cause of ARF characterized by progressive airflow limitation and chronic inflammation of the airways resulting in dyspnea, cough, and sputum production.[13] Nutritional therapy in COPD patients with ARF should focus on providing adequate energy to meet increased metabolic demands and prevent weight loss, which is associated with poorer outcomes in this population.[2]

Protein requirements in COPD patients with ARF are higher than in healthy individuals, and a protein intake of 1.5–2.0 g per kilogram of body weight per day is recommended to maintain muscle mass and promote anabolism.[7] Supplementation of specific micronutrients such as vitamin D, magnesium, and selenium may be necessary, as deficiencies in these nutrients are more prevalent in COPD patients.[8]

FUTURE DIRECTIONS AND RESEARCH IN NUTRITIONAL THERAPY FOR ARF PATIENTS

Personalized Nutrition

Personalized nutrition, which caters to dietary recommendations based on individual genetic, metabolic, and clinical characteristics, has the potential to improve patient outcomes in ARF.[14] Future research should explore the use of genomic, transcriptomic, and proteomic data to develop more precise and individualized nutritional strategies for patients with ARF.

Nutritional Biomarkers

The identification of novel biomarkers to assess nutritional status and monitor the response to nutritional therapy in ARF patients could improve clinical decision making and patient outcomes.[15] Future research should focus on the discovery and validation of nutritional biomarkers that can accurately predict the risk of malnutrition and guide the optimization of nutritional therapy in this patient population.

Long-term Outcomes of Nutritional Therapy

While the short-term benefits of nutritional therapy in ARF patients are well-established, the long-term outcomes such as survival, functional status, and quality of life are less clear.[15] Longitudinal studies are needed to assess the long-term effects of nutritional therapy on patient outcomes and identify potential areas for improvement in nutritional management.

ROLE OF NUTRITIONAL THERAPY IN WEANING FROM MECHANICAL VENTILATION

Weaning from mechanical ventilation is a critical step in the recovery of patients with ARF. Nutritional therapy can play a significant role in the weaning process by providing adequate energy and protein to support respiratory muscle function and prevent muscle wasting.[3]

Several factors can impact the success of weaning from mechanical ventilation including nutritional status, energy balance, and the presence of electrolyte imbalances[1] (Box 1).

BOX 1: Nutritional factors influencing weaning process.
- Hypokalemia
- Hypophosphatemia
- Hypomagnesemia
- Anemia
- Malnutrition

NUTRITIONAL SUPPORT IN EXTRACORPOREAL MEMBRANE OXYGENATION

Extracorporeal membrane oxygenation (ECMO) is a lifesaving intervention for patients with severe ARF who are unresponsive to conventional ventilatory support.[1] Nutritional support is crucial for ECMO patients to maintain adequate energy and protein balance and support immune function.

Enteral nutrition is the preferred method of nutritional support in ECMO patients, as it is associated with lower risks of complications and better outcomes compared to PN.[9] However, the initiation and advancement of EN in ECMO patients can be challenging due to hemodynamic instability, sedation, and the use of anticoagulants.[3]

Close monitoring of the patient's nutritional status, tolerance of EN, and the presence of gastrointestinal complications such as ileus and gastrointestinal bleeding is essential to optimize nutritional therapy in ECMO patients.[7]

NUTRITIONAL SUPPORT IN NONINVASIVE VENTILATION

Noninvasive ventilation (NIV) is an alternative to invasive mechanical ventilation for patients with ARF who have less severe hypoxemia or hypercapnia.[1] Nutritional support in NIV patients should focus on providing adequate energy and protein to support respiratory muscle function and prevent muscle wasting.[3]

Close monitoring of the patient's nutritional status, tolerance of EN, and the presence of gastrointestinal complications such as regurgitation and aspiration is essential to optimize nutritional therapy in NIV patients.[7]

NUTRITIONAL SUPPORT IN COVID-19-RELATED ARF

The coronavirus disease 2019 (COVID-19) pandemic has highlighted the importance of optimal nutritional support in patients with ARF. COVID-19 patients with ARF often have increased metabolic demands, systemic inflammation, and muscle wasting due to prolonged immobilization and critical illness.[16]

Early initiation of EN is recommended for mechanically ventilated COVID-19 patients with ARF, as it has been associated with improved outcomes and fewer complications compared to delayed feeding or PN.[16]

Protein requirements in COVID-19 patients with ARF are higher than in healthy individuals, and a protein intake of 1.5–2.0 g per kilogram of body weight per day is recommended to maintain muscle mass and promote anabolism.[16] Supplementation of specific micronutrients such as vitamin D, zinc, and selenium may be necessary, as deficiencies in these nutrients have been associated with increased severity and poorer outcomes in COVID-19 patients.[17]

PRACTICAL IMPLEMENTATION OF NUTRITIONAL THERAPY IN ARF (FLOWCHART 1)

The implementation of nutritional therapy in patients with ARF requires a multidisciplinary approach involving physicians, nurses, dietitians, and other healthcare professionals. The steps in **Flowchart 1** can help guide the successful implementation of nutritional therapy in ARF patients.

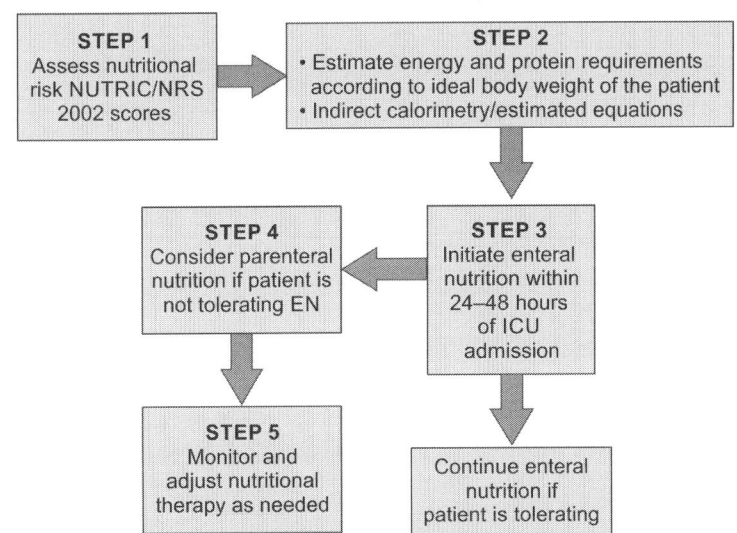

Flowchart 1: The steps involved in the implementation of nutritional therapy.

(EN: enteral nutrition; ICU: intensive care unit; NRS: Nutrition Risk Screening; NUTRIC: Nutrition Risk in Critically Ill)

EDUCATION AND TRAINING IN NUTRITIONAL THERAPY FOR ARF

Education and training in nutritional therapy for healthcare professionals involved in the management of patients with ARF is crucial to ensure the optimal delivery of care. This can be achieved through various approaches including formal education, continuing education programs, and multidisciplinary training sessions.

By investing in education and training, healthcare professionals can ensure the delivery of high-quality nutritional therapy for patients with ARF, ultimately improving clinical outcomes and patient quality of life.

CONCLUSION

Nutritional therapy is a critical component of the management of patients with ARF. Providing adequate and timely nutritional support can improve clinical outcomes, reduce complications, and shorten hospital stays. EN is the preferred method of nutritional support in these patients, while PN should be reserved for cases where EN is contraindicated or not tolerated. Accurate estimation of energy and protein requirements, supplementation of micronutrients, and close monitoring of the patient's clinical course and nutritional status are key elements in the successful management of ARF patients.

Future research should focus on the development of personalized nutritional strategies, the identification of novel nutritional biomarkers, and the evaluation of long-term outcomes of nutritional therapy in this patient population. Additionally, ethical considerations such as informed consent, patient autonomy, and balancing benefits and risks should be carefully addressed in the provision of nutritional therapy for patients with ARF. Education and training in nutritional therapy for healthcare professionals is crucial to ensure the optimal delivery of care and improve patient outcomes.

REFERENCES

1. MacIntyre N, Huang YC. Acute exacerbations and respiratory failure in chronic obstructive pulmonary disease. Proc Am Thorac Soc. 2008;5(4):530-5.
2. Schols AM, Slangen J, Volovics L, Wouters EF. Weight loss is a reversible factor in the prognosis of chronic obstructive pulmonary disease. Am J Respir Crit Care Med. 1998;157(6 Pt 1):1791-7.
3. Singer P, Berger MM, Van den Berghe G, Biolo G, Calder P, Forbes A, et al. ESPEN Guidelines on Parenteral Nutrition: intensive care. Clin Nutr. 2009;28(4):387-400.
4. Heyland DK, Cahill NE, Dhaliwal R, Wang M, Day AG, Alenzi A, et al. Enhanced protein-energy provision via the enteral route in critically ill patients: a single center feasibility trial of the PEP uP protocol. Crit Care. 2010;14(2):R78.
5. Arabi YM, Aldawood AS, Haddad SH, Al-Dorzi HM, Tamim HM, Jones G, et al. Permissive Underfeeding or Standard Enteral Feeding in Critically Ill Adults. N Engl J Med. 2015;372(25):2398-408.
6. Stapel SN, de Grooth HJ, Alimohamad H, Elbers PW, Girbes AR, Weijs PJ, et al. Ventilator-derived carbon dioxide production to assess energy expenditure in critically ill patients: proof of concept. Crit Care. 2015;19:370.
7. McClave SA, Taylor BE, Martindale RG, Warren MM, Johnson DR, Braunschweig C, et al. Guidelines for the Provision and Assessment of Nutrition Support Therapy in the Adult Critically Ill Patient: Society of Critical Care Medicine (SCCM) and American Society for Parenteral and Enteral Nutrition (ASPEN). JPEN J Parenter Enteral Nutr. 2016;40(2):159-211.

8. Berger MM, Reintam-Blaser A, Calder PC, Casaer M, Hiesmayr MJ, Mayer K, et al. Monitoring nutrition in the ICU. Clin Nutr. 2019;38(2):584-93.
9. Reintam Blaser A, Starkopf J, Alhazzani W, Berger MM, Casaer MP, Deane AM, et al. Early enteral nutrition in critically ill patients: ESICM clinical practice guidelines. Intensive Care Med. 2017;43(3):380-98.
10. Casaer MP, Mesotten D, Hermans G, Wouters PJ, Schetz M, Meyfroidt G, et al. Early versus late parenteral nutrition in critically ill adults. N Engl J Med. 2011;365(6):506-17.
11. Calder PC, Laviano A, Lonnqvist F, Muscaritoli M, Öhlander M, Schols A. Targeted medical nutrition for cachexia in chronic obstructive pulmonary disease: a randomized, controlled trial. J Cachexia Sarcopenia Muscle. 2018;9(1):28-40.
12. Chiumello D, Carlesso E, Brioni M, Cressoni M. Airway driving pressure and lung stress in ARDS patients. Crit Care. 2016;20:276.
13. Global Initiative For Chronic Obstructive Pulmonary Disease. (2023). GOLD REPORT. [online] Available from: https://goldcopd.org/ [Last accessed June, 2023].
14. Van Ommen B, van den Broek T, de Hoogh I, van Erk M, van Someren E, Rouhani-Rankouhi T, et al. Systems biology of personalized nutrition. Nutr Rev. 2017;75(8):579-99.
15. Wischmeyer PE. Tailoring nutrition therapy to illness and recovery. Crit Care. 2017;21(Suppl 3):316.
16. Martindale R, Patel JJ, Taylor B, Arabi YM, Warren M, McClave SA. Nutrition Therapy in Critically Ill Patients With Coronavirus Disease 2019. JPEN J Parenter Enteral Nutr. 2020;44(7):1174-84.
17. Carr A, Cullen K, Keeney C, Canning C, Mooney O, Chinseallaigh E, et al. Effectiveness of positive psychology interventions: A systematic review and meta-analysis. J Posit Psychol. 2021;16(6):749-69.

CHAPTER 31

Nutrition in the Critical Patient with Obesity

Anna Ferreira, Idiberto José, Zotarelli Filho, Durval Ribas Filho

INTRODUCTION

In the context of chronic diseases, it is observed that patients in the intensive care unit (ICU) are increasingly living with obesity, with an incidence of up to 40%.[1] Worldwide, it is estimated that 1.6 billion adults are overweight, and currently, at least 400 million are obese. In the United States, the number of individuals living with obesity has greatly increased in the last two decades. More than 16 million Americans are extremely obese.[2,3] Obesity is an important public health problem. Today, it is one of the main causes of preventable death. Recent research has determined that obesity-related medical cost in the United States is now $168,000 trillion per year or 17% of the total United States medical costs.[4,5]

In 2000, obesity with a body mass index (BMI) above 30 kg/m² was a disease with a global reach, increasing health risks.[6] As the prevalence of obesity continues to increase, the number of obese and obese morbid patients admitted to ICUs continues to increase as well. They are at higher risk of morbidity and mortality than nonobese patients. They will require specialized nutritional therapy that contributes to their overall recovery.[7,8]

The coronavirus disease 2019 (COVID-19) pandemic shows us the risks of obesity for the general population, the complex presentation, and the clinical needs of patients with obesity. Approximately, 50.8% of patients diagnosed with COVID-19 had obesity,[9-11] implying the worsening of obesity comorbidities. It is necessary to understand the mechanisms by which obese patients are at greater risk of developing severe forms of the disease, even death. In this sense, immunity plays a decisive role in severe acute respiratory syndrome coronavirus 2 (SARS-CoV-2) infection. The lack of regulation and the excessive immune response to the viral stimulus produce proinflammatory cytokines in an exacerbated way (cytokine storm), reaching the state of hyperinflammation, with consequent damage to various tissues of the obese.[11]

Also, studies highlight that obesity can implicate hypertension, cardiovascular diseases, dyslipidemia, type II diabetes, atherosclerosis, obstructive sleep, osteoarthritis, stroke, and some forms of cancer, among others. In people with a BMI between 18 and 25 kg/m² (ideal weight), there are about 8.0% of diabetics. In individuals with a BMI above 40 kg/m² (severe obesity), this percentage reaches 43.0%.[12]

According to the last assessment carried out by International Federation for the Surgery of Obesity and Metabolic Disorders (ISFO) in 2017, obesity is an important predictor for the development of several types of cancer, with increased risk with each BMI gain of 5 kg/m². One of the main causes of obesity is an imbalance in energy balance. International recommendations to reduce the incidence and prevalence of obesity are the adoption of a balanced diet and the regular practice of physical activity.[13]

Besides, available nutritional guidelines are inconsistent, presenting challenges for calculating caloric and protein needs, patients with obesity may be less likely to receive malnutrition screening, assessment, and diagnosis; stigma and bias may influence the quality of care provided; they may present with altered pharmacokinetics and/or response to supplementation; the excess adiposity may present a challenge to accurate nutrition-focused physical examination; bariatric equipment may not be available; sarcopenia may be underrecognized in this patient population; and the repositioning and ambulation may be more difficult for nursing staff to perform—all these points adding to the associated comorbidities.[14]

The objectives of nutritional therapy are to prevent morbidity and mortality directly attributable to macro- and micronutrient deficiency and to minimize the loss of lean body mass. There are clinical challenges in nutritional therapy to improve the anabolic of proteins, avoid the aggravation of the premorbid complications of obesity and hypoglycemia, avoid overfeeding, avoid further accumulation of fat mass, set nutritional goals, etc.[1,13]

Therefore, this chapter aims to describe the main considerations of nutritional importance as a fundamental basis for the treatment of critically ill and obese patients.

SCREENING AND ASSESSMENT

Malnutrition screening and assessment is a key challenge in patients with overweight and obesity, and it may not be routinely performed. Malnutrition as a diagnosis may be underestimated for these patients. In calculating nutritional risk, BMI cannot be considered the only indicator of poor outcomes, especially among critically ill patients with obesity.[14] Tools, such as the Malnutrition Universal Screening Tool (MUST), which include BMI as a risk marker, may be of limited value.[15-19] **Table 1** highlights the World Health Organization (WHO) classification for obesity based on BMI, evidencing the risk of diseases.[20]

In this context, regarding the cause of obesity, there is a complex relationship between biological, psychosocial, and behavioral factors, which include genetic composition, socioeconomic status, and cultural influences. In addition, obesity

TABLE 1: BMI analysis to classify obesity according to WHO.

Diagnosis	BMI (kg/m²)	Disease risk WC (cm)* Males ≤94 Females ≤80	Disease risk WC (cm)* Male >94 Female >80
Under weight	<18.5	–	–
Normal weight	18.5–24.9	–	–
Overweight	25–29.9	Augmented	Augmented
Moderate obesity	30–34.9	High	High
Severe obesity	35–39.9 ≥40	Very high Extremely high	Very high Extremely high

*The risk of disease may vary according to the distribution of fat in waist circumference (WC).
(BMI: body mass index; WHO: World Health Organization)

has been associated with microorganisms, epigenetics, increased maternal age, higher fertility, lack of sleep, endocrine disruptors, pharmaceutical iatrogenesis, and intrauterine and intergenerational effects.[14,17]

Comorbid conditions and their treatments may also be a factor in the development of obesity. To date, the best noninvasive interventions have been in food management and behavior change. The best results are associated with bariatric surgery. Drug therapy has limited efficacy, particularly in children. Genetic testing applies to a small group of obese patients.[14]

A J-shaped relationship between BMI and mortality was demonstrated, with overweight and moderate obesity being protective, compared with normal BMI or more severe obesity in ICU patients. Despite this protective effect on mortality, in the setting of critical illness, morbidity is impaired with an increased risk of respiratory and cardiovascular complications, requiring adapted management. Obesity is associated with an increased risk of infection, requiring adapted drug dosage and nutrition, and is associated with logistical and diagnostic challenges. Furthermore, negative attitudes toward obese patients (the social stigma of obesity) affect both healthcare professionals and patients.[21]

ENERGY AND PROTEIN NEEDS

There are still information gaps regarding the best nutritional treatment for patients with obesity and in a critical phase in the ICU.[22] Low muscle mass (sarcopenia) occurs mainly with aging and may be associated with critically ill patients and with high BMI.[23] Enteral nutritional therapy is the most indicated in any type of body constitution.[23-25]

In this context, analyzing caloric and protein needs in obese and sick patients is a challenge.

In addition, for metabolic syndrome, more rigorous monitoring of hyperglycemia and hyperlipidemia is required. International guidelines recommend calculating resting energy expenditure with indirect calorimetry in obese patients, but calculations often remain an estimate of energy expenditure.[22]

The guidelines of the American Society for Parenteral and Enteral Nutrition (ASPEN) recommend that 65–70% of resting energy expenditure be administered to individuals with obesity, recommending the use of 11–14 kcal/kg of actual weight/day (for BMI 30–50 kg/m^2) or 22–25 kcal/kg ideal body weight/day (for BMI >50 kg/m^2) to calculate this target **(Table 2)**.[24] The guidelines of the European Society for Clinical Nutrition and Metabolism (ESPEN)[22] recommend 20–25 kcal/kg of adjusted body weight/day without additional adjustments below resting energy expenditure in obese individuals **(Table 2)**. Still, the protein concentration for individuals with chronic diseases and obesity is also controversial. The ASPEN guidelines suggest a hypocaloric–hypercaloric diet with 2.0–2.5 g/kg ideal body weight/day,[24] while the ESPEN guidelines recommend 1.3 g/kg adjusted body weight/day **(Table 2)**.[22]

In addition, in obese individuals admitted to the ICU, the use of ketone bodies can reduce the percentage of protein oxidation that contributes to the basal metabolic rate. Therefore, energy storage in adipose tissue may reduce muscle wasting during critical illness.[26] In critically obese and elderly patients, a low-calorie, high-protein diet may increase blood urea concentrations.[27] The ESPEN guidelines recommend the assessment of lean body mass and nitrogen balance in obese patients, while no specific recommendations are provided for monitoring and managing glucose, urea, or triglycerides.[28]

TABLE 2: The ESPEN and the ASPEN guidelines for nutritional therapy in chronically ill and obese individuals.

	ESPEN guidelines[28]	ASPEN guidelines[29]
For calculating the energy target if measurement of REE is not possible		
In general	20–25 kcal/kg actual BW/day below 70% of REE should be given during "early" acute phase	25–30 kcal/kg actual BW/day
In obese	• Same as above, but calculated according to adjusted BW* • If REE measured, set target to 80–100% of REE after the early acute phase (within days 3–7)	• 11–14 kcal/kg actual BW/day if BMI 30–50 kg/m² • 22–25 kcal/kg ideal BW[†]/day if BMI >50 kg/m² • If REE measured, set target to 65–70% of REE
For calculating protein target		
In general	1.3 g/kg actual BW/day	1.2–2.0 g/kg actual BW/day
In obese	Same as above, but calculated with adjusted BW*	2.0–2.5 g/kg ideal BW[†]/day
For adjustment of nutritional therapy according to serum markers[‡]		
Glucose	Below 10 mmol/L (180 g/L), consider lowering carbohydrate administration, when >6 U insulin/h is needed for >24 hours	Below 10 mmol/L (180 g/L)
Urea	Consider lowering protein administration if >30 mmol/L; probably only justified if protein administration >1.5 g/kg BW/day	
Triglycerides	Investigate and consider lowering fat administration if >5.6 mmol/L	
Examples for calculating energy and protein targets in obese[§]		
Example 1: Male 120 kg, 185 cm ≥ BMI = 35.1 kg/m² (ideal BW[†] = 77 kg[†] and adjusted BW* 86–88 kg)		
Energy target	Calculated with adjusted BW* 25 kcal × 86–88 kg target = 2,150–2,200 kcal/day	Calculated with actual BW 14 kcal × 120 kg target = 1,680 kcal/day
Protein target	Calculated with adjusted BW* 1.3 g × 92–96 kg, target = 120–125 g/day	Calculated with ideal BW[†] 2.0–2.5 g × 77 kg, target = 154–193 g/day
Example 2: Female 140 kg, 165 cm ≥ BMI = 51.5 kg/m² (ideal BW[†]: 53 kg and adjusted BW* = 70–75 kg)		
Energy target	Calculated with adjusted BW* 25 kcal × 70–75 kg target = 1,750–1,875 kcal/day	Calculated with ideal BW[†] 25 kcal × 53 kg target = 1,325 kcal/day
Protein target	Calculated with adjusted BW* 1.3 g × 70–75 kg target = 91–98 g/day	Calculated with ideal BW[†] 2.0–2.5 g × 53 kg target = 106–133 g/day

*Adjusted BW = Ideal BW + 20–25% of difference between actual and ideal BW (actual BW − ideal BW).
[†]Ideal BW: For males: 0.9 × (height in cm − 100); for females: 0.9 × (height in cm − 106) suggested in ESPEN guidelines, no specific suggestion for calculating ideal BW in ASPEN guidelines.
[‡]No difference in guideline targets regardless of whether applied to normal weight or obese individuals.
[§]The upper level of suggested energy targets in kcal/BW/day is taken as a basis for calculations.
(ASPEN: American Society for Parenteral and Enteral Nutrition; BW: body weight; ESPEN: European Society for Clinical Nutrition and Metabolism; REE: resting energy expenditure)

MICRONUTRIENTS

Obesity is characterized by a nutritional imbalance with an inadequate intake of minerals, such as iron, calcium, magnesium, zinc, and copper, in addition to vitamin folate, vitamins A, D, and B_{12}.[30-33] It is known that micronutrients act as cofactors for the functioning of enzymes and modulation of metabolism,[31,34] causing health complications, such as birth defects, learning difficulties, immune dysfunction, cancer, cardiovascular diseases, defective defense mechanisms, osteoporosis, neurodegenerative disorders, malfunction of the intestinal microbiota, deterioration in the functionality of most organs and systems, and the aggravation of many diseases.[17]

Also, micronutrients play roles in fat and carbohydrate metabolism, glucose metabolic pathways, the insulin signaling cascade, and pancreatic β-cell function.[30,32,34,35] Thus, an unbalanced diet leads to nutritional deficiencies in obesity with low amounts of dietary fiber, protein, micronutrients, and phytochemicals.[30] Added to this, ultra-processed foods (UPFs) account for more than 60% of dietary energy intake and nearly 90% of added sugars in the US adult diets.[36-38]

Furthermore, obese patients have greater needs for zinc, magnesium, chromium, manganese, and vanadium due to the involvement of these minerals in the metabolism of carbohydrates and fats.[30,39] Thus, individuals with obesity are more likely to develop nutritional deficiencies.[32] Furthermore, increased adipose tissue and systemic inflammation may impair absorption, distribution, metabolism, and elimination of micronutrients.[30,31] In this sense, as an example, certain minerals and lipophilic vitamins such as vitamins D and A can be absorbed in adipose tissue, reducing bioavailability for metabolically active tissues.[31,32]

In this sense, individuals with obesity have deficiencies of water-soluble vitamins, such as thiamine (B1), folic acid, and ascorbic acid.[32] Also, elevated levels of triglycerides, cholesterol, and free fatty acids in the bloodstream of obese individuals may affect the distribution of protein-bound micronutrients (enzymes). Furthermore, minerals with chemical similarities to other compounds in the food matrix may compete for transport proteins or other absorption mechanisms.[30,31,39]

In this context, the authors Guan et al.[39] evaluated nutritional deficiencies in Chinese patients undergoing Roux-en-Y gastric bypass (RYGB) and sleeve gastrectomy (SG), showing severe vitamin D deficiency (78.8%), followed by vitamin B_1 (39.2%), vitamin B_6 (28.0%), folate (26.8%), vitamin C (18.0%), transferrin (11.6%), and phosphorus (11.5%). In a preoperative analysis of 200 candidates for bariatric surgery, the authors Pellegrini et al.[40] found that 85.5% of the patients had a deficiency of at least one micronutrient, highlighting the deficiency of vitamin D (74.5%), folate (33.5%), iron (32%), calcium (13%), vitamin B_{12} (10%), and albumin (5.5%).

Moreover, Asghari et al.[41] studied the micronutrient level of morbidly obese individuals for bariatric surgery and deficiencies were identified for vitamin D (53.6%), vitamin B_{12} (34.4%), and serum iron (10.2%). In another study carried out with 1,732 individuals with morbid obesity, the data showed a high frequency of micronutrient deficiency, with 63.2% of the patients presenting folic acid deficiency (<5.3 ng/mL), 97.5% in vitamin D (<75 nmol/L), 9.6% iron (ferritin <15 μg/L), 6.2% vitamin A (<1.05 μmol/L), and 5.1% vitamin B_{12} (<188 pg/mL).[42]

McKay et al.[31] found associations between increased BMI and low serum micronutrient levels in overweight and obese Australian adults compared to clinical micronutrient benchmarks. Significant relationships were found for vitamin D, folate, magnesium, and potassium.

GUIDELINES

Current guidelines recommend a low-calorie, high-protein nutritional regimen for patients with obesity and critical illness. The impact of advancing age presents unique challenges in that a higher protein intake is required to overcome the anabolic resistance associated with aging in the face of presumed decreased kidney function.[1]

According to ESPEN, previous guidelines for providing the best medical nutritional therapy for critically ill patients have been updated. These guidelines define who are at-risk patients, how to assess the nutritional status of a patient admitted to the ICU, how to define the amount of energy to supply, the route to be chosen, and how to adapt according to different clinical conditions. It also describes when to start and how to progress in managing an adequate supply of nutrients. Better determination of the amount and nature of carbohydrates, fats, and proteins is suggested. Special attention is paid to fatty acids, glutamine, and omega-3. Particular conditions often seen in intensive care, such as patients with dysphagia, frail patients, polytrauma patients, abdominal surgery, sepsis, and obesity, are discussed to guide the practitioner toward the best evidence-based therapy.[28]

Based on this and other evidence, the 2022 ASPEN/Society of Critical Care Medicine (SCCM) guidelines suggest a low-calorie, high-protein diet for patients with obesity.[29] Specifically, based on expert consensus, the guidelines state, "if available, an enteral formula with a low caloric density and a reduced nonprotein calorie:nitrogen (NPC:N) ratio should be used in the obese adult ICU patient."[43]

Notably, the 2022 ESPEN guidelines did not recommend any specific tool to be used in critically ill patients, and instead stated that "every critically ill patient who stays for more than 48 hours in the ICU should be considered at risk of malnutrition."[28] Meanwhile, the 2022 ASPEN and SCCM, as well as updated ASPEN guidelines do not address the topic.[26] None of the guidelines specifically highlight whether or how screening and assessment practices should differ for patients with obesity.

CONCLUSION

It was concluded that patients with chronic diseases in the ICU are increasingly obese. Obesity negatively alters the micronutrient status of individuals through an inadequate intake of minerals, such as iron, calcium, magnesium, zinc, and copper, as well as vitamins. Nutritional therapy can prevent morbidity and mortality directly attributable to macro- and micronutrient deficiencies and minimize body mass loss. International guidelines recommend measuring resting energy expenditure with indirect calorimetry in obese patients. There are still information gaps between the ASPEN and the ESPEN regarding optimal nutritional therapy for patients with obesity and critical illness.

REFERENCES

1. Dickerson RN, Andromalos L, Brown JC, Correia MITD, Pritts W, Ridley EJ, et al. Obesity and critical care nutrition: current practice gaps and directions for future research. Crit Care. 2022;26(1):283.
2. Flegal KM, Carroll MD, Ogden CL, Curtin LR. Prevalence and trends in obesity among US adults, 1999-2008. JAMA. 2010;303:235-41.

3. The Centers for Disease Control and Prevention. Overweight & Obesity. [online] Available from: http://www.cdc.gov/obesity [Last accessed August, 2023].
4. Mokdad AH, Marks JS, Stroup DF, Gerberding JL. Actual causes of death in the USA, 2000. JAMA. 2004;291(10):1238-45.
5. Cawley J, Meyerhoefer C. The medical care costs of obesity: An instrumental variables approach. Working Paper No. 16467. National Bureau of Economic Research. 2010.
6. Obesity: Preventing and managing the global epidemic. Report of a WHO consultation. World Health Organ Tech Rep Ser. 2000;894:i-xii, 1-253.
7. Nasraway Jr SA, Albert M, Donnelly AM, Ruthazer R, Shikora SA, Saltzman E. Morbid obesity is an independent determinant of death among surgical critically ill patients. Crit Care Med. 2006;34:964-70.
8. Alexopoulos AS, Fayfman M, Zhao L, Weaver J, Buehler L, Smiley D, et al. Impact of obesity on hospital complications and mortality in hospitalized patients with hyperglycemia and diabetes. BMJ Open Diabetes Res Care. 2016;4(1):e000200.
9. Barazzoni R, Bischoff SC, Busetto L, Cederholm T, Chourdakis M, Cuerda C, et al. Nutritional management of individuals with obesity and COVID-19: ESPEN expert statements and practical guidance. Clin Nutr. 2021;41(12):2869-86.
10. Zhang X, Lewis AM, Moley JR, Brestoff JR. A systematic review and meta-analysis of obesity and COVID-19 outcomes. Sci Rep. 2021;11(1):7193.
11. Noor FM, Islam MM. Prevalence and associated risk factors of mortality among COVID-19 patients: a meta-analysis. J Commun Health. 2020;45(6):1270-82.
12. Tutor AW, Lavie CJ, Kachur S, Milani RV, Ventura HO. Updates on obesity and the obesity paradox in cardiovascular diseases. Prog Cardiovasc Dis. 2023;78:2-10.
13. Bischoff SC, Barazzoni R, Busetto L, Campmans-Kuijpers M, Cardinale V, Chermesh I, et al. European Guideline on Obesity Care in Patients with Gastrointestinal and Liver Diseases—Joint ESPEN/UEG guideline. Clin Nutr. 2022;41(10):2364-405.
14. Pohlenz-Saw JAE, Merriweather JL, Wandrag L. (Mal)nutrition in critical illness and beyond: a narrative review. Anaesthesia. 2023;78(6):770-8.
15. National Institute for Health and Care Excellence (NICE). (2017). Nutrition support for adults: Oral nutrition support, enteral tube feeding, and parenteral nutrition. [online] Available from: https://www.nice.org.uk/guidance/cg32 [Last accessed August, 2023].
16. Gonzalez MC, Correia MITD, Heymsfield SB. A requiem for BMI in the clinical setting. Curr Opin Clin Nutr Metab Care. 2017;20(5):314-21.
17. Kesari A, Noel JY. Nutritional Assessment. In: StatPearls [Internet]. Treasure Island (FL): StatPearls Publishing; 2023.
18. Eisenberg D, Shikora SA, Aarts E, Aminian A, Angrisani L, Cohen RV, et al. 2022 American Society of Metabolic and Bariatric Surgery (ASMBS) and International Federation for the Surgery of Obesity and Metabolic Disorders (IFSO) Indications for Metabolic and Bariatric Surgery. Obes Surg. 2023;33(1):3-14.
19. Di Renzo L, Itani L, Gualtieri P, Pellegrini M, El Ghoch M, De Lorenzo A. New BMI cut-off points for obesity in middle-aged and older adults in clinical nutrition settings in Italy: a cross-sectional study. Nutrients. 2022;14(22):4848.
20. Duke T, AlBuhairan FS, Agarwal K, Arora NK, Arulkumaran S, Bhutta ZA, et al. STAGE (Strategic Technical Advisory Group of Experts). World Health Organization and knowledge translation in maternal, newborn, child and adolescent health and nutrition. Arch Dis Child. 2022;107(7):644-9.
21. Schetz M, De Jong A, Deane AM, Druml W, Hemelaar P, Pelosi P, et al. Obesity in the critically ill: a narrative review. Intensive Care Med. 2019;45(6):757-69.
22. Singer P, Blaser AR, Berger MM, Alhazzani W, Calder PC, Casaer MP. ESPEN guideline on clinical nutrition in the intensive care unit. Clin Nutr. 2019;38(1):48-79.
23. Ji Y, Cheng B, Xu Z, Ye H, Lu W, Luo X, et al. Impact of sarcopenic obesity on 30-day mortality in critically ill patients with intra-abdominal sepsis. J Crit Care. 2018;46:50-4.
24. McClave SA, Taylor BE, Martindale RG, Warren MM, Johnson DR, Braunschweig C, et al. Guidelines for the provision and assessment of nutrition support therapy in the adult critically ill patient: Society of Critical Care Medicine

(SCCM) and American Society for Parenteral and Enteral Nutrition (ASPEN). J Parenter Enteral Nutr. 2016;40:159-211.
25. Reintam Blaser A, Starkopf J, Alhazzani W, Berger MM, Casaer MP, Deane AM, et al. Early enteral nutrition in critically ill patients: ESICM Clinical Practice Guidelines. Intensive Care Med. 2017;43:380-98.
26. Goossens C, Vander Perre S, Van den Berghe G, Langouche L. Proliferation and differentiation of adipose tissue in prolonged lean and obese critically ill patients. Intensive Care Med Exp. 2017;5:16.
27. Dickerson RN, Medling TL, Smith AC, Maish GO 3rd, Croce MA, Minard G, et al. Hypocaloric, high-protein nutrition therapy in older vs younger critically ill patients with obesity. J Parenter Enteral Nutr. 2013;37:342-51.
28. Bischoff SC, Bager P, Escher J, Forbes A, Hébuterne X, Hvas CL, et al. ESPEN Guideline on Clinical Nutrition in Inflammatory Bowel Disease. Clin Nutr. 2023;42(3):352-79.
29. Adika E, Jia R, Li J, Seres D, Freedberg DE. Evaluation of the ASPEN Guidelines For Refeeding Syndrome Among Hospitalized Patients Receiving Enteral Nutrition: a retrospective cohort study. J Parenter Enteral Nutr. 2022;46(8):1859-66.
30. Astrup A, Bügel S. Overfed but undernourished: recognizing nutritional inadequacies/deficiencies in patients with overweight or obesity. Int J Obes. 2019;43:219-32.
31. McKay J, Ho S, Jane M, Pal S. Overweight and Obese. Australian Adults and Micronutrient Deficiency. BMC Nutr. 2020;6:12.
32. Lapik IA, Galchenko AV, Gapparova KM. Micronutrient status in obese patients: a narrative review. Obes Med. 2020;18:100224.
33. Huizar MI, Arena R, Laddu DR. The Global Food Syndemic: The Impact of Food Insecurity, Malnutrition and Obesity on the Health Span Amid the COVID-19 Pandemic. Prog Cardiovasc Dis. 2021;64:105-7.
34. Dapkekar A, Deshpande P, Oak MD, Paknikar KM, Rajwade JM. Getting more micronutrients from wheat and barley through agronomic biofortification. In: Gupta OP, Pandey V, Narwal S, Sharma P, Ram S, Singh GP (Eds). Wheat and Barley Grain Biofortification. Duxford, UK: Woodhead Publishing; 2020. pp. 53-99.
35. Kaur T, Rana KL, Kour D, Sheikh I, Yadav N, Kumar V, et al. Microbe-mediated biofortification for micronutrients: present status and future challenges. In: Rastegari AA, Yadav AN, Yadav N (Eds). New and Future Developments in Microbial Biotechnology and Bioengineering. Amsterdam, The Netherlands: Elsevier; 2020. pp. 1-17.
36. Gupta S, Hawk T, Aggarwal A, Drewnowski A. Characterizing ultra-processed foods by energy density, nutrient density, and cost. Front Nutr. 2019;6:70.
37. Khandpur N, Neri DA, Monteiro C, Mazur A, Frelut ML, Boyland E, et al. Ultra-processed food consumption among the paediatric population: an overview and call to action from the European Childhood Obesity Group. Ann Nutr Metab. 2020;76:109-13.
38. Malik VS, Hu FB. The Role of Sugar-Sweetened Beverages in the Global Epidemics of Obesity and Chronic Diseases. Nat Rev Endocrinol. 2022;18:205-18.
39. Guan B, Yang J, Chen Y, Yang W, Wang C. Nutritional deficiencies in chinese patients undergoing gastric bypass and sleeve gastrectomy: prevalence and predictors. Obes Surg. 2018;28:2727-36.
40. Pellegrini M, Rahimi F, Boschetti S, Devecchi A, De Francesco A, Mancino MV, et al. Preoperative micronutrient deficiencies in patients with severe obesity candidates for bariatric surgery. J Endocrinol Investig. 2021;44:1413-23.
41. Asghari G, Khalaj A, Ghadimi M, Mahdavi M, Farhadnejad H, Valizadeh M, et al. Prevalence of micronutrient deficiencies prior to bariatric surgery: Tehran Obesity Treatment Study (TOTS). Obes Surg. 2018;28:2465-72.
42. Krzizek EC, Brix JM, Herz CT, Kopp HP, Schernthaner GH, Schernthaner G, et al. Prevalence of micronutrient deficiency in patients with morbid obesity before bariatric surgery. Obes Surg. 2018;28:643-8.
43. Compher C, Bingham AL, McCall M, Patel J, Rice TW, Braunschweig C, et al. Guidelines for the provision of nutrition support therapy in the adult critically ill patient: The American Society for Parenteral and Enteral Nutrition. J Parenter Enteral Nutr. 2022;46(1):12-41.

CHAPTER 32

Nutrition in Critically Ill Patients with Liver Dysfunction and Failure

Keerti Brar, Rahul Harne, Sweta J Patel

INTRODUCTION

Cirrhotic patients are likely to be malnourished which by definition could include patients that are either undernourished or overnourished (obese). Increased severity of liver failure and a higher rate of complications are seen in patients with cirrhosis who are malnourished. It is imperative to provide cirrhotic patients a dedicated nutritional assessment with nutritional counseling and dietary advice. Nutritional management is vital to improve the survival and quality of life.

Deficiencies, excesses, or imbalances in intake of energy and/or nutrients are commonly seen in cirrhotic patients which put them at a higher risk of morbidity and mortality. Not only underweight, but also obese cirrhotic patients exhibit muscle mass depletion, also known as sarcopenic obesity. This could easily be clinically overlooked. Morbid obesity in itself is a strong contributor to morbidity and mortality in patients with cirrhosis. It is not a surprise that most of the data on malnutrition in cirrhosis focuses solely on undernutrition, but strong emphasis must be put on overnutrition as both contribute to poor outcome in decompensated cirrhosis.

PREVALENCE AND CAUSES OF MALNUTRITION IN CIRRHOSIS

Malnutrition, being one of the most common complications associated with cirrhosis, is reported in majority of patients with advanced decompensated cirrhosis (Child's C). It is a major contributor to hospitalizations and mortality before or after liver transplantation.

The pathogenesis and factors contributing to malnutrition are complex and multifactorial. Pathogenic factors are broadly categorized into three groups:[1]
1. First, inadequate intake due to anorexia, abnormal taste secondary to zinc deficiency, dietary restrictions advised by physicians, socioeconomic factors, alcohol intake, chronic encephalopathy, patient kept fasting for investigations, coexistent pancreatitis in alcoholics, ascites, and splenomegaly causing early satiety.
2. Second, contributing factor is poor absorption due to decreased bile salt pool, intestinal congestion secondary to portal hypertension, pancreatic insufficiency, and bacterial overgrowth.
3. Third, pathogenic factor is the patient being in a catabolic state (raised energy expenditure).

SCREENING FOR MALNUTRITION IN PATIENTS WITH CHRONIC LIVER DISEASE

Formulating a comprehensive nutritional assessment guide helps us in identifying protein-energy malnutrition and other macro- and micronutrient deficiencies which are commonly missed. Stepwise evaluation includes thorough history taking, physical examination, anthropometric assessment and finally reviewing laboratory parameters. Since no single parameter is adequate to diagnose protein-energy malnutrition due to lack of sensitivity and specificity, it is advisable to utilize a combination of tools to achieve greater clinical efficacy.[1,3]

If the patient provides a history of unintentional weight loss, it could be suggestive of significant degree of protein energy malnutrition. However, confounding factors such as hydration status and dietary habits, and extracellular fluid accumulation or diuresis must be kept in mind.

Physical examination targets are to identify signs of dehydration, fluid retention and sarcopenia and typical manifestations of micronutrient deficiencies.

There are certain screening tools available to quantify the nutritional status of patients with cirrhosis. These tools include:[1,3,4]

- Anthropometric measurements (mid-arm muscle circumference, mid-arm muscle area, and subscapular skinfold thickness)
- *Body mass index (BMI):* BMI is an inaccurate tool for nutritional assessment in cirrhotic patients with fluid overload (ascites and edema) as BMI will be falsely higher in these patients. To remove the effect of fluid overload, take postparacentesis body weight or the weight recorded before fluid retention (if known), or subtract a percentage of weight, based on the severity of ascites (5% for mild; 10% for moderate, and 15% for severe ascites), with an additional 5% subtraction for bilateral pedal edema (if present).
- Handgrip strength using a handheld dynamometer.
- *Subjective global assessment (SGA):* Highly effective in assessing malnutrition in cirrhosis.
- Physical frailty (evaluated by the fried frailty index)
- Short physical performance battery
- Whole body dual-energy X-ray absorptiometry (DEXA)
- Tetrapolar bioelectrical impedance analysis (BIA)
- Royal free hospital subjective global assessment (RFH-SGA)

Subjective global assessment is a widely used tool to evaluate cirrhotic patients for malnutrition, but it would be wise to remember that SGA could miss established sarcopenia in cirrhotic patients.

SARCOPENIA: EVALUATION AND OUTCOMES

Sarcopenia could be classified as either primary (age-related) or secondary (disease-associated); it is an innate part of malnutrition and is defined as reduction in muscle mass and function. The mechanisms leading to sarcopenia include decreased protein and calorie intake, alterations in amino acid profiles, endotoxemia, decreased mobility of patients, and hyperammonemia.

Quantification of the muscle loss can be done using computed tomographic assessment/estimation of the muscle mass at the level of L3 vertebra. As metabolic fluctuations in cirrhotic patients consistently impact Psoas and the paraspinal muscles, they serve as a confirmatory site for sarcopenia evaluation. One added benefit with this area is the minimal impact fluid status has on these muscles since it acts as a confounding factor. Sarcopenia could be routinely identified during computed tomography (CT) screening done for hepatocellular carcinoma, portal vein patency, and pretransplant workup.[7,11,12]

Muscle dimensions widely used to stratify cirrhotic sarcopenic patients are 50 cm^2/m^2 for men and 39 cm^2/m^2 for women; although, the exact range could vary based on country and center protocols.[11,12]

Presence of sarcopenia strongly indicates probability of poor outcomes and decreased survival in patients with cirrhosis. In addition, it is an independent predictor of mortality and morbidity in post liver transplant patients as it is a direct contributor to infections, increased ventilatory requirement and an increased duration of intensive care unit (ICU) stay. Encouraging supplemental nutrition, routine exercise, and physical activity along with anabolic steroids and ammonia correcting modalities could be of help.

NUTRITIONAL SCREENING

Nutritional screening helps in risk stratification of cirrhotic patients and provides a guide to further intervention.

Patients in the liver transplant waitlist with BMI <18.5 kg/m^2 or BMI >40 kg/m^2 along with patients who fall in the Child–Turcotte–Pugh (CTP) C category have overt malnutrition. These patients fall in the severe malnutrition category and require no further risk stratification, optimization of nutrition is the way ahead.

Patients with cirrhosis which do not fit the high risk of malnutrition bar need further evaluation. Three tools are present the armory of the clinician to consolidate findings of malnutrition, the Royal Free Hospital-Nutritional Prioritizing Tool (RFH-NPT), the Nutrition Risk Screening-2002 (NRS-2002) and the Liver Disease Undernutrition Screening Tool (LDUST) **(Table 1)**.

Most exemplary evidence-based tool for nutritional screening in cirrhosis is RFH-NPT. It classifies patients into low-, medium-, and high-risk. Complications in cirrhotic patients such as ascites, hepatorenal syndrome and hepatic encephalopathy are incorporated in the RFH-NPT scoring in the form of suggestive questions **(Flowchart 1)**.

Nutritional Requirements in Cirrhosis

Cirrhosis is a catabolic state wherein there is reduced protein synthesis along with over-emphasis on proteolysis; this physiological change occurs to fuel gluconeogenesis. This catabolic state explains the need for higher intake of total energy and proteins in patients with cirrhosis.

Resting energy expenditure (REE) in a healthy adult is 1 kcal/kg body weight/hour, that adds up to 24 kcal/kg/day. Although the gold standard to measure REE is indirect calorimetry, it is not readily accessible in most setups. A handheld calorimeter serves the same purpose and is more readily available.[2,5,6,8]

In cirrhotic yet hemodynamically stable patients, the total energy expenditure (TEE)

TABLE 1: Nutritional screening.

Nutritional screening	Overt malnutrition/high risk of malnutrition: • BMI of <18.5 kg/m^2 • BMI >40 kg/m^2 • Child–Pugh C disease
	Nutrition screening tests for other cirrhosis patients: • Royal Free Hospital-Nutritional Prioritizing Tool (RFH-NPT) • Nutrition Risk Screening-2002 (NRS-2002) • Liver Disease Undernutrition Screening Tool (LDUST)[1]

CHAPTER 32 | Nutrition in Critically Ill Patients with Liver Dysfunction and Failure

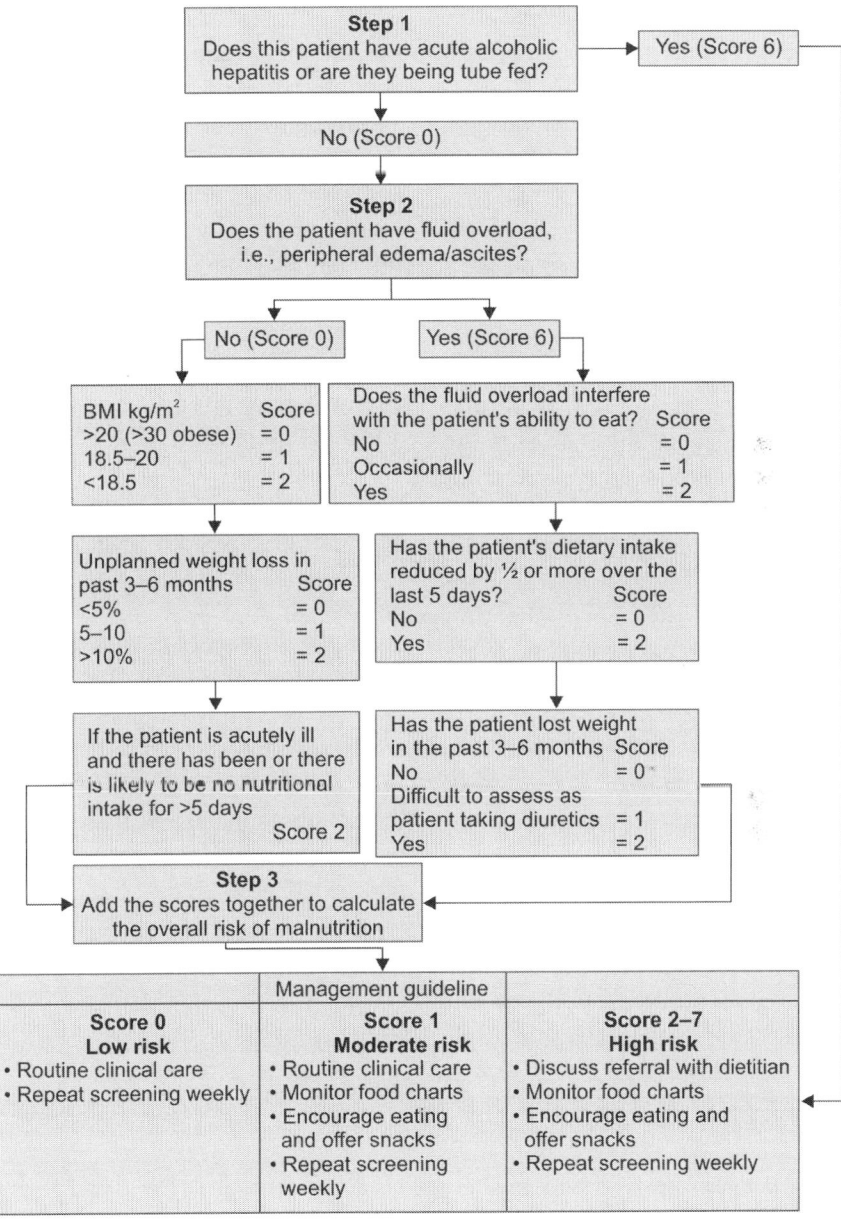

Flowchart 1: Royal Free Hospital-Nutritional Prioritizing Tool (RFH-NP).

for a sedentary lifestyle amounts to 1.3 times the estimated REE [i.e., 32 kcal/kg/day (range 30–35 kcal/kg/day)].

Total energy expenditure calculation mandates including the dry weight of the patient. Methods to derive dry weight in patients with ascites or edema are as follows: (i) Using preascites weight, (ii) Calculating ideal body weight (IBW) based on height; the ideal BMI for Indian population ranges from 18 to 22.9 kg/m^2, (iii) Postparacentesis weight, or (iv) empirically corrected bodyweight by subtracting a percentage of weight based on severity of ascites (mild, 5%; moderate, 10%; and severe, 15%). Additional 5% subtracted in patients with pedal edema.

Daily protein requirement in patients with cirrhosis is increased to 1.2 g/kg in the absence of malnutrition or 1.5 g/kg in the presence of malnutrition.

FRAILTY INDEX

Physical frailty accounts for multiple factors involved in patients' health and overall physical capacity and strength. Although sarcopenia is a critical component of frailty, frailty index also includes muscle function and the patient's strength and ease of functioning in day-to-day activities. Physical frailty plays an imperative role in post-transplant mortality, mortality after hospitalization, hospital length of stay, and overall recovery. Multiple frailty tools are in use which have prognostic utility. Some of the target based and performance reviewing tools in use are the liver frailty index (LFI), 6-minute walk test, and cardiopulmonary exercise **(Table 2)**.

RECOMMENDATIONS

Nutritional screening is vital in all patients with cirrhosis as malnutrition is a contributing factor to poor outcomes both pre- and posttransplant. Patients that fall in the Child Pugh-C category with BMI <18.5 kg/m^2 or a BMI >40 kg/m^2 are at increased risk of malnutrition and require aggressive assessment and intervention.

Dietary intake needs to be assessed on the ground of quality and quantity of food consumed. In addition, fluids intake, sodium intake, and number and timing of meals must be screened.

Decreasing protein intake is not advisable in patients with hepatic encephalopathy as it exacerbates sarcopenia. Patients with cirrhosis have good tolerance to vegetable and dairy proteins.

The recommended daily energy intake in this subset of patients is 30–35 kcal/kg/day of actual bodyweight. Ideal routine protein intake needs to be 1.2–1.5 g/kg/day of actual bodyweight.

If target protein intake is not achieved by routine diet, branched-chain amino acids (BCAA) as well as leucine-enriched amino acid supplements could be incorporated.[2,5]

Vitamin D deficiency is a major concern in this subset of patients, therefore, vitamin D levels must be checked and substitutes prescribed if required.

OBESITY IN CIRRHOSIS

Obesity is a common risk factor in illnesses such as diabetes, hypertension, chronic

TABLE 2: Liver frailty index (LFI)—components and formula.

Liver frailty index	Components: • *Dominant hand-grip strength:* The average of three attempts using a hand dynamometer • *Time to do five chair stands:* The time in seconds to stand up and down in a chair five times with the subject's arms folded across the chest • *Balance testing:* Measured as the number of seconds that the subject can balance in three positions (feet placed side to side, semi-tandem, and tandem) for a maximum of 10 seconds each
	Formula:[10] (−0.330 × gender-adjusted grip strength) + (−2.529 × number of chair stands per second) + (0.040 balance time) + 6

kidney disease, and cardiovascular disease which are poor prognostic factors in cirrhosis. It substantially increases risk of hepatocellular carcinoma, hepatic decompensation, and nonalcoholic steatohepatitis (NASH). There is a much higher chance of poor outcomes in both pre- and postoperative scenarios. Another factor to consider is the difficulty encountered in choosing a suitable live donor for morbidly obese patients since the risk of low graft to recipient ratio (GRWR) increases. In addition, risk of poor graft function and difficulty in postoperative care are concerns too.[9]

CONCLUSION

Cirrhotic patients are likely to be undernourished warranting thorough evaluation. Comprehensive nutritional assessment is a must as well as maintaining adequate protein and caloric intake.

REFERENCES

1. Puri P, Dhiman RK, Taneja S, Tandon P, Merli M, Anand AC, et al. Nutrition in Chronic Liver Disease: Consensus Statement of the Indian National Association for Study of the Liver. J Clin Exp Hepatol. 2021;11:97-143.
2. European Association for the Study of the Liver. Electronic address: easloffice@easloffice.eu; European Association for the Study of the Liver. EASL Clinical Practice Guidelines on nutrition in chronic liver disease. J Hepatol. 2019;70:172-93.
3. Sasidharan M, Nistala S, Narendhran RT, Murugesh M, Bhatia SJ, Rathi PM. Nutritional status and prognosis in cirrhotic patients. Trop Gastroenterol. 2012;33:257-64.
4. Alveras-da-Silva MR, Reverbelda Silveira T. Comparison between handgrip strength, subjective global assessment, and prognostic nutritional index in assessing malnutrition and predicting clinical outcome in cirrhotic outpatients. Nutrition. 2005;21:113-7.
5. Plauth M, Bernal W, Dasarathy S, Merli M, Plank LD, Schütz T, et al. ESPEN guideline on clinical nutrition in liver disease. Clin Nutr. 2019;38:485-521.
6. Mazurak VC, Tandon P, Montano-Loza AJ. Nutrition and the transplant candidate. Liver Transplant. 2017;23:1451-64.
7. Cruz-Jentoft AJ, Baeyens JP, Bauer JM, Boirie Y, Cederholm T, Landi F, et al. Sarcopenia: European consensus on definition and diagnosis: report of the European Working Group on Sarcopenia in Older People. Age Ageing. 2010;39:412-23.
8. Dasarathy S, Merli M. Sarcopenia from mechanism to diagnosis and treatment in liver disease. J Hepatol. 2016;65:1232-44.
9. Kumar N, Choudhary NS. Treating morbid obesity in cirrhosis: A quest of holy grail. World J Hepatol. 2015;7:2819-28.
10. Lai JC, Tandon P, Bernal W, Tapper EB, Ekong U, Dasarathy S, et al. Malnutrition, Frailty, and Sarcopenia in Patients With Cirrhosis: 2021 Practice Guidance by the American Association for the Study of Liver Diseases. Hepatology. 2021;74(3):1611-44.
11. Carey EJ, Lai JC, Wang CW, Dasarathy S, Lobach I, Montano-Loza AJ, et al. Fitness, Life Enhancement, and Exercise in Liver Transplantation Consortium. A multicenter study to define sarcopenia in patients with end-stage liver disease. Liver Transpl. 2017;23(5):625-33.
12. Giusto M, Lattanzi B, Albanese C, Galtieri A, Farcomeni A, Giannelli V, et al. Sarcopenia in liver cirrhosis: the role of computed tomography scan for the assessment of muscle mass compared with dual-energy X-ray absorptiometry and anthropometry. Eur J Gastroenterol Hepatol. 2015;27(3):328-34.

CHAPTER 33

Nutrition in Major Trauma and Burns

Khusrav Bajan, Shradha K Bajan

INTRODUCTION

Trauma and burns constitute inordinate patient conditions in the critical care unit needing specialized care. Since decades, nutrition has been a mainstay in the recovery and healing of critical care patients. Trauma due to road traffic accidents is the leading cause of death in India, and fourth leading cause reported worldwide.[1] India is the traumatic brain injury (TBI) capital of the world. Every 3 minutes, an Indian dies due to traffic accidents. In 2019, over 8.3 million burn cases were reported throughout the world, whereas India reports approximately 1 million burn cases every year.[2,3] With such high national and global burden of trauma and burn victims, it is imperative to identify critical treatment aspects, including medical, surgical, and adjunct interventions such as nutrition and early mobilization (physiorehabilitation), for positive outcomes and faster recovery of patients.

In trauma and burn patients, the extent of injuries proportionally increase metabolic rates which can last for over a year after injury. Consequently, the tremendous loss of lean body mass and malnutrition risk necessitates significant nutritional management. The hypermetabolism observed in trauma and burn patients are also associated with the intense tissue repair needs.[4,5] Though the physiological responses of stress and recovery phases are similar in trauma and burn cases, they are more severe in terms of basal energy expenditure, tissue damage, and stress in burn patients.[5] Therefore, as a nutritional management intervention, specific guidelines are prescribed for major trauma, severe burns, and other critically ill patients by many National and International Healthcare Societies. The European Society for Clinical Nutrition and Metabolism (ESPEN) and the American Society for Parenteral and Enteral Nutrition (ASPEN) are among the most recognized International Societies. The Indian Society for Parenteral and Enteral Nutrition (ISPEN), the Indian Society of Clinical Nutrition (INSCN), and the Indian Council of Medical Research–the National Institute of Nutrition (ICMR-NIN) are among the well-recognized National Societies for clinical research, quality control, and advanced education in clinical nutrition. It should be noted that all above guidelines do not have high evidence-based grades, and thus nutritional protocols should be tailored to the individual patient needs and physiological derangements **(Fig. 1)**.[6]

PHYSIOLOGICAL RESPONSES OBSERVED IN TRAUMA

In major trauma, there occurs an immediate cardiovascular response, followed by an inflammatory, immunological, and metabolic response **(Fig. 2)**. The inflammatory response may take few to several

Renal system
- Increased energy expenditure in chronic kidney failure
- Focus on hydration and electrolytes
- Loss of protein and micronutrients via RRT
- Calories via citrate in RRT

Preexisting malnutrition
- Early nutrition
- Micronutrient deficits
- Refeeding syndrome
- Outcome?

Obesity
- Diagnosis of malnutrition
- Substrate utilization
- Deranged metabolism
- Comorbidities and metabolic syndrome

Gastrointestinal tract
- Compromised anatomy with maldigestion and malabsorption
- Protection of GI anastomoses
- Loss of protein and micronutrients via open abdomen

Basic principles
- Every ICU-patient is at risk for malnutrition
- Regular screening for malnutrition
- Close monitoring and frequent adaptation of nutrition
- An early EN is preferred
- Micronutrients are mandatory if PN is necessary
- Individual adaptation

Central nervous system
- High risk for prolonged ICU-stay and iatrogenic malnutrition
- Dysphagia and aspiration
- Frequent GI dysmotility in deep sedation

Trauma/Burn
- High variability in energy expenditure
- Immunomodulating nutrients?

Sepsis/septic shock
- Early EN when hemodynamically stable (stable catecholamines and lactate)
- Metabolic and GI tolerance
- Disturbed substrate utilization

Cardiocirculatory system
- Frequent malnutrition and cachexia
- Prolonged ICU-stay and iatrogenic malnutrition
- Hemodynamic instability and variable volume demands
- GI-bleeding during systemic anticoagulation

Respiratory system
- Restrict fluids
- Avoid hyperalimentation
- Hypophosphatemia?

Elderly patients
- Malnutrition and micronutrient-deficits
- Comorbidities and frailty syndrome
- Anorexia and refusal to eat common
- Mobilization

Fig. 1: Key aspects of different trauma to be considered while deciding nutritional therapy.[6] (EN: enteral nutrition; GI: gastrointestinal; ICU: intensive care unit; PN: parenteral nutrition; RRT: renal replacement therapy)
Source: Adapted from Hill A, Elke G, Weimann A. Nutrition in the Intensive Care Unit—A Narrative Review. Nutrients. 2021;13(8):2851.

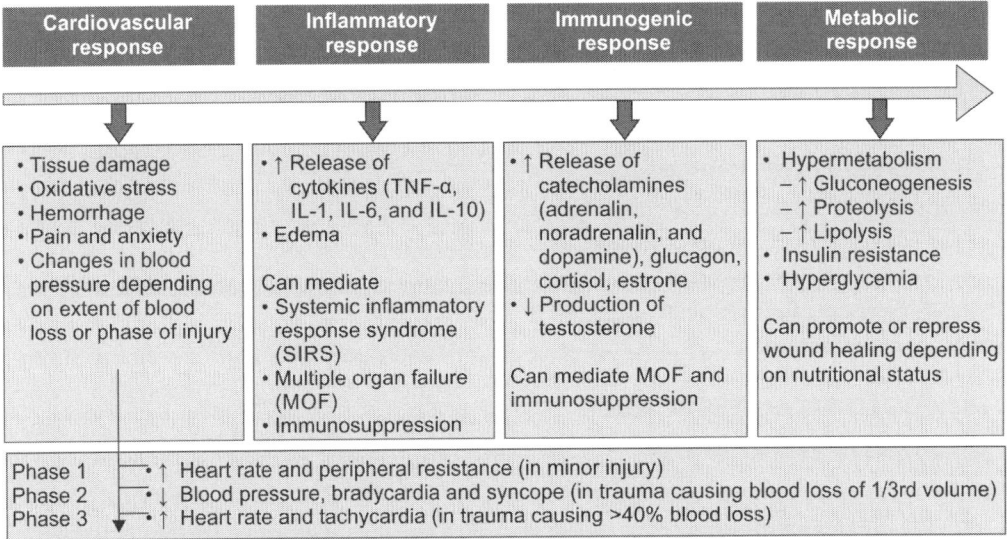

Cardiovascular response	Inflammatory response	Immunogenic response	Metabolic response

• Tissue damage
• Oxidative stress
• Hemorrhage
• Pain and anxiety
• Changes in blood pressure depending on extent of blood loss or phase of injury
	• ↑ Release of cytokines (TNF-α, IL-1, IL-6, and IL-10)
	• Edema
	
	Can mediate
	• Systemic inflammatory response syndrome (SIRS)
	• Multiple organ failure (MOF)
	• Immunosuppression
		• ↑ Release of catecholamines (adrenalin, noradrenalin, and dopamine), glucagon, cortisol, estrone
		• ↓ Production of testosterone
		
		Can mediate MOF and immunosuppression
			• Hypermetabolism
			  – ↑ Gluconeogenesis
			  – ↑ Proteolysis
			  – ↑ Lipolysis
			• Insulin resistance
			• Hyperglycemia
			
			Can promote or repress wound healing depending on nutritional status

Phase 1 — • ↑ Heart rate and peripheral resistance (in minor injury)
Phase 2 — • ↓ Blood pressure, bradycardia and syncope (in trauma causing blood loss of 1/3rd volume)
Phase 3 — • ↑ Heart rate and tachycardia (in trauma causing >40% blood loss)

Fig. 2: Physiological responses observed in trauma. (IL: interleukin; TNF: tumor necrosis factor)

hours for its onset depending on the extent of injury. Along with inflammatory cytokines, approximately 10-fold increase in catecholamines (adrenalin, noradrenalin, and dopamine) and corticosteroids are noted in trauma, which mediate stress as well as hypermetabolic response. The metabolism and tissue perfusion decreases for a short period in trauma patients, known as the "ebb phase" before entering the hypermetabolic and hyperdynamic state, known as the "flow phase".[7]

The flow phase increases whole-body oxygen consumption rate and causes >10% increase in resting energy expenditure (REE). This phase also determines the wound healing rate and depends largely on the nutritional status of patients. Particularly, the moderate or severe protein energy malnutrition impairs wound healing by interfering with new capillary formation, fibroblastic proliferation, production of proteoglycans, and collagen synthesis.[4,7] The loss of muscle mass occurs in trauma since the protein catabolism rate exceeds protein synthesis, where the catabolic products are used as substrates in wound healing mechanisms. The extent of injury thus determines the percent loss of muscle mass in trauma patients. In turn, the extent of muscle loss is linked to further physiological dysfunctions. For instance, reduced immune function is associated with 10% loss of muscle mass, whereas decreased wound healing and onset of severe infections are characteristic clinical representation observed at 20% and 30% loss of muscle mass, respectively. Muscle loss above 40% is fatal.[5]

PHYSIOLOGICAL RESPONSES OBSERVED IN BURNS

The intensity of pathophysiological responses in patients affected with up to 40% burns is similar to that of any other trauma. In severe cases, however, characterized by 40–80% burns, a hyperdynamic circulatory response exacerbates the length and intensity of stress, inflammation and hypermetabolism. It is characterized by 10–50-fold increase in cytokines, catecholamines, and corticosteroids, up to 100% increase in REE and substantially accelerated supraphysiological metabolic rates of gluconeogenesis, lipolysis, and proteolysis. Compared to trauma, burns has persistent and prolonged "flow phase" during hypermetabolic response **(Fig. 3)**, that lasts up to a year, resulting in increased catabolism leading to excessive muscle wasting and cachexia. It also aggravates stress-induced hyperglycemia which makes wound healing and graft acceptance an arduous task for the immune system. Typically, severely burned individuals lose approximately 25% of total body mass. The observed catabolism is highest in burns compared to trauma, surgical, and other critically ill patients **(Fig. 4)**. Consequently, insulin resistance, liver dysfunction, lowered immunity (increasing susceptibility to infection), and organ dysfunction are more profound in burns.[8,9]

CALORIE AND NUTRIENT REQUIREMENTS

The energy expenditure and calorie need in critically ill patients, affected with trauma or burns, can be measured using an indirect calorimetry. It uses the volume of oxygen consumption and carbon dioxide production as variables for calculation of metabolic rate and respiratory quotient of patients. Indirect calorimetry is also a universally accepted instrument for calculation of REE which is represented using the Weir's equation **(Box 1)**.[10] In addition, several formulas are derived specifically for calculating the calorie needs of burn patients, based on the extent of

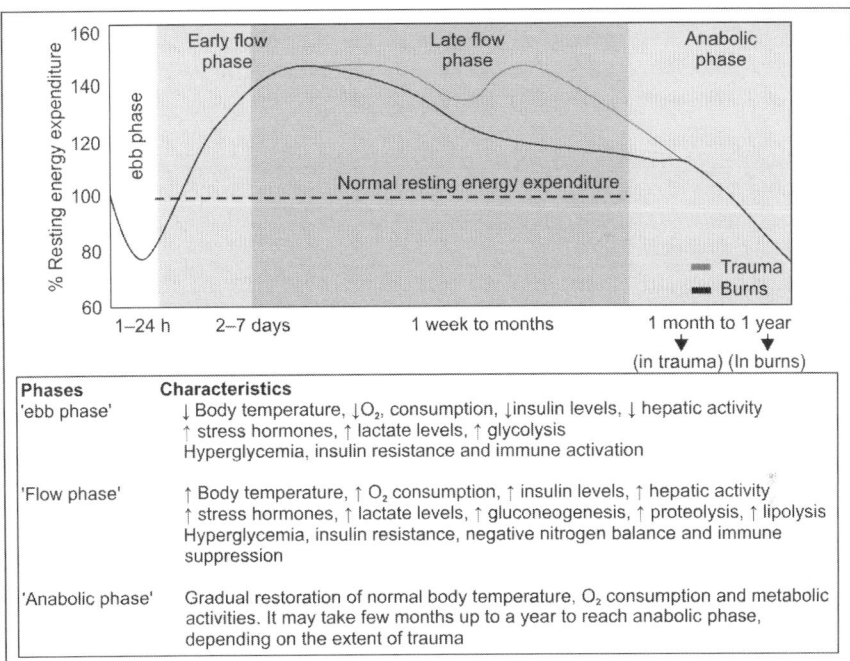

Fig. 3: Prolonged flow phase of metabolic response in burns compared to trauma.
Source: Adapted from Delsoglio M, Achamrah N, Berger MM, Pichard C. Indirect calorimetry in clinical practice. J Clin Med. 2019;8(9):1387.

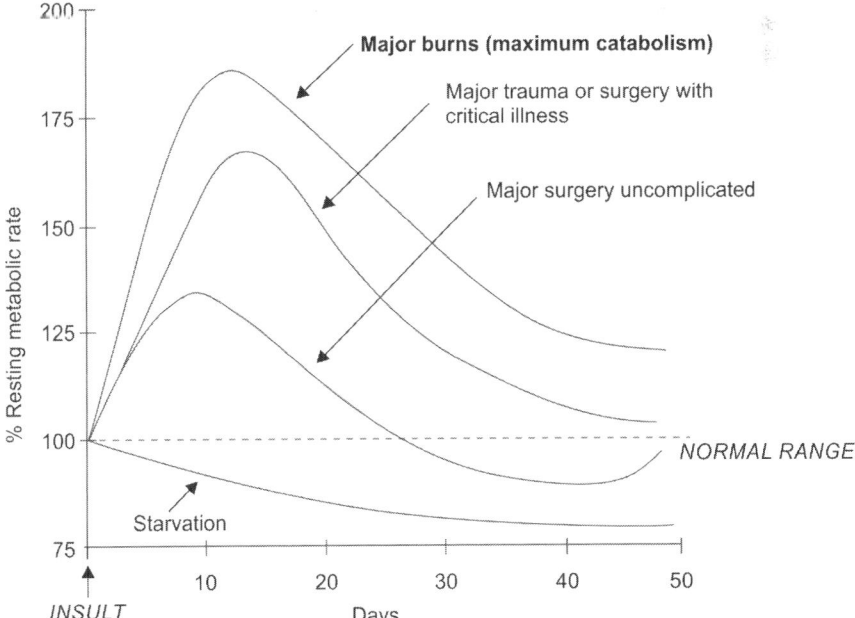

Fig. 4: Comparison of catabolic response in burns, trauma, ICU, and surgical patients.
Source: Adapted from https://www.plarecon.com/nutrition-burns/.

> **BOX 1:** Energy expenditure calculated using indirect calorimetry.
>
> $$\text{Metabolic rate (kcal/day)} = 1.44 \times (3.94 \times VO_2) + (1.11 \times VCO_2)$$
> $$\text{Respiratory quotient} = \frac{VCO_2}{VO_2}$$
> $$\text{Weir's equation [REE (kcal/day)]} = [(VO_2 \times 3.941) + (VCO_2 \times 1.11)] \times 1440$$
>
> Where, VO_2 is the volume of oxygen consumption and VCO_2 is the volume of carbon dioxide production. In practice, indirect calorimetry is an accurate method, but not always practical as it is cumbersome and not available in most critical care units.

(REE: resting energy expenditure)

> **BOX 2:** Equations for calculating calorie needs of burn patients.
>
> *Curreri equation* for estimation of calorie needs:
> = recommended dietary allowance + [25 × (TBSA)] (for age 1–3)
> = recommended dietary allowance + [40 × (TBSA)] (for age 4–15)
> = [25 × (weight in kg)] + [40 × (% TBSA)] (for age 16–59)
> = [20 × (weight in kg)] + [65 × (% TBSA)] (for age >60)
>
> *Harris–Benedict equation* for estimation of basal energy expenditure
> = 66.5 + [13.8 × (weight in kg)] + [5 × (height in cm)] – [6.76 × (age in years)] (for Men)
> = 655 + [9.6 × (weight in kg)] + [1.85 × (height in cm)] – [4.68 × (age in years)] (for Women)
>
> *Toronto equation* for acute burn care management:
> = 4,343 + [10.5 × (% TBSA)] + [0.23 × (calorie intake in last 24 h)] + [0.84 × (Harris–Benedict estimation)] + [114 × (temperature)] – [4.5 × (number of postburn days)]
>
> *Ireton–Jones equation* for acute burn care in ventilated, trauma, burn, or obese patients
> = 1,784 – [11 × (age in years)] + [5 × (weight in kg)] + (244 if male) + (239 if trauma) + (804 if burn) (for ventilated patients)
> = 629 – [11 × (age in years)] + [25 × (weight in kg)] – (609 if obese) (for nonventilated patients)
>
> Where, TBSA is the total body surface area burned.

(TBSA: total body surface area)

body surface area affected **(Box 2)**.[5] Precisely, the Toronto equation is more sensitive in estimating energy requirements during acute stages of burns and is highly recommended in monitoring nutritional requirements in burn patients.[11]

For nutritional management of trauma and burn patients, three key elements of metabolic support are targeted:
1. Hypermetabolic state
2. Muscle consumption
3. Stress hyperglycemia

The caloric requirements do not increase much post injury. Ideally, ESPEN (2019)[4] and ASPEN (2017)[12] recommend a low fat (>10% of nonprotein caloric needs) and high-protein diet along with regular carbohydrates intake for trauma as well as burn patients. The immune system is severely compromised in trauma and burns. To compensate for reduced immunity, immune-nutritional formulas containing vitamin and minerals along with calculated macronutrient limits are commonly used. Most common formulations consist of varied amounts of omega-3 fatty acids, glutamine, arginine, histidine, and vitamins A and C.[11] Though aggressive nutrition is recommended in early phase of burns, there is negligible supporting evidence to prove better outcomes. Few studies have reported negative effects of immune-nutrition in patients with sepsis and pneumonia. Hence, along with immune-nutritional diet, critical monitoring of patients is essential to prevent diet related complications.[13]

Timing of Nutritional Therapy

Trauma-induced intestinal mucosal damage decreases absorption of nutrients. At the same time, the hypermetabolic response leads to utilization of energy reserves for maintaining cellular and immune functions and promoting wound healing. Hence, nutritional support should be initiated ideally within 24 hours of injury.[13] In burns, ESPEN (2013)[14] recommends initiation of nutritional support within 12 hours. Newer guidelines, on the other hand, suggest *"Early but not very early enteral nutrition support"* in 24–48 hours.[4,11]

Routes of Nutrition Administration

The enteral route is preferred over parental route for administration of nutrients, since the latter is associated with complications such as overfeeding and liver dysfunction. The parental route also leads to decreased immune response, which increases mortality rate. On the other hand, the enteral route is safe and cost-effective alternative. It can utilize the nutrients more efficiently and thus preserves immune functions and prevents mucosal atrophy. The enteral route is recommended after shock resuscitation in hemodynamically unstable patients. Various advantages of enteral route are listed below.[13]

- It promotes gut-associated immune function by stimulating bowel functions and blood supply.
- It decreases bacterial translocation.
- It is associated with decreased incidences of hyperglycemia and hyperosmolarity.

Optimum Feeding

As described earlier in this chapter, insufficient calorie and protein intake leads to *"under-feeding"* and results in loss of muscle mass and risk of malnutrition that can induce immune dysfunctions, impair wound healing, and increase mortality. At the same time, aggressive nutrient supplements can lead to *"overfeeding"* causing critical complications such as hyperglycemia, fatty liver, hypercapnia, metabolic acidosis, azotemia, and respiratory insufficiency in trauma and burn patients. *"Refeeding syndrome"* is another potentially fatal outcome of aggressive fluids and electrolytes supplementation in malnourished patients. It is characterized by hypophosphatemia, abnormal fluid and sodium balance, thiamine deficiency, hypokalemia, hypomagnesemia along with changes in blood glucose, protein, and fat metabolism.[15] Hence, optimum feeding goals are achieved through continuous assessment and monitoring of several physical (body weight), biochemical (nitrogen balance and serum level of nutrients), and functional measures (exercise tolerance). However, objective assessment of nutritional support in these patients is challenging due to measurement of multiple variables. Clinical conditions such as obesity, diabetes, cardiovascular disease, and inflammatory conditions (arthritis) further challenge the nutritional assessment since predictive formulas overestimate the energy needs of these patients. Specific formulas for these conditions are rarely used in practice, and are almost never validated. Hence, it is necessary to follow standard nutritional guidelines by taking into account all possible variables. In addition, the patient's energy requirements should be regularly reassessed.[15-17]

Early Mobilization and Rehabilitation

In critically ill patients, factors such as bed rest, deep sedation, and neuromuscular blockade promote immobilized physical state in patients. Along with loss of muscle function and acute nerve damage, immobilization is identified as a major cause of intensive care unit-acquired weakness (ICU-AW). In a recent clinical trial, Zhou et al. 2020[18] reported a novel intervention, of early mobilization and rehabilitation combined with early nutrition, to prevent ICU-AW and reduce the length of hospital stay.

NUTRITIONAL SUPPORT FOR TRAUMA

The ESPEN (2019)[4] guidelines suggest that nutritional support is essential during the inflammatory as well as the metabolic phases in trauma. The early nutritional interventions reduce the secretion of catabolic hormones; thereby preserving body weight and muscle mass. Once the patient is hemodynamically stable, initiation of enteral nutrition is recommended 24–48 hours post-trauma.[11] Depending on the extent of trauma, ASPEN (2017)[12] recommends energy intake of 25–30 kcal/kg/day along with a protein intake of 1.2–2.0 g/kg/day. Immune-nutritional formulas containing arginine, glutamine, omega-3 fatty acids, selenium, and antioxidants are recommended in patients with TBI, but not recommended for routine use in patients with severe sepsis.[11,12] The immune-nutrition is associated with reduced incidences of nosocomial infections and length of hospital in critically ill patients.[11,12] The amount of macronutrients is calculated based on bodyweight to prevent stress-induced hyperglycemia. The recommended enteral nutrition in trauma and burns is represented in **Table 1**.

NUTRITIONAL SUPPORT FOR BURNS

As a result of more complex pathophysiological response of severely burned victims, designing a weight and formula-based predictive or standard nutritional therapy has proved to be highly inaccurate. The key challenges in nutritional support of severe burn patients are outlined below.

- The trace elements deficiencies develop early due to cutaneous exudative losses.
- The extensive non-nutritional therapies used to manage high-ambient temperature, extensive wounds (using anabolic steroids), and blood pressure (using nonselective β-blockers) tremendously interfere with the metabolic responses of the patient.
- Due to high-nutritional needs of burn patients, formula-based nutrition can be easily miscalculated resulting in overfeeding or underfeeding. Typically, overfeeding is associated with complications such as fatty liver (steatosis), azotemia, dehydration, metabolic acidosis, and hyperglycemia. In turn, these complications increase the risk of systemic infections. At the same time, it places a burden on the respiratory system which severely complicates the respiratory status (causing respiratory insufficiency) and makes ventilator weaning more challenging.[15]

For these reasons, the ESPEN (2019)[4] guidelines recommend highly specific artificial nutritional therapy for patients suffering major burns which are started as early as 24–48 hours post injury. Specifically, these therapies administer supranutritional amounts of vitamin C, zinc, copper, chromium, and selenium (*see* **Table 1**) along with calculated amounts of macronutrients

TABLE 1: Recommendations on enteral nutrition in trauma and burns for adults.

Guidelines	Nutrients	Trauma	Burns
ASPEN, 2017[12]	Macronutrients	• 25–30 kcal/kg/day calories • 1.2–2.0 g/kg/day proteins • 150 g of fat-free mass/day	• 25–35 kcal/kg/day calories • 1.5–2.0 g/kg/day proteins • 150 g of fat-free mass/day
	Vitamins	• Minimum essential dietary requirements for all vitamins	• 10–200 mg/kg/day vitamin C • Minimum essential dietary requirements for other vitamins
	Minerals	• 2.5–5 mg zinc • 0.3–0.5 mg/day copper • 60–100 µg/day manganese • 10–15 µg/day chromium • 20–60 µg/day selenium • 1.2–10 mg/day thiamine	• 3–5 mg zinc • 0.3–0.5 mg/day copper • 60–100 µg/day manganese • 10–15 µg/day chromium • 20–60 µg/day selenium • 1.2–10 mg/day thiamine

	Immunonutrition	• 0.2–0.3 g/kg/day glutamine
		• 0.1–0.2 g fish oil/kg/day (as source of omega-3-fatty acids)
		• Formulations containing:
		  1. Arginine and fish oil (severe trauma)
		  2. EPA/DHA supplement (for TBI)
			• 0.3–0.5 g/kg/day glutamine
			• Formulations containing antioxidants

ESPEN, 2019[4]	Macronutrients	• 1–5 g/kg/day low fats (<15% of total calorie intake) • 1.5–2 g/kg/day protein • *Not exceeding 5 mg/kg/min glucose in ICU and TBI patients*	• 1–5 g/kg/day low fats (<15% of total calorie intake) • 1.5–2 g/kg/day protein • 7 g/kg/day calorie
ESPEN, 2022[19]	Vitamins	• 1 g/day vitamin C • 1,000 IU/day vitamin E • 2.5–3.5 mg/day thiamine • 1.2 mg/day riboflavin • <12.5 ng/mL 25-hydroxy-vitamin D or 50 nmol/L vitamin D_3	• 66 mg/kg/h for 24 hours followed by 50–200 mg/kg/kg vitamin C • 1,000 IU/day vitamin E • 2.5–3.5 mg/day thiamine • 1.2 mg/day riboflavin • <12.5 ng/mL 25-hydroxy-vitamin D or 50 nmol/L vitamin D_3
	Minerals	• 50–150 mg/day selenium • 3–10 mg/day zinc • 3–20 mg/h for 10 hours up to 4 days for chromium • 1–3 mg/day copper • 150–300 µg iodine	• 375 mg/day selenium • 30–40 mg/day zinc • 35 mg/h for 10 hours up to 4 days for chromium • 1–3 mg/day copper • 150–300 µg iodine

	Immunonutrition	• 0.2–0.3 g/kg/d glutamine
		• 0.1–0.2 g/kg/day EPA + DHA
		• Formulations containing:
		  1. Selenium and antioxidants (TBI)
		  2. Glutamine, EPA/DHA, and antioxidants (severe trauma)
			• 0.3–0.5 g/kg/day glutamine
			• Formulations containing:
			  1. Glutamine and antioxidants
			  2. High-dose selenium and vitamin C

(ASPEN: American Society for Parenteral and Enteral Nutrition; DHA: docosahexaenoic acid; EPA: eicosapentaenoic acid; ESPEN: European Society for Clinical Nutrition and Metabolism; TBI: traumatic brain injury) to prevent deficiency-related complications. At the same time, aggressive nutrition during early phase of severe burn injury is avoided to prevent overfeeding and resulting complications. High doses of omega-3 enriched enteral formulas are not recommended for routine use in severe burns patients, since it can aggravate proinflammatory responses.[14]

ROLE OF ESSENTIAL MICRONUTRIENTS IN MANAGEMENT OF TRAUMA AND BURNS

The science of clinical nutrition takes into account the basics of nutrient role in cellular functions and immunity, possible complications and interfering factors, and evidence-based outcomes in patient management. Based on these primary factors, a decision can be made on whether a nutritional formula assists or complicates the recovery process. The role of essential macronutrients in management of trauma and burns is described below.[7,13]

Carbohydrates

Carbohydrates promote wound healing and also impart a protein-sparing effect (leading to decreased loss of muscle mass). Hence, it is an essential macronutrient required during recovery of trauma and burns. In excess, carbohydrates can lead to severe complications such as hyperglycemia, glycosuria, dehydration, conversion of glucose to fats, and respiratory problems. Hence, it is supplemented in optimal quantities and above conditions are critically monitored in patients regularly.

Proteins

The catabolic products of proteins aid in wound healing and immune functions. Hence, there is excessive loss of muscle proteins in critically injured patients. The protein requirement is much greater in severely burned patients due to the hormonal and proinflammatory response to burns. The supranormal amount of proteins administered in burn patients does not necessarily prevent catabolism of endogenous protein reserves. Instead, they promote protein synthesis and positive nitrogen balance. Thus, it minimizes the loss of lean body mass.

Fats

Though increased lipolysis occurs in hypermetabolic state, the utilization of fats for energy is suppressed during severe trauma and burns. The catabolized free-fatty acids undergo re-esterification and accumulate in liver causing fatty liver. Increased intake of fats is also associated with adverse immune functions. Hence, low-fat diet (<15% of total calories) containing omega-3 and omega-6 fatty acids is recommended by the most nutritional care guidelines for trauma and burns. Both omega-3 and omega-6 fatty acids promote proinflammatory immune response and prevent hyperglycemia. Thus, they are major components of immune-nutritional formulas recommended for trauma patients.

ROLE OF ESSENTIAL MICRONUTRIENTS IN MANAGEMENT OF TRAUMA AND BURNS[12-14]

Amino Acids

Amino acids play an important role in energy transport, wound healing, immune functions, cellular processes, and protein synthesis. The consumption of three essential amino acids such as glutamine, alanine, and arginine increases rampantly after trauma to compensate wound healing process. Hence, they are supplemented in generous amounts along with proteins during nutritional management of trauma and burns. The roles of these amino acids are outlined briefly below.

- Glutamine serves as a primary fuel for blood cells and administration of 25 g/kg/day reduces mortality, cardiac stress, infections, length of hospital stay, and improves protein anabolism, and positive nitrogen balance. In burn patients, glutamine mediates production of heat shock proteins and regulates hyperglycemia. It also prevents oxidative stress by mediating glutathione (antioxidant) production.
- Arginine stimulates production of T lymphocytes, natural killer cells, and improves resistance to infection (by accelerating nitric oxide synthesis). It is also essential in wound healing and immune responsiveness. In addition, it is linked with reduction of insulin resistance.

Vitamins

Like amino acids, vitamin consumption is also increased post-trauma to promote wound healing and immune functions. The roles of essential vitamins are outlined briefly below.

- Vitamin A promotes wound healing (in less time) and epithelial growth.
- Vitamin C is essential for cross-linking of collagen that further promotes wound healing. It is required in 20 times higher quantities in burn patients.
- Vitamin D prevents bone catabolism.
- Vitamin E reduces lipid peroxide levels in burn patients.

Minerals

Minerals are essential for optimal cellular functions. They are the backbone of the host defense mechanisms and biochemical processes activated during trauma and recovery phase. Overall, the mineral supplements reduce wound healing time, hospital stay, incidence of nosocomial infections, and patient mortality. Under normal conditions, they are required in minute quantities. During trauma, they are exhausted more rampantly compared to other nutrients due to the hypermetabolic response of trauma. The roles of essential minerals are outlined briefly below.

- Iron is an important cofactor in oxygen-carrying proteins. Its requirement increases during wound healing due to formation of new capillaries.
- Zinc is essential for DNA replication and lymphocyte function. Hence, it promotes both wound healing and immune functions.
- Selenium is essential for cell-mediated immunity.
- Copper is essential for optimum cardiac function and its deficiency is associated with arrhythmias. Copper also promotes wound healing (by promoting collagen synthesis) and immune functions.

MONITORING TO BE DONE WITH NUTRITIONAL THERAPY

Various cofactors are associated with successful nutritional interventions in trauma and burn patients. Hence, constant monitoring of various factors is necessary for optimal management of nutritional support. These factors are described briefly below.[11]

- Electrolytes should be strictly monitored in the patient on nutrition therapy.
- Enteral nutrition can trigger intestinal ischemia in hemodynamically unstable patients. Hence, peristalsis, gastrointestinal hypoperfusion, and mesenteric ischemia should be monitored in these patients before and after initiation of nutritional therapy.

- Vasopressors/inotropes may interfere with gut function and worsen with enteral nutrition. Hence, it should be monitored frequently. Drug-nutrient interaction should be regularly assessed.
- Enteral nutrition should be started within 24–48 hours, but it must be avoided in persistent shock.
- Nutritional assessment must be done for signs of malnutrition including cachexia, edema, muscle atrophy, and low body mass. Appropriate therapy with immune-nutrition and antioxidants should be prescribed and monitored regularly.
- In polytrauma and burns, nonprotein calorie to nitrogen ratio should be maintained between 150:1 and 100:1.
- The gastric residual volume (GRV) should be monitored every 6–8 hours and volume of 500 mL should be used as cut-off. Metoclopramide and erythromycin may be recommended in patients with intolerance and risk of aspiration.

NUTRITION AFTER DISCHARGE

Lastly, it is necessary that the patients continue to receive adequate nutrition after discharge. Simple measures that can be taken by patients include:[15-17]
- Regular monitoring of weight
- Continue resistance exercises to combat loss of muscle mass.
- Regular follow-up of nutritional assessments by physicians and dieticians
- Regular intake of prescribed medicines and immune enhancement formulas or diets.

CONCLUSION

Severe trauma and burns augment the nutritional requirements due to hypermetabolic physiological response and intense tissue repair needs. In these patients, the critical care nutrition should be individualized depending on the disease, its catabolic stage, and the loss of lean muscle mass. Along with optimum feeding goals, positive nitrogen balance and early mobilization help to fight the ICU-associated weakness. There is still no consensus on providing early versus late enteral and parental nutrition, and use of immune enhancing diets containing omega-3-fatty acids and glutamine. Thus, critical care nutrition remains a challenge in trauma and burns. There is a need to improve nutritional therapy in critically ill patients by generating knowledge which translates into lesser complications and better outcomes. Overall, critical care nutrition should be regarded as one of the many therapies such as intravenous fluids and antibiotics for better outcomes.

REFERENCES

1. Ram B, Thakur R. Measuring the burden of accidental injuries in India: a cross-sectional analysis of the National Sample Survey (2017–18). Humanit Soc Sci Commun. 2022;9:363.
2. World Health Organization. (2018). Fact sheet on Burns. [online] Available from: https://www.who.int/news-room/fact-sheets/detail/burns [Last accessed June, 2023].
3. Yakupu A, Zhang J, Dong W, Song F, Dong J, Lu S. The epidemiological characteristic and trends of burns globally. BMC Public Health. 2022;22:1596.
4. Singer P, Blaser AR, Berger MM, Alhazzani W, Calder PC, Casaer MP, et al. ESPEN guideline on clinical nutrition in the intensive care unit. Clin Nutr. 2019;38:48-79.
5. Clark A, Imran J, Madni T, Wolf SE. Nutrition and metabolism in burn patients. Burns Trauma. 2017;5:11.
6. Hill A, Elke G, Weimann A. Nutrition in the Intensive Care Unit—A Narrative Review. Nutrients. 2021;13(8):2851.

7. Genton L, Romand JA, Tyuy CP. Basics in Clinical Nutrition: Nutritional support in trauma. e-SPEN, Eur e-J Clin Nutr Metabol. 2010;5:e107-9.
8. Korkmaz HI, Flokstra G, Waasdorp M, Pijpe A, Papendorp SG, de Jong E, et al. The complexity of the post-burn immune response: an overview of the associated local and systemic complications. Cells. 2023;12(3):345.
9. Chourdakis M, Bouras E, Shields BA, Stoppe C, Rousseau AF, Heyland DK. Nutritional therapy among burn injured patients in the critical care setting: An international multicenter observational study on "best achievable" practices. Clin Nutr. 2020;39:3813-20.
10. Delsoglio M, Achamrah N, Berger MM, Pichard C. Indirect calorimetry in clinical practice. J Clin Med. 2019;8(9):1387.
11. Mehta Y, Sunavala JD, Zirpe K, Tyagi N, Garg S, Sinha S, et al. Practice Guidelines for Nutrition in Critically Ill Patients: A Relook for Indian Scenario. Indian J Crit Care Med. 2018;22(4):263-73.
12. Boullata JI, Carrera AL, Harvey L, Escuro AA, Hudson L, Mays A, et al. ASPEN safe practices for enteral nutrition therapy (Consensus Recommendation). JPEN J Parenter Enteral Nutr. 2017;41(1):15-103.
13. Smith-Ryan AE, Hirsch KR, Saylor HE, Gould LM, Blue MNM. Nutritional considerations and strategies to facilitate injury recovery and rehabilitation. J Athl Train. 2020;55(9):918-30.
14. Rousseau AF, Losser MR, Ichai C, Berger MM. ESPEN endorsed recommendations: Nutritional therapy in major burns. Clin Nutr. 2013;32:497-502.
15. Natarajan M, Sekhar DR. Nutrition in burns patient. IOSR J Dent Med Sci. 2015;14(3):38-54.
16. Gomes F, Schuetz P, Bounoure L, Austin P, Ballesteros-Pomar M, Cederholm T, et al. ESPEN guidelines on nutritional support for polymorbid internal medicine patients. Clin Nutr. 2018;37:336-53.
17. National Institute for Health and Clinical Excellence. Nutrition support for adults: oral nutrition support, enteral tube feeding and parenteral nutrition (Clinical Guidance 32). London, UK: National Collaborating Centre for Acute Care (UK) and National Institute for Health and Clinical Excellence; 2006.
18. Zhou W, Shi B, Fan Y, Zhu J. Effect of early activity combined with early nutrition on acquired weakness in ICU patients. Medicine (Baltimore). 2020;99(29):c21202.
19. Berger MM, Shenkin A, Schweinlin A. ESPEN micronutrient guideline. Clin Nutr. 2022;41:1357-424.

CHAPTER 34

Nutrition in Neurology and Neurosurgical Patients

Barkha Bindu, Amit Goyal, Indu Kapoor, Hemanshu Prabhakar

INTRODUCTION

Nutritional supplementation should be considered in all critically ill patients who are expected to stay in the ICU for >48 hours. Almost immediately after an acute neurological event, a hypercatabolic and hypermetabolic state ensues. Patients with neurological diseases are further prone to malnutrition owing to poor intake, increased metabolic demands, high metabolic rates, higher incidence of oropharyngeal dysphagia, cognitive dysfunction, etc. associated with these diseases.[1,2]

Data as well as recommendations regarding nutritional care in neurocritical care patients is scanty and mostly limited to patients with traumatic brain injury (TBI). General practice is therefore mostly based on data from general critical care patients.

METABOLIC RESPONSE TO CRITICAL ILLNESS

Critical illness leads to a stress response which affects all organ systems of the body. Acute neurological injury activates a cascade of neuroendocrine and adrenergic responses leading to a proinflammatory and hypercatabolic state, mediated by catecholamines, glucocorticoids and glucagon.[3] Gluconeogenesis and glycogenolysis lead to hyperglycemia along with increased skeletal protein catabolism and negative nitrogen balance.[4] This along with reduced oral intake leads to increased morbidity and mortality.[5]

Complex interactions between gut epithelium and immune system have been reported.[6] Critical illness shifts the normal gut microbiome toward a pathogenic one within hours of ICU admission.[7] Medications such as antibiotics, opioids, proton pump inhibitors further exacerbate this change.[8] Normal commensal microbiome of the gut helps in the metabolism of medications and nutrients and maintains mucosal barrier homeostasis. Critical illness related alteration of the microbiome increases the risk of bacterial translocation.[9,10] The microbiome has been shown to become progressively more pathogenic with increasing duration of ICU stay.[11]

Resting energy expenditure (REE) increases up to 200% of usual needs in up to two-thirds of patients with brain trauma in the first 2–4 weeks.[4] Patients with TBI have been shown to have altered energy metabolism and elevated nitrogen excretion for several weeks after injury leading to malnutrition.[12] Among patients with subarachnoid hemorrhage (SAH), incidence of vasospasm is reportedly higher as patients with higher grade SAH have elevated REE.[13] Therapies used in neurocritically ill patients such as use of barbiturates, sedatives, normothermia/hypothermia further alter metabolic demands.[3] Nutritional supplementation provides substrates to mitigate the damaging effects of hypermetabolism. Proper nutrition ensures preservation of lean body mass and prevents malnutrition.

NUTRITION ASSESSMENT IN ICU

No single tool can give a complete picture of a patients' nutritional status. Multiple monitoring strategies along with frequent evaluations are needed. Nutrition assessment in ICU is a two-step process:

1. *Step 1: Screening for malnutrition in ICU*—the American Society for Parenteral and Enteral Nutrition (ASPEN) and the Society of Critical Care Medicine (SCCM) recommend using a validated screening tool within 24–48 hours of admission to ICU.[14]

Some of the malnutrition screening tools used in ICU are subjective global assessment, malnutrition universal screening tool, nutritional risk screening,[15] mininutrition assessment, etc. More recently, the Nutrition Risk in the Critically Ill (NUTRIC) tool **(Table 1)** is being used in critically ill patients.[16]

Radiological tools include ultrasonography of quadriceps muscle (to measure muscle mass and changes during course of illness) and CT scan analysis of skeletal muscle density.

Malnutrition is associated with increased infections, mortality rate, and length of ICU stay in critically ill patients, thus requiring early identification of factors causing malnutrition and correcting them. The most common cause of malnutrition is imbalance between nutrition demand and supply, with underprescription of energy being the most common in critical care. **Box 1** lists the factors associated with malnutrition in critically ill patients.[17]

TABLE 1: NUTRIC (nutrition risk in the critically ill) score.

Variables	Range	Points
Age	<50 years	0
	50–<75 years	1
	≥75 years	2
APACHE-II	<15	0
	15–<20	1
	20–28	2
	≥28	3
SOFA	<6	0
	6–<10	1
	≥10	2
Comorbidities	0–1	0
	≥2	1
Days from hospital to ICU admission	0–<1	0
	≥1	1
IL-6	0–<400	0
	≥400	1

(APACHE: Acute Physiology and Chronic Health Evaluation; IL: interleukin; SOFA: Sequential Organ Failure Assessment)
Note: Total score is 10.

BOX 1: Factors associated with malnutrition in critically ill patients.

Reduced nutrition supply:
- Delayed initiation
- Slow advancement
- *Under-prescription*: Erratic calculation of energy expenditure
- Interruption to enteral feed (intolerance, surgical or diagnostic procedures)
- Parental nutrition

Increased demand:
- NUTRIC score ≥5
- Sepsis
- Trauma
- Burn
- APACHE >10

Gastrointestinal intolerance:
- Surgical patients
- High vasopressor support
- Gastrointestinal bleeding

Increased susceptibility to undernutrition:
- Age ≥70 years
- BMI <18.5
- NRS ≥3
- ICU stay >48 hours

(APACHE: Acute Physiology and Chronic Health Evaluation; NRS: Nutritional Risk Screening; NUTRIC: Nutrition Risk in the Critically Ill)

2. *Step 2: Assessment of current nutritional status*—screening for risk of malnutrition must be followed by a systematic assessment of nutrition status of the patient.[14] It helps to identify patients who will benefit from nutritional therapy. **Table 2** gives list of factors that need to be considered when assessing nutritional status of a patient. **Table 3** describes tools used for assessment of nutritional status.

TABLE 2: Factors to be considered during assessment of nutritional status.

Factors	Remarks
Comorbidities	Diabetes, hypertension, renal failure, and liver failure
Abnormal gastrointestinal function	Gastrointestinal function may be affected by autonomic nervous dysfunction
Dysphagia	May be due to neurological disorder or oropharyngeal muscle weakness
Change in body composition	• Loss of muscle mass • Edema

TABLE 3: Tools used for assessment of nutritional status.

Tools	Remarks
Anthropometry	• Simple and inexpensive • Can be performed bedside
Body mass index (BMI)	• Weight (kg)/Height^2 (m) • BMI <20 is associated with high mortality
Skin-fold thickness	Measured at biceps, triceps, subscapular region, and iliac crest using skin-fold calipers
Mid-arm circumference	Measured at midpoint of the line joining acromion and olecranon processes, in nondominant upper limb
Percentage weight loss	[(Usual bodyweight—actual bodyweight)/actual bodyweight)] × 100 Significant if >5%, 7.5%, and 10% at 1, 3, and 6 months respectively
Subjective global assessment (SGA)	Takes into account: anorexia, functional capacity, gastrointestinal symptoms, weight loss over 6 months, and visual assessment of subcutaneous fat and muscle mass
Serum albumin and prealbumin levels	• Simple and widely available • Unreliable, as they may increase in acute illness • Prealbumin has shorter half-life, gets affected earlier in malnutrition states
Serum ketones	• Indicator of starvation when present without hyperglycemia • Presence of urinary ketones suggests reduced oral intake over several days prior to admission as well as risk of refeeding syndrome
Transferrin level	• Has short half-life • Sensitive indicator of visceral protein status
Nitrogen balance	• Measure of the severity of protein catabolism and adequacy of nutrition • Estimated from urinary nitrogen excretion in 24 hours • Negative nitrogen balance implies inadequate protein intake and increased protein catabolism • Goal of nutrition supplementation is to maintain a positive nitrogen balance

ASSESSMENT OF CALORIC REQUIREMENT

The recent ASPEN guidelines for provision of nutrition support therapy in adult critically ill patients have made certain recommendations that are mentioned in **Table 4**.[18]

Several methods are used for assessment of caloric requirements in ICU.

- **Predictive equations** have traditionally been used to estimate a patients' REE and to set caloric targets. These equations are commonly derived from Harris–Benedict equation (HBE) or Ireton–Jones equation. However, these equations do not take into account the dynamic changes in a patients' condition, making them unreliable for use in ICU. They also require multiplication with a stress factor in certain situations.
- **Fixed weight-based calculations** of energy and protein requirements show an overall accuracy of only 40% in predicting energy expenditure.[19] An average build

TABLE 4: ASPEN guidelines for nutrition therapy in adult critically ill patients.

Questions	Recommendation
In adult critically ill patients, does provision of higher versus lower energy intake impact clinical outcomes?	No significant difference in clinical outcomes was found between patients with higher versus lower levels of energy intake. We suggest feeding between 12–25 kcal/kg (i.e., the range of mean energy intakes examined) in the first 7–10 days of ICU stay
In adult critically ill patients, does provision of higher as compared to lower protein intake impact clinical outcomes?	There was no difference in clinical outcomes in the relatively limited data. Due to a paucity of trials with high-quality evidence, we cannot make a new recommendation at this time beyond the 2016 guideline suggestion for 1.2–2.0 g/kg/day
In adult critically ill patients who are candidates for EN, does similar caloric intake by PN versus EN as the primary feeding modality in the first week of critical illness impact clinical outcomes?	There was no significant difference in clinical outcomes. Since similar caloric intake provided as PN is not superior to EN and no differences in harm were identified, we recommend that either PN or EN is acceptable
In adult critically ill patients receiving EN, does provision of supplemental PN, as compared to no supplemental PN during the first week of critical illness impact clinical outcomes?	There was no significant difference in clinical outcomes. Based on findings of no clinically important benefit in providing supplemental PN early in the ICU admission, we recommend not initiating supplemental PN prior to day 7 of ICU admission
In adult critically ill patients receiving PN, does provision of mixed oil lipid injectable emulsions (ILE) [i.e., medium chain triglycerides, olive oil, fish oil (FO), mixtures of oils], as compared to 100% soybean oil ILE, impact clinical outcomes?	Due to limited statistically or clinically significant differences in key outcomes, we suggest that either mixed oil ILE or 100% soybean oil ILE be provided to critically ill patients who are appropriate candidates for initiation of PN, including within the first week of ICU admission
In adult critically ill patients receiving PN, does provision of FO containing ILE, as compared to non-FO containing ILE, impact clinical outcomes?	Due to finding only one outcome with a significant difference that was not supported by data covering the other key downstream outcomes, we suggest that either fish oil- or non-fish oil-containing ILE be provided to critically ill patients who are appropriate candidates for initiation of PN, including within the first week of ICU admission

(ASPEN: American Society for Parenteral and Enteral Nutrition; EN: enteral nutrition; PN: parenteral nutrition)

TABLE 5: Indirect calorimetry.

Advantages	Disadvantages
Noninvasive technique	• Costly, labor intensive • Uncommonly used in clinical practice • Needs especially trained clinicians to perform and interpret the measurements
Provides real-time information of energy requirements	Needs to be repeated routinely as conditions change to ensure that the measurements accurately reflect patient's current metabolic state and prevent under or overfeeding
Useful in circumstances when equations for predicting REE are unreliable	May be limited in mechanically ventilated patients needing high-positive pressure and oxygen settings, in those requiring noninvasive mechanical ventilation, continuous renal replacement therapy, extracorporeal membrane oxygen (ECMO) exchange, and chest tubes with poor seals

(REE: resting energy expenditure)

and middle-aged patient in ICU typically needs 25–30 kcal/kg/day [including calories from dietary carbohydrates, proteins, intravenous fluids, propofol infusion (1.1 kcal/mL)] of energy, 1–2 g/kg/day of protein, 30–35 mL/kg/day of fluids along with vitamins, minerals, and trace elements replacement.

- Indirect calorimetry (IC) is the gold standard for determining energy requirements in critically ill patients.[14] It uses the amount of oxygen and carbon dioxide consumed and provides a measurement of REE. The results are then extrapolated over a 24-hour time period.[20] **Table 5** gives advantages and disadvantages of IC. It must be noted that IC, when done repeatedly over a period of duration, may be more accurate in estimating REE rather than extrapolating values from a single IC assessment.[21]

COMPONENTS OF NUTRITION

Nutrition in ICU should be tailored to include adequate macronutrients as well as micronutrients to achieve optimal energy targets, fulfill preexisting deficiencies, and immune modulation. This can be achieved by standard polymeric formula feeds or blended kitchen tube feed. However, blended kitchen feeds have associated limitations of microbial contamination, inconsistent nutrients supply (16–50%), higher osmolality, and viscosity.[22,23]

Macronutrients

Protein

Protein provides 5.3 kcal/g. Various guidelines recommend total protein intake of 1–2 g/kg/day in all critically ill patients.[14,22,24] Several commercial formula feeds do not provide adequate proteins in comparison to the calorie content. However, new products with higher protein to calorie ratio are now available. Optimal timing of increasing protein intake is also debated. Initial catabolic phase of injury is associated with increased muscle protein degradation, requiring high protein intake to reduce the negative protein balance. Various retrospective studies have shown varying effect of early high protein intake on survival rate, though overall low-protein intake has been associated with high mortality rate.[25,26] A recent trial has shown that high-protein intake during late phase of critical illness has no significant impact on preservation of muscle mass in long-term immobilized ICU patients.[27]

Lipid

Lipid provides 9.3 kcal/g. The upper limit for intravenous lipid is described as 1 g/kg/day.[24] Calories from lipid should be limited to 40% of total calories including nonnutritional lipid calories (propofol infusion).[28] A close watch on lipid metabolism is required. Increased triglyceride with low high-density lipoprotein is associated with reduced survival in critically ill patients.

Carbohydrate

Carbohydrate provides 3.75 kcal/g in vivo. The remaining energy requirements should be given as carbohydrate. Excessive carbohydrate-based energy is associated with hyperglycemia, increased CO_2 production, and increased insulin requirements with no advantage on protein sparing. The upper limit for carbohydrate intake in ICU is described as 5 mg/kg/min.[24] A higher glucose/lipid ratio improves nitrogen balance.

Micronutrients

Micronutrients including vitamins (such as E, C, and β-carotene) and trace elements (such as copper, manganese, zinc, iron, and selenium) play an important role as catalyst in various enzyme reactions in metabolic pathways. They are also essential for immunity and antioxidant defense, endocrine function, DNA synthesis, gene repair, and cell signaling.[24] Compared to standard polymeric formula feeds (contain these micronutrients), patients on parental nutrition (PN) need supplementation of these micronutrients since these are not added to maintain the stability of PN solutions. These should also be prescribed to patients receiving blended kitchen feeds. Repletion of micronutrients is also recommended in conditions like systemic inflammatory response syndrome (SIRS) due to leakage into interstitial compartment and patients on renal replacement therapy (particularly copper and selenium).[24,29] Selenium monotherapy in high dose following initial loading dose has shown to reduce mortality in critically ill patients.[30]

Immunonutrition

While earlier meta-analysis suggested potential benefits of immune-modulating nutritional supplementation with reduction in infection and length of hospital stay, the current guidelines do not recommend routine use of immune-modulating enteral formulas in all critically ill patients.

Glutamine

Glutamine is a normal component of proteins and serves as a metabolic fuel in rapidly proliferating cells. It is endogenously synthesized by skeletal muscles and liver. Glutamine supplementation may reduce bacterial translocation from gut, decrease proinflammatory cytokines, and improve immune cell function. Plasma glutamine levels have been observed to be low in critical illness.[31] Additional enteral glutamine is not recommended in all critically ill patients except burn and trauma patients.[14,24] Glutamine supplementation may be considered in patients on renal replacement therapy due to associated losses,[24] or in patients exclusively on parental nutrition.[32] Higher plasma glutamine levels in critically ill patients with multiorgan failure has shown to increase mortality in REDOXS trial.[33]

Arginine

Arginine is a conditionally essential amino acid. It has a role in protein biosynthesis, proline, and collagen synthesis (wound healing), and regulation of T-cell function (immune-modulation).[34] Arginine deficiency in sepsis can impair nitric oxide (NO) production with impaired microcirculation. On the other hand, arginine supplementation leads to increased NO production with risk of hemodynamic instability in septic shock.[35] Therefore, potential role of arginine supplementation has been extensively studied in sepsis. Clinically, arginine infusion has not shown improvement in local perfusion but is safe with regard to hemodynamic stability in septic shock.[34,36] Parental arginine also leads to reduced protein catabolism in critically ill. Current guidelines give weak recommendation for consideration of arginine supplementation in TBI and perioperative period.[14]

Omega-3 Fatty Acids

A daily intake of 500 mg of eicosapentaenoic acid (EPA) and docosahexaenoic acid (DHA) is recommended for healthy person. Fatty acids (FA) have anti-inflammatory properties and are available for both enteral and parental route. Current guidelines have reviewed omega-3 FA supplementation of EN and PN separately. Omega-3 FA enriched enteral formulas have shown improvement in PO_2/FiO_2 ratio in patients with ALI and acute respiratory distress syndrome (ARDS), but that can be affected by multiple factors including ventilator settings, patient's position, and fluid status.[24] Routine use of omega-3 FA enriched enteral formulas is not recommended. However within nutritional doses, continuous administration rather than bolus doses has shown to improve ventilator days and length of stay.[14,24] In patients requiring PN, lipid emulsions enriched with EPA and DHA have shown reduction in ventilator days and infection rate.

Antioxidants

Level of antioxidant vitamins (E and C) and minerals (cooper, selenium, and zinc) are reduced in conditions of SIRS, ARDS, burns and trauma, and can lead to depressed immunity, compromised wound healing and increased morbidity/mortality. The ASPEN guidelines recommend combination of antioxidant vitamins and minerals in safe doses.[14] The European Society for Clinical Nutrition and Metabolism (ESPEN) recommends that antioxidants in higher doses (exceeding 10 times the dietary reference intake) should not be administered without proven deficiency.[24]

INITIATION, ADVANCEMENT, AND MONITORING OF NUTRITION

Current evidence in adult critically ill patients suggests that early enteral nutrition (EN) is the best practice and leads to improved clinical outcomes. Clinical practice guidelines by the SCCM,[14] ASPEN, and the ESPEN,[24] all recommend early EN within 48 hours of admission in critically ill adult patients. Many experts believe that early feeding helps to improve gut permeability and increased blood flow, thus decreasing complications of the inflammatory stress response. However, evidence in critically ill neurological patients is lacking. Evidence in this patient group is limited to few studies supporting EN in TBI,[37] spinal cord injury (SCI), and stroke.[38,39] Comparison between EN and PN in brain injured patients has shown PN to be associated with less mortality and infection.[40]

Whether to administer calories as per estimated REE or not is controversial. Several studies have shown either no harm or benefit from underfeeding.[41] The Enteral Nutrition in Adult Critically Ill Patients (EPaNIC) trial showed that matching caloric requirements to REE by supplementing EN with PN in patients who could not meet caloric goals by EN feeds alone, led to worse outcomes in terms of time to recovery and complications.[42] It is common practice nowadays to feed a patient "sufficiently" while preventing both undernutrition and overfeeding.

While choosing between EN and PN in a patient, enteral route must be preferred wherever possible. Absence of bowel sounds has no predictive value regarding the extent of ileus or the success or failure of EN. EN is associated with lesser infectious complications, greater feasibility, and lower costs than PN.[43]

The decision regarding when to start oral feeds is also important. Swallow tests and video fluoroscopic swallow studies have been described for detection of dysphagia. Simple bedside algorithms using National Institutes of Health Stroke Scale (NIHSS) and Glasgow Coma Scale (GCS) scores may also be used with good success.

In critically ill adults, EN must begin as soon as medically and surgically appropriate. The rate of enteral infusion is advanced as tolerated toward goal of 80% of measured energy and protein requirements over the next 7-10 days.[14] Studies in neurological patients suggest that establishment of nutrition protocols may be beneficial. For example, unless contraindicated, all ICU patients with GCS <11 should have automatic orders for placement of postpyloric enteral access, radiological confirmation of proper placement of feeding tube and EN formula feed to be initiated at a standard rate until a nutritional assessment is done.[44] Authors also suggest that incremental rates of EN should be avoided in neurological patients because they may tolerate target rates of EN infusion from the beginning itself. In case of intolerance, EN rate should be lowered

> **BOX 2:** Key factors for successful enteral nutrition.
> - Obtain early postpyloric access, preferably within 24 hours.
> - Initiate enteral nutrition early, preferably within 48 hours.
> - Increase rate of enteral nutrition as tolerated to reach target quickly.
> - Use a systematic method of estimating caloric and protein requirements.
> - When necessary, use prokinetic agents and bowel regimen early in feeding to facilitate tolerance.
> - Take into account additional sources of energy such as propofol.
> - Manage glycemic levels.
> - Assess patients with dysphagia to prevent aspiration.
> - Adjust calorie and protein according to phase of illness and metabolic parameters.

and then systematically increased to reach target rate.[44] Bowel regimens and need for prokinetic agents should be assessed upon admission or initiation of nutrition to prevent complications such as distention, gastroparesis, and constipation that are often associated with acute illness and use of anesthetic/analgesic agents in neurocritically ill patients. **Box 2** enumerates key factors for successful nutrition support.[44]

The practice of measuring gastric residual volumes (GRV) should be discouraged. GRV has not been shown to correlate with incidence of pneumonia, regurgitation, or aspiration.[14] Patients on vasopressors with symptoms of feed intolerance such as abdominal distension, increased nasogastric tube output, hypoactive bowel sounds, decreased gut motility, metabolic acidosis, base deficit, etc. should be monitored for signs of ischemic bowel. EN should be held until condition improves.[14]

Nutrition must include appropriate quantities of energy, protein, fluid, electrolyte, mineral, micronutrients, and fiber.

Immunonutrients include glutamine, arginine, omega-3 FA, vitamins, and nucleotides. The disease stage, gastrointestinal tolerance, likely duration of nutritional support and the risk of developing refeeding syndrome all must be taken into account.[45]

Regarding glycemic control in neurocritical care units, studies have showed that although some benefits cannot be excluded among special subgroups of patients, intensive sugar control increases the risk of hypoglycemia greatly and has no mortality benefit against a moderate sugar control strategy of 110–180 mg%. Blood sugar levels > 200 mg% should be avoided.[46]

TYPES OF NUTRITIONAL SUPPLEMENTATION

Nutrition can be supported either enterally or parenterally. Type of neurological condition and its effect on resting and total energy expenditure decide the route of nutrition. **Table 6** gives common complications associated with EN and PN.

Enteral Nutrition

The gastrointestinal tract is the preferred route for nutrition supplementation. A functioning gastrointestinal tract reduces bacterial translocation and improves gut mucosal integrity and enzymatic activity. Tube feeding is the commonly practiced technique in critically ill patients.[47] The route of enteral nutrition may be nasogastric, nasojejunal, or via percutaneous endoscopic gastrostomy. None of them has been shown to have any significant benefits over the other.[48]

Common obstacles to early initiation of EN are feeding intolerance, altered gut motility, acute pancreatitis, gastrointestinal hemorrhage, enterocolitis, complete mechanical bowel obstruction, high output enterocutaneous fistula, etc. Specific to neurological patients, factors such as raised intracranial pressure, impaired swallow, altered level of consciousness, use of medications such as barbiturates, opioids, vasopressors, and overall poor neurological function also impair enteral nutrition.[44]

Standard enteral formulas do not resemble whole food diets. Whole food-based nutrition therapy may be beneficial but has

TABLE 6: Common complications associated with enteral or parenteral nutrition.

Enteral nutrition

Gastrointestinal	• Nausea and vomiting • Abdominal distention • Aspiration • Infection, *Clostridium difficile* enterocolitis • Diarrhea
Metabolic	• Hyperglycemia • Refeeding syndrome • Electrolyte imbalance • Overhydration
Enteral tube related	• Malposition • Colonic perforation, peritonitis • Ulceration • Accidental removal • Sinusitis • Strictures

Parenteral nutrition

Central line related	• Pneumothorax • Infection • Arrhythmias
Metabolic	• Early volume overload • Hyperglycemia • Refeeding syndrome • *Electrolyte disturbances:* Hypokalemia, hypophosphatemia, hypomagnesemia, hyperchloremic metabolic acidosis • Vitamin, mineral, trace elements deficiency • Steatosis, cholestasis • Acute pancreatitis • Bone demineralization

higher risk of infection.[49] Most commercially available enteral formula feeds provide 1 kcal/mL of feed absorbed.

Enteral feeds are usually supplied in two forms.
1. *Polymeric formulations:* They are composed of intact proteins, carbohydrates, complex fats with added vitamins, minerals, and trace elements. They are lactose-free and fiber is added to maintain structural integrity of enterocytes.
2. *Elemental preparations:* These preparations may be helpful in malabsorption states since they contain nutrients in readily absorbable forms. Carbohydrates are present in the form of mono or disaccharides, fats in the form of medium chain FA and proteins in the form of peptides or amino acids.

Parenteral Nutrition

For patients with adequate baseline nutritional status on admission, guidelines suggest that supplemental parenteral nutrition (PN) should be considered after 7–10 days of inadequate intake via oral or enteral route (<60% of requirements).[14] However, PN is recommended as soon as possible following ICU admission when oral or enteral routes are not feasible and patient is at high risk of severe malnutrition on initial assessment. Parenteral nutrition is also employed in patients who have failure of enteral nutrition, who are not expected to start enteral feeding within 5–7 days and when enteral feeding alone is leading to undernutrition.

The osmolality of parenteral nutrition decides whether the solution will be administered through central venous catheter or peripheral intravenous line. A dedicated port must be used for administration with minimal interruptions in administration.

Before starting PN, always rethink the decision to start PN over EN, decide about total caloric requirements and consider the risk of refeeding syndrome. In patients at risk of refeeding syndrome, PN is initiated at 50% of daily caloric requirement. **Table 7** gives a general example of how PN can be planned in an average build middle-aged patient in ICU.

TABLE 7: Typical plan of parenteral nutrition in an average build, middle-aged patient in ICU.

Component	Calculation
Dextrose	1,000 mL of 25% dextrose contains 250 g dextrose that provides 850 kcal
Protein	1–2 g/kg bodyweight
Lipid	200 mL of 20% lipid contains 40 g lipid that provides 400 kcal

Plan of PN for a 70 kg, middle aged patient in ICU

Requirements:
Nonprotein caloric requirement = 70 kg × 25 kcal/kg/day = 1,750 kcal/day
Protein requirement = 70 kg × 1 g/day = 70 g/day
Fluid requirement = 70 kg × 35 mL/kg/day = 2,450 mL/day

Plan:
1,500 mL of 25% dextrose contains 375 g dextrose that provides 1,275 kcal
250 mL of 20% lipid contains 50 g lipid that provides 500 kcal
So, 1,775 nonprotein kcal can be supplied in 1,750 mL fluid
700 mL of 10% amino acid contains 70 g protein
So, a total of 1,775 nonprotein kcal and 70 g protein can be supplied in 2,450 mL/day of fluid

(PN: parental nutrition)

Parenteral nutrition solution is a sterile emulsion consisting of proteins in the form of soluble mixture of essential and non-essential amino acids, fat as intralipid formed of soya with chylomicron sized particles and carbohydrates in the form glucose. Micronutrient supplementation is important. Electrolytes and minerals are therefore added to the emulsion. Daily monitoring of electrolytes, complete blood count, intake and output, and weekly prealbumin level monitoring is required.

Ketogenic Therapy

A ketogenic diet is a high fat, low carbohydrate, adequate protein diet. Increased ketogenesis from lipid metabolism mimics the metabolic effect of fasting. Apart from being an energy substrate, ketones also have potential beneficial effects of activating antioxidant defenses, mitochondrial biogenesis, autophagy, and anti-inflammatory pathways, which may be helpful in recovery from critical illness.[50,51] In clinical practice, ketogenic diet has been in use as an adjunctive treatment for super-refractory status epilepticus. Potential benefits of ketogenic diet in TBI may include increased ATP production, better glycemic control, and antiepileptic effect.[52] Patients on ketogenic diet require careful monitoring of blood glucose and ketones.

NUTRITION THERAPY IN NEUROCRITICAL CARE

Routine use of specialty/disease-specific formulae is not recommended in all critically ill patients.

Traumatic Brain Injury

Early feeding may reduce inflammatory response in patients with TBI and has been associated with significant reduction in 2-weeks mortality and incidence of early-onset ventilator associated pneumonia.[53] It is recommended to initiate enteral feeding at the earliest, once the patient is hemodynamically stable.[24,53,54] Transpyloric jejunal feeding is associated with reduced residual gastric volume and is recommended to reduce the incidence of ventilator-associated pneumonia.[53] Optimal energy and protein intake have been associated with reduced 2-week mortality. Protein up to of 1.2–2 g/kg/day is given.[14] Strict glycemic control is associated with higher incidence of hypoglycemic episodes and is not recommended.[53] Immune-modulating nutrition supplementation has demonstrated reduction in infectious complication in TBI patients.[14]

Stroke

Prior to initiating feeding, all patients with stroke should be screened for dysphagia to reduce the risk of pneumonia.[54] Early enteral nutrition (<72 hours) reduces long-term mortality.[55] In patients anticipated to have long-term persistent dysphagia (>28 days) or reduced consciousness, percutaneous gastrostomy tube feeding should be considered.[54] Blood glucose level must be maintained between 140 and 180 mg/dL.[54] Nutritional supplements should be considered for patients who are malnourished or at risk of malnourishment.[2,54,56]

Spinal Cord Injury

Early enteral nutrition is recommended in SCI.[57] In patients with SCI, lower metabolic rate and dysregulated endometabolic milieu increase the risk of neurogenic obesity and cardiometabolic disorder.[58] Neurogenic obesity is associated with sarcopenia and muscle atrophy. Therefore, a low caloric-high nutrition density diet is optimal for these patients. Academy of Nutrition and Dietetics Evidence Analysis Library (ANDEAL) recommends a minimum protein intake of 0.8–1 g/kg/day in patients with SCI.[59] Protein requirement is increased in presence of pressure sores and infections. For patients with chronic SCI, US Department of Agriculture (USDA) recommends high fiber intake (22–34 g/day) which is higher than the recommendations of ANDEAL (15 g/day).[60]

Chronic Neurological Disorder

Patients with chronic neurological disorders are at increased risk of malnutrition due to associated dysphagia, gastroparesis, depression, and cognitive impairment. This requires frequent monitoring of nutritional and vitamin status (vitamin D, B_{12}, and folate).

Parkinson's Disease

Various predictors of malnutrition in Parkinson's disease (PD) include old age, higher levodopa dose, anxiety and depression, and living alone.[2] All PD patients with Hoehn and Yahr stage >III, BMI <20 kg/m^2, drooling, and cognitive decline should be screened for dysphagia. Side effects of anti-Parkinson's drugs may also influence nutritional status of these patients. Levodopa can cause hyperhomocysteinemia and requires supplementation of vitamin B. Levodopa also competes with large amino-acids for intestinal absorption and is advised to consume at least 30 minutes prior to meals. The ESPEN recommends protein-redistribution dietary regimen (low protein-breakfast and lunch, no protein restriction dinner) to maximize levodopa absorption and efficacy in patients experiencing motor fluctuations.[2]

Amyotrophic Lateral Sclerosis

In amyotrophic lateral sclerosis (ALS) patients, malnutrition is an independent risk factor for survival. Weight stabilization (BMI: 25–35 kg/m^2) is recommended to improve mobilization. Energy requirement in all ALS patients is estimated based on clinical condition and ventilator requirement (approximately 30 kcal/kg bodyweight in nonventilated patients, 25–30 kcal/kg bodyweight in patients with noninvasive ventilation and 30–35 kcal/kg bodyweight in patients on positive pressure ventilation) and adapted to weight evolution.[2] All patients with ALS should be screened for dysphagia. Nutritional supplementation is recommended in patients with deficiencies and weight loss.

Multiple Sclerosis

The ESPEN recommends a diet lower in saturated fat and higher in polyunsaturated fatty acids (PUFA) along with ensuring adequate vitamin D level for the prevention of multiple sclerosis (MS). This may be based on the immunomodulatory and anti-inflammatory properties of PUFA as well as their role as compounds of the myelin membrane. Supplementation with omega-6 FA may reduce the number and severity of relapses.

■ REFEEDING SYNDROME

Refeeding syndrome is a clinical manifestation resulting after restarting nutrition therapy after a period of starvation. Starvation is associated with depletion of intracellular electrolytes (phosphate, potassium, magnesium, and calcium) store even though serum electrolytes level may appear normal. When nutrition is restarted, availability of carbohydrate leads to insulin-dependent intracellular influx of electrolytes resulting in rapid decrease in serum levels. Severe hypophosphatemia may present with confusion, delirium, seizures, respiratory failure, cardiac failure, and rhabdomyolysis. At risk, patients must be identified and feeding started with 25-50% calorie requirement and advanced as quickly as tolerated over 24-48 hours while monitoring for refeeding syndrome.[14] Risk of refeeding is higher with initiation of parental nutrition compared to enteral nutrition. Serum electrolytes should be monitored carefully and supplemented while restarting nutrition therapy.

OVERFEEDING

Overfeeding results in uremia, hyperglycemia, hyperlipidemia, hypercapnia, and fluid overload. It has been associated with poor outcome. It has also been suggested that permissive underfeeding may be beneficial than aggressive full feeding.[61] It is important to include nondietary calories (such as propofol infusion and intralipids) while calculating total calorie intake.

UNDERFEEDING

Recently, idea of permissive underfeeding (moderate amount of nonprotein calories) has erupted against full feeding in early acute phase of illness. This idea is based on the belief that initial phase of illness is associated with inflammation, insulin resistance, and feed intolerance. Brief starvation may also be important to preserve autophagy. Various studies have shown that patients receiving full feeding had worse outcome compared to those receiving permissive underfeeding. However, these studies were methodologically flawed.[61,62] A meta-analysis found no differences in ICU and overall mortality, length of stay, duration of mechanical ventilation, and infectious complications between underfeeding and full feeding in patients with ARDS.[63] Permissive underfeeding avoids the risk of overfeeding, hyperglycemia, feed intolerance, and refeeding syndrome. If protein goals are met, slow advancement in total calorie intake may be afforded in selected patients.

CONCLUSION

Patients with neurologic diseases are prone to develop malnutrition owing to decreased intake, disease-related changes in resting energy expenditure, and effect of drug therapy. A well-structured nutrition plan is important in these patients. Malnutrition in these patients can increase morbidity and impair positive rehabilitative outcome. Early and adequate nutrition is an important determinant of outcome and recovery in neurologically injured patients. Both enteral and parenteral routes can be employed. Enteral route is preferred and a balanced diet containing trace elements, vitamins, and minerals must be used. Blood sugars kept <180 mg% as in the general ICU population is safe.

REFERENCES

1. Chapple LS, Deane AM, Heyland DK, Lange K, Kranz AJ, Williams LT, et al. Energy and protein deficits throughout hospitalization in patients admitted with a traumatic brain injury. Clin Nutr. 2016;35:1315-22.
2. Burgos R, Breton I, Cereda E, Desport JC, Dziewas R, Genton L, et al. ESPEN Guideline Clinical Nutrition in Neurology. Clin Nutr. 2018;37:354-96.
3. Kurtz P, Rocha EEM. Nutrition therapy, glucose control, and brain metabolism in traumatic brain injury: a multimodal monitoring approach. Front Neurosci. 2020;14:190.
4. Dickerson RN. Nitrogen balance and protein requirements for critically ill older patients. Nutrients. 2016;8:226.

5. Foley N, Marshall S, Pikul J, Salter K, Teasell R. Hypermetabolism following moderate to severe traumatic acute brain injury: a systematic review. J Neurotrauma. 2008;25:1415-31.
6. Rea K, Dinan TG, Cryan JF. The microbiome: a key regulator of stress and neuroinflammation. Neurobiol Stress. 2016;4:23-33.
7. Hayakawa M, Asahara T, Henzan N, Murakami H, Yamamoto H, Mukai N, et al. Dramatic changes of the gut flora immediately after severe and sudden insults. Dig Dis Sci. 2011;56:2361-5.
8. Lankelma JM, Cranendonk DR, Belzer C, de Vos AF, de Vos WM, van der Poll T, et al. Antibiotic-induced gut microbiota disruption during human endotoxemia: a randomized controlled study. Gut. 2017;66:1623-30.
9. Fay KT, Ford ML, Coopersmith CM. The intestinal microenvironment in sepsis. Biochim Biophys Acta Mol Basis Dis. 2017; 1863(10 Pt B):2574-83.
10. Lyons J, Coopersmith CM. Pathophysiology of the gut and the microbiome in the host response. Pediatr Crit Care Med J. 2017;18 (3 suppl 1):S46-9.
11. Yeh A, Rogers MB, Firek B, Neal MD, Zuckerbraun BS, Morowitz MJ. Dysbiosis across multiple body sites in critically ill adult surgical patients. Shock. 2016;46:649-54.
12. Abdelmalik PA, Dempsey S, Ziai W. Nutritional and bioenergetic considerations in critically ill patients with acute neurological injury. Neurocrit Care. 2017;27:276-86.
13. Kofler M, Schiefecker AJ, Beer R, Gaasch M, Rhomberg P, Stover J, et al. Enteral nutrition increases interstitial brain glucose levels in poor-grade subarachnoid hemorrhage patients. J Cereb Blood Flow Metab. 2018; 38:518-27.
14. McClave SA, Taylor BE, Martindale R, Warren MM, Johnson DR, Braunschweig C, et al. Guidelines for the provision and assessment of nutrition support therapy in the adult critically ill patient: Society of Critical Care Medicine (SCCM) and American Society for Parenteral and Enteral Nutrition (ASPEN). J Parenter Enter Nutr. 2016;40:159-211.
15. Kondrup J, Rasmussen HH, Hamberg O, Stanga Z; Ad Hoc ESPEN Working Group. Nutritional risk screening (NRS 2002): a new method based on an analysis of controlled clinical trials. Clin Nutr. 2003;22:321-36.
16. Heyland DK, Dhaliwal R, Jiang X, Day AG. Identifying critically ill patients who benefit the most from nutrition therapy: the development and initial validation of a novel risk assessment tool. Crit Care. 2011;15:R268.
17. Osooli F, Abbas S, Farsaei S, Adibi P. Identifying critically ill patients at risk of malnutrition and underfeeding: a prospective study at an academic hospital. Adv Pharm Bull. 2019;9:314-20.
18. Compher C, Bingham AL, McCall M, Patel J, Rice TW, Braunschweig C, et al. Guidelines for the Provision of Nutrition Support Therapy in the Adult Critically ill Patient: The American Society for Parenteral and Enteral Nutrition. J Parenter Enteral Nutr. 2022;46:12-41.
19. Neelemaat F, van Bokhorst-de van der Schueren MA, Thijs A, Seidell JC, Weijs PJ. Resting energy expenditure in malnourished older patients at hospital admission and three months after discharge: predictive equations versus measurements. Clin Nutr. 2012;31:958-66.
20. Delsoglio M, Achamrah N, Berger MM, Pichard C. Indirect calorimetry in clinical practice. J Clin Med. 2019;8:1387.
21. McClave SA, Martindale RG, Kiraly L. The use of indirect calorimetry in the intensive care unit. Curr Opin Clin Nutr Metab Care. 2013;16:202-8.
22. Mehta Y, Sunavala JD, Zirpe K, Tyagi N, Garg S, Sinha S, et al. Practice guidelines for nutrition in critically ill patients: a relook for Indian scenario. Indian J Crit Care Med. 2018;22:263-73.
23. Sullivan MM, Sorreda-Esguerra P, Santos EE, Platon BG, Castro CG, Idrisalman ER, et al. Bacterial contamination of blenderized whole food and commercial enteral tube feedings in the Philippines. J Hosp Infect. 2001;49:268-73.

24. Singer P, Blaser AR, Berger MM, Alhazzani W, Calder PC, Casaer M, et al. ESPEN guideline on clinical nutrition in the intensive care unit. Clin Nutr. 2019;38:48-79.
25. Bendavid I, Zusman O, Kagan I, Theilla M, Cohen J, Singer P. Early Administration of Protein in Critically Ill Patients: A Retrospective Cohort Study. Nutrients. 2019;11:106.
26. Koekkoek WACK, van Setten CHC, Olthof LE, Kars JCNH, van Zanten ARH. Timing of PROTein INtake and clinical outcomes of adult critically ill patients on prolonged mechanical VENTilation: The PROTINVENT retrospective study. Clin Nutr. 2019;38:883-90.
27. Dresen E, Weißbrich C, Fimmers R, Putensen C, Stehle P. Medical high-protein nutrition therapy and loss of muscle mass in adult ICU patients: a randomized controlled trial. Clin Nutr. 2021;40:1562-70.
28. Charriere M, Ridley E, Hastings J, Bianchet O, Scheinkestel C, Berger MM. Propofol sedation substantially increases the caloric and lipid intake in critically ill patients. Nutrition. 2017;42:64-8.
29. Ben-Hamouda N, Charriere M, Voirol P, Berger MM. Massive copper and selenium losses cause life-threatening deficiencies during prolonged continuous renal replacement. Nutrition. 2017;34:71-5.
30. Manzanares W, Dhaliwal R, Jiang X, Murch L, Heyland DK. Antioxidant micronutrients in the critically ill: a systematic review and meta-analysis. Crit Care. 2012;16:R66.
31. Rodas PC, Rooyackers O, Hebert C, Norberg A, Wernerman J. Glutamine and glutathione at ICU admission in relation to outcome. Clin Sci. 2012;122:591-7.
32. Weimann A, Braga M, Carli F, Higashiguchi T, Hubner M, Klek S, et al. ESPEN practical guideline: Clinical nutrition in surgery. Clin Nutr. 2021;40:4745-61.
33. Heyland DK, Elke G, Cook D, Berger MM, Wischmeyer PE, Albert M, et al. Glutamine and antioxidants in the critically ill patient: a post hoc analysis of a large-scale randomized trial. J Parenter Enteral Nutr. 2015;39:401-9.
34. Patel JJ, Miller KR, Rosenthal C, Rosenthal MD. When is it appropriate to use arginine in critical illness? Nutr Clin Pract. 2016;31:438-44.
35. Luiking YC, Poeze M, Deutz NE. Arginine infusion in patients with septic shock increases nitric oxide production without haemodynamic instability. Clin Sci. 2015;128:57-67.
36. Luiking YC, Poeze M, Deutz NE. A randomized-controlled trial of arginine infusion in severe sepsis on microcirculation and metabolism. Clin Nutr. 2020;39:1764-73.
37. Grahm TW, Zadrozny DB, Harrington T. The benefits of early jejunal hyperalimentation in the head-injured patient. Neurosurgery. 1989;25:729-35.
38. Haddad SH, Arabi YM. Critical care management of severe traumatic brain injury in adults. Scand J Trauma Resusc Emerg Med. 2012;20:12.
39. Sabbouh T, Torbey MT. Malnutrition in stroke patients: risk factors, assessment, and management. Neurocrit Care. 2018;29:374-84.
40. Rapp RP, Young B, Twyman D, Bivins BA, Haack D, Tibbs PA, et al. The favorable effect of early parenteral feeding on survival in head-injured patients. J Neurosurg. 1983;58:906-12.
41. Rice TW, Mogan S, Hays MA, Bernard GR, Jensen GL, Wheeler AP. Randomized trial of initial trophic versus full-energy enteral nutrition in mechanically ventilated patients with acute respiratory failure. Crit Care Med. 2011;39:967-74.
42. Casaer MP, Mesotten D, Hermans G, Wouters PJ, Schetz M, Meyfroidt G, et al. Early versus late parenteral nutrition in critically ill adults. N Engl J Med. 2011;365:506-17.
43. Desai SV, McClave SA, Rice TW. Nutrition in the ICU: An evidence-based approach. Chest. 2014;145:1148-57.
44. Zarbock SD, Steinke D, Hatton J, Magnuson B, Smith KM, Cook AM. Successful enteral nutritional support in the neurocritical care unit. Neurocrit Care. 2008;9:210-6.

45. Tripathy S, Mishra P, Dash SC. Refeeding syndrome. Indian J Crit Care Med. 2008; 12:132-5.
46. McCormick M, Hadley D, McLean JR, Macfarlane JA, Condon B, Muir KW. Randomized, controlled trial of insulin for acute post stroke hyperglycemia. Ann Neurol. 2010;67:570-8.
47. Bajwa SJS, Gupta S. Controversies, principles and essentials of enteral and parenteral nutrition in critically ill-patients. J Med Nutr Nutraceutical. 2013;2:77-83.
48. Davies AR, Morrison SS, Bailey MJ, Bellomo R, Cooper DJ, Doig GS, et al. ENTERIC Study Investigators, ANZICS Clinical Trials Group. A multicenter, randomized controlled trial comparing early nasojejunal with nasogastric nutrition in critical illness. Crit Care Med. 2012;40:2342-8.
49. Tavarez T, Roehl K, Koffman L. Nutrition in the neurocritical care unit: a new frontier. Curr Treat Options Neurol. 2021;23:16.
50. de Cabo R, Mattson MP. Effects of intermittent fasting on health, aging, and disease. N Engl J Med. 2019;381:2541-51.
51. Gunst J, Casaer MP, Langouche L, Van den Berghe G. Role of ketones, ketogenic diets and intermittent fasting in ICU. Curr Opin Crit Care. 2021;27:385-9.
52. Omori NE, Woo GH, Mansor LS. Exogenous Ketones and Lactate as a Potential Therapeutic Intervention for Brain Injury and Neurodegenerative Conditions. Front Hum Neurosci. 2022;16:846183.
53. Carney N, Totten AM, O'Reilly C, Ullman JS, Hawryluk GWJ, Bell MJ, et al. Guidelines for the Management of Severe Traumatic Brain Injury, Fourth Edition. Neurosurgery. 2017;80:6-15.
54. Powers WJ, Rabinstein AA, Ackerson T, Adeoye OM, Bambakidis NC, Becker K, et al. Guidelines for the Early Management of Patients With Acute Ischemic Stroke: 2019 Update to the 2018 Guidelines for the Early Management of Acute Ischemic Stroke: A Guideline for Healthcare Professionals From the American Heart Association/American Stroke Association. Stroke. 2019;50:e344-e418.
55. Dennis MS, Lewis SC, Warlow C, FOOD Trial Collaboration. Effect of timing and method of enteral tube feeding for dysphagic stroke patients (FOOD): a multicentre randomized controlled trial. Lancet. 2005; 365:764-72.
56. Wirth R, Smoliner C, Jäger M, Warnecke T, Leischker AH, Dziewas R; DGEM Steering Committee. Guideline clinical nutrition in patients with stroke. Exp Transl Stroke Med. 2013;5:14.
57. Blaser AR, Starkopf J, Alhazzani W, Berger MM, Casaer MP, Deane AM, et al. ESICM Working Group on Gastrointestinal Function. Early enteral nutrition in critically ill patients: ESICM clinical practice guidelines. Intensive Care Med. 2017;43:380-98.
58. Yahiro AM, Wingo BC, Kunwor S, Parton J, Ellis AC. Classification of obesity, cardiometabolic risk, and metabolic syndrome in adults with spinal cord injury. J Spinal Cord Med. 2020;43:485-96.
59. Academy of Nutrition and Dietetics. (2009). Spinal Cord Injury (SCI) Guidelines. [online] Available from: https://www.andeal.org/topic.cfm?cat=3485 [Last accessed July, 2023].
60. Farkas GJ, Sneij A, Gater DR Jr. Dietetics After Spinal Cord Injury: Current Evidence and Future Perspectives. Top Spinal Cord Inj Rehabil. 2021;27:100-8.
61. Patel JJ, Martindale RG, McClave SA. Controversies surrounding critical care nutrition: an appraisal of permissive underfeeding, protein, and outcomes. J Parenter Enteral Nutr. 2018;42:508-15.
62. McClave SA, Codner P, Patel J, Hurt RT, Allen K, Martindale RG. Should we aim for full enteral feeding in the first week of critical illness? Nutr Clin Pract. 2016;31: 425-31.
63. Franzosi OS, von Frankenberg AD, Loss SH, Nunes DSL, Vieira SRR. Underfeeding versus full enteral feeding in critically ill patients with acute respiratory failure: a systematic review with meta-analysis of randomized controlled trials. Nutr Hosp. 2017;34: 19-29.

35. Nutrition in Solid Organ Transplantation and Immunocompromised Patients

Pooja Tyagi, Sweta J Patel, Jagadeesh KN

INTRODUCTION

The transplant patients are on the rise with rising awareness and more and more transplant surgeries happening across the globe for failing organs. Solid organ transplant comprises liver, kidney, heart, lung, and pancreas. Peritransplant nutrition is an important arena, which needs its due importance as it impacts the overall outcome of such patients. Pretransplant sarcopenia negatively impacts postoperative outcomes. Malnutrition adds to increased morbidity, mortality, and cost in post-transplantation period. Providing adequate nutrition in these subsets of patients is challenging. Nutrition planning in such patients should consider the pretransplant nutritional status, immunosuppressant medications, infections, wound healing, grafted organ function, metabolic and surgical complications, and providing support to other organs.

DIFFERENT TERMINOLOGY IN CANCER MALNUTRITION[1] (FIG. 1)

Disease-related malnutrition: The inflammatory response of underlying disease leads to anorexia, tissue breakdown, weight loss, altered body composition, and decreased physical function.

Cachexia: Multifactorial wasting syndrome, inclusive of involuntary weight loss with ongoing skeletal muscle mass loss with or without loss of fat mass.

Precachexia: Early clinical and metabolic signs preceding involuntary loss of weight and muscle.

Sarcopenia: Low lean body mass, muscle mass loss, fatigue is common, and limited physical activity.

Sarcopenia obesity: Low lean body mass in obese individuals. Due to excess fat and

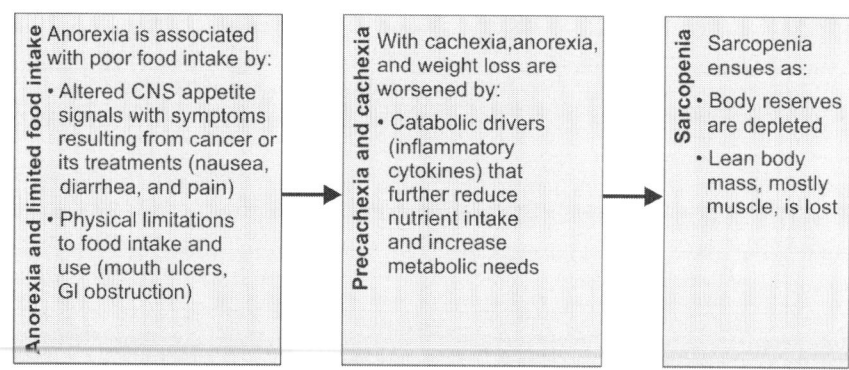

Fig. 1: Different terminologies in cancer malnutrition. (CNS: central nervous system; GI: gastrointestinal)

CHAPTER 35 | Nutrition in Solid Organ Transplantation and Immunocompromised Patients

extracellular water, muscle mass loss is often overlooked. It is an important predictor of adverse outcome.

Cancer Cachexia[1] (Fig. 2)

The three stages of cancer cachexia being precachexia, cachexia, and refractory cachexia.

Cancer-related Malnutrition[1]

It is a multimodel process, as several factors work in combination to decrease food intake, increase energy and protein needs, decrease physical activity, and altered metabolism in different tissues (Figs. 3 and 4).

- *Immune response and systemic inflammation:* Cancer patients report symptoms related to poor intake, weight loss, decreased physical activity, fatigue, and depression. These symptoms are related to systemic inflammation and unregulated immune response.
- *Spillover of cytokines derived from tumor causes worsening of inflammation:* Proinflammatory cytokines disrupt metabolism of carbohydrates, protein, and fats throughout the body.
- *Hypoxia stress in tumor microenvironment:* A growing tumor outpaces its blood supply, causes hypoxia in healthy tissues,

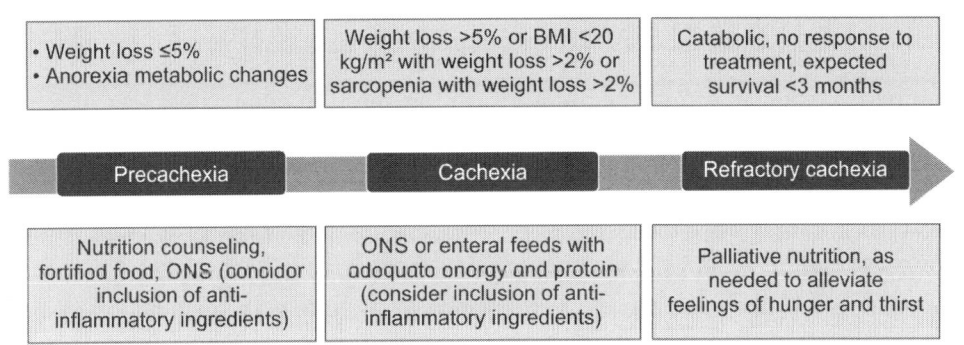

Fig. 2: Cancer cachexia. (BMI: body mass index; ONS: oral nutritional supplements)

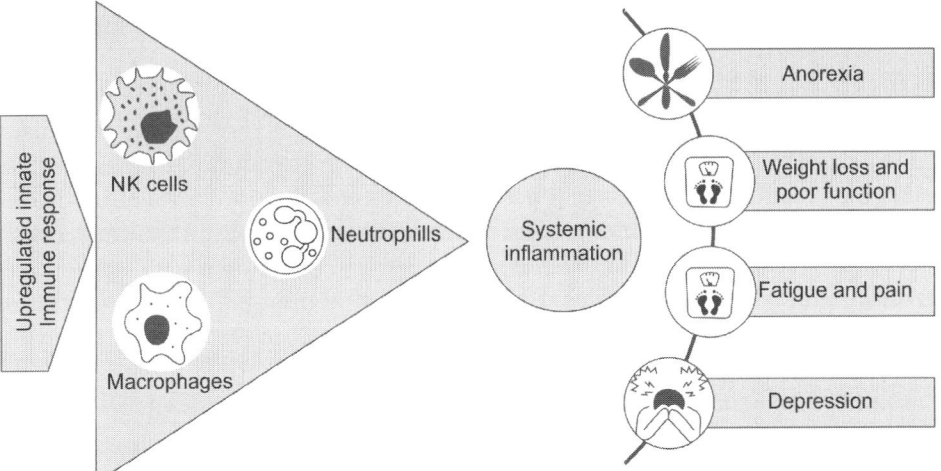

Fig. 3: Systemic inflammation: Upregulated innate immune response.

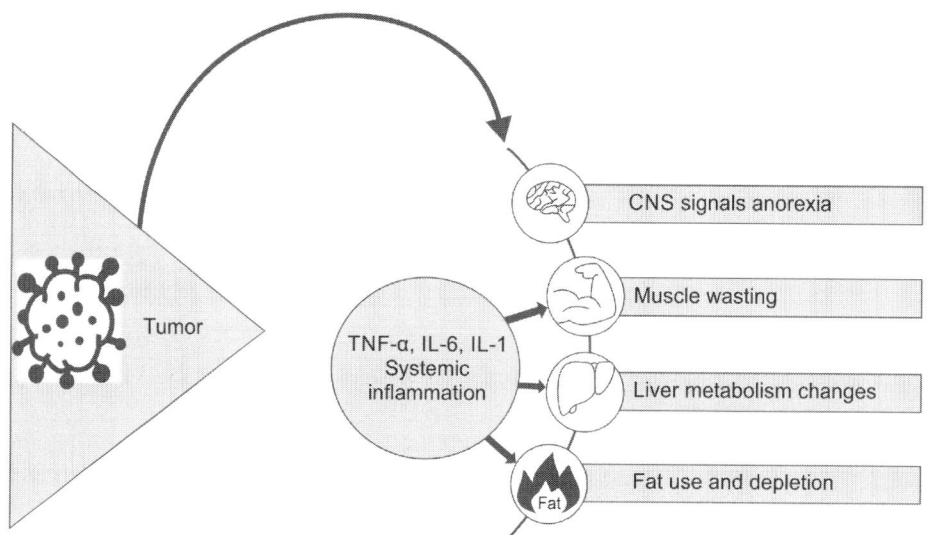

Fig. 4: Cancer-related malnutrition—Systemic inflammation. (CNS: central nervous system; IL: interleukin; TNF: tumor necrosis factor)

leading to hypoxia. Tumor metabolism now relays on anaerobic metabolism, glycolysis and less on oxidative phosphorylation, thus protection against reactive oxygen species is reduced.

- *Indirect effects of tumor and its management:* Poor intake also results from cancer treatment such as chemotherapy, radiation or surgery leading to pain, mouth ulcers, difficulty while chewing, nausea, and others.

NUTRITIONAL ASSESSMENT

The nutritional assessment of transplant patients begins in the pretransplant period, which includes history, physical examination, anthropometric measurements, and laboratory tests **(Table 1)**. Both extremes, malnutrition and obesity have negative impact in post-transplantation period.

In pretransplantation stage, nutritional status, age, weight, gender, metabolic abnormalities, specific organ failure, comorbids, losses, and malabsorption and goals to achieve are to be taken into consideration **(Table 2)**.

In the immediate post-transplantation stage, nutrition support[2] is essential to prevent infection, promote wound healing, meet metabolic demands, and promote immune response **(Table 3)**.

The complications associated with organ transplantation such as infection, rejection, wound healing, optimal glycemic control, immunosuppressant regimen side effects, surgery related, and other organ dysfunction needs specific and planned nutrition program.

Kidney Transplant Patients

The most common organ being transplanted is kidney. Most common causes leading to chronic renal failure and leading to renal transplant are polycystic kidney disease, chronic glomerulonephritis, chronic IgA nephropathy, drug, and dye-induced chronic renal failure. Protein energy malnutrition seen in chronic renal failure patients is due to numerous factors such as anorexia, nutrient loss during dialysis, impaired glucose control, nephrotic dyslipidemia and abnormalities related to metabolism of potassium,

CHAPTER 35 | Nutrition in Solid Organ Transplantation and Immunocompromised Patients

TABLE 1: Nutrition assessment in pretransplantation.

History (determines cause, extent, and duration of deficiencies)	• Obtain medical history related to organ failure and complications • Dietary history and use of nutritional supplements (vitamins, minerals, and herbal) • Gastrointestinal symptoms • Drug-nutrient interaction • Assess for psychosocial support
Physical assessment (determines general nutrition and assesses degree of deficiencies)	• Look for appropriate weight • Any fluid retention or ascites • Any apparent muscle wasting • Alertness of patient • Look for pallor and jaundice • Examine nails, hair, and oral cavity • Examine skin for color and texture
Subjective global assessment (SGA)	*SGA scale:* • Well-nourished • Moderately malnourished • Severely malnourished
Biochemical parameters of nutritional status (non-nutritional factors are to be excluded)	• Serum albumin • Serum transferrin • Prealbumin • Retinal-binding proteins • Creatinine height index • 24-hour urine nitrogen • 3-methyl histidine excretion • Total body potassium • Serum proteins and urine nitrogen levels are affected by non-nutritional factors (fluid status, liver, and kidney functions) • Immune competence tests (TLC, skin test antigen) are influenced by immunosuppressive drugs
Immune competence	• Hypersplenism • Decrease total lymphocytes and CD8 cells • Skin anergy tests
Anthropometric measurements (objective measure to evaluate and monitor progress)	• Body mass index (BMI) • Midarm muscle circumference • Skin-fold thickness
Handgrip dynamometry	• Hand-grip strength dynamometry • Useful if monitored serially over time by single observer • Hand grip is indirect measure of protein stores • 6-minute walk test
Indirect calorimetry	Nonprotein respiratory quotient
Bioelectrical impedance	Direct segmental multifrequency bioelectrical analysis
Others	• Dual energy X-ray absorptiometry • In viva neutron activation analysis • Deuterium isotope dilution • Psoas muscle cross-sectional area

(TLC: total lymphocyte count)

TABLE 2: Pretransplant nutrition recommendations (Based on dry weight).

Calories	
Weight maintenance	• 1.2–1.3 times BEE (basal energy expenditure) • 30 kcal/kg
Weight gain	• 1.5 times BEE • 35–40 kcal/kg
Weight loss	Create deficit of 500–1,000 cal/day
Proteins	
Maintenance	0.8–1.2 g/kg/day
Replenishing stores	1.3–2.0 g/kg/day
Dialysis	• *HD:* 1.2–1.5 g/kg/day • *CRRT:* 2 g/kg/day • *Peritoneal dialysis:* 1.5 g/kg/day
Hepatic encephalopathy (HE)	• Determine cause of HE • *Increase proteins:* Maintenance or repletion • Add branched chain amino acids enriched supplements
Vitamins	
Vitamin A deficiency	Caused by steatorrhea, alcoholism, decreased retinal binding proteins in renal failure
Vitamin B_6, B_{12}, niacin, thiamine deficiencies	Seen in alcoholism
Vitamin C deficiency	Due to dietary restrictions and losses during dialysis
Vitamin D deficiency	Poor diet, steatorrhea, steroid use in cirrhotic liver
Vitamin E and K deficiency	Steatorrhea, antibiotics
Folate deficiency	Alcoholism and dialysis patients
Minerals	
Calcium	• Urinary losses with steroids • GI losses with steatorrhea • Abnormal vitamin D, calcium, and phosphorus metabolism in renal diseases
Copper	Decreased excretion with biliary obstruction/Wilson disease
Iron	• Chronic bleed • Renal diseases—decreased erythropoietin and dialysis losses • Liver diseases—excess iron stores in hemachromatosis
Magnesium	• Loss with diuretic and in alcoholism • Decreased excretion in renal failure
Phosphorus	• Alcohol and steroid use • Increased in renal failure
Potassium	• Hypokalemia—diuretic and insulin use • Hyperkalemia—potassium sparing diuretic and renal diseases
Sodium	Needs restrictions, depends on fluid status, and blood pressure
Zinc	• Loss due to diarrhea, diuretic, and alcohol • Decreased excretion in renal failure • Low levels in patients on dialysis

(CRRT: continuous renal replacement therapy; HD: hemodialysis)

CHAPTER 35 | Nutrition in Solid Organ Transplantation and Immunocompromised Patients

TABLE 3: Nutrition in post-transplant period (Based on dry weight).

	Kidney	Liver	Heart	Lung	Pancreas
Protein					
Short term	1.3–2 g/kg/day	1.5–2 g/kg/day	1.3–1.5 g/kg/day	1–1.5 g/kg/day	1.3–2 g/kg/day
			<2.5 g/kg/day (infection, repletion)	1.5–2 g/kg/day (repletion)	
Long term	0.8–1 g/kg/day	0.8–1 g/kg/day	1–1.3 g/kg/day	1–1.3 g/kg/day	0.8–1 g/kg/day
Kilocalories					
Short term	30–35 kcal/kg	30–35 kcal/kg	35 kcal/kg	35 kcal/kg	30–35 kcal/kg
Maintenance	25–30 kcal/kg	25–30 kcal/kg	25–30 kcal/kg	25–30 kcal/kg	25–30 kcal/kg
Fat					
Short term	30–50% nonprotein kcal	25–35% nonprotein kcal	<30% kcal <300 mg cholesterol, <7% from saturated fats	<30% kcal <300 mg cholesterol, <7% from saturated fats	30–50% nonprotein kcal
Maintenance	<30% total kcal <300 mg cholesterol, 7–10% calories from saturated fats	25–30% total kcal, <300 mg cholesterol, <7% from saturated fats	<300 mg cholesterol, 7–10% calories from saturated fats	<300 mg cholesterol, 7–10% calories from saturated fats	<300 mg cholesterol, 7–10% calories from saturated fats
Carbohydrate					
Short term	50–70%	50–70%	50–70%	50–70%	50–70%
Maintenance	45–50% of total calories 25–30 g fibers/day	50% of total calories, 25–30 g fibers/day	50–60% total calories 25 g fibers/day	50–60% total calories 25 g fibers/day	45–50% total calories
Electrolytes and minerals	No added salt, monitor potassium, phosphorus, magnesium, calcium 1–1.5 g/day	No added salt, monitor potassium, phosphorus, magnesium, calcium 1–1.5 g/day	No added salt, monitor potassium, phosphorus, magnesium, calcium 1–1.5 g/day	No added salt, monitor potassium, phosphorus, magnesium, calcium 1–1.5 g/day	No added salt, monitor potassium, phosphorus, magnesium, calcium 1–1.5 g/day
Vitamin D	Supplements	Supplements	Supplements	Supplements	Supplements

phosphorus, and calcium. The patient on dialysis can lose protein up to 2–8 g/day on hemodialysis and 5–12 g/day on peritoneal dialysis.[3] These patients need 1.2–1.3 g/kg/day (dry weight), of which 50% containing essential amino acids of high biologic value.[4]

In post-transplant period, 4–20% patients develop new onset of diabetes (NODPT).[5] Most commonly implicated medication is steroid which is a part of immunosuppressant regimen. The common side effects being hyperglycemia and weight gain. Impaired glucose control delays wound healing, increase infection risk and dehydration thus affecting the transplanted kidney function.

In post-transplant period, protein losses via dialysis do not occur and potassium and phosphorus restrictions may not be needed. On an average, a 10% weight gain is seen in first post-transplant year due to better diet, improved metabolism and less of nutrient losses. BMI >28 kg/m^2 in post-transplantation is associated with increased mortality,[6] also increased risk for metabolic syndrome and cardiovascular diseases such as coronary artery disease, hypertension, diabetes, and stroke.

Liver Transplant Patients

The liver is the major metabolic organ, central to biochemical pathways involved in metabolism of carbohydrates, proteins, fat, and vitamins. The common reasons for which liver transplant happens are decompensated chronic liver disease with varied etiologies, acute liver failure, primary biliary cirrhosis, primary scleroising cirrhosis, and hepatocellular carcinoma. Those with chronic liver diseases may have poor nutritional status in pretransplant period, majorly attributed to poor intake, anorexia, hypermetabolic state, and decreased nutrient absorption. Malnutrition occurs in 34–84% in alcoholic cirrhotic and 27–87% of nonalcoholic cirrhosis.[3]

Nutrition in Pretransplant Period

The primary goal in pretransplant phase is to provide adequate nutrition so as to prevent further muscle breakdown and nutrient losses and correct vitamin and mineral deficiencies.[7] Since DDLT occurs in short notice period, an early aggressive postoperative nutrition support is initiated, as there may not be time to build nutrition before surgery. Unlike in LDLT, an early planned nutrition program pertaining to individual needs can be executed.

Enteral nutrition (EN) either through gastric or jejunal routes is preferred when oral intake is inadequate or not possible. The importance of EN lies in the fact it provides nutrition while maintaining gut mucosa integrity and gut barrier, barrier against translocation of luminal microorganisms into portal circulation through antigenic stimulation to gut associated lymphoid tissue and also it is inexpensive, associated with less complications and decreased length of stay in hospital in comparison with parenteral nutrition (PN)[8] **(Table 4)**.

The parenteral nutrition (PN) is indicated when patient is moderate to severely malnourished and is not able to take adequate energy intake orally or enterally due to gastrointestinal dysfunction related to gastrointestinal bleed, ileus, or intestinal obstruction.[9]

Any fasting period amounts to regular blood sugar monitoring and dextrose infusions if need be as these patients have low glycogen stores.

Carbohydrates: It should cover 50–60% of nonprotein energy requirements, essentially provided by glucose. Excess glucose shall result in hyperglycemia, lipogenesis, and increased carbon dioxide production.[9] Altered glucose homeostasis is common in liver diseases, thus vigilant glucose monitoring is needed to avoid both hypoglycemia and hyperglycemia. The glucose intake up to 2 g/kg/day is advocated.

Lipids: These patients are usually deficient in essential fatty acids and their polyunsaturated fatty acids derivatives, which are associated with low survival rates.

TABLE 4: Routes of nutrition support therapy.

Oral	• Liquid diet—start when patient passes flatus • Normal diet—when bowel movement is present • Carbohydrates controlled diet—when hyperglycemia is present • Sodium restriction—in severe fluid retention • Fluid restriction—in presence of hyponatremia	Monitor bowel sounds, intake and output, edema, ascites and serum sodium
Tube feed	• Formula/commercial feeds • Polymeric, high nitrogen formula • High-fiber formula—in presence of diarrhea or constipation • Concentrated formula—in volume overload • Semielemental/polypeptide formula—in presence of indigestion	Monitor weight, intake, and output, laboratory—sodium, glucose, potassium, phosphorus, magnesium, calcium, and carbon dioxide
TPN	• *Dextrose:* 70% nonprotein calories • *Lipids:* 30% nonprotein calories • *Amino acids:* 10–15% • Vitamin and trace elements supplements daily • Insulin if blood sugars elevated	Monitor weight, intake, and output, laboratory—sodium, glucose, potassium, phosphorus, magnesium, calcium, and carbon dioxide

(TPN: total parenteral nutrition)

Lipids supplements are provided in emulsion forms and should account for 40–50% of nonprotein energy requirements.[10] Lipids being essential nutrient in malnourished, dietary fat should not be restricted unless true fat malabsorption conditions are encountered. Lipid intake is limited to 1 g/kg/day, considering dry prehospital weight.

Protein: A fine balance between protein as nutrient needs to counter catabolic state and avoid hyperammonemia has to be taken into consideration, when providing adequate nutrition. Initial protein intake of at least 1 g/kg/day is warranted and subsequent measurement of 24 hours urine urea nitrogen to assess for catabolic state is done. If tolerated, protein intake can be gradually increased to 1.8–2 g/kg/day.[11]

Other Supplements

Branched-chain amino acids (BCAAs)—leucine, isoleucine, and valine, these are not metabolized in liver. BCAAs lead to glutamine production and induce hepatocyte growth factor secretion.

It is reported oral BCAAs supplements in preoperative period leads to reduced incidence of bacteremia and sepsis in postoperative period. They lower ammonia levels, improve glucose tolerance, and aid in liver regeneration and immune function.

Micronutrient: Several micronutrients' deficiencies are commonly seen in liver disease such as folate, thiamine, and pyridoxine, which may be associated with increased brain levels of ammonia.

Vitamin A, B_{12}, calcium, and phosphorus are other noted deficiencies, vitamin K deficiency leads to coagulation derangements. Increased oxidative stress is seen in these subsets of patients due to deficiencies of vitamin C, E, and selenium.

Zinc and magnesium are also deficient due to decreased absorption and increased urinary excretion. Vitamin D supplements are added as it aids in immune tolerance of liver allograft.

Nutrition in post-transplant period: The post-transplant nutrition goals are aimed at to provide adequate nutrition to treat catabolism and promote healing, achieve optimal glucose levels, monitor and treat dyselectrolytemia, and replenish nutrient stores.

The malnutrition associated with liver disease does not get corrected in post-transplant period, specifically sarcopenia. Even though liver function improves, bodyweight is regained, but body composition alterations persist. The poor muscle mass can persist up to a year or more. During long-term follow-up, overweight and obesity is seen in liver recipients.

These patients have significant improvement in their diet in post-transplant period as factors contributing to less dietary intake, catabolic state, and nutrient losses are taken care of. The calories intake improved from 27 to 32 kcal/kg/day, protein intake from 0.8 to 1.3 g/kg/day has been seen in pre- and post-transplant period.[12] On long-term follow-up, patients with overweight and obesity correlated with increased dietary intake.

Even after the transplantation, the energy and protein requirements remain high for weeks. The increased metabolism seen in post-transplant period is reflective of pretransplant metabolism and steroid use. The metabolism normalizes in up to 4 months' time post-transplantation. In immediate post-transplantation, protein intake of 1.5–2 g/kg/day is recommended to promote wound healing and hepatocyte recovery due to high-protein catabolism on initial 2 weeks' post-transplantation. While 25–30 kcal/kg/day in nonprotein energy requirements should be aimed, considering metabolic and inflammatory status of the patients. Increased REE remains for long time in post-transplantation.

The total body water is decreased and there is increase in body fat, overweight, and hypercholesterolemia is seen on long-term follow-up.

Nutritional status in post-transplantation is affected by allograft function, even if allograft functions well, some nutritional disturbances do not normalize.

Vitamin A and zinc deficiencies improve in immediate post-transplantation.

The nutrition support in immediate transplantation is usually started after 24 hours of transplant surgery. The oral route is preferred whenever feasible. In severely malnourished, those who cannot take adequate oral diet should be started on enteral feeding, gradual build-up of energy intake should be aimed, hence avoiding refeeding syndrome.

Heart Transplantation

The chronic heart failure either due to cardiomyopathy or ischemic heart disease is a common cause for heart transplantation. Nausea and anorexia associated with chronic heart failure lead to malnutrition, further leading to cardiac cachexia when there is loss of cardiac muscle mass.[13,14] The salt and water retention in chronic heart failure, as a mechanism to maintain blood pressure, diverts blood flow to vital organs, hence reduced blood flow in skin and gut. Reduced blood flow to gut leads to hypomotility, delayed gastric emptying, and malabsorption leading to weight loss and muscle wasting.[14] The congested lung, liver, and spleen are due to salt and water retention. Increased morbidity and mortality are seen with visceral muscle wasting and loss of fatty tissue. The small frequent nutrient dense meals should be encouraged, sodium is restricted to <2 g/day and fluid is restricted to 2 L/day.

In post-transplantation, low cholesterol and low saturated fat diet is advised. Indirect calorimetry should be used to determine energy needs. Weight-gain up to 10 kg can be seen in initial 12 months after transplantation leading to new onset of diabetes and metabolic syndrome. The incidence of new onset of diabetes ranges from 4 to 40% in heart transplant patients.[5] Weight reduction in obese patients improves overall well-being.

Lungs Transplantation

Cystic fibrosis, emphysema, severe chronic obstructive pulmonary disease (COPD), interstitial lung disease, and bronchiectasis are common indications for lung transplantation. Cachetin, a hormone seen in chronic infections such as cystic fibrosis and bronchiectasis, causes muscle wasting and loss of muscle mass.[14] Increased effort to breathe in chronic respiratory illnesses leads to hypermetabolism, inflated chest leads to early satiety. Protein energy malnutrition impairs immune response, increasing susceptibility to lung infections.[15] The calorie needs are calculated through indirect calorimetry.[16] Frequent small nutrient dense feeds are encouraged. The pancreatic insufficiency associated with cystic fibrosis leads to glucose intolerance and diabetes; hence, optimal glucose levels are to be maintained and also fat-soluble vitamins and pancreatic enzymes are supplemented.

In post-transplantation, five to six frequent energy dense, high calorie, and high protein supplement along with pancreatic enzymes are to be included in diet. Underweight is associated with poor survival in post-transplant period. Those patients who gain weight in post-transplantation have favorable outcome. The incidence of new onset of diabetes post-transplantation is seen in 30–35% patients.[5] The optimal weight gain should be aimed at and no added salt helps to control hypertension, calcium, magnesium, and vitamin D supplements are to be provided.

Pancreas Transplantation

Type 1 diabetes mellitus is the most common reason for pancreas transplantation. Nearly 75% of pancreas transplantation happen along with renal transplantation due to associated diabetic nephropathy.[17] The BMI >30 kg/m^2 is associated with post-transplant failure while BMI <27 kg/m^2 supports post-transplant wound healing.[3] Soon after transplantation, glucose levels normalize. A diet consisting of well-controlled fat and calories are aimed to maintain healthy weight goals. Calcium, magnesium, and vitamin D need to be supplemented and no added salt to be advised to control hypertension.

PROBLEMS RELATED TO IMMUNOSUPPRESSIVE MEDICATIONS

The common immunosuppressant drugs employed in these patients are corticosteroids, calcineurin inhibitors (tacrolimus and cyclosporine), sirolimus, and everolimus.[13]

- *Hypertension and fluid retention:* Corticosteroids cause stimulation of mineralocorticoid receptors leading to sodium retention and volume expansion, as a result hypertension occurs, these patients need dietary sodium restrictions and weight management.
- *Hyperglycemia:* Corticosteroids stimulate gluconeogenesis, and inhibit glucose uptake into muscles, peripheral tissues, and adipose tissues. Tacrolimus decreases glucose-mediated insulin release, and sirolimus causes insulin resistance by impairing insulin-mediated suppression of hepatic glucose production.

- *Hyperlipidemia:* Sirolimus alters insulin pathway to alter lipoprotein lipase activity leading to hypertriglyceridemia, increase in very low-density lipoprotein. Corticosteroids cause redistribution of body fat. Glucose and triglycerides accumulate in response to high-insulin levels. The dietary fat in these patients should include less of saturated fats and low cholesterol, more of polyunsaturated and monounsaturated fatty acids.
- *Hyperkalemia:* Cyclosporine causes hyperkalemia by decreasing activity of renin-angiotensin aldosterone pathway, and decreasing excretion of potassium and impaired tubular response to aldosterone. Dietary restrictions of potassium are warranted.
- *Hypomagnesemia:* Calcineurin inhibitors cause intracellular shift of magnesium and less of reabsorption occurs in tubules. Magnesium supplements are essential.
- *Osteoporosis:* Corticosteroids increase excretion of calcium, decrease absorption, and inhibit bone formation. Meanwhile calcineurin inhibitors affect calcium transportation in distal tubule. Calcium and vitamin D supplements are essential.
- *Gastrointestinal symptoms:* Nausea, vomiting, diarrhea, and abdominal pain can occur due to calcineurin inhibitors, and dose adjustments may be needed to relieve symptoms.
- *Weight gain and obesity:* An obesity paradox has been observed in some transplant patients, wherein obese patients have better survival before transplantation but after transplantation they have more complications, higher healthcare costs, and worst outcomes, while those who are underweight before transplantation have poor survival due to less lean muscle mass. Corticosteroids use in pretransplantation is responsible for weight gain. In post-transplantation, obesity is associated with delayed graft function, increased wound infections and overall higher hospital cost. Weight management with watch on calorie intake and regular exercise should be performed.

FOOD AND IMMUNOSUPPRESSIVE DRUG INTERACTIONS (TABLES 5 AND 6 AND BOXES 1 TO 3)

The following foods should be avoided as they affect absorption of immunosuppressive drugs by modulating P450 cytochrome activity:
- Grapefruit
- Papaya
- Star fruit
- Pomegranate
- Black pepper

TABLE 5: Foods to regulate potassium levels.

Potassium-rich foods (>200 mg/serving):		
Bananas	Mango	Avocado
Oranges/Orange juice	Papaya	Brussels sprouts
Cantaloupe	Potatoes	Nuts
Honeydew	Tomato sauce	Peanut butter
Prunes	Spinach	Beans
Raisins	Kale	Lentils
Lower-potassium foods (<100 mg/serving):		
Apple sauce	Carrots	
Green beans	Bagel	
Frozen green peas	Waffle	
Raspberries, blueberries, strawberries	Cranberry juice, apple juice, grape juice	
Watermelon	Hummus	
Cucumbers	Bread, whole wheat or white	
Oatmeal	Cheese	
Rice, white or brown	Spaghetti/macaroni, cooked	
English muffin		

- Cranberry juice
- Black tea, beer, and wine
- Kava and licorice roots
- Olive oil
- Herbal tea
- Green tea extract
- St John's wort
- Astragalus.

The following health supplement/herbal products affect absorption of immunosuppressive drugs, hence these should be avoided:

- Ginseng
- Garlic in supplements form
- Ginger in supplements form
- Evening primrose oil

BOX 1: Food rich in protein.

Protein-rich food:
- Lean meat (beef, pork, or lamb), turkey, chicken, and fish
- Eggs, egg whites, or egg substitutes
- Low-fat milk, cheese, and yogurt
- Beans and lentils
- Soy and tofu products

TABLE 6: Foods rich in phosphorus and magnesium.

Phosphorus-rich foods (>100 mg/serving):

Chocolate	Beans*
Granola	Lentils*
Beef or veal	Milk or yogurt (low-fat/fat-free)*
Pork loin	Oatmeal*
Bran*	

Magnesium-rich foods (50–150 mg/serving):

Okra (frozen)	Pumpkin seeds*
Tofu	Bran*
Chocolate	Black beans*
Brown rice	Trail mix*
Halibut*	Avocado*
Spinach*	Artichokes*
Soybeans*	

*These foods are rich in potassium.

BOX 2: Foods to regulate fat intake.

Foods to increase:
- Lean cuts of animal protein (turkey, chicken, beef, pork, buffalo, and elk)
- Fish and seafood
- Low-fat dairy (cheese, milk, and yogurt)
- Healthy fats (nuts, seeds, flaxseed, soft margarine, oils: olive, canola, and peanut)
- Fresh fruits and vegetables
- Legumes and lentils
- Whole grain bread, pasta, and crackers

Reduce or eliminate:
- High fat meat (heavily marbled beef, ribs, wings, bacon, and sausage)
- High fat dairy (whole milk, 4% milk cheese, whole milk yogurt, and butter)
- Pastries, pies
- Fried foods

BOX 3: Tips to prevent weight gain, lose weight, and maintain healthy weight.

- Increase physical activity after you have been cleared to start exercising from your doctor.
  - Your goal is to exercise for at least 150 min/week.
  - You may break up your exercise sessions into 10–15 minutes intervals.
  - Move around any way that you can. Every bit of movement counts.
  - Plan or schedule exercise into each day.
- Eat three balanced meals at regular times with 4–5 hours between meals.
- Eat at least five servings of fruits and vegetables each day.
- Eat a half plate of vegetables/fruit, one-quarter grain/starchy foods and one-quarter lean protein (chicken, fish, pork, or turkey).
- Do not drink your calories. Sweetened soda pop, juices, and other beverages add unnecessary calories.
- Limit high calorie snack foods (candy, cakes, cookies, crackers, and sun chips).
- Choose cooking methods that do not increase the fat content of foods.
  - Healthy cooking methods include grilling, baking, boiling, broiling, poaching, and steaming.
  - Avoid frying and deep frying.

Nutrition Algorithm in Solid Organ Transplant Patient

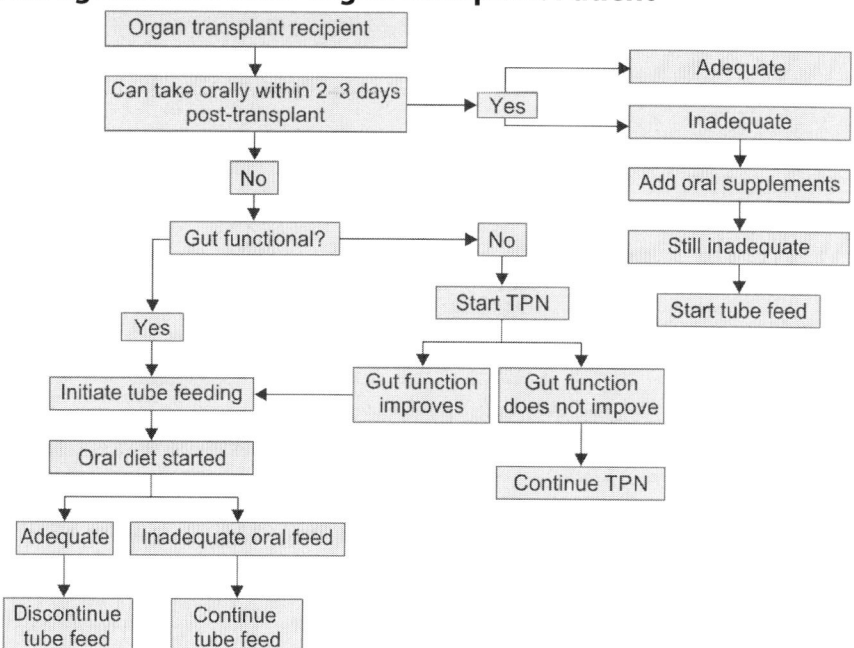

CONCLUSION

The nutrition therapy should be considered an important adjunct to clinical therapies. Peritransplant nutrition support therapy should be aimed at, nutrition support should begin in pretransplant period itself, and nutritional assessment should be carried out, it may not always be correct but use of various parameters to assess nutrition is useful. Pretransplant malnutrition and sarcopenia negatively impacts post-transplant outcomes. Peritransplant nutrition support is indispensable to improve post-transplant outcomes.

REFERENCES

1. Arends J, Baracos V, Bertz H, Bozzetti F, Calder PC, Deutz NEP, et al. ESPEN group recommendations for action against cancer related malnutrition. Clin Nutr. 2017;36(5):1187-96.
2. Hasse JM. Nutrition assessment and support of organ transplant recipients. J Parenter Enteral Nutr. 2001;25(3):120-31.
3. Boudi FB, Lam HD, Talavera F, Sudan DL, Shapiro R (2020). Nutritional requirements of adults before transplantation. Medscape. [online] Available from: https://emedicine.medscape.com/article/431031-overview [Last accessed June, 2023].
4. American Diabetic Association (2010). Chronic Kidney Disease: Evidence-based Nutrition Practice Guideline. [online] Available from: https://www.andeal.org/vault/pq137.pdf [Last accessed June, 2023].
5. Pham PTT, Pham PMT, Pham SV, Pham PAT, Pham PCT. New onset diabetes after transplantation: an overview. Diabetes Metab Syndr Obes. 2011;4:175-86.
6. Ward HJ. Nutritional and metabolic issues in solid organ transplantation, target for future research. J Ren Nutr. 2009;19(1):111-22.
7. Cabré E, Abad-Lacruz A, Núñez MC, González-Huix F, Fernández-Bañares F, Gïl A, et al. The relationship of plasma PUFA deficiency with survival in advanced liver cirrhosis, multivariate analysis. Am J Gastroenterol. 1993;88(5):718-22.
8. Kaido T, Mori A, Ogura Y, Hata K, Yoshizawa A, Iida T, et al. Impact of enteral nutrition using

new immune modulating diet after liver transplantation. Hepatogastroenterolgy. 2010;57(104):1522-5.

9. Baskin WN. Acute complications associated with bedside placement of feeding tubes. Nutr Clin Pract. 2006;21(1):40-55.

10. McClave SA, Taylor BE, Martindale RG, Warren MM, Johnson DR, Braunschweig C, et al. Society of Critical Care Medicine; American Society for Parenteral and Enteral Nutrition. Guidelines for Provision and Assessment of Nutrition Support Therapy Adult Critically ill, SCCM and American Society for Parenteral and Enteral Nutrition. J Parenter Enteral Nutr. 2016;40(2):159-211.

11. Seyan AS, Hughes RD, Shawcross DL. Changing face of hepatic encephalopathy, role of inflammatory and oxidative stress. World J Gastroenterol. 2010;16(27):3347-57.

12. Merli M, Giusto M, Riggio O, Gentili F, Molinaro A, Attili AF, et al. Improvements of nutritional status in malnourished cirrhotic patients one year post liver transplant. e-SPEN Eur e-J Clin Nutr Metab. 2011;6(3):e142-7.

13. Malik SM, deVera ME, Fontes P, Shaikh O, Ahmad J. Outcome after liver transplant in NASH cirrhosis. Am J Transplant. 2009;9(4):782-93.

14. Hasse JM, Blue LS. Comprehensive guide to transplant nutrition. Am Diab Assoc. 2002;264.

15. Singer LG, Brazelton TR, Doyle RL, Morris RE, Theodore J; International Lung Transplant Database Study Group. Weight gain after lung transplant. J Heart Lung Transplant. 2003;22(8):894-902.

16. Handu D, Moloney L, Wolfram T, Ziegler P, Acosta A, Steiber A. Academy of Nutrition and Dietetics Methodology for Conducting Systematic Reviews for the Evidence Analysis Library. J Acad Nutr Diet. 2016;116(2):311-8.

17. Kaufman DB. Pancreas transplant overview. Medscape. 2013.

CHAPTER 36

Nutritional Support in a Critically Ill Parturient

Sunil T Pandya, Nishanth Aasuri

■ INTRODUCTION

Pregnancy is a physiologically demanding period, requiring an increased intake of essential nutrients to support both the mother's health and the developing fetus. Adequate nutrition plays a vital role in promoting maternal recovery, preventing complications, and supporting optimal fetal development.[1] Most women adapt physiologically with a minimal need for supplementation other than with a few minerals and vitamins. When a pregnant woman becomes critically ill, her nutritional needs become more crucial and may be unable to meet this nutritional challenge. Parturient will require medical intervention to overcome nutritional deficiencies especially when the critical illness is prolonged, nutritional support by the enteral or parenteral route will become obstetrically necessary.

This chapter focuses on the importance of nutritional support in a critically ill pregnant mother, highlighting key considerations and interventions.

The first half of pregnancy is considered to be the *anabolic phase*. During this period, there is predominant influence of progesterone and aldosterone resulting in the maternal accumulation and storage of fat, protein, minerals, and fluid account for most of the maternal weight gain.

The catabolic phase predominates during the latter half of pregnancy. This phase is under the influence of the stress hormones, the human placental lactogen, cortisol, estrogen, and deoxycorticosterone leading to the depletion of the maternal glycogen, fat, and protein stores to provide glucose, free fatty acids, and free amino acids for the fetal accumulation of fat and protein and for placental growth.[2]

The fetal growth primarily depends on the fetal fat depots which are important storage sites for high-calorie-density tissue, fat-soluble vitamins, and essential fatty acids necessary for brain growth and metabolism in the perinatal period. The free amino acids are fundamental building blocks for organ development and enzyme synthesis. Any aberration of this process may compromise fetal growth.

Thus, the altered metabolism in pregnancy along with added stress of critical illness makes the scenario more complex and complicated.[3] The target is not only to nurture the critically ill mother but also to provide adequate calories to growing fetus during antepartum period and to consider additional calories needed for lactation during postpartum critical illness.

The hormonal milieu or environment in a critically ill parturient is characterized by a decrease in the ratio of insulin to glucagon, increased catecholamine levels, and insulin resistance. The critically ill parturient increases the rate of gluconeogenesis, proteolysis, acute phase protein production, lipolysis, and oxygen consumption. A host of cytokine and eicosanoid mediators also are present, creating an inflammatory response and the energy expenditure is increased on average by about 25%.[4] Changes in maternal hormone secretion lead to changes in the utilization of carbohydrates, fats, and proteins during pregnancy. The growing fetus requires a continual supply of glucose and amino acids for growth and hormone produced by placenta, human choriogonadotropin, is thought to encourage maternal tissue to make greater use of lipid for energy production and increase the availability of glucose and amino acids for the fetus. Changes in hormonal levels help to ensure that maternal lean tissues are conserved and are not used to provide energy or amino acids for the fetus.

NUTRITIONAL ASSESSMENT, ENERGY, AND MACRONUTRIENT REQUIREMENTS

In critically ill pregnant women, a comprehensive nutritional assessment is essential to determine their specific needs. This assessment should include a thorough medical history, anthropometric measurements, biochemical markers, and a detailed evaluation of the mother's current condition. Factors such as gestational age, underlying medical conditions, and the severity of illness should also be considered. The energy requirements of a critically ill pregnant mother are influenced by various factors, including the severity of illness, gestational age, maternal body mass index (BMI), and metabolic response to injury.

Indirect calorimetry or predictive equations can be used to estimate energy expenditure accurately. However, adjustments may be necessary based on the individual's condition.

Energy Requirements

Sufficient energy is required to ensure the delivery of full term, a healthy baby. This energy is required to deposit energy in the form of new tissues such as fetus, placenta, and amniotic fluid, extra maternal fat deposits, increased energy requirements for tissue synthesis, increased oxygen consumption by maternal organs, and increased energy requirements for products of conception.

Calculating daily requirements of critically ill parturient is complex. In the normal singleton pregnancy, the average total extra energy necessary to meet the metabolic demands of the fetus, placenta, and uterus is about 80,000 kcal, or about 300 kcal/day above maternal basal needs. In multi-fetal pregnancy, the placental mass is larger and this results in an increase in placental steroid and hormonal production. Thus, twin pregnancy has been described as a state of "accelerated starvation", in which the development of starvation ketosis occurs at a more rapid rate than in singleton pregnancy. The increase in resting energy expenditure (REE) can result in a 40% increase in caloric requirements for women with a twin pregnancy.

Routinely 25 kcal/kg (ideal bodyweight) is what is recommended. Upon this 650 kcal/day (0-6 months) and 520 kcals/day (6-12 months) are added during pregnancy and lactation to sustain the fetal growth and lactational needs respectively. Another important factor that has to be considered is the weight gain during pregnancy.

Average-sized female, energy requirements are 2,200–2,800 kcal/day. As per ICMR, for an Indian woman with prepregnancy weight of 55 kg and a weight gain of 10–12 kg: an average of +350 kcal is recommended.[5] Calorie requirements in various trimesters are:

1st trimester—+85 kcal/day, 2nd trimester—+280 kcal/day, 3rd trimester—+270 kcal/day.

Studies on BMR at different stages of pregnancy showed gradual increase from 5 to 10%, 25% increase respectively.

IMPACT OF CRITICAL ILLNESS, GOALS AND ASSESSMENT OF RESTING ENERGY EXPENDITURE

The relationship between the REE increase in diseased states is depicted in **Figure 1**.[6] The REE increases by 70–200% of normal in diseased states like major burns, sepsis, polytrauma and elective surgeries.

Thus, provision of inadequate nutritional support in a critically ill parturient results in immune dysfunction, weak respiratory muscles and difficulty in weaning, lowered ventilatory capacity, ventilator dependency, increased infection risk, and loss of lean body mass.

Hence, the goals of nutritional support is initial assessment to identify the parturient at risk for increased morbidity and mortality due to poor nutritional status. Once assessed, following goals are met with: provision of substrate for metabolic functions, positive nitrogen balance, prevent any deficiency, improve immune function, improve organ functions, modify stress response, and prevent metabolic complications.

ASSESSMENT OF PARTURIENT AT RISK OF MALNOURISHMENT

Assessment is same as in nonpregnant cohorts except for the need to consider the physiological demands of macro- and micronutrients as per the disease condition and gestational state.

Anthropometric measurements including height, bodyweight, skin-fold thickness, etc. are unreliable. Biochemical data includes assessment of total serum proteins, serum albumin (index of visceral and somatic protein stores), transferrin, and ceruloplasmin.

Limitations of biochemical indicators are physiologic overhydration state, decreased synthesis (exaggerated in liver disease like

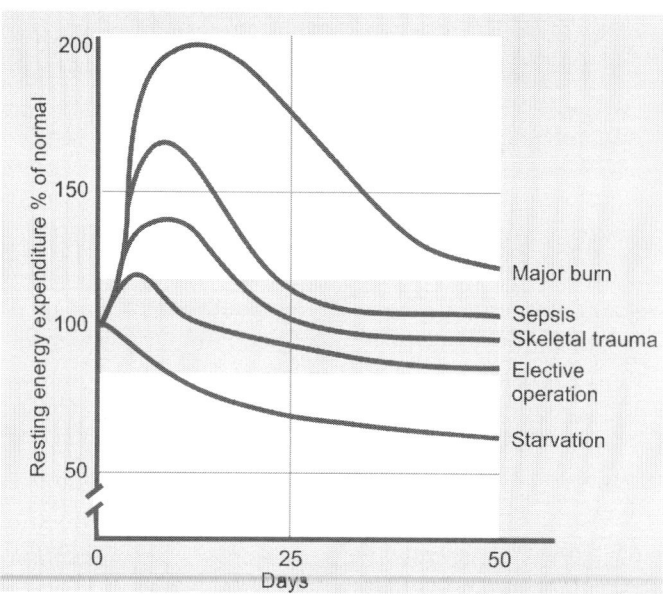

Fig. 1: The relationship between the resting energy expenditure increase in diseased states.

acute fatty liver in pregnancy, etc.), increased loss (burns, large wounds, etc.). Other indicators such as serum transferrin (half-life is 8 days), thyroid-binding prealbumin (half-life is 2 days), retinol-binding protein (half-life is 12 hours), and fibronectin (half-life is 12 hours) are also less reliable in predicting malnutrition.

"Subjective global assessment" using clinical parameters (history and physical examination) and other assessments include BMI <18.5, recent weight loss >10% of usual bodyweight, poor intake >5 days, and hyperemesis gravidarum.

Conventional energy requirement assessment tools such as Harris–Benedict equation, indirect calorimetry can be extrapolated during pregnancy. Indirect calorimetry underestimates calorie needs by 10–15% in patient at rest, is expensive and time-consuming, and is unreliable at higher FiO_2 (>60%). Adjustments in "energy requirements" such as activity factor, disease factor and thermal factor to be applied as in nonpregnant patients.

Simple Assessment

Most critically ill patients including the pregnant need 25–35 kcal/kg bodyweight. **Table 1** shows the calorie needs as per the BMI and use of actual or adjusted bodyweight.

TABLE 1: BMI and calorie needs calculation.

BMI	Kcal/Day	Bodyweight to be considered
<15	35–40	• *BMI:* 18.5–25 and underweight parturient: Consider actual bodyweight • *Overweight parturient:* Consider adjusted bodyweight Adjusted bodyweight = IBW + (Actual bodyweight – IBW) × 25%
15–19	30–35	
20–25	20–29	
26–29	15–17	
>29	15	

(BMI: body mass index; IBW: ideal bodyweight)

COMPONENTS OF DIET

It includes macronutrients (carbohydrate, proteins, and fats), micronutrients (minerals and vitamins), and fluids (30–50 mL/kg plus losses).

Carbohydrates

Carbohydrates constitute the primary source of energy which provides 3.4 kcal/g of energy which is available as monohydrate dextrose. Carbohydrates constitute 60–75% of the total calories. Requirements for starch, sugar, and nonstarch polysaccharides are not increased. Constipation is common in all stages of pregnancy. No data is available to suggest any alteration in percentage of fats and carbohydrates in critically ill obstetric patients. However, carbohydrate intake should be sufficient to meet energy needs and prevent protein catabolism. Complex carbohydrates, such as whole grains, fruits, and vegetables, are preferred over simple sugars. Monitoring and maintaining blood glucose levels within an appropriate range is crucial, especially in women with preexisting diabetes or gestational diabetes.

Adverse effects of excessive carbohydrates include increase minute ventilation, CO_2 production, increased respiratory quotient (RQ) thus leading to increased O_2 consumption, lipogenesis, and hyperglycemia.

Hence, in parturients with diabetes or respiratory failure, appropriate adjustments and monitoring of RQ should be done.

Proteins

Protein requirements are increased in critically ill pregnant women to promote tissue repair, support immune function, and maintain nitrogen balance. The recommended protein intake is generally 1.2–2.0 g/kg of bodyweight/day, but it can vary depending on the severity of illness and underlying conditions. Protein requirements increase during pregnancy from each trimester.[3,7] Rate of accumulation of nitrogen rises 10-fold over the course of pregnancy with apparently no rise in nitrogen balance. There is a reduction in urea synthesis and fall in urea concentration in last trimesters in pregnancy. This suggests that maternal breakdown of amino acids may be suppressed representing a mechanism for protein sparing. Evidence also shows that protein may be stored in early pregnancy and used at a later stage to meet the demand of growing fetus.

The critically ill patient experiences an increase in muscle proteolysis that is resistant to the usual attenuating effect of feeding. This proteolysis is thought to occur in order to mobilize amino acids from muscle to be used in the viscera for gluconeogenesis, acute phase protein synthesis. Another unique aspect of protein metabolism in critically ill patient is nitrogen balance and is independent of energy balance, while in case of healthy adults nitrogen balance can be achieved only when energy balance and adequate protein intake are achieved. Proteins are considered as building blocks of the body. A dose 0.8–2 g/kg/day is needed depending on the clinical requirement. Proteins are not considered in the calculation of calories. Specialized amino acids—branched chain and essential amino acids which are used in liver failure, are more expensive, and have not shown to improve outcome. Adverse effects of excess proteins intake include azotemia in pregnant patients with kidney injury.

Table 2 depicts the protein needs in various diseased states, similar to nonpregnant patients.

TABLE 2: Protein requirements in normal and diseased states.

Condition	Requirement
Normal	0.75–1 g/kg/day
Critically ill patient	1–1.5 g/kg/day
AKI not on dialysis	0.8–1 g/kg/day
AKI on dialysis	1.2–1.4 g/kg/day
Burns/sepsis	1.5–2 g/kg/day
CVVHD	1.7–2 g/kg/day

Fats

Lipids constitute 30–40% of total calories. There is no evidence on additional lipids requirements during pregnancy. Fat intake should be limited to a moderate level, primarily consisting of healthy unsaturated fats. Including omega-3 fatty acids, found in fatty fish, flaxseeds, and walnuts, may provide additional benefits, including anti-inflammatory effects.

Pregnant women need adequate dietary intake of essential fatty acids (EFA) and their longer chain derivatives which are necessary for development of brain and central nervous system activity of fetus.[8] Long chain n-3 fatty acid during pregnancy may have beneficial effect on birthweight and duration of pregnancy and was advocated to decrease the incidence of preterm labor and preeclampsia.[9] Docosahexaenoic acid, a type of omega-3 fatty acids, has shown some promise in terms of better outcomes in neonatal visual and neural testing.[10,11] The adverse effects of lipids are egg allergy, hypertriglyceridemia, decreased cell mediated immunity, limit to <1 g/kg/day in critically ill immunosuppressed patients, can derange LFTs.

Micronutrient and Vitamin Requirements

Adaptive response helps to meet the increased demands for nutrients irrespective of nutritional status of mother. Such responses include increased absorption of iron, calcium, copper, and zinc and reduced urinary excretion of some nutrients including riboflavin and amino acids. Increased requirements for several micronutrients during pregnancy including thiamine, riboflavin, folate, and vitamins A, C, and D.

Critically ill pregnant women may require supplementation with micronutrients and vitamins to prevent deficiencies and support recovery. A daily multivitamin and mineral supplement specifically formulated for pregnant women can help to meet these requirements. Additionally, specific micronutrients such as iron, folic acid, calcium, and vitamin D should be monitored and supplemented as needed, based on individual deficiencies and clinical recommendations.

Role of immune-nutrition in critically ill parturients is limited. There are no clear recommendations. They can be considered in patients undergoing abdominal surgery during pregnancy, especially malnourished patients (both preoperatively and postoperatively), ICU patients with APACHE scores of 10–20 but not higher; and patients with multiple trauma.

ENTERAL AND PARENTERAL NUTRITION

Enteral nutrition, delivered through a tube directly into the gastrointestinal tract, is the preferred route of nutritional support when feasible in critically ill pregnant women. It helps to maintain gut integrity, stimulates digestion, and reduces the risk of infection. Early initiation of enteral nutrition is associated with improved clinical outcomes and a reduced risk of complications.

However, the impact of the physiological changes in pregnant women are likely to reject enteral feed and develop constipation due to relaxant effects of progesterone on bowel smooth muscles. There are increased chances of aspiration due to relaxant effect of lower esophageal sphincter and enlarging uterus compressing the stomach may render enhanced aspiration risk especially those who require noninvasive ventilation.

In cases where enteral nutrition is contraindicated or inadequate, parenteral or supplemental parenteral nutrition may be necessary.

Parenteral nutrition involves delivering nutrients intravenously and is typically reserved for patients who cannot tolerate enteral feeding or require additional supplementation. Close monitoring of metabolic parameters and complications is necessary when administering parenteral nutrition. Monitoring during total parenteral nutrition (TPN) should include daily weights, strict input–output, urine sugar and ketones, serum glucose (every 6–12 hours), daily urea and electrolytes, liver function assessment and calcium, phosphorous, magnesium, and albumin (2–3 times/week), weekly nitrogen balance, and fetal growth assessment (every 2–4 weeks). Complications due to TPN includes *catheter-related issues like* pneumothorax, arterial laceration, mediastinal hematoma, malposition, brachial plexus/phrenic nerve palsy, catheter sepsis, subclavian vein thrombosis/right arterial thrombosis, and hydrothorax/chylothorax. Metabolic issues due to TPN can be deficiencies of vitamins, minerals, electrolytes, trace metals, or essential fatty acids; hypoglycemia; hepatic dysfunction and fatty infiltration; carbon dioxide retention; and over and underhydration. Other complications include bowel atrophy, cholecystitis, heparin-related complications (e.g., hemorrhage, thrombocytopenia, and osteopenia), and *neonatal issues like* maternal diabetes syndrome (e.g., macrosomia and postnatal hypoglycemia), and growth restriction.[12]

MONITORING NUTRITIONAL STATUS[13-27]

Nutritional assessment also challenging in patients as weight gain due to pregnancy and albumin decrease due to pregnancy cannot be used as a reliable predictor. Indicators such as prealbumin and serum transferrin are preferred for follow-up for assessment of the response to nutritional support, but have their own limitations, as has already been discussed. The response to nutrition should be assessed regularly by nitrogen balance. The nitrogen balance evaluates somatic protein status. It is inaccurate in acute kidney injury.

Another way to monitor adequacy of nutritional support is measuring "respiratory quotient". RQ = Vol CO_2 released/Vol O_2 absorbed. Vol CO_2 = 200 mL/min and Vol O_2 = 250 mL/min, resulting in 0.8 respiratory ratio.

Values of 0.84–0.86 desired range/Mixed fuel utilization. 0.6–0.7 indicates starvation or underfeeding. 0.9–1.0 indicates carbohydrate metabolism. 1.0+ indicates overfeeding or lipogenesis.

DISEASE-SPECIFIC NUTRITION

Acute Kidney Injury

Parturients with AKI do not restrict protein in patients with renal insufficiency as a means to avoid or delay initiating dialysis therapy. High-concentrated fluid restricted diet is necessary. Standard ICU requirements for protein (1.2–2 g/kg) and energy (25–30 kcal/kg/day) should be followed. Patients on hemodialysis and continuous renal replacement therapy (CRRT) should receive proteins up to 2.5 g/kg/day.

Respiratory Failure

Fluid-restricted high-calorie enteral diet is recommended with acute respiratory failure especially in a state of fluid overload. RQ should be closely monitored. Serum phosphate also should be closely monitored and supplemented. It helps in improving diaphragmatic function and respiratory muscle strength. Adequate amount of protein is required for respiratory muscle endurance.

Liver Failure

Standard enteral nutrition is preferred. Dry weight is used instead of actual weight in patients with cirrhosis, hepatic failure due to ascites, edema, intravascular volume depletion, and hypoalbuminemia. Protein restriction should be avoided. Use intact protein or peptide-based formulas. 1–1.2 g/kg/day of proteins. There is no evidence of further benefit of branched chain amino acids rather than aromatic amino acids in patients on coma grades who are already on first-line therapy with luminal acting antibiotics and lactulose.

Pancreatitis

Pancreatitis is a state of acute inflammation with severe catabolic response. Frequent assessment of feeding tolerance and enteral is preferred to parenteral. Allow oral diet in mild pancreatitis, if not able to tolerate orally, nasojejunal feeds are advised. If not able to reach the required target by 7 days, consider starting parenteral nutrition. Peptide-based formulas with low lipid diets and usage of prokinetics are suggested. Probiotics are harmful. Data is lacking to recommend starting immune enhancing formula in pancreatitis.

Obesity

Enteral nutrition should be started within 24 hours of admission for obese patients with BMI >40. High protein with permissive underfeeding/hypocaloric diets are recommended to preserve lean body mass, mobilize fat stores and minimize metabolic complications of overfeeding. Energy goal should be 60–70% of target calories which promotes steady weight loss, while infusing proteins to maintain neutral nitrogen balance. There is lack of evidence for immunomodulating diet in obese population. Additional monitoring of hyperglycemia, hyperlipidemia, hypercapnia, fluid overload and hepatic fat accumulation is needed for the obese ICU patient receiving EN.

Sepsis

Sepsis is a higher catabolic state with requirement of vasopressors and fluids in the early stage which avoids the need for early enteral nutrition. It is preferable to start enteral nutrition as early as possible preferably within 24–48 hours of diagnosis of sepsis once the patient is hemodynamically stable and vasopressors are minimal.

Trauma

Early enteral nutrition is recommended unless there are any absolute contraindications. Caloric requirements are up to 25 kcal/kg/day initially and proteins requirement up to 1.5–2 g/kg/day. Arginine-containing immune-modulating supplements should be considered in trauma.

Burns

Burns is a state of severe catabolism with high-energy requirements. Adequate nutrition helps in wound healing and improving the immunity to combat infections. Diet with high carbohydrate and low fat is suggested due to decreased utilization of fats after burn injury. The protein requirements increase up to 1.5–2 g/kg/day to compensate for losses. Special formulas used for burns patients include the CURRIE formula which includes the percentage of burns and Galveston's equation.

■ BREASTFEEDING AND LACTATION

Promoting breastfeeding and lactation is crucial for critically ill pregnant women who have delivered their babies. Breast milk provides optimal nutrition and immune protection for the newborn. If the mother is unable to breastfeed directly due to critical illness, techniques such as pumping and storing breast milk should be encouraged to ensure the baby receives the benefits of breast milk.

■ CONCLUSION

Nutritional support is an integral component of care for critically ill pregnant women. Adequate energy, macronutrients, micronutrients, and vitamins play a crucial role in promoting maternal recovery and supporting optimal fetal development.

■ REFERENCES

1. Lakoff KM, Feldman JD. Anorexia nervosa associated with pregnancy. Obstet Gynecol. 1972;39:699-701.
2. Long CL, Schaffel N, Geiger JW, Schiller WR, Blackmore WS. metabolic response to injury and illness. Estimation of energy and protein needs from indirect calorimetry and nitrogen balance. J Parenter Enteral Nutr. 1979;3:452-6.
3. Compher C, Bingham AL, McCall M, Patel J, Rice TW, Braunschweig C, et al. Guidelines for the provision and assessment of nutrition support therapy in adult critically ill patient. Society of critical care medicine and American society for Parenteral and enteral nutrition. (ASPEN). J Parenter Enteral Nutr. 2016;40:159-211.
4. Butte N, King JC. Energy requirements during pregnancy and lactation. Public Health Nutr. 2005;8(7A):1010-27.

5. Lain KY, catalano PM. Metabolic changes in pregnancy. Clin Obstet Gynaecol. 2007; 50(4):936-48.
6. Frankenfield DC, Wiles CE, Bagley S, Siegel JH. Relationships between resting and total energy expenditure in injured and septic patients. Crit Care Med. 1995;22:1796-804.
7. Lewin GA, Schachter HM, Yuen D, Merchant P Mamaladze V, Tsertsvadze A. Effects of Omega 3 Fatty Acids On Child And Maternal Health. Evid Rep Technol Assess. 2005;118:1-11.
8. Kaiser L, Allen LH. Position of the American dietetic association: nutrition and lifestyle for a healthy pregnancy outcome. J Am Diet Assoc. 2008;108:553-61.
9. Al MDM, van Houwelingen AC, Hornstra G. Long chain polyunsaturated fatty acids, pregnancy and pregnancy outcome. Am J Clin Nutr. 2000;71:285-91.
10. Allen KG, Harris MA. The role of n-3 fatty acids in gestation and parturition. Exper Biol Med. 2001;226:498-506.
11. Kris-Etherton PM, Innis S. Position of the American dietetic association and dietetics of Canada: dietary fatty acids. J Am Diet Assoc. 2007;107:1599-611.
12. Tang B, Michael J. Tang MJ, Phelan JP. Nutritional Support. In: Phelan JP, Pacheco LD, Foley MR, Saade GR, Dildy III GA, Belfort MA (Eds). Critical Care Obstetrics, 6th Edition. United States: Wiley Blackwell; 2019.
13. Mowery NT, Dortch MJ, Dossett LA, Norris PR, Diaz JJ Jr, Morris JA Jr, et al. Insulin resistance despite glucose control is associated with mortality in critically ill surgical patients. J Intensive Care Med. 2009;24:242-51.
14. Casaer MP, Mesotten D, Hermans G, Wouters PJ, Schetz M, Meyfroidt G, et al. Early versus late Parenteral nutrition in critically ill adults. N Eng J Med. 2011;365:506-17.
15. Royal College of Obstetrician and Gynaecology. (2011). Maternal collapse in pregnancy and puerperium. (Green-top Guideline No. 56). [online] Available from: https://www.rcog.org.uk/guidance/browse-all-guidance/green-top-guidelines/maternal-collapse-in-pregnancy-and-the-puerperium-green-top-guideline-no-56/ [Last accessed June, 2023].
16. Preiser JC, Ichai C, Orban JC, Groeneveld AB. Metabolic response to the stress of critical illness. Br J Anaesthesia. 2014;113(6):945-54.
17. Martindale RG, McClave SA, Vanek VW, McCarthy M, Roberts P, Taylor B, et al. Guidelines for the provision and assessment of nutrition support therapy in the adult critically ill patient: Society of Critical Care Medicine and American Society for Parenteral and Enteral Nutrition: Executive Summary. Crit Care Med. 2009;37:1757-61.
18. Cox JT, Phelan ST. Nutrition during pregnancy. Obstet Gynaecol Clin N Am. 2008;35:369-83.
19. Makrides M, Duley L, Olsen SE. Marine oil, and other prostaglandin precursor, supplementation for pregnancy uncomplicated by preeclampsia or IUGR. Cochrane Data Base Rev. 2006;(3):CD003402.
20. Price LC, Slack A, Nelson-Piercy C. Aims of obstetric critical care management. Best Pract Res Clin Obstet Gynaecol. 2008;22:775-99.
21. Fall C. Fetal and maternal nutrition in cardiovascular disease: diet, nutrition and emerging risk factors. Br Nutr Foundation task force. 2005;177-95.
22. Bucher HC, Guyatt GH, Cook RJ, Hatala R, Cook DJ, Lang JD, et al. Effect of calcium supplementation on pregnancy induced hypertension and preeclampsia: a meta-analysis of randomised controlled trials. J Am Med Assoc. 1996;275:1113-7.
23. Mendieta Zeron H, Gabrela H, Layton CF. The adiponectin/leptin ratio is a useful tool to evaluate the metabolic status in an obstetric ICU. Rom J Int Med. 2013;51(2):107-13.
24. Galbán C, Montejo JC, Mesejo A, Marco P, Celaya S, Sánchez-Segura JM, et al. An immune enhancing enteral diet reduces mortality rate and episodes of bacteremia in septic intensive care unit patients. Crit Care Med. 2000;28:643-8.
25. Drover JW, Dhaliwal R, Weitzel L, Wischmeyer PE, Ochoa JB, Heyland DK. Perioperative use of Argentine-supplemented diets: a systemic review of the evidence. J Am Coll Surg. 2011;212:385-99, 399.e1.
26. Hall JC, Dobb G, Hall J, de Sousa R, Brennan L, McCauley R. A prospective randomised trial of enteral glutamine in critical illness. Intensive Care Med. 2003;29:1710-6.
27. Heyland D, Muscedere J, Wischmeyer PE, Cook D, Jones G, Albert M, et al. A randomised trial of glutamine and antioxidants in critically ill patients. N Engl J Med. 2013;368:1489-97.

SECTION 6: Special Issues in Critical Illness

37. **Immunonutrition in the Critically Ill**
    William Manzanares, Gil Hardy

38. **Dysglycemia in Critical Illness**
    Shweta Ram Chandankhede, Balguri Mukesh Kumar

39. **Refeeding Syndrome in Critically Ill Adults: Preemptive Strategies**
    Krishnan Sriram, Chitra Mahesh

40. **Nutrition in Severe Hemodynamic Failure and in Noninvasive Ventilation**
    Khalid Ismail Khatib, Subhal Bhalchandra Dixit

41. **Gut Microbiome in Critical Illness**
    B Ruvinder Reddy

42. **Evaluation of Sarcopenia in Critical Illness**
    Deeksha Kapoor

43. **Feeding Options in Patients with Intra-abdominal Hypertension**
    Sunil Karanth, Mahesha P

44. **Nutrition and Wound Healing**
    Sónia Maria Cabral

CHAPTER 37

Immunonutrition in the Critically Ill

William Manzanares, Gil Hardy

INTRODUCTION

Immunity defines the ability of the host to mount a successful attack on an invasive organism and its toxic products, such that destruction of the organism and its product is achieved with minimal damage to the host's tissues. Nutrition therapy can affect different physiological processes, including those that regulate the immune system.[1] Moreover, nutrition indirectly impacts the immune system by regulating the composition and function of the microbiota, which controls the host response to nutrition. Also, in seriously ill patients, malnutrition and immune dysfunction are common features. Malnutrition may have a direct effect on the lymphoid system, reflected by thymic atrophy and reduced organ weights (compared with those of normal children) of tonsils, lymph nodes and spleen. This would suggest alterations in cell mediated immunity.[2] So far, many studies have shown that up to 50% of patients in both surgical and medical departments are malnourished at hospital admission.[3]

Critical illness is often associated with a physiological immunosuppression leading to increased secondary infections, increased morbidity, and a high risk of mortality.[4] Impaired host immunity has been increasingly related to protein–energy malnutrition, which is known to depress antibody production, the functions of phagocytes, T-cells, and levels of plasma complement. The disciplines of nutrition and immunology are, therefore, closely interrelated, with current interest surrounding specific dietary components which may influence and correct immune dysfunction.[1] The relationship between nutritional status and immune function is, therefore, a complex subject. In critically ill patients, particularly in those with trauma and undergoing major surgery, dietary intervention with nutrients able to enhance immune function has been the subject of controversy and continuous debate.[4,5] These nutrients named immune-modulating nutrients or immunonutrients in so-called immune enhancing diets (IEDs), are arginine (ARG), glutamine (GLN), omega-3 fatty acids, nucleotides, and antioxidant micronutrients (vitamins and trace elements)[5,6] **(Table 1)**.

Immunonutrition is considered as the nutritional strategy characterized by the administration of IEDs by enteral route, mostly in surgical intensive care unit (ICU) patients. In contrast, pharmaconutrition is another nutritional strategy where high-dose individual macro- or micro-nutrients are provided intravenously, individually, or in various combinations and studied to understand their effects on underlying metabolism, inflammation, immunity, and relevant clinical outcomes.[7]

TABLE 1: Immune-enhancing diets. Composition in immune-modulating nutrients (Arginine, Glutamine, EPA/DHA, and antioxidant micronutrients).

Enteral formula, company	Arginine g/100 cc	Glutamine g/100 cc	Fish oils (EPA/DHA) g/100 cc	Antioxidant micronutrients
Impact Enteral, Nestle	1.3	—	0.30	Vitamins A, D, E, K, C, B_1, B_2, B_6, B_{12}, Se, Cu, Zn, Mo, Cr, I, F
Pivot 1.5, Abbott	1.3	7.6	0.37	Vitamins A, D, E, K, C, B_1, B_2, B_6, B_{12}, Se, Cu, Zn, Mo, Cr
Perative, Abbott	0.85	—	0.16	Vitamins A, D, E, K, C, B_1, B_2, B_6, B_{12}, Se, Cu, Zn, Mo, Cr, I
Inmunex Plus, Megalabs	7.0	5.7	0.35	Vitamins A, D, E, K, C, B_1, B_2, B_6, B_{12}, Se, Cu, Zn, Mo, Cr, I, F
Atempero, Vegenat	0.40	—	0.27	Vitamins A, D, E, K, C, B_1, B_2, B_6, B_{12}, Se, Cu, Zn, Mo, Cr, I, F

(DHA: docosahexaenoic acid; EPA: eicosapentaenoic acid)

According to current knowledge, the administration of specific enriched enteral nutrition (EN) formulas with immune and metabolic modulating nutrients can modulate the inflammatory response and the immune system, improving clinical outcomes in specific patient populations (trauma, and perioperative).[4,5] Despite the rationale for the use of IEDs in the ICU, the different variable compositions of IEDs and different dosages of individual immunonutrients in commercial enteral formulas can be a possible explanation for the inconclusive and contradictory results published among recent clinical trials.

Moreover, IEDs have identifiable pharmacological effects upon the immune system at supraphysiological doses but unlike drugs, there may not be immediately measurable changes in physiological or pathological conditions. Therefore, on clinical grounds they are justifiably classified as pharmaconutrients rather than drugs. Finally, IEDs and individual immune nutrients have three primary targets: (1) mucosal barrier function, (2) cellular defense function, and (3) local and systemic inflammation.[5]

IMMUNE-ENHANCING DIETS IN THE CRITICALLY ILL: SUMMARY OF CURRENT RECOMMENDATIONS

Disease-related malnutrition (DRM) in surgical patients is often associated with an increased incidence of postoperative infectious complications, morbidity, and mortality. In severe trauma or surgery, lymphocytes decrease both in number and in responsiveness. This may suggest an impaired ability to duplicate and differentiate.[8] Considerable increases in blood polymorph numbers are encountered in the 24 hours postoperatively, following the stress-related cortisol release. Subset distributions of T- and B-cells are altered and largely contribute to the apparently reduced immunocompetence of these patients. Most IEDs consist of more than one nutraceutical and are administered enterally, but few studies have addressed the stability/compatibility of these combinations. Moreover, there are controversial issues relating to clinical evaluations of IED. Isonitrogenous controls are rarely used, small sample sizes result in unreliable statistics so that conclusions are sometimes difficult to interpret.[9]

According to current evidence, the IEDs could have a place in the following clinical conditions: (1) perioperative in elective gastrointestinal (GI) surgery, particularly in those previously malnourished patients, (2) surgery for head and neck cancer with concomitant DRM, (3) blunt and penetrating torso trauma, (4) severe head injury, especially those patients with traumatic brain injury, (5) severe burns, (6) surgical patients on mechanical ventilation (MV) at high risk of secondary infection.[5]

The use of IEDs containing nutrients such as eicosopentaenoic acid (EPA), docosahexaenoic acid (DHA), GLN ARG, and nucleotides have been extensively evaluated in surgical ICU patients, where current evidence is more robust in showing clinical benefits.[4-6] In a very elegant meta-analysis by Drover et al.[10], the authors showed that the use of IEDs given postoperatively reduced infections (RR = 0.78; 95% CI: 0.64-0.95; $p = 0.01$) and hospital stay (WMD = -2.23; 95% CI, -3.80 to -0.65; $p = 0.006$), although overall mortality was not modified. Similarly, Mazaki et al.[11] in a systematic review and meta-analysis exploring the effects of immuno-enhancing enteral and parenteral nutrition for GI surgery that included 74 trials and almost 7,600 patients found a significant reduction in overall complications including infections, anastomotic leaks, sepsis, and mortality.

However, in severe acute pancreatitis, IEDs have not shown positive clinical effects, compared to standard EN formulas and thus IEDs are not currently recommended.[6] Nevertheless, immunonutrition has been shown to have a place in severe trauma patients including those after traumatic brain injury (TBI).[6] Similarly, based on the heterogeneity of the clinical populations studied and the inconsistency in the outcomes, in medical ICU patients, these formulas have shown no outcome benefits, and therefore, these IEDs are not routinely recommended in critically ill patients.[5]

Recently, a multicenter Spanish observational study[12] including 61 patients receiving an IED showed higher mean energy and protein intake, as well as better 28-day survival (85.2% vs. 73.3%; $p = 0.014$). Also, the multivariate analysis showed a lower need for vasopressor support (OR: 0.49; 95% CI: 0.26-0.91; $p = 0.023$) and continuous renal replacement therapies (OR: 0.13; 95% CI: 0.01-0.65; $p = 0.049$) in those patients who received IEDs, independently of the severity of the disease. Nonetheless, the authors did not find any difference in most laboratory parameters, except for a trend toward lower triglyceride levels ($p = 0.045$) in those who received IEDs.[12]

Glutamine

Glutamine is the most abundant free amino acid in circulation (500-900 µmol/L) under normal circumstances: skeletal muscle GLN constitutes >60% of the total free amino acid pool.[13] Under conditions of critical illness or with GI disorders, GLN levels may not be adequate to meet demands and become conditionally essential.[14,15]

During stress or after major surgery, plasma, and muscle GLN concentrations are significantly decreased, reflecting the increased demand of these immune cells, which cannot always be met by protein breakdown. There is also a significant negative correlation between GLN levels and interleukin 6 (IL-6) production.[16,17]

In healthy individuals, GLN is considered a nonessential amino acid because it is synthesized within the skeletal muscles and the lungs. Animal and human studies, however, have shown that GLN is not only an important nutrient but an energy substrate precursor for purine and pyrimidine synthesis. Resting lymphocytes and macrophages utilize L-glutamine for fuel at a rate comparable to that of glucose. Indeed, Newshome et al. have demonstrated that within the intestine, GLN is the preferred major fuel source, rather than glucose, for enterocytes and for the immune cells in the gut-associated lymphoid tissue (GALT),[16,17] where in healthy volunteers, 40–50% of administered GLN is consumed by cells of the intestine[18] and a similar percentage of available GLN is metabolized in EN patients.[19] Its synthesis and release from muscle are, therefore, physiologically and immunologically important. Indeed, it may be rate limiting for the maintenance of plasma GLN levels and hence uptake by the cells of the immune system, gut, and endothelium.[20]

It also serves as a fuel source for immunocytes such as lymphocytes and macrophages, as well as a precursor for glutathione (GSH), a major intracellular antioxidant.[21] *In vitro* L-GLN added to lymphocytes in culture increases the rate of proliferation, presumably by supplying a pool of precursors for the synthesis of nucleotides. GSH expression is high in the intestinal mucosa, and the reduced activity of this antioxidant causes mucosal degradation, diarrhea, and malabsorption. Moreover, GLN promotes heat shock protein (HSP) responses, which is protective during cellular stress through prevention of cell damage and death in the splanchnic bed and other organs.[22]

Over the past three decades, GLN has been a topic of debate and the most extensively discussed nutrient in the field of immunonutrition and pharmaconutrition. Historically, clinical benefits with L-GLN, mostly administered by the parenteral route, were small single-center studies. Initial meta-analyses, of these trials concluded that high-dose L-GLN supplementation led to significant reduction in hospital infections, mortality, ICU, and overall hospital length of stay (LOS). Nevertheless, the largest randomized controlled trial (RCT) using enteral and parenteral alanyl-glutamine dipeptide plus intravenous and enteral antioxidant micronutrients (including high-dose selenium), the Reducing Deaths due to OXidative Stress (REDOXS) study,[23] which was designed to bring higher-quality evidence into the field of pharmaconutrition was surprisingly negative. Unfortunately, the REDOXS trial[23] showed several methodological weaknesses. First, the study had a randomization problem, where fixed supraphysiological doses of glutamine dipeptides (rather than L-GLN alone) were administered to all patients, irrespective of weight, age, or sex,—a significant proportion of whom did not have hypoglutaminemia (nor were necessarily "hyposelenemic"). Second, the nutrition support regimen was also inadequate: Energy intakes of most patients were very low; the study group received much higher protein from an unbalanced amino acid mixture, which the patient's already compromised livers had to oxidize, whereas nitrogen intake was much lower in the controls. Another multicenter study, the MetaPlus trial[24] randomized 301 ventilated patients in 14 ICUs to DIPEP-enriched EN versus an isocaloric diet and noted increased 6-month mortality in the GLN dipeptides-supplemented medical ICU patients.

It is still not clear what caused the unfavorable outcome for patients in the

GLN dipeptides supplemented patients, but the REDOXS subgroup of North American patients, for which plasma GLN concentrations were available, showed that high plasma concentrations were not the reason. It is noteworthy that both GLN and Alanine (ALA) are involved in gluconeogenesis but to date no one has reported or commented upon the equally high ALA levels resulting from dipeptides supplementation.

In burn patients, GLN levels decrease after injury, which has been associated with increased morbidity and mortality.[25,26] Over the past years, several small trials have evaluated the effect of enteral GLN in burn patients suggesting a reduction in overall mortality and hospital LOS. Consequently, it has been estimated that almost 50% of mechanically ventilated burn patients receive enteral GLN.[27] However, the recently published REENERGIZE study[28] did not find any clinical benefits nor any reduction in hospital discharge time. This study randomized 1,200 patients with deep second- or third-degree burns affecting ≥10% to ≥20% of total body-surface area to receive 0.5 g/kg BW enteral GLN or placebo within 72 hours after hospital admission. The median time to discharge alive from the hospital was 40 days in the GLN group and 38 days in the placebo group ($p = 0.17$). Additionally, 6 month-mortality was 17.2% in the GLN group and 16.2% in the placebo group.[28] After the REENERGIZE publication, Ortiz Reyes et al. conducted a systematic review and meta-analysis including 12 RCTs.[29] The authors concluded that although single-center trials showed a significant reduction in mortality and secondary infections,[29] the main findings were that enteral GLN did not affect mortality (RR = 0.65, 95% CI: 0.33–1.28; $p = 0.21$), infectious complications (RR = 0.83; 95% CI: 0.63–1.09; $p = 0.18$), or other secondary outcomes of adult burns patients.

Arginine

L-Arginine is a dibasic conditionally essential amino acid included in IEDs that is important for normal lymphocyte function, such as proliferation and the expression of normal T-cell receptors, and is additionally involved in multiple metabolic pathways, such as synthesis of nitric oxide, and production of polyamines and hydroxyproline.[4,5,30] ARG is essential for growth and is required for synthesis of collagen for wound repair.[5] It may also be essential in hypermetabolic and septic states. In several animal models involving malignant lesions, supplementation of an enteral diet with ARG improved the response of peripheral lymphocytes to mitogens and retarded tumor growth.[31] Critical illness is characterized by ARG depletion, which has several consequences such as low NO production, poor wound healing, endothelial dysfunction, ischemic reperfusion injury, and immunosuppression.[32] The metabolic route of ARG is dependent on the underlying pathophysiology of the individual.[5] ARG is the substrate for 2 myeloid cell enzymes that are upregulated during immune activation: inducible NO synthase (iNOS) and arginase. Sepsis is characterized by the release of T-helper 1 cytokines, which preferentially induce inducible nitric oxide (NO) expression, increasing NO production and therefore, amplifying the systemic inflammation.[33] In addition, NO is directly bactericidal and used by leukocytes and macrophages to destroy pathogens. Furthermore, NO produces vasodilatation, arterial hypotension, lipid peroxidation, and alterations in gene expression. Otherwise, trauma and major surgery patients appear to generate Th2 responses, which is responsible for arginase activation and thus, synthesis of ornithine (ORN) which can be used to synthesize polyamines and proline, which are needed for wound healing.[4,5]

High levels of arginase are expressed in myeloid cells after trauma or surgery, which suggest that IEDs rich in ARG may overcome arginase-mediated T-cell suppression. An obvious shortcoming is the lack of ARG-specific data, as many investigations have utilized enteral cocktails that contain other immunonutrients. Current recommendations suggest ARG supplementation in IEDs at a daily dose no greater than 30 g (the usual suggested daily dose is 15–30 g) in surgical patients in the preoperative and postoperative period, hemodynamically stable trauma patients, and TBI.[5,34] Nevertheless, recommendations for the use of ARG-containing IEDs for the medical ICU population is inconclusive, as no clinical benefits regarding mortality infectious complications or hospital LOS have been demonstrated in this subset of ICU patients.[4-6]

LIPIDS AND IMMUNE FUNCTION: THE ROLE OF OMEGA-3 POLYUNSATURATED FATTY ACIDS

Lipids are a dense source of nonprotein energy and provide essential polyunsaturated fatty acids (PUFAs) that also exhibit immunomodulatory properties. Thus, omega-3 fatty acids show anti-inflammatory properties, omega-6 are pro-inflammatory, and omega-9 monounsaturated (MUFA) are immune neutral.[35,36] Eicosapentaenoic acid (EPA) and docosahexaenoic acid (DHA), omega-3 PUFAs mostly found in fish oil (FO) have been provided enterally or parenterally as constituents of IEDs to critically ill patients with acute respiratory distress syndrome (ARDS). Gamma-linolenic acid (GLA), an omega-6 PUFA present in borage oil, has been coadministered enterally.[37] EPA and DHA replace arachidonic acid (AA) in the phospholipid membrane; thus, AA concentration is reduced, and production of the highly inflammatory AA-derived eicosanoids (2-series prostaglandins and thromboxane's, and 4-series leukotrienes) is decreased. Also, EPA is a precursor of less inflammatory eicosanoids such as PGE3 and LTB5, as well as 5-series leukotrienes.[38,39] Also, small bioactive lipid mediators termed "specialized proresolving mediators" such as maresins, protectins, and resolvins may be the bioactive component of omega-3 fatty acids and are powerful proresolvers of inflammation through endogenous pathways.[40] EPA and DHA have also been shown to downregulate expression of nuclear factor-kappa B, intracellular adhesion molecule 1, and E-selectin, which reduces local and systemic inflammation.[5,38,39]

Several RCTs have been conducted over the past 25 years with the aim to evaluate the potential benefits of FO on clinical outcomes in ARDS patients. In 2016, the American Society for Parenteral and Enteral Nutrition (ASPEN) and the Society of Critical Care Medicine[6] did not make a recommendation about the use of inflammation-modulating diets enriched with EPA and GLA in ARDS. More recently, the ESPEN Expert Group[41] have supported the administration of FO in critically ill patients, although no specific recommendation in ARDS patients was made. In 2019, Langlois et al.[42] demonstrated that omega-3 PUFAs, particularly when they are provided in combination with GLA and antioxidants as a continuous enteral infusion, are associated with a significant improvement in gas exchange. Nonetheless, this immunomodulatory strategy did not influence any clinical outcomes in the overall analysis, although this meta-analysis showed that omega-3 PUFAs plus GLA and antioxidants may be able to significantly improve pulmonary gas exchange and are associated with a trend toward reduced ICU LOS and MV duration in critically ill patients with ARDS.[42] Moreover, enteral FO produced a significant reduction in mortality, but the mortality effect was mostly driven from clinical trials published before 2011, with almost 50% of the effect derived from the earlier studies. Finally, the authors concluded that further well-powered clinical trials are warranted and should aim at evaluating how EPA, DHA provided in enterally fed patients can modulate the ARDS pathophysiology.[42] Subsequently, Koekkoek et al.[43] after aggregating 24 trials, enrolling 3,574 patients, found no significant effects of enteral FO supplementation on 28-day ICU or hospital mortality. However, ICU LOS and MV duration were significantly reduced in patients receiving enteral FO. Also, subgroup analysis revealed a significant reduction in 28-d mortality, ICU LOS, and duration of MV in patients with ARDS but not in other subgroups. Thus, according to this systematic review of the literature, enteral FO administration cannot be recommended for ICU patients, as so far, strong evidence showing clear clinical benefits was not found.[6,25] Similarly, the Cochrane database Systematic Review[44] found that IED with EPA, DHA, and antioxidant micronutrients may produce little or no difference in all-cause mortality between groups.

It is still uncertain if this type of enteral diets improve the duration of mechanical ventilator days and ICU LOS or oxygenation at day 4 due to the very low quality of evidence.

Therefore, given conflicting data, current guidelines are not able to make a strong recommendation concerning the routine use of enteral formulations with an anti-inflammatory lipid profile-containing FO and borage oil in ARDS patients.

ANTIOXIDANT MICRONUTRIENTS: VITAMINS AND TRACE ELEMENTS

Oxidative stress is recognized as a major promoter of systemic inflammation, which can lead to multiple organ dysfunction (MOD).[45] Different micronutrients exhibit antioxidant properties either directly (vitamins) or indirectly (trace elements) via antioxidant enzymes.[46] Regarding the antioxidant cascade, there are multiple physiological interactions between antioxidant micronutrients, so the best combination with the right dose remains unproven, as it has not yet been defined.[46] Antioxidant micronutrients mediate the actions of reactive oxygen species, which cause damage to DNA, lipids, and proteins. These free radicals are scavenged by GSH, which plays an important role in the regulation of vitamin regeneration and detoxification. GSH, working in synergy with vitamins E and C (ascorbic acid), accounts for most of the natural antioxidant capacity of human plasma. Ascorbic acid regenerates α-tocopherol (the active form of vitamin E) in an energy-dependent process involving NADPH via GSH.[47] Oxidative stress and hence low GSH levels[48] may occur through inadequate dietary intake of vitamins, selenium, and the GSH precursor amino acids, or by excess production of oxygen and hydrogen peroxide.[49] Maintaining good GSH status may, therefore, provide a survival advantage in humans[50] by decelerating the aging process.

Over the past three decades, many observational studies have evaluated the status of antioxidant micronutrients in different critically ill patient populations.[51-53] These studies showed that trace elements (selenium, copper, and zinc) and vitamin availability decrease early and rapidly during critical illness. In addition, micronutrient status at the onset of critical illness has shown to be a biomarker of illness severity. Various micronutrients appear to have immune-stimulating properties. Vitamin A supplementation in mice can reduce the immunosuppression caused by UV radiation and restore antibody production in vitamin A-deficient rats and vitamin C is an important antioxidant which enhances the nitrogen-dependent blastogenesis of lymphocytes.[54] Furthermore, vitamin E is known to stimulate immunoglobulin production and have an enhancing effect on humoral and cellular immunity.[54]

In preterm infants, zinc deficiency causes reduced T-cell counts, lymphocyte response, natural killer (NK) cell activity and phagocyte dysfunction, which can be corrected by zinc supplements, facilitating recovery of the immune system.[55] Iron is essential for the optimal function of NK cells, neutrophils, and lymphocytes.[56] Copper deficiency has been seen to suppress lymphocyte function,[57] and selenium which also acts as an antioxidant via its cofactor role in GSH peroxidase, enhances lymphocyte activity.[58] The clinical significance of micronutrient supplementation either singly or in combination requires further investigation.

In 2012, a systematic review and meta-analysis, by Manzanares et al.[59] found that antioxidant micronutrients may be associated with significantly reduced mortality in the critically ill. Moreover, this meta-analysis showed that supplementation with high-dose vitamins and trace elements might improve clinical outcomes in those ICU patients at high risk of death, such as seriously ill patients with sepsis and septic shock.[59] In contrast, the two largest multicenter immunonutrition RCTs, the REDOXS study[23] that utilized a factorial 2 × 2 study to supplement glutamine and selenium plus an antioxidant cocktail including selenium, zinc, vitamins C and E, and beta-carotene, and the MetaPlus clinical trial,[24] critiqued earlier, showed unexpected negative results.

Recently, the ESPEN guideline on micronutrients[60] recommended that adequate micronutrients be supplied to all orally or enterally fed patients, starting early during nutritional therapy. Unfortunately, laboratory assessment of vitamins and trace elements status in the acute care setting is uncommon, so the current guidelines do not recommend monitoring micronutrients as a clinical routine.[60] Nevertheless, in the ICU, if clinical symptoms and a concomitant measurement of C-reactive protein (CRP) suggest the possibility of micronutrient deficiencies, we recommend consideration should be given to prescribing and monitoring higher supplementation of the critically ill with micronutrients.

CONCLUSION

Nutrition therapy can affect different physiological processes including those that regulate the immune system. Critical illness is often associated with a physiological immunosuppression leading to increased secondary infections, increased morbidity, and a high risk of mortality. Impaired host immunity has been increasingly related to protein—energy malnutrition, which is known to depress antibody production, the functions of phagocytes, T-cells, and levels of plasma complement. In this context, immunonutrition as a specialized nutrition strategy aimed at improving intestinal barrier and cellular defense functions, and modulating local and systemic inflammation has been extensively studied over the past three decades. Current evidence shows clinical benefits when IEDs are administered in surgical ICU patients and major trauma patients. Understanding the pharmacokinetics/dynamics, functions, interactions, and metabolism of individual immune modulating nutrients included in IED formulations could promise better prognosis for the critically ill, immune compromised patients who are fighting invading organisms trying to overwhelm their normal immune processes.

REFERENCES

1. Collins N, Belkaid Y. Control of immunity via nutritional interventions. Immunity. 2022;55:210-23.
2. Smythe PM, Schonland M, Brereton-Stiles GG, Mafoyane A, Schonland M, Coovadia HM, et al. Thymolymphatic efficiency and depression of cell mediated immunity in protein calorie malnutrition. Lancet. 1971;2:939-43.
3. Van Vilet IM, Gomes-Neto AW, de Jong MFC, Jager-Wittenaar H, Navis GJ. High prevalence of malnutrition both on hospital admission and predischarge. Nutrition. 2020;77:110814.
4. Pierre JF, Heneghan AF, Lawson CL, Wischmeyer PE, Kozar RA, Kudsk KA. Pharmaconutrition review: Physiological mechanism. JPEN J Parenter Enteral Nutr. 2013;37:51S-65S.
5. McCarthy MS, Martindale R. Immunonutrition in critical illness. What is the role? Nutr Clin Pract. 2018;33:348-58.
6. McClave S, Taylor BE, Martindale RG, Warren MM, Johnson DR, Braunschweig Carol, et al. Guidelines for the provision and assessment of nutrition support therapy in the adult critically ill patient: Society of Critical Care Medicine (SCCM) and American Society for Parenteral and Enteral Nutrition (ASPEN). JPEN J Parenter Enteral Nutr. 2016;40:159-211.
7. Manzanares W, Heyland DK. Pharmaconutrition with arginine decreases bacterial translocation in an animal model of severe trauma. Is a clinical study justified? The time is now. Crit Care Med. 2012;40:350-1.
8. Polk HC, George CD, Welhausen SR, Cost K, Davidson PR, Regan MP, et al. A systematic study of host defence processes in badly injured patients. Arch Surg. 1988;204:282-99.
9. Oltermann MH, Rassas TN. Immunonutrition in a multidisciplinary ICU population. JPEN J Parenter Enteral Nutr. 2001;25:S30-5.
10. Drover JW, Dhaliwal R, Weitzel L, Wischmeyer PE, Ochoa JB, Heyland DK. Perioperative use of arginine-supplemented diets: a systematic review of the evidence. Am J Coll Surg. 2011;212:385-99.
11. Mazaki T, Ishii Y, Murai I. Immunoenhancing enteral and parenteral nutrition for gastrointestinal surgery: a multiple treatments meta-analysis. Ann Surg. 2015;261:662-9.
12. Lopez Delgado JC, Grau Carmona T, Trujillano Cabello J, García-Fuentes C, Mor-Marco E, Bordeje-Laguna ML, et al. The effects of enteral immunonutrition in the intensive care unit: Does it impacts on outcomes? Nutrients. 2022;14:1904.
13. Brosnan JT. Interorgan amino acid transport and its regulation. J Nutra. 2003;133(suppl 1):2068S-72S.
14. Lacey JM, Wilmore DW. Is glutamine a conditionally essential amino acid? Nutr Rev. 1990;48:297-309.
15. Parry Billings M, Evans J, Calder PC, Newsholme EA. Does glutamine contribute to immunosuppression after major burns? Lancet. 1990;336:523-5.
16. Newsholme EA, Parry-Billings M. Properties of glutamine release from muscle and its importance for the immune system. J Parent Nutr. 1990;14:635-75.

17. Parry-Billings M, Baigrie RJ, Lamont PM, Morris PJ, Newsholme EA. Effects of major and minor surgery on plasma glutamine and cytokine levels. Ann Surg. 1992;127:1239-40.
18. Hanna M, Kudsk K. Nutritional and pharmacological enhancement of gut-associated lymphoid tissue. Can J Gastroenterol. 2000;14(suppl D):145D-51D.
19. Li J, Kudsk K, Janu P, Renegar K. Effect of glutamine-enriched total parenteral nutrition on small intestinal gut-associated lymphoid tissue and upper respiratory tract immunity. Surgery. 1997;121:542-9.
20. Hardy G, Hardy IJ. Can glutamine enable the critically ill to cope better with infection? JPEN J Parenter Enteral Nutr. 2008;32:489-91.
21. Luo M, Bazargan N, Griffith DP, Estívariz CF, Leader LM, Easley KA, et al. Metabolic effects of enteral versus parenteral alanyl-glutamine dipeptide administration in critically ill patients receiving enteral feeding: a pilot study. Clin Nutr. 2008;27:297-306.
22. Singleton KD, Serkova N, Beckey VE, Wischmeyer PE. Glutamine attenuates lung injury and improves survival after sepsis: role of enhanced heat shock protein expression. Crit Care Med. 2005;33:1206-13.
23. Heyland D, Muscedere J, Wischmeyer PE, Cook D, Jones G, Albert M, et al. A randomized trial of glutamine and antioxidants in critically ill patients. N Engl J Med. 2013;368:1489-97.
24. van Zanten A, Sztark F, Kaisers UX, Zielmann S, Felbinger TW, Sablotzki AR, et al. High-protein enteral nutrition enriched with immune-modulating nutrients vs standard high-protein enteral nutrition and nosocomial infections in the ICU: a randomized clinical trial. JAMA. 2014;312:514-24.
25. Singer P, Blaser AR, Berger MM, Alhazzani W, Calder PC, Casaer MP, et al. ESPEN guideline on clinical nutrition in the intensive care unit. Clin Nutr. 2019;38:48-79.
26. Zhou Y-P, Jiang Z-M, Sun Y-H, Wang X-R, Ma E-L, Wilmore D, et al. The effect of supplemental enteral glutamine on plasma levels, gut function, and outcome in severe burns: a randomized, double blind, controlled clinical trial. JPEN J Parenter Enteral Nutr. 2003;27:241-5.
27. Oudemans-van Straaten HM, Bosman RJ, Treskes M, van der Spoel HJ, Zandstra DF, et al. Plasma glutamine depletion and patient outcome in acute ICU admissions. Intensive Care Med. 2001;27:84-90.
28. Heyland DK, Wibbenmeyer L, Pollack JA, Friedman B, Turgeon AF, Eshraghi N, et al. A randomized trial of enteral glutamine for treatment of burn injuries. N Engl J Med 2022; 387:1001-10.
29. Ortiz Reyes L, Lee ZY, Han Lew CC, Hill A, Jeschke MG, Turgeon AF, et al. The efficacy of glutamine supplementation in severe adults burn patients: a systematic review with trial sequential meta-analysis. Crit Care Med. 2023;51.
30. Ochoa JB. Arginine deficiency caused by myeloid cells: importance, identification, and treatment. In: Makrides M, Ochoa JB, Szajewska H (eds). 77th Nestlé Nutrition Institute Workshop, The Importance of Immunonutrition. Panama. (Oct-Nov 2012). Ser. Nestec Ltd. Vevey/S Karger AG Basel. 2013;77:29-45.
31. Barbul A. Arginine and immune function. Nutrition. 1990;6:53-62.
32. Visser M, Vermeulen MA, Richir MC, Teerlink T, Houdijk APJ, Kostense PJ, et al. Imbalance of arginine and asymmetric dimethylarginine is associated with markers of circulatory failure, organ failure and mortality in shock patients. Br J Nutr. 2012;10:1458-65.
33. Galban C, Montejo JC, Mesejo A, Marco P, Celaya S, Sánchez-Segura JM, et al. An immune enhancing enteral diet reduces mortality and episodes of bacteriemia in septic ICU patients. Crit Care Med. 2000;28:643-8.

34. Patel JJ, Miller KR, Rosenthal C, Rosenthal MD. When is it appropriate to use arginine in critical illness? Nutr Clin Pract. 2016;31: 438-44.
35. Calder PC. Polyunsaturated fatty acids, inflammation, and immunity. Lipids. 2001; 36:1007-24.
36. Singer P, Shapiro H, Theilla M, Anbar R, Singer J, Cohen J. Anti-inflammatory properties of omega-3 fatty acids in critical illness: novel mechanisms and an integrative perspective. Intensive Care Med. 2008;34:1580-92.
37. Pontes-Arruda A, Aragao AM, Albuquerque JD. Effects of enteral feeding with eicosapentaenoic acid, gamma-linolenic acid, and antioxidants in mechanically ventilated patients with severe sepsis and septic shock. Crit Care Med. 2006;34: 2325-33.
38. Stapleton RD, Matin JM, Mayer K. Fish oil in critical illness: mechanisms and clinical applications. Crit Care Clin. 2010;26:501-14.
39. Bulger EM, Maier RV. Lipid mediators in the pathophysiology of critical illness. Crit Care Med. 2000;28(Suppl 4):N27-36.
40. Vanzant E, Loftus T, Kamel A, Carmichael E, Rosenthal MD. Nutritional impact of omega 3 fatty acids and metabolites in acute and chronic critical illness. Curr Opin Clin Nutr Metab Care. 2022;25:75-80.
41. Calder P, Adolph M, Deutz NE, Grau T, Innes JK, Klek S, et al. Lipids in the intensive care unit: Recommendations from the ESPEN Expert Group. Clin Nutr. 2018;37:1-18.
42. Langlois PL, D´Arafon F, Hardy G, Manzanares W. Omega-3 polyunsaturated fatty acids in critically ill patients with acute respiratory distress syndrome: A systematic review and meta-analysis Nutrition. 2019;61: 84-92.
43. Koekkoek K, Panteleon V, van Zanten AR. Current evidence on omega-3 fatty acids in enteral nutrition in the critically ill: a systematic review and meta-analysis. Nutrition. 2019;59:56-68.
44. Dushianthan A, Cusack R, Burgess VA, Grocott MP, Calder PC. Immunonutrition for acute respiratory distress syndrome (ARDS) in adults. Cochrane Database Syst Rev. 2019;1(1):CD012041.
45. Lovat R, Preiser JC. Antioxidant therapy in intensive care. Curr Opin Crit Care. 2003;9:266-70.
46. Berger MM, Manzanares W. Micronutrients early in critical illness, selective or generous, enteral, or intravenous? Curr Opin Clin Nutr Metab Care. 2021;4:165-75.
47. Alexander JW, Saito H, Ogle CK, Trocki O. The importance of lipid type in the diet. Ann Surg. 1986;204:1-8.
48. Pasatiempo AM, Bowman TA, Taylor C, Moss AC. Vitamin A depletion and repletion: effects on antibody response to capsular polysaccharide of strep pheymonniae. J Clin Nutr. 1989;49:501-51.
49. Sinkeldem EJ, De Groot AP, van den Berg H. The effect of pyridoxine on the number of lymphocytes in the blood of rats fed caramel colour. Food Chem Toxic. 1988;26: 195-203.
50. Oh C, Narkano K. Reversal by ascorbic acid of suppression by endogenous histamine of rat lymphocyte blastogenesis. J Nutr. 1988; 118:639-44.
51. Forceville X, Vitoux D, Gauzit R, Combes A, Lahilaire P, Chappuis P. Selenium, systemic immune response syndrome, sepsis and outcome in critically ill patients. Crit Care Med. 1998;26:1536-44.
52. Manzanares W, Biestro A, Galusso F, Torre MH, Mañay N, Pittini G, et al. Serum selenium and glutathione peroxidase-3 activity: biomarkers of systemic inflammation in the critically ill. Intensive Care Med. 2009;35:882-9.
53. Stoppe C, Shälte G, Rossaint R, Coburn M, Graf B, Spillner J, et al. The intraoperative decrease of selenium is associated with the postoperative development of multiorgan dysfunction in cardiac surgical patients. Crit Care Med. 2011;39:1879-85.

54. Haberal M, Harmalogu E, Bora S, Oner G, Bilgin N. The effects of vitamin E on immune regulation after thermal injury. Burns. 1988; 14:388-93.
55. Fraken PJ, Gershwin EM, Good RA, Prasad A. Interrelationships between zinc and immune function. Fed Proc. 1986;45:1474-9.
56. Watabayashi Y, Sigimoto M, Ishiyama T, Hirose S. Effect of iron on T-cell colony formation in patients with iron deficiency anaemia. Acta Haematol Jpn. 1988;51:691-7.
57. Mulhern Sa, Koller LD. Severe or marginal copper deficiency results in a graded reduction in immune status in mice. J Nutr. 1989;118:1041-7.
58. Larsen HJ, Overnes G, Moksnes K. Effect of selenium on sheep lymphocyte responses to mitogens. Res Vet Sci. 1988;45:11-5.
59. Manzanares W, Dhaliwal R, Jiang X, Murch L, Heyland DK. Antioxidant micronutrients in the critically ill: a systematic review and meta-analysis. Crit Care. 2012;16:R66.
60. Berger MM, Shenkin A, Schweinlin A, Amrein K, Augsburger M, Biesalski HK, et al. ESPEN micronutrient guideline. Clin Nutr. 2022;41:1357-424.

CHAPTER 38

Dysglycemia in Critical Illness

Shweta Ram Chandankhede, Balguri Mukesh Kumar

INTRODUCTION

Dysglycemia referred as abnormality in the blood glucose stability is a very common occurrence in the intensive care unit (ICU). Critical illness is a state of stress and severe physiological abnormalities due to trauma, infections, use of steroids, and nutritional problems. Dysglycemia can manifest as hyperglycemia, hypoglycemia, or blood glucose variability and has significant adverse effects on patient outcomes.[1] It is prevalent not only in diabetic patients but also in nondiabetic patients admitted to the ICU.[2] A significant percentage of the population in the community suffers from chronic dysglycemia, which is underdiagnosed and is associated with the worst outcomes and complications during ICU admission. It is of paramount importance to consider the history, nutritional status, preadmission glycemic values, and glycosylated hemoglobin in such cases.[3,4]

Ever since the publication of the Leuven study in 2001, the measurement of plasma glucose and insulin therapy has become a standard of practice in the ICU setting. The variability of the results in the subsequent large trials led to many controversies regarding the ideal range of blood glucose levels in critical illness.[1,5] Dysglycemia management in critically ill patients needs a holistic and individualized approach to seek the right balance between the glycemic target and minimizing the complications of overenthusiastic management.

Maintaining hemostasis of blood glucose is very important for proper functioning and depends on various factors like absorption, breakdown, and metabolism of glucose, fats, and amino acids as well as gluconeogenesis. A harmony between the metabolic function of various tissues and hormones like insulin, epinephrine, glucagon, and glucocorticoids is crucial to stabilize the blood glucose levels.[2]

Dysglycemia is the abnormality in the blood glucose level due to abnormal hemostasis of blood glucose due to a combination of multiple factors such as physiological, pathological, and therapeutic factors.

There are four types of dysglycemia in critically ill patients **(Fig. 1)**.
1. Stress hyperglycemia
2. Hypoglycemia
3. Glycemic variability (GV)
4. Time in the target range (TITR).

STRESS HYPERGLYCEMIA

It is a type of hyperglycemia typically seen in critically ill patients with or without prior history of diabetes. It is either due to an endogenous response to extreme stress caused by systemic inflammation or exogenous factors like the use of steroids, catecholamines,

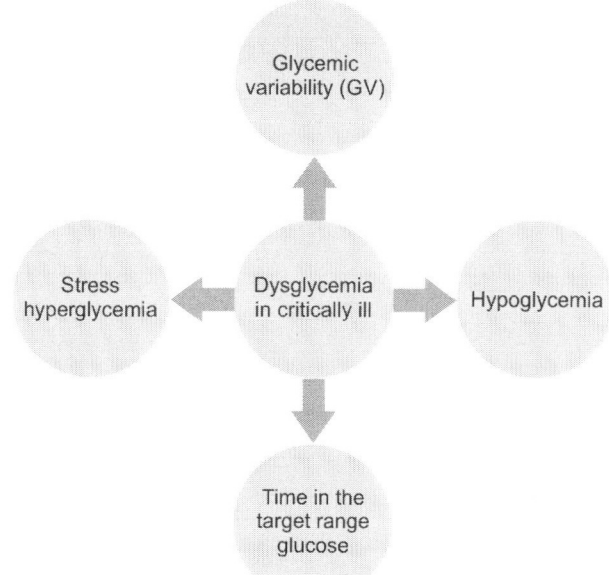

Fig. 1: Types of dysglycemia.

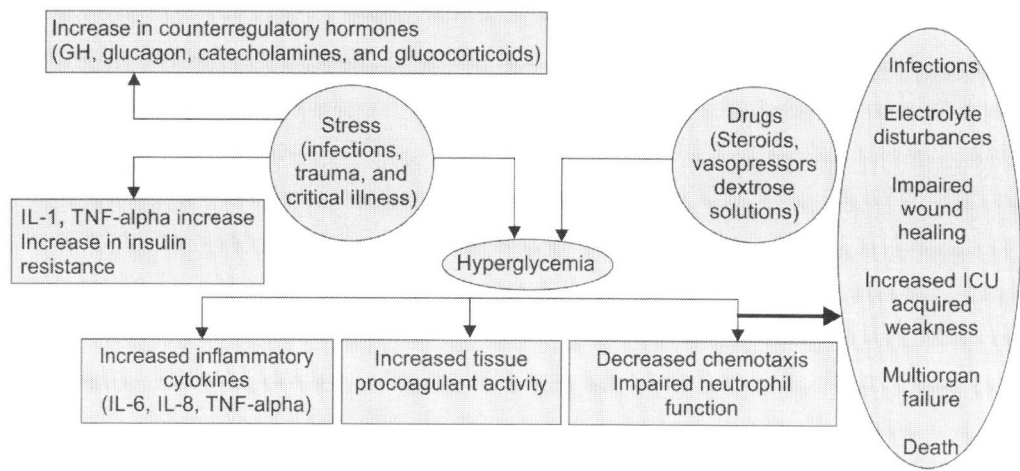

Fig. 2: Pathophysiology of hyperglycemia in intensive care unit (ICU). (GH: growth hormone; IL: interleukin; TNF: tumor necrosis factor)

glucose, and antibiotics in the ICU.[5] It is generally transient in nature and recovers once the triggering factor is eliminated. In diabetics, it is referred as elevated blood glucose levels above 180–220 mg/dL, whereas in nondiabetic patients, it is referred as blood glucose levels above 140 mg/dL.[6]

Pathophysiology of Stress Hyperglycemia (Fig. 2)

Critical illness is characterized by systemic inflammation, which leads to physiological stress response by elevation of the endogenous catecholamine levels. At first, it is a protective and adaptive mechanism for survival by providing a substrate for energy.[6] In severe state the counterregulatory hormones such as glucagon, cortisol, catecholamines, and growth hormone antagonize insulin leading to neoglucogenesis, glycogenolysis, and peripheral insulin resistance.[1,5]

Stress hyperglycemia is much more severe in critically ill diabetic patients as compared to nondiabetic patients due to preexisting insulin resistance and hyperglucagonemia. It is commonly seen in patients with sepsis and multiorgan dysfunction, cardiac surgery, trauma, and neurosurgical patients.[6]

Stress hyperglycemia ratio is the ratio of blood sugar levels at admission and estimated average sugar levels calculated from hemoglobin A1c (HbA1c) (HbA1c × 1.59–2.59). Roberts et al. in their study have shown that stress hyperglycemia ratio rather than stress hyperglycemia is associated with increased mortality and morbidity.[7]

HYPOGLYCEMIA

The incidence of hypoglycemia in critically ill patients is quite high and can be either related to the disease or intensive insulin therapy. It is commonly seen in patients with hepatic dysfunction, sepsis, and renal dysfunction.[5]

The American Diabetes Association (ADA) defines hypoglycemia as a blood glucose level <70 mg/dL and classifies it into three levels **(Table 1)**.[8,9]

TABLE 1: Levels of hypoglycemia by the American Diabetes Association.

Level	
Level 1	70 to ≥54 mg/dL
Level 2	<54 mg/dL
Level 3	A clinical event characterized by altered mental or physical status requiring assistance for the treatment of hypoglycemia

In the early stage, there is increased endogenous glucose production through glycogenolysis and gluconeogenesis as well as reduced endogenous insulin secretion as a response to hypoglycemia. Further drop in blood glucose leads to endogenous glucagon secretion and adrenaline secretion, which further reduces the insulin secretion and tissue sensitivity to insulin and increases the utilization of glycogenic substrate. Later as the disease progresses, all these mechanisms fail and can cause severe hypoglycemia leading to severe neurological damage.[2,10]

Causes of Hypoglycemia in ICU[2]

Causes hypoglycemia in ICU include:
- Insulin overdose
- Insulin nutrition mismatch
- Severe sepsis
- Hepatic failure
- Adrenal insufficiency
- Renal failure (prolonged insulin action)

Several observational studies and randomized controlled trials (RCTs) including the landmark NICE-SUGAR (Normoglycemia in Intensive Care Evaluation–Survival Using Glucose Algorithm Regulation) study have correlated hypoglycemia with increased mortality.[11-14] Real-time continuous glucose monitoring (RT CGM)-based glucose monitoring studies have shown that CGM is a promising tool to alert physicians regarding impending hypoglycemia.[15-18] Insulin-related hypoglycemia can be prevented by titration of insulin infusion based on anticipated feeding interruptions, medications change (e.g., steroid cessation), and drug adjustments in accordance with kidney and liver function.

GLYCEMIC VARIABILITY

In critically ill patients, the plasma glucose levels may fluctuate significantly. This may lead to a spectrum of glycemic values from low to high keeping mean values similar. Owing to this the glycemic control may differ even though the mean values are same.[1]

Glycemic variability can be defined as the tendency or propensity of a patient to develop repeated excursions of plasma glycemia over a relatively short period of time, which exceeds the range expected for a normal physiological response.[5,19]

Glycemic variability can be assessed using the following tools:[5,8]
- Standard deviation (SD) of glucose
- Coefficient of variation of glucose
- Mean amplitude of glycemic excursion (MAGE)
- Glycemic lability index (change in glucose level over a period of 4 weeks).

Even if mean glucose is same in two different patients, their glycemic control and fluctuations in glucose levels may vary. This can be identified by GV.[20-22] High GV causes oxidative stress leading to endothelial dysfunction in diabetics, an increase in apoptosis of cells in nondiabetics rendering them more vulnerable to infections.[1,6]

Various studies have shown an increase in mortality in patients with high GV. Chao et al. noticed that MAGE >65 mg/dL on the first day of ICU is associated with an increase in 30-day mortality.[23]

TIME IN THE TARGET GLUCOSE RANGE

It is the percentage of time during which patients' plasma glucose levels remain in the target range. It is affected by hyperglycemia, hypoglycemia, and GV.[8] Various studies have shown that time in range (TIR) >50–80% is required for better patient outcomes **(Box 1)**. The ADA recommends TIR >70%. Lanspa et al. have shown reduction in mortality if TIR

BOX 1: Beneficial effects of time in range >50–80%.
- Increased survival
- Reduced organ failure
- Shorter duration of mechanical ventilation
- Shorter intensive care unit stay
- Reduced susceptibility to infections
- Lower incidence of postoperative complications

>80% for blood glucose target of 70–139 mg/dL, more specifically for patients with well-controlled diabetes mellitus (DM).[24] Cardiac surgery patients had an increase in sternal wound infections when TIR was <80%.[25] In Glucontrol study RCT, TIR >50% was associated with better survival.[26] Krinsley and Preiser in their study have seen that mortality of nondiabetic patients is more if TIR is <80%, whereas in diabetic patients TIR was not associated with mortality.[27] It is therefore important to protocolize good glycemic control, prevention of GV, and control TIR for better outcomes.[5]

CONSEQUENCES OF DYSGLYCEMIA IN CRITICALLY ILL PATIENTS

Dysglycemia can impact the outcomes negatively in critically ill patients whether they are known diabetics or nondiabetics.[1] Following are the consequences of dysglycemia:
- Increased mortality
- Impaired immune response
- Organ dysfunction
- Delayed wound healing
- Higher risk of complications like hospital-acquired infections
- Prolonged ICU stay
- Increased healthcare cost.

GLUCOSE MONITORING IN ICU

Blood glucose level is the fifth vital parameter that needs to be monitored in ICU. The ADA recommends to measure HbA1c level in all patients with hyperglycemia (>140 mg/dL) in ICU if not done in the preceding 3 months.[28] Although blood gas analyzers are more accurate for precise measurement of glucose levels, it is more feasible to use point-of-care Food and Drug Administration (FDA)-approved capillary glucometer in ICU. These glucometer measurements can be fallacious in anemia, erythrocytosis, abnormal arterial O_2 tension, edema, and poor perfusion.[29,30]

Frequency of Blood Glucose Measurements in ICU

In critically ill patients without glycemic instability, blood glucose levels need to be measured every 4-6 hours.[31] In less sick patients on oral diet, it should be measured before meals. In patients on insulin infusion, glucose levels need to be measured every 30 minutes to 2 hours.

FEASIBILITY AND VALIDITY OF CONTINUOUS GLUCOSE MONITORING IN ICU

Continuous glucose monitoring is a glucose monitoring system, which measures glucose levels either in interstitial fluid or in the venous blood. In ICU, RT CGM is preferable.[32]

COMPONENTS OF CONTINUOUS GLUCOSE MONITORING

The components of CGM are as:
- Tiny needle biosensor
- Transmitter
- Monitor

Continuous glucose monitoring can be integrated into the closed loop system and allow for automated delivery of insulin (ADI).[33] Its use has been particularly increased during the coronavirus disease 2019 (COVID-19) pandemic, primarily to avoid repeated exposure to the infected patients.[34]

CGM use in ICU settings is not FDA approved. Clinical trials evaluating CGM in hospitalized patients [Manual versus Automated moNitoring Accuracy of GlucosE II (MANAGE II)] used intravascular CGM systems and preliminary data suggest that CGM can improve glycemic management.[35] Glucoscout and OptiScanner are advanced intravascular CGM systems that are commonly used in hospital settings.[36]

Advantages of Continuous Glucose Monitoring[18,37]

Advantages of CGM are:
- Better tight glucose control in the ICU without increasing the risk of hypoglycemia by adjusting insulin infusions more rapidly
- RT monitoring helps in quick response
- Better monitoring of glycemic metrics such as GV and TITR
- Less labor intensive
- Reduced need for blood sampling and thus patient discomfort
- Decreased exposure of the staff to highly contagious patients
- Individualization of treatment plan tailored to needs of patient.

Limitations of Continuous Glucose Monitoring

Limitations of CGM include:
- Continuous glucose monitoring systems based on interstitial fluid glucose measurements have a lag time when compared to blood glucose levels
- Requires frequent calibrations
- Its use in patients with anasarca has not been validated
- Need to be changed every 7-14 days
- High cost
- Technical failures can arise due to malfunctioning of CGM sensors and equipment.

GLYCEMIC TARGETS IN ICU (TABLE 2)

The patient population in the ICU is heterogeneous with regards to age, gender, comorbidities, current sickness, and its severity. Many studies have been done to know "what is the glycemic target for best outcomes in ICU patients?" Despite of number of trials, glycemic targets in patients with preexisting diabetes whether previously well-controlled or poorly controlled, nondiabetic patients, surgical and nonsurgical patients as well as trauma patients in the ICU is still an area of debate and active research.

A recent retrospective analysis has shown that effect of hyperglycemia on mortality in patients with and without diabetes is different. Time-weighted average (TWA) glucose levels of 80–120 mg/dL in nondiabetic patients and 90–150 mg/dL in diabetic patients had lesser risk of mortality. It was observed that glucose variability had a flattened response in diabetics.[38]

In a retrospective observational study, patients with HbA1c <7% at admission had greater risk of mortality with increase in mean blood glucose levels compared to HbA1c >7%. This implies that patients with preexisting uncontrolled diabetes may require less stringent glucose targets.[39]

MANAGEMENT OF DYSGLYCEMIA IN ICU

Managing dysglycemia in ICU is crucial as it impacts the outcomes and the recovery. It needs an individualized and holistic approach (**Fig. 3**). Titrated insulin therapy, appropriate nutrition, appropriate management of sepsis as well as adjustment of corticosteroids are important in managing dysglycemia in ICU. Insulin is the mainstay of therapy, which can be given either in the form of infusion or fixed doses according to the severity of the illness. Oral hypoglycemic agents are avoided in critically ill patients as they may

TABLE 2: Recommendation of glycemic targets.

Society/Guidelines	Target glucose	Category of patients
ADA[9]	• 140–180 mg/dL • 110–140 mg/dL • (if can be achieved without hypoglycemia) • >250 mg/dL	• Critically ill patients • Postsurgical and postcardiac surgery patients • Terminally ill with short-life expectancy
SSG[40]	144–180 mg/dL	Sepsis
SCCM[41]	150–180 mg/dL	Critically ill
ACP[42]	140–200 mg/dL	• Surgical ICU • Medical ICU
ESC[43]	• <200 mg/dL • Avoid hypoglycemia • Less stringent targets	• STEMI—acute phase • Advanced cardiovascular disease • Older age • Longer DM status • Multiple comorbidities

(ACP: American College of Physicians; ADA: American Diabetes Association; DM: diabetes mellitus; ESC: European Society of Cardiology; ICU: intensive care unit; SCCM: Society of Critical Care Medicine; SSG: surviving sepsis guidelines; STEMI: ST-elevation myocardial infarction)

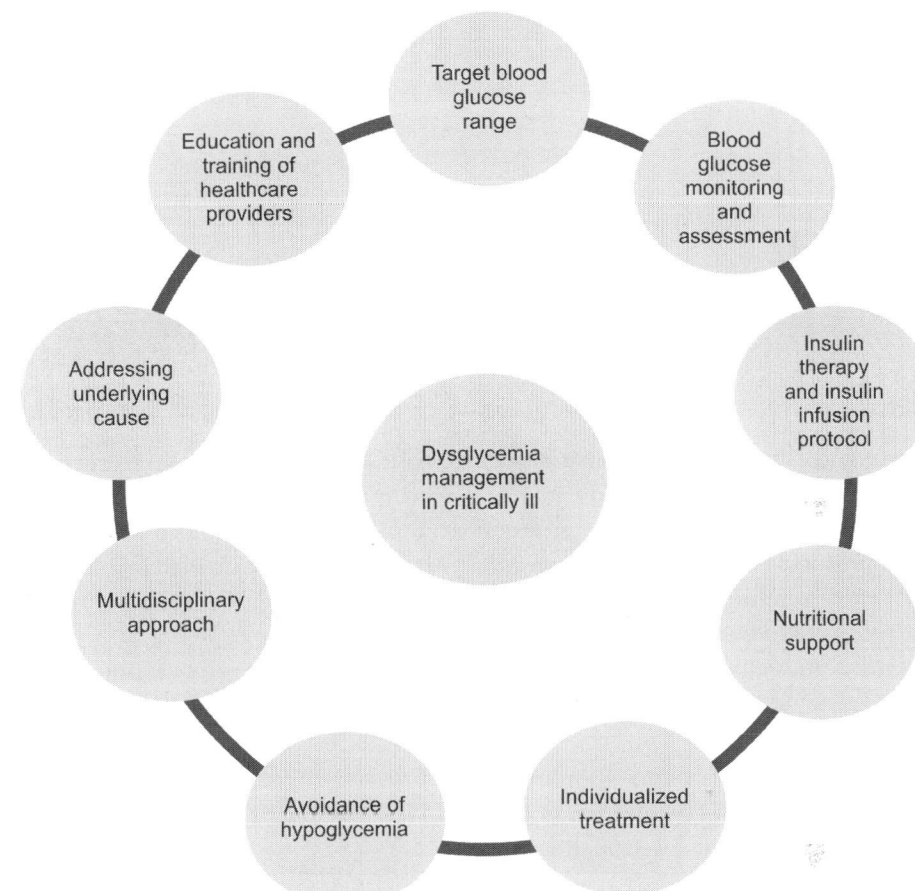

Fig. 3: Overview of dysglycemia management in critically ill patients.

have unpredictable pharmacokinetics and pharmacodynamics due to the presence of shock, kidney dysfunction, and liver dysfunction. Metformin can cause lactic acidosis in patients with renal failure.[44] Sodium-glucose cotransporter-2 (SGLT2) inhibitors can cause euglycemic diabetic ketoacidosis and dehydration. Its use in patients with ketonemia, prolonged fasting, and planned surgical procedures should be avoided. Contrarily its use may be judicious in patients with heart failure.[45] Sulfonylureas can cause severe hypoglycemia and should be avoided.[46]

INSULIN THERAPY IN ICU

Insulin therapy should be initiated in cases of persistent hyperglycemia. The ADA recommends insulin administration using validated written or computerized protocols **(Flowchart 1)**.

INSULIN INFUSION PROTOCOL IN ICU

Many standard ICUs have their own protocol for insulin infusion. Computerized protocols called electronic glucose management systems (eGMS) like Endo Tool, Glucommander,

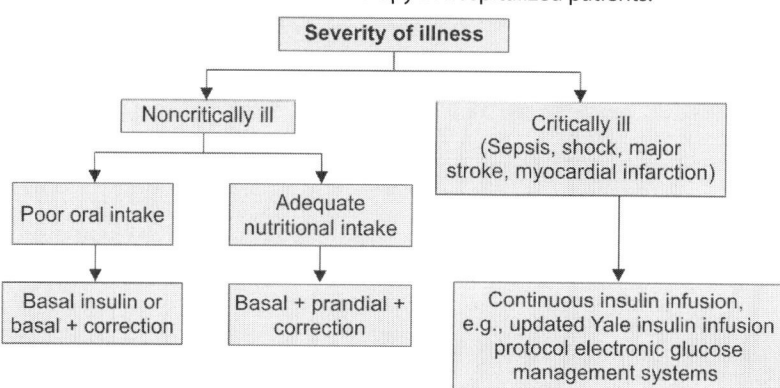

Flowchart 1: Insulin therapy in hospitalized patients.

GlucoCare, and GlucoStabilizer have been in use in ICUs for more than a decade.[47] Studies comparing written versus computer generated protocols have shown improved outcomes with computer-based protocols.[48] The rates of hypoglycemia were lower when computerized protocols were used.[49] eGMS may fail in patients on glucocorticoids as insulin requirements increase.

The following important points should be included in the protocol for insulin infusion:
- Method and frequency of blood glucose measurements
- Method of preparation of insulin solution
- Data interpretations for adjustment of insulin infusion.

Insulin protocols for mere hyperglycemia and diabetic emergencies (ketoacidosis, nonketotic hyperosmolar coma) should be different.

The updated Yale insulin infusion protocol is a widely used protocol for insulin infusion.[50]

Salient Features of the Yale Protocol

- Insulin infusion solution should be prepared to obtain concentrations of 1 unit regular human insulin per 1 mL 0.9% NaCl.
- The infusion tubing should be primed with 20 mL of the insulin solution.
- Blood glucose should be measured every hour initially and later second hourly when the preceding three readings are within the target range.
- Initial bolus and infusion rate calculated as blood glucose divided by 100, this value should be rounded off to the nearest 0.5 units.
- If nutrition abruptly stopped, decrease the infusion rate by 50%.
- Insulin infusion rate should not exceed 20 U/h without decreasing the carbohydrate load, especially in obese patients.

Insulin Dosage

The amount of insulin requirement depends upon:
- Insulin resistance of that patient
- Patient's body mass index (BMI)
- Patient's nutritional support
- Drugs (glucocorticoids, vasopressors)

The prandial insulin dose in patients on enteral nutrition can be calculated as 1 unit of insulin for every 10–15 g carbohydrate intake, whereas in patients on total parenteral nutrition, the dose is 1 unit human regular insulin for 10 g dextrose.

TRANSITION FROM INTRAVENOUS TO SUBCUTANEOUS INSULIN

Once the patient's clinical status and glycemic stability improve, the intravenous insulin should be changed to subcutaneous insulin. Subcutaneous basal insulin dose should be administered 2 hours before discontinuation of *intravenous* insulin infusion to avoid hyperglycemia and rebound hypoglycemia.

Dose calculation: Mean insulin infusion rate (M) in the preceding 6 hours should be calculated.

$$M \times 24 = X \text{ units/day}$$

About 70–85% of this dose is the estimated first day's total insulin requirement. Subsequent doses should be calculated based on patients' clinical status. This can partly (50%) be administered as basal dose and the remaining (50%) as prandial dose.

NUTRITIONAL SUPPORT

Adequate and timely nutrition is an important aspect in the treatment of dysglycemic patients in the ICU. Nutrition plays an important role not only in management but also in the prevention of dysglycemia in ICU patients. A proper nutrition program in the critically ill patients can maintain stable glucose levels, prevent complications, and hasten recovery.

Following are the important aspects of nutrition in critically ill dysglycemic patients given by practice guidelines for enteral nutrition management.[51]

- Continuous feeding is better than bolus feeding as it minimizes dysglycemic episodes.
- Formulated feeds with low glycemic index or low glycemic load are preferred.
- Formulated feeds with low glycemic index with consideration of the protein and electrolyte content are important in critically ill patients with renal or liver dysfunction.
- Complex and slowly digestible carbohydrate-containing feeds are preferable for glycemic optimization in critically ill patients.
- High protein digestibility-corrected amino acid score proteins are preferred as they help in minimizing GV.
- Disease-specific nutrition plays an important role in the management of dysglycemia in ICU patients.
- Multidisciplinary approach to nutrition with the involvement of nurses, dieticians, pharmacologist, and doctors is important.
- Assessment of nutritional practices by healthcare workers, frequent training sessions, and reassessment should be protocolized by every hospital for managing dysglycemia in critically ill patients.

CONCLUSION

Dysglcemia has a wide spectrum from hyperglycemia, GV to hypoglycemia in critically ill patients. It is a common occurrence in diabetic and nondiabetic patients in the ICU, which significantly impacts the outcomes. A structured program which is individualized according to the need of the patient with the help of a multidisciplinary team and the use of advanced new technologies like CGM can be very beneficial for critically ill patients in improving the glycemic balance and thus outcomes.

REFERENCES

1. Anshu J, Yatin M. Dysglycemia in ICU Patients. J Cardiac Crit Care TSS. 2022: 40-2.
2. Wu Z, Liu J, Zhang D, Kang K, Zuo X, Xu Q, et al. Expert consensus on the glycemic management of critically ill patients. J Intensive Med. 2022;2(3):131-45.
3. Balintescu A, Palmgren I, Lipcsey M, Oldner A, Larsson A, Cronhjort M, et al. Prevalence and impact of chronic dysglycemia in intensive care unit patients-A retrospective cohort study. Acta Anaesthesiol Scand. 2021;65(1):82-91.

4. Sarvin S, Mahmoodpoor A. (2017). Dysglycemia in Critically Ill Patients: Common Problems and Future Direction. Advances in Bioscience and Clinical Medicine, 5(3), 1-2. doi:https://doi.org/10.7575/aiac.abcmed.17.05.03.01.
5. Aramendi I, Burghi G, Manzanares W. Dysglycemia in the critically ill patient: current evidence and future perspectives. Rev Bras Ter Intensiva. 2017;29(3):364-72.
6. Silva-Perez LJ, Benitez-Lopez MA, Varon J, Surani S. Management of critically ill patients with diabetes. World J Diabetes. 2017;8(3):89-96.
7. Roberts GW, Quinn SJ, Valentine N, Alhawassi T, O'Dea H, Stranks SN. Relative Hyperglycemia, a Marker of Critical Illness: Introducing the Stress Hyperglycemia Ratio. J Clin Endocrinol Metab. 2015;100(12):4490-7.
8. Alhatemi G, Aldiwani H, Alhatemi R, Hussein M, Mahdai S, Seyoum B. Glycemic control in the critically ill: Less is more. Cleve Clin J Med. 2022;89(4):191-9.
9. ElSayed NA, Aleppo G, Aroda VR, Bannuru RR, Brown FM, Bruemmer D, et al. Glycemic Targets: Standards of Care in Diabetes-2023. Diabetes Care. 2023;46(Suppl 1):S97-S110.
10. Lacherade JC, Jacqueminet S, Preiser JC. An overview of hypoglycemia in the critically ill. J Diabetes Sci Technol. 2009;3(6):1242-9.
11. Egi M, Bellomo R, Stachowski E, French CJ, Hart GK, Taori G, et al. Hypoglycemia and outcome in critically ill patients. Mayo Clin Proc. 2010;85(3):217-24.
12. Hermanides J, Bosman RJ, Vriesendorp TM, Dotsch R, Rosendaal FR, Zandstra DF, et al. Hypoglycemia is associated with intensive care unit mortality. Crit Care Med. 2010;38(6):1430-4.
13. Krinsley JS, Grover A. Severe hypoglycemia in critically ill patients: risk factors and outcomes. Crit Care Med. 2007;35(10):2262-7.
14. Finfer S, Liu B, Chittock DR, Norton R, Myburgh JA, McArthur C, et al. NICE-SUGAR Study Investigators. Hypoglycemia and risk of death in critically ill patients. N Engl J Med. 201220;367(12):1108-18.
15. Longo RR, Elias H, Khan M, Seley JJ. Use and Accuracy of Inpatient CGM During the COVID-19 Pandemic: An Observational Study of General Medicine and ICU Patients. J Diabetes Sci Technol. 2022;16(5):1136-43.
16. Davis GM, Spanakis EK, Migdal AL, Singh LG, Albury B, Urrutia MA, et al. Accuracy of Dexcom G6 Continuous Glucose Monitoring in Non-Critically Ill Hospitalized Patients with Diabetes. Diabetes Care. 2021;44(7):1641-6.
17. Baker M, Musselman ME, Rogers R, Hellman R. Practical implementation of remote continuous glucose monitoring in hospitalized patients with diabetes. Am J Health Syst Pharm. 2022;79(6):452-8.
18. Wright JJ, Williams AJ, Friedman SB, Weaver RG, Williams JM, Hodge E, et al. Accuracy of Continuous Glucose Monitors for Inpatient Diabetes Management. J Diabetes Sci Technol. 2022:19322968221076562.
19. Braithwaite SS. Glycemic variability in hospitalized patients: choosing metrics while awaiting the evidence. Curr Diab Rep. 2013;13(1):138-54.
20. Akirov A, Diker-Cohen T, Masri-Iraqi H, Shimon I. High Glucose Variability Increases Mortality Risk in Hospitalized Patients. J Clin Endocrinol Metab. 2017;102(7):2230-41.
21. Atamna A, Ayada G, Akirov A, Shochat T, Bishara J, Elis A. High blood glucose variability is associated with bacteremia and mortality in patients hospitalized with acute infection. QJM. 2019;112(2):101-6.
22. Subramaniam B, Lerner A, Novack V, Khabbaz K, Paryente-Wiesmann M, Hess P, et al. Increased glycemic variability in patients with elevated preoperative HbA1C predicts adverse outcomes following coronary artery bypass grafting surgery. Anesth Analg. 2014;118(2):277-87.
23. Chao WC, Tseng CH, Wu CL, Shih SJ, Yi CY, Chan MC. Higher glycemic variability within the first day of ICU admission is associated with increased 30-day mortality in ICU patients with sepsis. Ann Intensive Care. 2020;10(1):17.

24. Lanspa MJ, Krinsley JS, Hersh AM, Wilson EL, Holmen JR, Orme JF, et al. Percentage of Time in Range 70 to 139 mg/dL Is Associated With Reduced Mortality Among Critically Ill Patients Receiving IV Insulin Infusion. Chest. 2019;156(5):878-86.
25. Omar AS, Salama A, Allam M, Elgohary Y, Mohammed S, Tuli AK, et al. Association of time in blood glucose range with outcomes following cardiac surgery. BMC Anesthesiol. 2015;15(1):14.
26. Penning S, Chase JG, Preiser JC, Pretty CG, Signal M, Mélot C, et al. Does the achievement of an intermediate glycemic target reduce organ failure and mortality? A post hoc analysis of the Glucontrol trial. J Crit Care. 2014;29(3):374-9.
27. Krinsley JS, Preiser JC. Time in blood glucose range 70 to 140 mg/dL >80% is strongly associated with increased survival in non-diabetic critically ill adults. Crit Care. 2015;19(1):179.
28. Pasquel FJ, Gomez-Huelgas R, Anzola I, Oyedokun F, Haw JS, Vellanki P, et al. Predictive Value of Admission Hemoglobin A1c on Inpatient Glycemic Control and Response to Insulin Therapy in Medicine and Surgery Patients With Type 2 Diabetes. Diabetes Care. 2015;38(12):e202-3.
29. Mann EA, Salinas J, Pidcoke HF, Wolf SE, Holcomb JB, Wade CE. Error rates resulting from anemia can be corrected in multiple commonly used point-of-care glucometers. J Trauma. 2008;64(1):15-20.
30. Tang Z, Louie RF, Payes M, Chang KC, Kost GJ. Oxygen effects on glucose measurements with a reference analyzer and three handheld meters. Diabetes Technol Ther. 2000;2(3):349-62.
31. Moghissi ES, Korytkowski MT, DiNardo M, Einhorn D, Hellman R, Hirsch IB, et al. American Association of Clinical Endocrinologists and American Diabetes Association consensus statement on inpatient glycemic control. Diabetes Care. 2009;32(6):1119-31.
32. Chen C, Zhao XL, Li ZH, Zhu ZG, Qian SH, Flewitt AJ. Current and Emerging Technology for Continuous Glucose Monitoring. Sensors (Basel). 2017;17(1):182.
33. Freckmann G, Link M, Kamecke U, Haug C, Baumgartner B, Weitgasser R. Performance and Usability of Three Systems for Continuous Glucose Monitoring in Direct Comparison. J Diabetes Sci Technol. 2019;13(5):890-8.
34. Chow KW, Kelly DJ, Rieff MC, Skala PA, Kravets I, Charitou MM, et al. Outcomes and Healthcare Provider Perceptions of Real-Time Continuous Glucose Monitoring (rtCGM) in Patients With Diabetes and COVID-19 Admitted to the ICU. J Diabetes Sci Technol. 2021;15(3):607-14.
35. Righy Shinotsuka C, Brasseur A, Fagnoul D, So T, Vincent JL, Preiser JC. Manual versus Automated moNitoring Accuracy of GlucosE II (MANAGE II). Crit Care. 2016;20(1):380.
36. Pasquel FJ, Lansang MC, Dhatariya K, Umpierrez GE. Management of diabetes and hyperglycaemia in the hospital. Lancet Diabetes Endocrinol. 2021;9(3):174-88.
37. Faulds ER, Jones L, McNett M, Smetana KS, May CC, Sumner L, et al. Facilitators and Barriers to Nursing Implementation of Continuous Glucose Monitoring (CGM) in Critically Ill Patients With COVID-19. Endocr Pract. 2021;27(4):354-61.
38. Fong KM, Au SY, Ng GWY. Glycemic control in critically ill patients with or without diabetes. BMC Anesthesiol. 2022;22(1):227.
39. Egi M, Bellomo R, Stachowski E, French CJ, Hart GK, Taori G, et al. The interaction of chronic and acute glycemia with mortality in critically ill patients with diabetes. Crit Care Med. 2011;39(1):105-11.
40. Evans L, Rhodes A, Alhazzani W, Antonelli M, Coopersmith CM, French C, et al. Surviving Sepsis Campaign: International Guidelines for Management of Sepsis and Septic Shock 2021. Intensive Care Med. 2021;47(11):1181-247.
41. Jacobi J, Bircher N, Krinsley J, Agus M, Braithwaite SS, Deutschman C, et al. Guidelines for the use of an insulin infusion for the management of hyperglycemia in critically ill patients. Crit Care Med. 2012;40(12):3251-76.

42. Qaseem A, Chou R, Humphrey LL, Shekelle P; Clinical Guidelines Committee of the American College of Physicians. Inpatient glycemic control: best practice advice from the Clinical Guidelines Committee of the American College of Physicians. Am J Med Qual. 2014;29(2):95-8.
43. Ibanez B, James S, Agewall S, Antunes MJ, Bucciarelli-Ducci C, Bueno H, et al. 2017 ESC Guidelines for the management of acute myocardial infarction in patients presenting with ST-segment elevation: The Task Force for the management of acute myocardial infarction in patients presenting with ST-segment elevation of the European Society of Cardiology (ESC). Eur Heart J. 2018;39(2):119-77.
44. Luft FC. Lactic acidosis update for critical care clinicians. J Am Soc Nephrol. 2001;12 Suppl 17:S15-9.
45. Levine JA, Karam SL, Aleppo G. SGLT2-I in the Hospital Setting: Diabetic Ketoacidosis and Other Benefits and Concerns. Curr Diab Rep. 2017;17(7):54.
46. Kagansky N, Levy S, Rimon E, Cojocaru L, Fridman A, Ozer Z, et al. Hypoglycemia as a predictor of mortality in hospitalized elderly patients. Arch Intern Med. 2003;163(15):1825-9.
47. Salinas PD, Mendez CE. Glucose Management Technologies for the Critically Ill. J Diabetes Sci Technol. 2019;13(4):682-90.
48. Newton CA, Smiley D, Bode BW, Kitabchi AE, Davidson PC, Jacobs S, et al. A comparison study of continuous insulin infusion protocols in the medical intensive care unit: computer-guided vs. standard column-based algorithms. J Hosp Med. 2010;5(8):432-7.
49. Rabinovich M, Grahl J, Durr E, Gayed R, Chester K, McFarland R, et al. Risk of Hypoglycemia During Insulin Infusion Directed by Paper Protocol Versus Electronic Glycemic Management System in Critically Ill Patients at a Large Academic Medical Center. J Diabetes Sci Technol. 2018;12(1):47-52.
50. Shetty S, Inzucchi SE, Goldberg PA, Cooper D, Siegel MD, Honiden S. Adapting to the new consensus guidelines for managing hyperglycemia during critical illness: the updated Yale insulin infusion protocol. Endocr Pract. 2012;18(3):363-70.
51. Mehta Y, Mithal A, Kulkarni A, Reddy BR, Sharma J, Dixit S, et al. Practice Guidelines for Enteral Nutrition Management in Dysglycemic Critically Ill Patients: A Relook for Indian Scenario. Indian J Crit Care Med. 2019;23(12):594-603.

CHAPTER 39

Refeeding Syndrome in Critically Ill Adults: Preemptive Strategies

Krishnan Sriram, Chitra Mahesh

INTRODUCTION

Refeeding syndrome (RFS) is a recognized complication of nutrition therapy, masquerading as dysfunction of various organ systems. The very expression "syndrome" indicates that immediate and delayed manifestations may vary from patient to patient. It requires an astute clinician to suspect RFS and to take aggressive preventive measures as fatality may occur, often erroneously ascribed to other causes. It is likely that clinicians who are not involved in critical care may not even be aware of this entity, especially the importance of phosphorus (P) and thiamine.

Several recent reviews on this subject, as well as chapters in this textbook, provide detailed discussions about electrolyte and metabolic management. This chapter concentrates on practical and pragmatic approaches to the prevention and early detection of the serious complications of RFS in critically ill adult patients with a focus on Asian countries. RFS may occur even when clinicians practice evidence-based nutrition therapy with all good intentions to benefit patients.

DEFINITIONS

Refeeding syndrome is described as "a range of metabolic and electrolyte alterations, occurring because of reintroduction and/or increased provision of calories after a period of decreased or absent caloric intake" as suggested in the American Society for Parenteral and Enteral Nutrition (ASPEN) 2020 consensus.[1]

The ASPEN recommendations further expand the diagnosis criteria for RFS to a decrease of more than 10–20% in any one of the three major electrolyte components of RFS—P, potassium (K), and/or magnesium (Mg). They also add organ dysfunction due to a decrease of any of the above or thiamine deficiency. They specify a 5-day window for the purposes of standardizing definitions, although a shorter period is also valid to document RFS and to implement urgent corrective measures.

It is often mentioned that the definitions of RFS are vague. We recommend using the more current ASPEN recommendations for documenting the diagnosis, and for future publications, in preference to the much earlier and often quoted the National Institute of Health and Care Excellence 2006 guidelines.[2] The latter has a low sensitivity and specificity, especially in low-income countries.[3]

HISTORIC PERSPECTIVE

As frequently mentioned, RFS was first described in detail in prisoners after World War II. There are even earlier reports in victims of famine who experienced unexpected morbidity and mortality after access to good nutritional repletion was subsequently possible. Since then, numerous reports crept into the medical literature. In fact, there are historic reports of death during "feast after famine", some dating to 2000 years ago. The death of Charlotte Brontë, an English poet and novelist, in 1885, during recovery from hyperemesis gravidarum (HG), earlier ascribed to other causes, is now considered to be due to RFS.

With the easy availability of both enteral (including oral) and parenteral nutrition (PN) products and the increased experience with access devices, detection of RFS became well recognized. Interesting case reports have highlighted the importance of suspecting RFS.[4] This was coupled with an enthusiasm to provide a modality of therapy that the patient has not received for several days prior to seeking medical attention but resulted in serious and sometimes fatal electrolyte and metabolic disturbances.

INCIDENCE

The exact incidence of RFS is unclear due to various earlier definitions but has been reported to be as high as 80%, although one cannot be sure of this figure as the criteria for making the diagnosis has varied. The inclusion of P and thiamine deficiencies as components of RFS increases the actual reported incidence. A recent meta-analysis involving 35 observational studies emphasized that the incidence of RFS is higher in intensive care unit (ICU) patients.[5] Suffice it to conclude that RFS occurs commonly in critically ill patients.

PATHOPHYSIOLOGY

Endogenous glucose production in critical illness increases with decreased glucose clearance, attributing to reduced insulin secretion and increased resistance. The multiple mechanisms are involved—systemic inflammation, release of counterregulatory hormones, including glucagon and catecholamines, and alterations in the hypothalamic-pituitary axis. Contributing iatrogenic factors include vasopressors and corticosteroids, often needed in the critically ill and hemodynamically unstable patient. Multiple organ systems are involved, including the liver, kidneys, brain, skeletal muscles, and even adipose tissues.[6]

The management strategies to control hyperglycemia involve administration of insulin. This results in intracellular shift of the traditional intracellular ions, K, P, and Mg, whose functions are interrelated. The differences between the intracellular and extracellular levels of these ions are responsible for the various perturbations that occur in RFS.

An increase of sodium (Na) and water retention leads to a decrease in excretion of both, leading to rapid fluid overload leading to congestive heart failure, which can be fatal.[7] The effects on the heart are not only due to electrolyte imbalances but also thiamine deficiency.

RISK FACTORS

The risk factors (in alphabetic order) include acquired immunodeficiency syndrome, alcohol-use disorder (especially for thiamine deficiency), anorexia nervosa, advanced age, cancer, chemotherapy, cirrhosis, dysphagia, diabetes mellitus, esophageal dysmotility, HG, inflammatory bowel disease, malabsorptive states, neurologic impairments, obesity and postbariatric surgery, pancreatic insufficiency, prolonged fasting for any reason followed by unplanned surgical procedures, renal failure on renal replacement therapy, short bowel syndromes, and trauma, although this list is not all-inclusive.[8]

Trauma, especially those with a high injury severity score, and burns have been recognized as significant risk factors due to associated hypophosphatemia.[9] Severe head injury is also a risk factor due to urinary losses of K, Mg, P, and calcium (Ca) noted even at admission as a direct result of cranial trauma, and subsequently due to mannitol, often used to decrease intracranial pressure.[10]

The obese patient with unsuspected sarcopenia is especially at high risk. We have reported an obese patient where enteral nutrition (EN) was initiated at very low rates, yet developed severe hypophosphatemia, leading to respiratory failure and ventilatory support.[11]

Pregnancy with hyperemesis, HG, is a unique condition with a high risk for RFS. The availability of soft-bore polyurethane nasojejunal feeding tubes in the late 1980s resulted in increased use of EN in this condition. Soon afterward, several reports crept into the literature of unexpected and unexplained deaths during recovery; some were recognized to be due to hypophosphatemia, and some suspected even decades ago due to thiamine deficiency.

Renal insufficiency, either acute kidney injury or chronic kidney disease, is often associated with elevated levels of K, Mg, and P. However, as seen in several case reports, the risk of RFS is still substantial if nutrition support is initiated concomitantly with renal replacement therapy.

Several authors have called for risk stratification for early detection and therefore by default preventive steps to minimize the complications of RFS. Many of these recommendations are not specific to critical care.[12] We do not believe that this is always necessary in the management of RFS in critically ill patients, and in fact may make the clinician complacent when dealing with patients classified as low risk. Weight (preadmission or actual) does not factor in when dealing with critically ill patients. Anthropometric measures are of little use and physical examination is unreliable. Subnormal electrolyte levels are more dangerous in elderly patients and in those with other comorbidities and polypharmacy. RFS may occur even in patients with short periods of starvation or suboptimal calorie intake. Obviously, premorbid period of starvation cannot be considered in emergency surgery or trauma. As RFS may have fatal outcomes, it is imperative that all critically ill patients should be considered as being at risk, irrespective of a perceived benefit of risk stratification. The lack of benefit from risk stratification and strict adherence to protocols have not been shown to be beneficial in other areas of critical care, such as management of sepsis and hypotension, provided the intervention is appropriate.

There are no predictive biomarkers for RFS risk assessment. Hypophosphatemia and hypomagnesemia have been shown to predict RFS in prospective studies involving ICU patients.[13]

Unsuspected thiamine deficiency warrants special mention. Thiamine is an essential water-soluble vitamin with a half-life of 9–18 days, deficiencies of which are often observed in patients with alcohol-use disorders but may also occur in other individuals with no identifiable risk factors.

CLINICAL MANIFESTATIONS BY ORGAN SYSTEMS[14]

As can be appreciated from the list mentioned further, RFS can present in numerous ways, involving one or more organ systems, and often mimicking other medical conditions, with significant overlap in presenting signs and symptoms, many due to thiamine deficiency rather than electrolyte imbalances.

Cardiovascular system: Arrhythmias, congestive heart failure, bradycardia, prolongation of QT interval, and other electrocardiogram (EKG) abnormalities including Torsades de Pointes are the common causes of sudden death.[15] Life-threatening EKG changes may sometimes occur without a prior warning.

Respiratory system: Tachypnea, hypoxia, dependence on ventilatory support, and poor diaphragmatic muscle function.

Gastrointestinal system: Gastroparesis, emesis, ileus, abdominal pain mimicking ischemic bowel, and constipation.

Hepatic: Steatosis and acute liver failure.

Neurologic: Encephalopathy, neuropathy, Guillain–Barré-like syndromes (lower motor neuron paralysis), cranial nerve palsies, central pontine myelinolysis, and Wernicke's encephalopathy (confusion, disorientation, delirium, or even coma, may be permanent and fatal).

Eye: Nystagmus, ophthalmoplegia, pupillary abnormalities, and optic neuropathy.

Auditory: Tinnitus and hearing loss.

Musculoskeletal: Myalgia and rhabdomyolysis.

Metabolic: Mixed acid–base abnormalities, metabolic acidosis, and respiratory alkalosis.

Hematologic: Thrombocytopenia, anemia, and hemolysis.

Renal: Acute tubular necrosis, brown-colored urine indicating rhabdomyolysis, and nephrogenic diabetes mellitus.

Mucocutaneous: Glossitis, cheilosis, and skin rashes—if present at the time of ICU admission, may point to thiamine deficiency.

CLINICAL MANIFESTATIONS BY SPECIFIC DEFICIENCY

P: Shifting of oxygen-dissociation curve of hemoglobin to the left, tissue hypoxia, rhabdomyolysis, hemolysis, respiratory depression, dependence on ventilator, leukocyte dysfunction, and cardiac dysfunction, including decreased stroke volume and paralysis. Hypophosphatemia is clearly associated with higher mortality.[16]

Thiamine:[17] Thiamine deficiency manifests itself in multiple ways including unexplained metabolic acidosis, mental changes, Wernicke's encephalopathy, ophthalmoplegia, abdominal pain ("gastrointestinal beriberi"), and congestive heart failure ("wet beriberi"). Thiamine plays multiple roles in metabolism, including conversion of lactate to pyruvate and Krebs cycle. Other pathways and enzymes include the pentose phosphate pathway and nicotinamide adenine dinucleotide (NAD) pathways, involved in multiple metabolic processes. Thiamine is closely involved with phosphorous metabolism. The diverse signs and symptoms noted in thiamine deficiency constitute a diagnostic dilemma, often leading to unnecessary investigations, which could be possibly avoided by preemptive administration, as discussed further.

K: Cardiac arrythmias are common; ileus, delayed gastric emptying, nausea and emesis, weakness and paralysis, rhabdomyolysis, and respiratory failure.

Mg: Cardiac arrythmias, altered mental status leading to coma, weakness and tremors, tetany and convulsions, gastrointestinal symptoms including nausea and emesis, and increased perception of pain.

PREVENTIVE STRATEGIES

The risk of RFS can be attenuated by initiating nutrition therapy, both EN and PN, at low rates of infusion, as has been recommended in major guidelines.[18] The benefits of trophic EN are noted even when providing 50-60% of the calculated requirements. Initiation at 15-20 kcal/kg/day is ideal. If risks for RFS are recognized to be high, even lower rates of 5-10 kcal/kg/day are safer. Restricted caloric intake has been clearly shown to decrease the risk of RFS in critically ill patients, in a randomized multicenter trial.[19] There is no convincing evidence to suggest that the routine use of indirect calorimetry will decrease the risk of RFS.

Calorie intake is gradually increased over the next several days, 4-7 days, but it is difficult to predict how this can be achieved in an individual patient, as it depends on fluid balance, tolerance, and maintenance of euglycemia and safe electrolyte levels. A stepwise increase of 200-300 kcal every 2-3 days seems ideal. Recent recommendations to provide less protein during the initial stages of critical illness fall well in line with providing hypocaloric feeding. During the early phases of critical illness, initiation of nutrition therapy involves a low-protein intake of 0.8 g/kg/day subsequently increased to >1.2 g/kg/day or more.[20] Preventive strategies form the cornerstone of management of RFS.[21]

Serum levels of electrolytes do not always concomitantly reflect intracellular levels of P, K, and Mg. Electrolyte abnormalities are common during initiation of nutrition therapy in ICUs.[22] Prophylactic supplementation of these electrolytes within safe limits will often be needed to maintain or improve serum levels after initiation of nutrition therapy.[23]

More recently, the routine administration of thiamine in all critically ill patients for the first 3-5 days, while EN or PN is being increased, has been strongly recommended.[20]

The routine monitoring by EKG during the risk period for developing RFS and until electrolyte imbalances have been adequately corrected is recommended.

CORRECTION AND REPLACEMENT STRATEGIES

Although we are encouraged to limit blood sampling in the critically ill patient, the management of RFS is one exception; the frequency of testing depends on the specific deficiency that is being corrected, and the urgency of the same. Monitoring can be effectively done using point-of-care testing, thus minimizing the risk of iatrogenic anemia. Correction of glucose levels and of other electrolytes must be done slowly and cautiously to avoid the risk of effects on the brain due to rapid overcorrection. In order to avoid over- or undercorrection, it is necessary to obtain serum levels periodically, every few hours **(Table 1)**. Detailed discussions on safe correction of electrolyte abnormalities and glucose level control can be accessed from several sources,[24] from other chapters in this textbook, and will be summarized further **(Table 2)**. Medical facilities dealing with seriously ill patients, including trauma and outpatient management of cancer, are well advised to assure adequate stocks of parenteral Na, phosphate, and thiamine for emergency use.

- *Glucose levels:* Dysglycemia should be the initial abnormality to be addressed, generally requiring continuous insulin infusions. This will invariably result

TABLE 1: Electrolyte replacement guidelines for adult intensive care units.

Potassium replacement (normal laboratory range: 3.5/5.0 mEq/L)

Potassium level	Replace with
<2.5 mEq/L	120 mEq IVPB* with or without 40 mEq PO/NG
2.5–2.9 mEq/L	80 mEq IVPB*
3.0–3.5 mEq/L	40 mEq IVPB* or PO

Magnesium replacement (normal laboratory range: 1.8–2.7 mg/dL)

Magnesium level	Replace with
1.0–1.4 mg/dL	4 g IVPB**
1.5–1.8 mg/dL	2 q IVPB**

Note for potassium replacement:
- Recheck potassium level 1 hour post infusion and repeat dosing if needed.
- Serum magnesium levels must be in the normal range to effectively replete serum potassium.

*Recommended peripheral venous line maximum infusion rate 10 mEq/h
Recommended central venous line maximum infusion rate 20 mEq/h
Consider more dilute preparation if patient has peripheral access only and/or if patient is experiencing burning with infusion.

Note for magnesium replacement: Recheck magnesium level in 4 hours or more and repeat dosing if needed.
**Recommended infusion rate 1 g/h
(IVPB: intravenous piggyback; PO/NG: per os/nasogastric)

TABLE 2: Phosphorous replacement (normal laboratory range: 2.5–4.5 mg/dL).

Phosphorus level	Potassium level	Replace with (IV replacement)
<1.2 mg/dL	<4 mEq/L	Potassium phosphate 45 mmol IVPB*
<1.2 mg/dL	>4 mEq/L	Sodium phosphate 45 mmol IVPB*
1.2–1.7 mg/dL	<4 mEq/L	Potassium phosphate 30 mmol IVPB*
1.2–1.7 mg/dL	>4 mEq/L	Sodium phosphate 30 mmol IVPB*
1.8–2.5 mg/dL	<4 mEq/L	Potassium phosphate 15 mmol IVPB*
1.8–2.5 mg/dL	>4 mEq/L	Sodium phosphate 15 mmol IVPB*
Phosphorus level		**Replace with (PO replacement)**
1.8–2.5 mg/dL	Potassium acid phosphate	• *500 mg tablet:* Phosphorous 114 mg (3.68 mmol) and potassium 144 mg (3.7 mEq) per tablet • *Dose:* 1,000 mg qid × 4 doses (total 29.4 mmol phosphorous and 29.6 mEq potassium)

Recheck phosphorous level 1–2 hours post infusion and repeat dosing if needed.
3 mmol of potassium phosphate contains 4.4 mEq of potassium.
3 mmol of sodium phosphate contains 4 mEq of sodium.
*Recommended infusion rate 5 mmol/h
(IV: intravenous; IVBP: intravenous piggyback; PO: per os)

in transport of electrolytes into the cell, necessitating corrective measure concomitantly.
- *Dysnatremia:* Both hyper- and hyponatremia are associated with increased mortality in critically ill patients. Serum levels must be interpreted with the fluid status in mind, as hyponatremia is invariably due to excess water rather than Na restriction. The management of dysnatremia, and narrowing down the precipitating factors, is complex and is

beyond the scope of this chapter but is accessible from other sources.[25] The Na content of scientific EN formulas is indicated in the package inserts in milligrams (mg), while serum Na levels as well the content in parenteral fluids is reported in milliequivalents (mEq). 1 g or 1,000 mg of elemental Na is equivalent to 43.5 mEq of Na, while 1 g of table salt (NaCl) contains only 17.5 mEq of elemental Na. Restriction of Na or fluids is not recommended by the ASPEN 2020 recommendations. Fluid restriction, recommended for other reasons in the management of critically ill patients, is also of benefit in the prevention and management of RFS.

- *Other electrolytes* (**Tables 1 and 2**): It is preferable to use the parenteral route for replacement of electrolytes, although depending on the serum levels and the perceived urgency and risks, clinicians may elect to selectively use the oral or enteral route, whenever possible, either entirely or to supplement parenteral replacement. Other causes of electrolyte imbalances, such as endocrine or medications, not specifically related to initiation of nutrition therapy, must also be considered, and addressed appropriately. In addition to metabolic derangements that cause electrolyte imbalances, several medications affect the renal handling of electrolytes and hydrogen ions. The replacement strategies suggested have to be modified in renal insufficiency.
  - *P:* Parenteral replacement is ordered in millimoles (mmol) as the Na or K form.
  - *K:* Replacement must consider the acid–base status as alkalosis will be reflected by low levels. Correction of hypokalemia will involve steps to correct the alkalosis and hypomagnesemia.
  - *Mg:* Parenteral and oral/enteral orders are entered in grams. 1 g of magnesium sulfate ($MgSO_4 \cdot 7H_2O$) contains 8 mEq or 4 mmol of elemental Mg.

- *Thiamine:* It is liberally used in critically ill patients, especially in unexplained lactic acidosis and sensorium changes. Recent publications strongly recommend the routine use of 100–300 mg intravenous (IV) thiamine in all ICU patients, while EN is advanced.[20] When hypophosphatemia is also identified, higher dosage of 500–1,000 mg IV of thiamine is recommended. If EN feeding is fairly well tolerated, parenteral route of administering thiamine may not be essential and enteral or oral administration may suffice, either as an individual preparation or combination with other vitamins. Laboratory testing to ascertain whole-blood thiamine level or body stores is not needed; tests are expensive or not available, except from specialized reference laboratories and results may not be immediately available.

Role of Nutrition Support Teams in Refeeding Syndrome

Although clinicians with experience in nutrition therapy are generally familiar with RFS, this may not always be true. Many non-intensivists may not even be aware of this entity. An urgent need to make clinicians aware of the role of thiamine in nutrition support and the risk of RFS was emphasized in 2014.[26] An even earlier publication reported that RFS was underdiagnosed and undertreated and many clinicians were not even aware of this entity and stressed the importance of a nutrition support team.[27,28]

A team approach, well summarized in a recent publication,[29] involving several disciplines increases the detection of RFS and by default early interventions. The importance of implementation science in nutrition support is a burgeoning field of interest.

OUTCOMES

The large multicenter EFFORT trial, which looked as the "The Effect of early nutritional support on Frailty, Functional Outcomes, and Recovery of malnourished medical inpatients", clearly showed that RFS is associated with poor outcomes and that a specific nutrition-focussed treatment plan is beneficial.[30] However, there are very few studies that directly look at the overall outcome of interventions in RFS. A study involving 13 ICUs in New Zealand and Australia, referenced earlier, showed that calorie restriction, with an associated decrease in RFS, resulted in a 60- and 90-day improvement in survival rate, although the length of hospitalization was longer.[19] Another study showed that overall mortality at 6 months was less when permissive hypocaloric feeding decreasing RFS was used.[31] These two studies clearly inform us that hypocaloric feeding improves outcomes in RFS.

SPECIAL CONSIDERATIONS AND QUESTIONS

- *Is RFS more common with EN or PN?:* The logical question is whether EN is less of a risk for RFS when compared to PN. In PN, except for very high glucose levels after initiation, the infusion rate may not require urgent revisions. EN on the other hand is always initiated at low rates and advanced only when tolerance and other factors have been considered. This suggests that RFS may be less with EN than with PN. However, one publication suggests just the opposite.[32] The explanation offered is that EN causes a greater increase in glucagon-like peptide 1 (GLP-1) levels, resulting in higher levels of insulin when compared to PN.

- *Does fat emulsion cause problems during refeeding?:* RFS has traditionally been associated with glucose metabolism and associated disturbance of intracellular electrolytes. There is one case report of refeeding with parenteral fat emulsion, resulting in cardiogenic shock.[33] In this patient, predetermined to be at risk for RFS, calories were increased carefully in a stepwise manner, and no electrolyte abnormalities were noted. Cardiac hypercontraction resulted in shock which promptly reversed when the fat emulsion infusion was discontinued.

- *Does protein intake affect RFS?:* A higher protein intake during the early stages of nutrition support is associated with refeeding hypophosphatemia.[34] From a practical point of view, the nonprotein calorie:nitrogen ratio is always kept within range for both EN and PN, making the amount of protein intake a less important factor in precipitating RFS. ASPEN recommendations do not mention protein restriction as a strategy in the management of RFS.

- *Do we need to correct electrolyte levels to normal levels prior to initiation of EN or PN?:* National Institute of Clinical Excellence guidelines advise that electrolyte corrections can be initiated at the same time as cautious, low-volume nutrition therapy.[2] However, the intensivist may elect to replace electrolytes first in situations where the level is dangerously low and a delay in initiating nutrition support is unlikely to affect outcomes.

- *Do vitamin deficiencies other than thiamine contribute to RFS?:* Although it

is imperative to include multivitamins in the provision of nutrition therapy, there is no information on the role of specific vitamins, except for thiamine.
- *Do trace element deficiencies contribute to RFS?:* Although essential trace elements (Zn, Se, Cu, Cr, and Mn) need to be part of any kind of nutrition therapy,[35] there is no information that deficiency of any of these directly contribute to RFS. Zn is needed for numerous crucial enzymatic functions. Se is important for cardiac function, deficiency manifests as myositis with muscle pain and cardiac failure, in addition to a role in thyroid hormone secretion. There is no evidence that megadoses of any vitamin or trace element, over and above the recommended daily allowances, are needed in ICU patients.[36]

Recent recommendations include parenteral iron (Fe) as an additional trace element in critical illness, using hepcidin levels to guide therapy. However, we recommend not using Fe for the first 7 days of refeeding, as this may exacerbate hypokalemia and hypophosphatemia.
- *Should hypocalcemia be treated if identified in RFS?:* The symptoms of hypocalcemia include carpopedal spasm, laryngospasm, seizures, and prolonged QT interval. Ionized Ca levels better reflect Ca status as nonionized levels are influenced by serum albumin levels. The normal range of ionized Ca is 4.8–5.6 mg/dL or 1.2–1.4 mmol/L. Levels of ionized Ca <3 mg/dL require urgent IV Ca, assuring that Mg levels are also corrected. Suggested infusion is 1–2 g of Ca gluconate, equivalent to 90–180 mg of elemental Ca, in 50 mL of 5% dextrose or normal saline, infused over 10–20 minutes, never more rapidly, and repeated if necessary.

CONCLUSION

We have provided information to manage RFS by maintaining a high level of clinical suspicion, in turn leading to early implementation of corrective strategies **(Flowchart 1)**. While nutrition therapy is of paramount importance in the care of critically ill patients, it is equally important to minimize iatrogenic complications. A thorough appreciation of the pathophysiology of critical illness, including dysglycemia, electrolyte abnormalities, acid–base imbalances, and the role of micronutrients especially thiamine, will result

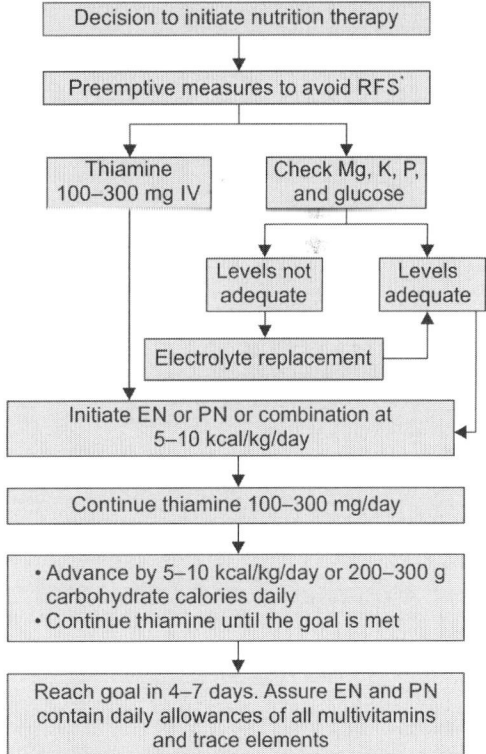

Flowchart 1: Stepwise approach for prevention, early detection, and interventions in RFS.

*Irrespective of weight-related parameters, duration of prior suboptimal intake and medical/surgical history (EN: enteral nutrition; IV: intravenous; PN: parenteral nutrition; RFS: refeeding syndrome)

in the ability to provide optimal nutrition therapy with minimal complications. Nutrition therapy, both EN and PN, should be initiated cautiously in the critically ill patient, advancing in a stepwise matter over several days, depending on volume status, cardiac and respiratory parameters, and correction of glucose and electrolyte levels.

REFERENCES

1. Silva JSV, Seres D, Sabino K. ASPEN (American Society for Parenteral and Enteral Nutrition) consensus recommendations for refeeding syndrome. Nutr Clin Pract. 2020;35:178-95.
2. National Institute for Health and Care Excellence. (2006). Nutrition support in adults—Clinical guideline: Oral nutrition support, enteral tube feeding, and parenteral nutrition. Available from: www.nice.org.uk/page.aspx?o=cg032 [Last accessed August, 2023].
3. Buitendag J, Variawa S, Davids R, Ahmed N. Refeeding syndrome in surgical patients post initiation of artificial feeding, a prospective cohort study in a low-income country. Clin Nutr ESPEN. 2021;46:21-215.
4. McCray S, Parrish CR. Refeeding the malnourished patient: Lessons learned. Nutritional Issues in Gastroenterology. 2016,Series155:56-66.
5. Cioffi I, Ponzo V, Pelligrini M, Evangelista A, Bioletto F, Ciccone G, et al. The incidence of the refeeding syndrome: a systematic review and meta-analysis of literature. Clin Nutr. 2021;40:3688-701.
6. Al-Yousif N, Rawal S, Jurczak M, Mahmud H, Shah FA. Endogenous glucose production in critical illness. Nutr Clin Pract. 2021;36:344-59.
7. Mehanna HM, Moledina J, Travis J. Refeeding syndrome: What it is, and how to prevent and treat it. BMJ. 2008;336:1495-8.
8. Krutkyte G, Wenk L, Odermatt J, Schuetz P, Stanga Z, Friedli N. Refeeding syndrome: a critical reality in patients with chronic disease. Nutrients. 2022;14:2859.
9. Boyd A, Gervasio J, Harris S, Blair M, Whitten J, Foster D, et al. Redefining refeeding syndrome in trauma patients. Crit Care Med. 2019;47:848.
10. Polderman KH, Bloemers FW, Girbes ARJ. Hypomagnesemia and hypophosphatemia at admission in patients with severe head injury. Crit Care Med. 2000;28:2022-5.
11. Patel U, Sriram K. Acute respiratory failure due to refeeding syndrome and hypophosphatemia induced by hypocaloric enteral nutrition. Nutrition. 2009;25:364-7.
12. Friedli N, Stanza Z, Culkin A, Crook M, Laviano A, Sobotka L, et al. Management and prevention of refeeding syndrome in medical patients: an evidence-based and consensus-supported algorithm. Nutrition. 2018;47:13-20.
13. McKnight CL, Newberry C, Sarav M, Martindale R, Hurt R, Daley B. Refeeding syndrome in the critically ill: A literature review and clinician's guide. Curr Gastroenterol Rep. 2019;21(11)58.
14. Boetang AA, Sriram K, Meguid MM, Crook M. Refeeding syndrome: Treatment considerations based on collective analysis of literature case reports. Nutrition. 2020;26:156-67.
15. Crook MA. Cardiac abnormalities in the refeeding syndrome. Nutrition. 2017;35:146-7.
16. Blaser AR, Gunst J, Ichai C, Casaer MP, Benstoem C, Besch G, et al. Hypophosphatemia in critically ill adults and children—a systematic review. Clin Nutr. 2021;40:1744-54.
17. Sriram K, Manzanares W, Joseph K. Thiamine in nutrition therapy. Nutr Clin Pract. 2012;27:41-50.
18. McClave SA, Taylor BE, Martindale RG, Warren MM, Johnson DR, Braunschweign C, et al. Guidelines for the provision and assessment of nutrition support therapy in the adult crucially ill patient: Society of Critical Care Medicine (SCCM) and American Society of Parenteral and Enteral Nutrition (ASPEN). JPEN J Parenter Enteral Nutr. 2016;40:159-221.

19. Doig GS, Simpson F, Heighes PT, Bellomo R, Chesher D, Caterson ID, et al. Restricted versus continued standard caloric intake management of refeeding syndrome in critically ill adults: a randomized, parallel-group, multicenter single-blind controlled trial. Lancet Respir Med. 2015;3:943-52.
20. Preiser J-C, Arabi YM, Berger M, Casaer M, McClave S, Montejo-González JC, et al. A guide to enteral nutrition in intensive care units: 10 expert tips for the daily practice. Critical Care. 2021;25:424.
21. Friedli N, Odermatt J, Reber E, Schuetz P, Stanga Z. Refeeding syndrome: an update and clinical advice for prevention, diagnosis, and treatment. Curr Opin Gastroenterol. 2020;36:136-40.
22. Blaser AR, van Zanten ARH. Electrolyte disorders during initiation of nutrition therapy in the ICU. Curr Opin Nutr Metab Care. 2021;24:151-8.
23. Gallagher D, Parker A, Samavat H, Zelig R. Prophylactic supplementation of phosphate, magnesium, and potassium for the prevention of refeeding syndrome in hospitalized individuals with anorexia nervosa. Nutr Clin Pract. 2022;37:328-43.
24. Siparsky N. Overview of postoperative electrolyte abnormalities. [online] Available from: https://www.uptodate.com/contents/overview-of-postoperative-electrolyte-abnormalities [Last accessed August, 2023].
25. Seay NW, Lehrich RW, Greenberg A. Diagnosis and management of disorders of body tonicity—hyponatremia and hypernatremia: Core Curriculum 2020. Am J Kidney Dis. 2020;75(2):272-82.
26. Crook MA, Sriram K. Thiamine deficiency: The importance of recognition and prompt management. Nutrition. 2014;30:953-4.
27. Gariballa S. Refeeding syndrome: a potentially fatal condition but remains underdiagnosed and undertreated. Nutrition. 2008;24:604-6.
28. Panteli JV, Crook MA. Refeeding syndrome still needs to be recognized and managed appropriately. Nutrition. 2009;25:130-1.
29. Baraccos A, Schwartz DB, Bistrian BR, Guenter P, Mueller C, Chernoff R, et al. Nutrition support teams: Institution, evolution, and innovation. Nutr Clin Pract. 2023;38:10-26.
30. Scheutz P, Fehr R, Baechli V, Geiser M, Deiss M, Gomes F, et al. Individualised nutrition support in medical in patients at nutritional risk: a randomised clinical trial. Lancet. 2019;393:2312-21.
31. Olthof E, Koekkoek WACK, van Setten C, Kars JCN, van Blokland D, van Zanten ARH. Impact of caloric intake in critically ill patients with and without refeeding syndrome: a retrospective study. Clin Nutr. 2017;37:1609-17.
32. Zeki S, Culkin A, Gabe SM, Nightingale JM. Refeeding hypophosphatemia is more common in enteral than parenteral feeding in adult in-patients. Clin Nutr. 2011;30:365-8.
33. Sakamoto Y, Kioka H, Hashimoto R, Takeda S, Momose K, Ohtani t, et al. Cardiogenic shock caused by midventricular obstruction during refeeding. Nutrition. 2017;35:148-50.
34. Singerland-Boot R, Roojakkers E, Koekkoek K, van Blokland D, Arbous S, van Zanten A. Macronutrient intake and outcomes of ICU patients with refeeding hypophosphatemia. Clin Nutr ESPEN. 2023;55:191-9.
35. Blaauw R, Osmond E, Sriram K, Ali A, Allard JP, Ball P, et al. Parenteral provision of micronutrients to adult patients: An expert consensus paper. JPEN J Parenter Enteral Nutr. 2019;43(Suppl 1):S5-23.
36. Gudivada KK, Kumar A, Sriram K, Baby J, Shariff M, Sampath S, et al. Antioxidant micronutrient supplementation for adult critically ill patients: a Bayesian multiple treatment comparison meta-analysis. Clin Nutr ESPEN. 2022;47:78-88.

CHAPTER 40

Nutrition in Severe Hemodynamic Failure and in Noninvasive Ventilation

Khalid Ismail Khatib, Subhal Bhalchandra Dixit

INTRODUCTION

Patients with circulatory or respiratory failure are critically ill patients suffering from organ failures due to various etiologies. There treatment comprises correcting the impaired pathophysiology, supplementing the lost function of the organs artificially and allowing sufficient time for the damaged organ to heal. Nutrition may not be of utmost priority in the thinking of treatment teams and hence is often neglected. Starting immediate nutrition or delaying it is an important dilemma which must be tackled, so as to help to improve patient outcomes.

NUTRITION IN SEVERE HEMODYNAMIC FAILURE

Early enteral nutrition (EN) should be started in critically ill patients and it has been shown to reduce infectious complications in such patients.[1,2] Patients having severe hemodynamic failure are a special class of patients in whom nutrition needs to be thought about very carefully. These patients may be on varying doses of vasopressors (dopamine, noradrenaline, adrenaline, and vasopressin), inotropes (dobutamine, levosimendan, and milrinone) among other drugs. There are various changes and pathophysiologic modifications to the splanchnic circulation owing to the original disease process, sepsis per se and the therapy used. The physician has to keep in mind the risk benefit ratio when thinking about starting early EN in these patients.[3-5] Some data from the start of this century suggests that giving very low amounts of feeding in such patients (so-called "trickle feeding") may be feasible in patients on vasopressors, even those on high doses.[6] There are few randomized controlled trials (RCTs) on the risk/benefit of EN in patients with severe hemodynamic failure. Several observational studies in the 1st decade and early part of 2nd decade of this century have alluded to the possibility of these patients developing severe complications like bowel ischemia and necrosis when exposed to EN.[7-9] However, establishing a causality between early EN and bowel complications in these studies is fraught with problems. Just because there is an association which does not mean it is the cause.

The NUTRIREA-2 study was conducted in 2018 to study the effects of giving early EN or giving early parenteral nutrition (PN) in seriously ill patients who are on mechanical ventilation and had shock.[10] The amount or dose of EN and PN was calculated to match the energy expenditure (normocaloric goal of nutrition) of these patients. The study found no difference in the 28th-day mortality between the groups given early EN or PN. But, there was an increase in gastrointestinal (GI) symptoms (vomiting and diarrhea) and GI complications (bowel ischemia and colonic pseudo-obstruction) in the early enteral group. The findings of this study demonstrate that isocaloric or normocaloric EN should be avoided in patients with hemodynamic instability. However, the best approach (whether providing lower amounts of EN or not giving EN at all) is not clear. A recent Cochrane review of 11 RCTs comprising a sizable number of patients (approximately 600) has not been able to conclusively demonstrate the benefit of early EN in reducing infectious complications in critically ill patients (general medical, surgical, trauma, and burns ICU patients).[11] Another RCT comparing early EN versus PN in critically ill patients (CALORIES trial) did not show any reduction in infectious complications or mortality in the early EN group.[12] Many questions related to these patients are being studied in various trials, including low dose (hypocaloric or trophic) nutrition and no enteral nutrition.[13-15]

Approach to Feeding in Patients with Severe Hemodynamic Failure[1,2]

Hence, on reviewing the existing data, the following approach should be adopted:
- In patients with shock which is stabilized with low/moderate dose or decreasing doses of vasopressors (Epinephrine ≤5 µg/min, norepinephrine ≤5 µg/min, dopamine ≤10 µg/kg/min, vasopressin ≤0.04 units/min, and MAP >60 mm Hg), EN may be started at low dose (hypocaloric or trophic).
- EN should be delayed in patients who are being actively resuscitated and those on high doses of vasopressors.
- When EN has been started in patients on vasopressors, its dose should be increased slowly (over 3–5 days) and carefully with monitoring for GI intolerance or unexplained worsening shock.

NUTRITION IN NONINVASIVE VENTILATION

Noninvasive ventilation (NIV) is used in the treatment of patients with respiratory failure and has been found to be useful in respiratory failure due to many etiologies. It is especially useful in acute exacerbation of chronic obstructive pulmonary disease (COPD), acute cardiogenic pulmonary edema, in weaning from invasive ventilation, among others.

Feeding the patients on NIV has always been an issue with no clearcut guidelines. The fact that malnourished patients have high mortality which has to be counterbalanced with the fact that the physicians are worried about aspiration on NIV.

Reasons for Underfeeding Patients on NIV

- Patients on NIV can deteriorate and require invasive mechanical ventilation anytime during their initial few days and so keeping them nil per oral seems to be a safer strategy.
- Placing a nasogastric (NG) tube will increase the leak through the mask and contribute to NIV failure.
- Gastric insufflation during NIV application increases the diaphragmatic dysfunction and increases the risk of vomiting and aspiration.
- Disconnection of NIV for oral feeding may result in failure of NIV therapy as patients may have deterioration of their baseline condition.

In a recent French multicenter observation study, >60% patients were starved for first 48 hours and <2.6% patients were fed enterally.[16] In this study, enterally fed patients had higher mortality. The NutritionDay ICU audit was carried out worldwide and >10,000 patients were included. Of these, 47% patients were on mechanical ventilation and 6.2% of these patients were on NIV. 40% of patients were not fed on the 1st day of mechanical ventilation and 20% on the 2nd day.[17]

The use of NIV for prevention of reintubation after extubation is being used extensively in certain subset of patients. Macht et al. showed that patients have some degree of swallowing dysfunction postextubation and this is a risk factor for aspiration, nosocomial infections, and increased mortality.[18]

Approach to Feeding in Patients on NIV

- If the patients are not malnourished at the time of admission, then keeping them underfed or nil-per-oral is a feasible strategy for a maximum of 48 hours.
- If the patient's nutritional status is poor at the time of admission, then attempts should be made to feed the patient. The route of feeding should be selected very carefully as certain studies have shown increased mortality after enteral route of feeding.[19]
- The risk of gastric insufflation can be decreased by improving the patient-ventilator synchrony and by titrating the pressures so that the leak is reduced.
- Parenteral nutrition should not be started as the first choice of nutritional support as it has been shown to increase mortality in intubated patients.
- Specialized NIV mask with NG tube hole or perhaps a helmet device, where available, can be used in select population. But, they are costly and not easily available.

CONCLUSION

Patients requiring NIV due to acute or acute-on-chronic respiratory failure have a high prevalence of malnutrition.[20] When considering the need, route, and quantity of nutrition on NIV, patient safety should be of paramount importance. This should determine all aspects of nutrition in these critically ill patients with single or multiorgan failure. Ability to achieve nutrition targets should be improved by careful considerations of impediments to nutrition delivery and attempts to overcome them.

REFERENCES

1. Reintam Blaser A, Starkopf J, Alhazzani W, Berger MM, Casaer MP, Deane AM, et al. Early enteral nutrition in critically ill patients: ESICM clinical practice guidelines. Intensive Care Med. 2017;43:380-98.
2. Taylor BE, McClave SA, Martindale RG, Warren MM, Johnson DR, Braunschweig C, et al. Guidelines for the provision and assessment of nutrition support therapy in the adult critically ill patient: Society of Critical Care Medicine (SCCM) and American Society for Parenteral and Enteral Nutrition (ASPEN). Crit Care Med. 2016;44: 390-438.
3. Berger MM, Reintam-Blaser A, Calder PC, Casaer M, Hiesmayr MJ, Mayer K, et al. Monitoring nutrition in the ICU. Clin Nutr. 2019;38:584-93.
4. Arabi YM, McClave SA. Enteral nutrition should not be given to patients on vasopressor agents. Crit Care Med. 2020;48:119-21.
5. Wischmeyer P. Enteral nutrition can be given to patients on vasopressors. Crit Care Med. 2020;48:122-5.
6. Berger MM, Berger-Gryllaki M, Wiesel PH, Revelly JP, Hurni M, Cayeux C, et al. Intestinal absorption in patients after cardiac surgery. Crit Care Med. 2000;28:2217-23.
7. Melis M, Fichera A, Ferguson MK. Bowel necrosis associated with early jejunal tube feeding: a complication of postoperative enteral nutrition. Arch Surg. 2006;141:701-4.
8. Marvin RG, McKinley BA, McQuiggan M, Cocanour CS, Moore FA. Nonocclusive bowel necrosis occurring in critically ill trauma patients receiving enteral nutrition manifests

no reliable clinical signs for early detection. Am J Surg. 2000;179:7-12.
9. Mancl EE, Muzevich KM. Tolerability and safety of enteral nutrition in critically ill patients receiving intravenous vasopressor therapy. JPEN J Parenter Enter Nutr. 2013; 37:641-51.
10. Reignier J, Boisramé-Helms J, Brisard L, Lascarrou JB, Ait Hssain A, Anguel N, et al. NUTRIREA-2 trial investigators; clinical research in intensive care and sepsis (CRICS) group. Enteral versus parenteral early nutrition in ventilated adults with shock: a randomised, controlled, multicentre, open-label, parallel-group study (NUTRIREA-2). Lancet. 2018;391:133-43.
11. Fuentes Padilla P, Martinez G, Vernooij RW, Urrutia G, Roqué I Figuls M, Bonfill Cosp X. Early enteral nutrition (within 48 h) versus delayed enteral nutrition (after 48 h) with or without supplemental parenteral nutrition in critically ill adults. Cochrane Database Syst Rev. 2019;2019:10.
12. Harvey SE, Parrott F, Harrison DA, Bear DE, Segaran E, Beale R, et al. Trial of the route of early nutritional support in critically ill adults. N Engl J Med. 2014;371:1673-84.
13. Patel JJ, Kozeniecki M, Peppard WJ, Peppard SR, Zellner-Jones S, Graf J, et al. Phase 3 pilot randomized controlled trial comparing early trophic enteral nutrition with "no enteral nutrition" in mechanically ventilated patients with septic shock. JPEN J Parenter Enter Nutr. 2020;44:866-73.
14. Shah FA, Kitsios GD, Zhang Y, Morris A, Yende S, Huang DT, et al. Design of the study of early enteral dextrose in sepsis: a pilot placebo-controlled randomized clinical trial. JPEN J Parenter Enter Nut. 2020;44:541-7.
15. El-Kersh K, Jalil B, McClave SA, Cavallazzi R, Guardiola J, Guilkey K, et al. Enteral nutrition as stress ulcer prophylaxis in critically ill patients: a randomized controlled exploratory study. J Crit Care. 2018;43:108-13.
16. Terzi N, Darmon M, Reignier J, Ruckly S, Garrouste-Orgeas M, Lautrette A, et al. Initial nutritional management during noninvasive ventilation and outcomes: a retrospective cohort study. Crit Care. 2017;21(1):293.
17. Bendavid I, Singer P, Theilla M, Themessl-Huber M, Sulz I, Mouhieddine M, et al. NutritionDay ICU: a 7 year worldwide prevalence study of nutrition practice in intensive care. Clin Nutr. 2017;36:1122-9.
18. Macht M, Wimbish T, Clark BJ, Benson AB, Burnham EL, Williams A, et al. Postextubation dysphagia is persistent and associated with poor outcomes in survivors of critical illness. Crit Care. 2011;15:R231.
19. Kogo M, Nagata K, Morimoto T, Ito J, Sato Y, Teraoka S, et al. Enteral nutrition is a risk factor for airway complications in subjects undergoing noninvasive ventilation for acute respiratory failure. Respir Care. 2017; 62:459-67.
20. Sharma G, Venkataraman R, Rajagopal S, Ramakrishnan N, Abraham BK, Savio RD. Nutrition therapy in patients requiring noninvasive ventilation in the intensive care unit: Feasibility, tolerance, and complications. Indian J Respir Care. 2021; 10:289-93.

CHAPTER 41

Gut Microbiome in Critical Illness

B Ravinder Reddy

Bacteria are, and always have been the dominant forms of life on earth!
— **Stephen Jay Gould, Full House**

■ INTRODUCTION

Humans have a diverse group of microorganisms, comprising mainly of viruses, bacteria, fungi, archaea (primitive single-celled organisms), and even protozoa. Even though viruses, which also include bacteriophages, constitute the maximum number of microorganisms, bacteria actually are the most dominant "live" forms of microorganisms in humans. Bacteria are present on every niche of the external surfaces (skin, hair, and nails) as well as within the body—mouth, saliva, gastrointestinal tract (GIT), respiratory tract, breasts, genital tract, seminal fluid, and eyes, as commensals (from Medieval Latin *commensalis* for "sharing a table"). The ratio of bacteria to human cells in an average man is reported at 1.3:1, with a slight preponderance of microbial cells in females, in view of relatively reduced number (by 10%) of red cells. Therefore, the revised estimate stands at 39 trillion bacteria, which marginally outnumber the human cells.[1] An average bacterium (like an *Escherichia coli*) has a mass of 10–12 g (about a trillionth of a gram), and together, all the microbes weigh about 1–2 kg. These are made of approximately 1,000 diversely different species, and each species has about 2,000 unique genes, yielding an estimated 2 million microbial genes, which overwhelm the human genes (about 20,000), and enable humans to live in a microbe-dominated milieu. Human microbiome varies with the anatomical location. GIT, especially the colon, is the largest reservoir of microbiota (microorganisms) and microbiome (microbial genes), followed by skin, oral cavity, respiratory, and genital tract.[2] In the last two decades, there has been a tremendous progress in the classification and identification of genes specific to bacteria. This was achieved by sequencing their genetic profiles, including virulence- and antibiotic resistance-genes, as well as the metabolic pathways by 16S ribosomal RNA (rRNA), next-generation sequencing, and by shotgun metagenomics. Based on these sequencing and studies, gut microbiome has been classified into various phyla. Human gut microbiome comprises four prominent phyla, composed of *Firmicutes* (the most predominant phyla, at 60–75%), followed by Bacteroidetes (30–40%), which together constitute over 90% of the gut phyla. The remaining are *Actinobacteria* and *Proteobacteria* **(Fig. 1)**. *Firmicutes* phyla are largely gram-positive bacteria, about 95% of them comprise *Clostridium* genera (anaerobic, gram positive). The other prominent genera include

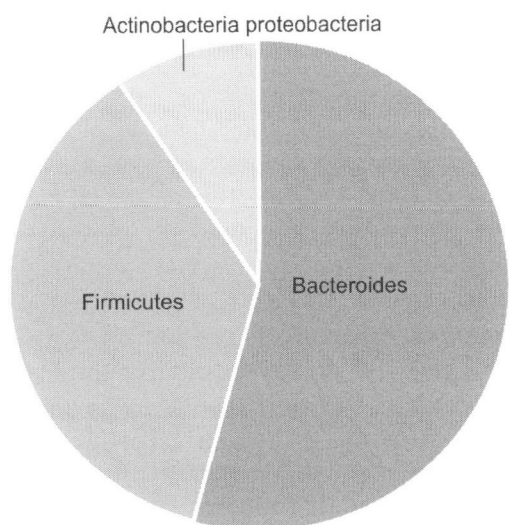

Fig. 1: Prevalence of common phyla of gut microbiome.

Staphylococcus, Streptococcus, Enterococcus, and *Lactobacillus*. Bacteroidetes make up the next common phyla, made up of gram-negative gut commensals, and the common genera comprise *Bacteroides, Porphyromonas, Prevotella,* and *Flavobacterium*. *Actinobacteria* are less frequent and composed of gram-positive bacteria, and *Bifidobacterium* species represent the most prominent genera, followed by *Corynebacterium, Mycobacteria,* and *Actinomyces*. Proteobacteria phyla are composed exclusively of gram-negative organisms, which include pathogenic genera, such as *Escherichia, Pseudomonas, Klebsiella, Salmonella, Helicobacter,* and *Legionella*. In addition to the huge bacterial phyla, a minor component of commensals is formed by species of archaea and as well as fungi. The notable fungal species are composed of *Saccharomyces* and *Candida*. Intestinal viruses too form an essential component of gut microorganisms, comprised predominantly of bacteriophages, which constitute a major part of gut virome. A recent study of the human gut microbiome has disclosed hundreds of newly discovered species, which expanded our understanding of the gut microbiome, and their role in homeostasis and dysbiosis.[3,4]

GUT MICROBIOME

The composition of human microbiota and microbiome depends on various factors. It is thought that the developing fetus is exposed to maternal microbial metabolites at the placental interface. Fragments of bacterial DNA (deoxyribonucleic acid) were also identified from amniotic fluid by 16S rRNA sequencing. Though this notion is still debatable, it is assumed that the origin of microbiome perhaps is initiated before birth. Mode of delivery plays a role in the initial formation of microbiome. A vaginal delivery exposes the newborn to the beneficial and diverse maternal microbes from vagina and fecal matter; a cesarean section exposes the baby to the less diverse microbes from the mother's skin, and the relatively sterile hospital environment. The immature gut microbiome of the newborn is reinforced by breast milk, which is a complex biofluid. It contains vital elements like milk proteins, such as lactalbumin, lactoferrin; secretory antibodies, the secretory immunoglobulin A (SIgA); and the complex human milk oligosaccharides (HMO), which act as prebiotics, especially for the *Bifidobacterium* species. These bioactive molecules, Igs, HMOs, and milk microbiota are deficient in the milk made by processed milk powder, hence lack the significant benefits of breast milk. Thus, breastfeeding enables the proliferation of the early gut commensals, and provides an excellent immune protection, which is a crucial factor for healthy development. Further expansion of microbiome, its configuration, and diversity depend on myriad factors like diet, especially during the weaning period, geographical locations, exposure to other humans, pets, antibiotics, and other medications, and reaches the adult composition by about 3 years of age.[5,6]

A "healthy" gut microbiome is made up of diverse species of microbiome, whose composition is predominantly made of phyla belonging to the dominant commensals, and at densities, which are crucial for digestive and immunological homeostasis. A crucial aspect is microbial fermentation of dietary fiber in the colon, resulting in the production of bioactive metabolites—the short-chain fatty acids (SCFAs). The three most common ones are butyrate, propionate, and acetate. In healthy adults, an adequate intake of dietary fiber from 25 to 30 g/day generates SCFAs that provide up to 5–10% of the energy requirements and act as fuel for the colonic epithelium (especially by butyrate). SCFAs modulate immune responses, regulate appetite, glucose, and cholesterol metabolism. A key function of SCFAs is the anti-inflammatory effect by inhibition of nuclear factor kappa-B (NF-κB), which reduces the production of inflammatory mediators, especially tumor necrosis factor alpha (TNF-α), and elicits an antioxidant and antineoplastic effects.[7]

GASTROINTESTINAL TRACT AND INTESTINAL EPITHELIUM

The GIT is a multifaceted structure, which measures about 7–9 meter, and with an average surface area of about 250 m^2 (equivalent to a tennis court) and is a central organ for digestion and absorption of nutrients, water, and electrolytes; it produces endocrine and paracrine hormones and gastrointestinal peptides. The intestinal epithelium is a complex and an intricate assembly of diverse cells, which apart from digestive functions is involved in innate and acquired immune responses and achieves immune homeostasis, despite being home to the maximum number of microbial species in the body.

Intestinal epithelium is made up of highly specialized cells, arranged in a single layer and consists of absorptive epithelial cells (which are most abundant and involved in nutrient absorption), enteroendocrine cells (EECs—secrete cholecystokinin, glucagon-like peptide-1, and 2, peptide-YY, neurotransmitters, and other neuropeptides), goblet cells (produce mucins forming the mucus layer), Paneth cells [produce antimicrobial peptides (AMPs); intestinal epithelial lymphocytes (IELs), which are a type of T lymphocytes interacting with luminal bacteria, and microfold cells (M cells) are present in the epithelium overlying the Peyer's patches (PP), which sense and transport antigens to the lymphoid cells)], tuft cells (are least in number, involved in the elimination of parasites and modulate immune responses), and stem cells and transit amplifying cells (TACs), both of which are located in the epithelial crypts and renew the epithelium every 5–7 days.[8] Along with the commensal microbes, this single layer, composed of highly specialized epithelial cells, and with its underlying lamina propria [containing lymphoid tissues and various immune cells: dendritic cells (DCs), macrophages, and regulatory T cells (T$_{regs}$)] and smooth muscle layers constitute the various barriers to maintain the intestinal integrity. They are microbial barrier, chemical barrier, physical barrier, immunological barrier, and smooth muscle layers **(Table 1)**. Microbial barrier is formed mainly by the resident commensals, which aid in the digestion of nutrients, regulation of immune responses, and production of various bioactive molecules such as SCFA, amino acids, and vitamins. The chemical barrier

Type of intestinal barrier	Components of barrier	Functions
Microbial barrier	Commensal bacteria (gut microbiota and microbiome)	Digestion, immune responses, and production of various metabolites
Chemical barrier	• Mucus and glycocalyx layers • Various AMPs	Microbial killing and modulation of inflammatory responses
Physical barrier	Epithelial cells, tight and adhesion cell junctions	Prevent microbial adhesion and translocation of microbes and toxins
Immune barrier	• Intestinal epithelial lymphocytes • Lamina propria, dendritic cells	Innate and acquired immune responses, tolerance and surveillance
Muscle layers	Smooth muscles (muscularis externa and muscularis interna)	Involved in peristalsis and propulsion of gut contents

TABLE 1: Various barriers of intestinal integrity.

(AMPs: antimicrobial peptides)

is made up of mucins (secreted by goblet cells), glycocalyx (secreted by the absorptive epithelial cells), AMPs (secreted by Paneth cells), and contains defensins, lysozymes, histatins, and other peptides, which kill or inhibit pathogenic microorganisms. Intestinal epithelial and their tight junctions, together with the mucus layer, constitute the physical (or anatomical) barrier, which prevents microbial adhesion, and translocation from the lumen. The lamina propria forms the immunological barrier, which contains lymphoid tissues, immune cells, including DCs, macrophages, and plasma cells, and constitutes the largest immune organ in the body. In close association with the commensals, they regulate innate defenses, acquired immune responses, immune tolerance, and surveillance. The smooth muscle layers are essential in peristalsis and in propulsion activities. Gut microbiome also produces neurotransmitters. Dopamine is produced by bacterial species of the genus *Bacillus*, serotonin by the genera *Enterococcus* and *Escherichia*, norepinephrine by the genera *Bacillus* and *Escherichia*, and gamma-aminobutyric acid (GABA) by the genus *Bifidobacterium*. These various neurotransmitters influence the endocrine, immune, and enteric nervous systems, as illustrated by the gut–brain axis, having afferents and efferents signals via the vagus nerve, which interact with hypothalamus-pituitary-adrenal axis. The gut–brain axis has an impact on appetite, cognition, memory, mood, sleep, pain, mental stress, and physical activities. Thus, the intestinal epithelium plays a pivotal role in physiological and immunological homeostasis.[9,10]

GUT MICROBIOME AND IMMUNE HOMEOSTASIS

Diet plays the most pivotal role in nature and composition of gut microbiome. Intake of food is potentially accompanied by a microbial load, majority of which is destroyed by gastric acid. Microbes that resist the effects of acidic pH, along with the nutrients, interact with the small intestinal villi. Partially digested nutrients and especially microbial antigens are constantly sampled by M cells and DCs, which in turn interact with T cells within the PP. The mucus layer overlying the PP is thinner to facilitate this "crosstalk" between antigens and immune cells.

Antigenic exposure most often initiates a tolerogenic response, wherein T_{regs} secrete anti-inflammatory cytokines [like interleukin-10 (IL-10) and transforming growth factor-beta] and modulate the immune responses. On the contrary, antigens from pathogenic bacteria trigger innate lymphoid cells (ILCs), natural killer (NK) cells, and naïve T cells and induce a cytotoxic response by activating macrophages, neutrophils, CD8$^+$ and Th17 cells, and secretion of inflammatory mediators [IL-6, TNF-β, and interferon gamma (IFN-γ)] and induce phagocytosis and formation of neutrophil extracellular traps (NETs), resulting in killing the microbes and has the potential to damage the intestinal barrier integrity. On the other hand, certain gut commensals like the segmented filamentous bacteria (SFB) activate a different subset of Th17 cells, which dampen inflammatory responses, thus moderating immune responses, reiterating the modulatory role of gut microbiome in healthy states. Commensal gut microbiome is also involved in enabling B cells activation in the production of diverse types of SIgA, which are essential for immune tolerance, as well as enable phagocytosis of the pathogenic bacteria by macrophages, in concurrence with complement proteins. SIgA is also involved in immune tolerance by reducing the inflammatory actions of other Igs and boosting symbiosis with other commensal bacteria. (Description of the various immune cells, their activations, and responses along with alterations in the metabolic pathways are mentioned in chapter).

Detrimental diet, infections, stress, antibiotics, and other medications can result in serious disruption of healthy gut commensals, causing gut dysbiosis. Antigens from these pathogenic microbes can activate epithelial cells, DCs, and macrophages, and trigger an effector T-cell response by inducing CD4$^+$ and CD8$^+$ cytotoxic activation, with release of proinflammatory molecules (TNF-α, IFN-γ, IL-6, IL-17, IL-12, and IL-23) with the recruitment of neutrophils, resulting in severe tissue destruction, injury to the gut mucosa, with a significant loss in intestinal integrity.[11-13]

CRITICAL ILLNESS, SEPSIS, AND GUT MICROBIOME

A healthy gut microbiome is crucial for immune regulation and inhibits the growth and proliferation of pathogenic bacteria, especially the anaerobic species. Various illnesses can significantly change the composition of intestinal commensals, resulting in gut dysbiosis. This disruption can lead to the expansion and amplification of pathogenic microbes called pathobiome. Acute conditions such as severe trauma, serious infections, major surgery, cardiac arrest, etc., can disturb the gut immune homeostasis within a few hours, and lead to a rapid development of pathobiome, which is associated with an increase in pathogenic bacteria and a significant reduction in normal commensals. A critically ill patient has significant biochemical and metabolic alterations. Exposure to medications such as antibiotics, opioid derivatives, sedatives, catecholamines, vasopressors, proton pump inhibitors, metformin, statins, nonsteroidal anti-inflammatory drugs (NSAIDs), and others accelerates gut dysbiosis. Antibiotics acutely alter the gut microbiome—they reduce the bacterial diversity considerably and enable rapid proliferation of multidrug-resistant organisms (MDROs) such as *methicillin-resistant Staphylococcus aureus (MRSA), vancomycin-resistant enterococci (VRE), carbapenem-resistant* Entero-bacterales *(CRE), multiresistant Acinetobacter,*

Klebsiella, Pseudomonas, and *Clostridium difficile*. Additionally, mechanical ventilation, reduced or total lack of oral feeds, artificial nutritional interventions, and alterations in the gastrointestinal transit time have the potential to exponentially intensify the intestinal pathobiome. Reduction in the colonic commensals results in decreased production of SCFAs, which promotes a pro-inflammatory state, dysmotility, cell death, and immune dysregulation. A reduction in the mucosal SIgA enables expansion of pathogenic microbiome, and thus increasing the risk of developing ventilatory-associated pneumonia and hospital-acquired infections. Severe reduction in the mucus layer of the intestine, and/or even disappearance of specific beneficial microbes (*Faecalibacterium prausnitzii*, etc.), accelerates the proliferation of gut dysbiosis, damage to the paracellular tight junctions, resulting in a leaky gut and enabling translocation of pathogenic microbiome, along with their toxins to the systemic circulation significantly induce dysfunctions of respiratory system, cardiovascular system, renal, hepatic, and hematological systems.[14,15]

Therefore, in critical illness, the density and diversity of "healthy" gut microbiome are grossly reduced, or in severe cases, they even disappear completely. Simultaneously, there is an expansion and proliferation of pathobiome, thus demonstrating a link between alterations in the gut microbiome to the maladaptive immune responses and clinical outcomes. Gut is therefore considered as the driver of sepsis and organ failure. Given the high incidence of mortality of sepsis the world over, swift pathobiome identification and sequencing by metagenomics and prompt attempts to repopulate the gut with "healthy" microbiome with specific prebiotics, probiotics, SCFAs, or even dietary fiber are potential options to improve the clinical outcomes in critical illness and sepsis.

CONCLUSION

Gut microbiome plays a crucial role in many physiological functions, including various metabolic pathways, immune-inflammatory pathways and immunoregulation. Various factors, and especially diet and lifestyle are involved in the biogenesis and composition of gut microbiota. The biochemical molecules along with the genome of these trillions of intestinal microorganisms interact with various axes, the predominant of which are gut-liver axis and gut-brain axis, in addition to maintaining to the integrity of the single-layered intestinal epithelium. In various disease states including critical illnesses, there is a significant distortion of the commensal microorganisms, resulting in gut dysbiosis with expansion of pathogenic organisms. Therefore, attempts to modulate gut microbiota by diet, prebiotics and probiotics offers a targeted mode of therapy to decrease the impact of pathobiome in many disease-states including the critically ill.

REFERENCES

1. Sender R, Fuchs S, Milo R. Are we really vastly outnumbered? Revisiting the ratio of bacterial to host cells in humans. Cell. 2016;164(3):337-40.
2. Gilbert JA, Blaser MJ, Caporaso JG, Jansson JK, Lynch SV, Knight R. Current understanding of the human microbiome. Nat Med. 2018;24(4):392-400.
3. Scholz M, Ward DV, Pasolli E, Tolio T, Zolfo M, Asnicar F, et al. Strain-level microbial epidemiology and population genomics from shotgun metagenomics. Nat Methods. 2016;13(5):435-8.
4. Leviatan S, Saar Shoer, Rothschild D, Gorodetski M, Segal E, et al. An expanded

reference map of the human gut microbiome reveals hundreds of previously unknown species. Nat Commun. 2022;13(1):3863.
5. Ganal-Vonarburg SC, Hornef MW, Macpherson AJ. Microbial-host molecular exchange and its functional consequences in early mammalian life. Science. 2020;368(6491):604-7.
6. Stewart CJ. Diet-microbe-host interaction in early life. Science. 2023;381(6653):38A-38C.
7. Reddy BR. Noncaloric benefits of carbohydrates. Nestle Nutr Inst Workshop Ser. 2015;82:27-33.
8. Okumura R, Takeda K. Roles of intestinal epithelial cells in the maintenance of gut homeostasis. Exp Mol Med. 2017;49(5):e338.
9. Turner JR. Intestinal mucosal barrier function in health and disease. Nat Rev Immunol. 2009;9(11):799-809.
10. Liu L, Huh JR, Shah K. Microbiota and the gut-brain axis: Implications for new therapeutic designs in the CNS. EBioMedicine. 2022;77:103908.
11. Omenetti S, Bussi C, Metidji A, Iseppon A, Lee S, Tolaini M, et al. The Intestine Harbors Functionally Distinct Homeostatic Tissue-Resident and Inflammatory Th17 cells. Immunity. 2019;51(1):77-89.
12. Sansonetti PJ. War and peace at mucosal surfaces. Nat Rev Immunol. 2004;3(12):953-64.
13. Dickson RP. The microbiome and critical illness. Lancet Respir Med. 2016;4(1):59-72.
14. Miniet AA, Grunwell JR, Craig M. Coppersmith CM. The microbiome and the immune system in critical illness. Curr Opin Crit Care. 2021;27(2):157-63.
15. Szychowiak P, Villageois-Tran K, Patrier J, Timsit JF, Ruppé É. The role of the microbiota in the management of intensive care patients. Ann of Intensive Care. 2022;12(1):3.

Evaluation of Sarcopenia in Critical Illness

Deeksha Kapoor

INTRODUCTION

Low muscle mass is an important prognostic factor in predicting outcomes in various medical conditions. This chapter focuses on muscle loss encountered in patients with critical illness, its evaluation, and its impact on outcomes. Before discussing the evaluation of sarcopenia in critical illness, it is important to understand the concept of sarcopenia and identify what constitutes as critical illness. Further on, the chapter aims to discuss the evaluation of muscle loss in the critically ill and the outcomes associated with muscle wasting.

What is sarcopenia?

Sarcopenia is a phenomenon of progressive decline in skeletal muscle mass and function.[1] It involves a structural component, i.e., loss of muscle area, volume, myosteatosis and a physiological element, i.e., loss of muscle strength and function. Primary sarcopenia is age-related, whereas secondary sarcopenia may be associated with various factors such as malnutrition, malignancy, or chronic conditions.[1,2] Assessment of sarcopenia should include evaluation of muscle strength, muscle mass, and physical performance.[1] However, it is difficult to assess physical performance and strength in critically ill patients and most assessment of sarcopenia is limited to radiological means.

What is critical illness?

When a certain disease condition worsens to the extent of causing deranged hemostasis, it is referred to as critical illness. Is it often accompanied by life-threatening organ dysfunction, needing organ support, and thereby associated with high mortality and morbidity. Such a clinical state predisposes to loss of muscle mass which further worsens the patient's clinical situation, creating a vicious cycle of progressive sarcopenia and clinical worsening.

What is intensive care unit-associated weakness (ICU-AW)?

This condition is described by a conglomeration of circumstances associated with neuromuscular dysfunction occurring because of admission into the ICU and severe illness.[3] This condition is triggered by critical illness, while the severity of the primary underlying condition may not contribute so much to ICU-AW. The important pathophysiological pathways in the development of ICU-AW include an inflammatory response, and disturbed protein hemostasis, leading to neuroaxonal degeneration, muscle wasting, and changes in muscle histology.[3,4] During critical illness, the prolonged immobilization, negative protein balance, and altered neuroendocrine response lead to muscle wasting. Muscle dysfunction is contributed by circulatory disturbances, deranged oxygenation of tissue, mitochondrial impairment, and ion-channel membrane disruption.[5]

Intensive care unit-associated weakness includes symmetrical weakness of bilateral limbs. It develops because of axonal polyneuropathy and myopathy and more frequently affects bilateral lower limbs.[6,7] It also results in weakness of the respiratory muscles leading to delayed weaning from mechanical ventilation, prolonging ICU, and hospital stay. ICU-AW may be considered a secondary form of sarcopenia.[6,7] Evidence suggests that about half the patients admitted to ICU with critical illness develop ICU-AW.

What is the relevance of sarcopenia in the critically ill patient?
Sarcopenia is expected to be associated with poor outcomes in various clinical scenarios, especially in critically ill patients. Sarcopenia gets exaggerated in critically ill patients because of prolonged immobilization and systemic inflammation.[8,9] The prevalence of sarcopenia in critically ill patients ranges between 30 and 70%.[10,11] Critically ill patients can lose up to 15% muscle mass within a week and about 2% of muscle mass per day.[12] It has also been shown that about half the patients who are critically ill have ICU-AW. The documented rate of loss of muscle mass depends on the modality and site of assessment of the muscle. Muscle depletion starts early, within the 1st week of critical illness and is worse for patients with multiorgan dysfunction.[13] Muscle loss has been found to be associated with increased length of ICU stay, higher ICU mortality and higher hospital mortality and higher readmission rates.[14-17] Patients on mechanical ventilation who have low skeletal muscle mass have a risk of mortality increased by 25% compared to patients with normal muscle mass.

How is sarcopenia evaluated in critically ill patients?
The well-validated tools for measuring muscle mass include the assessment of body composition with computed tomography (CT) scans, magnetic resonance imaging (MRI) studies, dual-energy X-ray absorptiometry (DEXA), musculoskeletal ultrasound and bioelectrical impedance analysis (BIA). The typical functional tests involve measuring muscle strength by means of a handgrip test and a gait-speed test. These methods have severe limitations while assessing muscle mass and strength in the critically ill because of their clinical instability, the need for mechanical ventilatory support and the time-consuming and resource-intensive nature of these investigations.

RADIOLOGICAL METHODS FOR ESTIMATING MUSCLE MASS

Radiological methods such as CT, DEXA, ultrasonography, etc., have traditionally been used to study patients' muscle mass. The definition of sarcopenia depends on the radiological method, the group of muscles studied, the parameter being studied, and the outcome of interest. There is no standardized way of assessing muscle mass in ICU patients, multiple methods exist and have their unique advantages and disadvantages.

- *Computed tomography:* Axial CT imaging provides a precise estimate of the body composition. Lean muscle mass can be assessed quantitatively by measuring cross-sectional muscle area or muscle volume and qualitatively by assessing muscle density in Hounsfield units. Axial image at the level of the third lumbar vertebrae is the most commonly used level to obtain muscle mass measurements. Multiple studies suggest that measurement of the psoas muscle at the level of L3–L4 vertebra correlates well with whole-body muscle mass.

CT-assessed low muscle mass has been found to be associated with higher mortality rates, higher time on the ventilator and more time spent in ICU.[18,19] In another prospective study, CT-assessed low-muscle mass was associated with an increased rate of hospital-acquired pneumonia.[20] Muscle quality also has an impact on patient outcomes and can be analyzed by studying muscle density (expressed in Hounsfield units) on CT scans. When muscle mass is replaced by intramuscular lipids, the muscle density is reduced on plain CT images. In fact, low-muscle density, independent of muscle quantity has been found to have an impact on 6-month outcomes.[21,22] This observation parallels results from a recent Indian study suggesting a higher impact of muscle density on post-operative outcomes following pancreatic surgery than the impact of depleted muscle mass.[22]

Limitations of using CT-guided assessment of muscle mass in critically ill patients are many. Performing a CT requires moving the patient to a radiology suite, which is not justified in patients who are hemodynamically unstable or have respiratory decompensation. Moreover, performing a CT scan merely for the assessment of muscle mass, may not be justified. The data of sarcopenia in critically ill patients, using CT scans, is generated from patients who underwent an abdominal CT for reasons other than assessment of sarcopenia. Such patients are generally sicker and have a higher illness severity score. An inherent bias exists in such data as certain groups of patients are overrepresented. The routine use of CT assessment for following up muscle mass loss is, therefore, not justified.

- *Ultrasonography:* Musculoskeletal ultrasonography (MKUS) using a linear probe, with frequencies between 2 and 20 MHz, is a readily available technique to assess muscle mass in ICU patients.[23] This is probably the most commonly used method to assess muscle mass in patients admitted to ICU. The test does not involve shifting patients to a radiology suite, or repeated radiation exposure and can be used bedside to monitor the progression of muscle mass loss in various muscle groups. Muscle mass loss ranging from 8 to 30% has been reported within 7–10 days of ICU admission.

Like CT assessment, MKUS involves the assessment of muscle quantity and quality. Muscle mass is quantified by assessing the muscle thickness or the cross-sectional area of an individual muscle or a muscle group. Muscle quality is studied by the muscle's echogenicity. The most commonly studied muscle group on MKUS is the quadriceps muscle. Other muscles which can be easily assessed on MKUS are rectus femoris, quadriceps, and biceps brachii. It has been suggested that muscles of the lower limb undergo atrophy sooner than the muscles of the upper limb during critical illness. Atrophy of the rectus femoris muscle has also been studied as a predictor of outcomes and was found to be associated with difficulty in weaning from the ventilator as well as a longer length of ICU stay.[24,25] Evidence also suggests that critically ill patients with sepsis develop muscle wasting in a more rapid fashion and is associated with architectural abnormalities. Muscle echogenicity assesses muscle quality and quantifies the fatty infiltration or the intramuscular glycogen storage in lower limb muscles. Muscle tissue containing more glycogen produces a darker image on MKUS.[23] As catabolism sets in, healthy muscle is replaced by fibrotic fatty muscle, increasing its echogenicity. This can be studied using high-frequency ultrasound, which in critically ill patients has been found to be associated with prolonged ICU stay.[26] MKUS has the advantage of being a noninvasive, bedside investigation, and can be used to follow up on the status of muscle mass loss or quality worsening and assess the change in the muscle quality with nutritional interventions, exercises, and rehabilitation.

Other important parameters of muscle function can also be studied on MKUS. The muscle structure and architecture are important for the force or resistance a muscle can generate. The angle between the axis of the entire muscle and the muscle fibers is called pennation angle—this angle is responsible for the force generated by the muscle and is influenced by the extent of fibrosis, myonecrosis, and accumulation of fluid in the fascial planes. Pennation angle of the muscle the vastus lateralis has been shown to increase with edema and inflammation in patients admitted in ICU and has been associated with length of stay in the ICU.

Musculoskeletal ultrasonography has certain limitations. There can be significant interobserver variability, especially with respect to the amount of compression required to assess the muscle and the anatomical landmark of muscle assessment. These variations in methodology make standardization of the results an extremely cumbersome task. Nevertheless, MKUS is a useful bedside tool to monitor and follow muscle mass loss and the impact of interventions.

- *Bioelectrical impedance analysis*: This technique uses a low amplitude alternating electrical current at multiple or single radiofrequencies to study the conductance of electric current across fluid and tissue. Air-filled spaces, bones, and fatty tissues are poor conductors. On the contrary, muscle and blood are excellent conductors. Two parameters are studied while calculating impedance—"resistance" which is the opposition to the flow of current across the tissue, and "reactance" which is the delay in conduction caused by cell membranes, nonionic substances, and tissue interfaces. During illness when edema increases, resistance and reactance have been shown to correlate with the severity of the illness.

  Multiple techniques of BIA are available, like single-frequency BIA, multiple-frequency BIA, and spectroscopy. Studies of BIA have reported mixed results in predicting outcomes. Though some studies have suggested the predictive potential of BIA in predicting mortality in patients admitted to ICU, the use of this technology in critically ill patients is limited.[27,28]

- *Dual-energy X-ray absorptiometry*: DEXA uses two X-ray beams of different energy levels to differentiate between fat and muscle and can be used to assess generalized or regional loss of muscle mass.[29,30] The most accepted parameter using a DEXA scan is the appendicular lean mass index, which has been shown to correlate with body cell mass which is the metabolically active part of the fat-free mass and is responsible for the resting metabolism of the patient. Though DEXA

SERUM BIOMARKERS FOR EVALUATING SARCOPENIA

The use of serum biomarkers for muscle growth or loss is controversial and poorly standardized. Multiple molecular pathways exist which modulate muscle growth. An imbalance between myogenic and myogenesis inhibitors during critical illness tips the balance toward increased muscle loss in these patients.[31] Markers responsible for muscle growth include bone morphogenetic proteins, follistatin, brain-derived neurotrophic factors, and irisin. The muscle growth inhibitors include transforming growth factor beta, activins A and B, growth and differentiation factor 15, and myostatin.[32] The increased oxidative and inflammatory response during critical illness, hypercatabolic state, increased insulin resistance, decreased mobility and decreased nutritional intake, and compromised absorption stimulate the muscle growth inhibitors causing increased muscle loss.[32,33]

Serum Creatinine

Serum creatinine has been used as a marker of sarcopenia. It is a marker of glomerular filtration rate (GFR), and its concentration is one of the final products of muscle catabolism. As it is produced primarily by skeletal muscle, it can be used to estimate muscle mass when kidney functions are stable.[34] Therefore, creatinine varies with body composition and can influence the estimation of the GFR, underestimating GFR in patients with a high muscle mass and overestimating GFR in patients with low muscle mass. Multiple factors can influence creatinine levels including protein intake, fluid resuscitation, heart failure, and sepsis, or rhabdomyolysis. Nevertheless, creatinine levels have been observed to decrease by 10–25% in critically ill patients with no evidence of acute kidney injury within 1 week of hospitalization. Although this fall in creatinine levels may be attributed to muscle mass loss, serum creatinine levels remain an imperfect biomarker for sarcopenia in the critically ill because of the confounding effect of associated clinical conditions.

Cystatin C

All nucleated cells produce cystatin C and release it into the circulation. Muscle mass does not influence the levels of cystatin C and this protein has been used to estimate the GFR. As it undergoes glomerular filtration, it is neither secreted nor absorbed into the circulation. Cystatin C is also used to assess sarcopenia, as a component of the sarcopenia index (SI) [(serum creatinine/serum cystatin C) × 100]. SI has been shown to correlate with muscle mass and is a predictor of in-hospital and 90-day mortality in patients without acute kidney injury.[35]

SARCOPENIA INDEX

Sarcopenia index has been used to estimate muscle mass in different groups of critically ill patients and has been shown to strongly correlate with worse clinical outcomes. It accounts for two different markers of glomerular filtration with different cellular origins—creatinine and cystatin C. As mentioned previously, creatinine is an endogenous marker of GFR and a final product of muscle catabolism, the production of which is relatively constant provided the muscle mass remains stable. Cystatin C, on the other hand, is a low-molecular weight protein produced by all nucleated cells, therefore, the impact of muscle mass on cystatin C is less than that on creatinine. Therefore, in a patient with stable kidney function, the difference between these two can be used to assess skeletal muscle mass, exploiting the differential cellular origin of these molecules. SI is defined by the formula (serum creatinine/serum cystatin C) × 100. A low SI–low serum creatinine in comparison with cystatin C, therefore, points toward a low muscle mass.[36] SI has been shown to correlate well with muscle mass as calculated on abdominal CT scans, using the muscle surface area of paraspinal muscles to calculate sarcopenia. SI was also found to be a predictor of hospital and 90-day mortality rates, and a low SI was shown to be predictive of prolonged mechanical ventilation in critically ill patients.[35]

The prevalence of malnutrition can be up to 50% in critically ill patients. To quantify the nutritional status of ICU patients, a modified NUTRIC (Nutritional Risk in Critically Ill Score) score has been developed and validated. It is a composite score of the patient's age, severity of illness, number of days from hospital admission to ICU admission, and comorbid conditions.[37] Higher scores have been shown to be associated with higher 6-month mortality rates. In another retrospective study, SI was shown to correlate well with the modified NUTRIC score and actually performed better as a screening tool for malnutrition in critically ill patients. A low SI (<43) was shown to be associated with a significantly higher risk of mortality (HR = 2.61, 95% CI: 1.06–6.48, p = 0.038).[38] SI has also been shown to be a predictor of chemotherapy-induced toxicity in lung cancer patients.[39]

Sarcopenia index has emerged as an easily useable tool for assessment of sarcopenia. It has many benefits such as low cost, ease of calculation, correlation with muscle mass, and a clinically relevant impact on outcomes. Nevertheless, it has certain disadvantages and can be reliably used only in patients with stable kidney function. Sole dependence on SI to assess muscle mass makes lead to erroneous judgment and it may be the best to use it in collaboration with some other techniques as well.

What all Outcomes are Affected by Muscle Depletion in Critically Ill Patients?

Muscle loss has been associated with increased mortality rate, length of ICU stay, and increased time to wean from the ventilator.

- Patients with multiorgan failure have a higher rate of muscle loss than patients with single-organ failure.[13]
- A significantly higher rate of change in the cross-sectional area of the rectus femoris has been seen in patients requiring mechanical ventilation compared with those without mechanical ventilation.[40] Another study reported that patients who lost >10% of the thickness of the quadriceps femoris at day 7 had a higher chance to remain on mechanical ventilation.[16]
- Loss of >10% of rectus femoris area was also associated with an increased length of ICU and hospital stay.[14]
- Critically ill patients with sarcopenia have an increased risk of mortality compared to nonsarcopenic patients (OR = 2.28, 95% CI: 1.83–2.83, p < 0.001).[41] These results are reported from a recent meta-analysis analyzing data from 3,249 patients. Some of the studies used in this meta-analysis did not show a significant contribution of sarcopenia to mortality and this discrepancy was attributed to the small sample size of these studies.[11,42-44]

CONCLUSION

- Sarcopenia is progressive decline in skeletal muscle mass and function, which involves loss of muscle volume, fatty infiltration and loss of muscle strength and function.
- Assessment of sarcopenia involves evaluation of muscle strength, muscle mass and physical performance.
- Intensive care unit-associated weakness is neuromuscular dysfunction occurring because of admission in the ICU because of critical illness. Prolonged immobilization, negative protein balance and altered neuroendocrine response lead to muscle wasting.
- Muscle wasting is associated with worse clinical outcomes, like, higher mortality and readmission rates, in critically ill patients.
- Sarcopenia is assessed by estimation of muscle mass or volume using CT scans, MRI, DEXA, musculoskeletal ultrasound and bioelectrical impedance analysis. Functional tests include handgrip and gait-speed tests.
- There is no standardized way of assessing muscle mass, multiple methods exist, each with their unique advantages and disadvantages.
- Musculoskeletal ultrasound is probably the most common way of assessing muscle mass in patients admitted to ICU. Muscle mass is quantified as per the muscle thickness or cross-sectional area and quality by assessing the muscle's echogenicity.
- Certain serum biomarkers can be used for the evaluation of sarcopenia, their use, however, is controversial and methods of assessment poorly standardized. The markers for muscle growth are bone morphogenetic proteins, follistatin, brain-derived neurotrophic factors and irisin. Muscle growth inhibitors include transforming growth factor beta, activins A and B, growth and differentiation factor 15 and myostatin.
- Since creatinine is primarily a product of muscle metabolism, it has been used to estimate muscle mass when the kidney functions are stable. Cystatin C is another protein which is produced by all nucleated cells and has been used to assess sarcopenia, as a component of the sarcopenia index.

REFERENCES

1. Cruz-Jentoft AJ, Bahat G, Bauer J, Boirie Y, Bruyère O, Cederholm T, et al. Sarcopenia: revised European consensus on definition and diagnosis. Age Ageing. 2019;48(1):16-31.
2. Dhillon RJS, Hasni S. Pathogenesis and Management of Sarcopenia. Clin Geriat Med. 2017;33(1):17-26.
3. Schefold JC, Bierbrauer J, Weber-Carstens S. Intensive care unit-acquired weakness (ICUAW) and muscle wasting in critically ill patients with severe sepsis and septic shock. J Cachexia Sarcopenia Muscle. 2010;1(2):147-57.
4. Weber-Carstens S, Deja M, Koch S, Spranger J, Bubser F, Wernecke KD, et al. Risk factors in critical illness myopathy during the early course of critical illness: a prospective observational study. Crit Care. 2010;14(3):R119.
5. Puthucheary ZA, Astin R, Mcphail MJW, Saeed S, Pasha Y, Bear DE, et al. Metabolic phenotype of skeletal muscle in early critical illness. Thorax. 2018;73(10):926-35.
6. Vanhorebeek I, Latronico N, Van Den Berghe G. ICU-acquired weakness. Intensive Care Med. 2020;46(4):637-53.
7. Thille AW, Boissier F, Muller M, Levrat A, Bourdin G, Rosselli S, et al. Role of ICU-acquired weakness on extubation outcome among patients at high risk of reintubation. Crit Care. 2020;24(1):86.

8. Toptas M, Yalcin M, Akkoc İ, Demir E, Metin C, Savas Y, et al. The Relation between Sarcopenia and Mortality in Patients at Intensive Care Unit. BioMed Res Int. 2018;2018:1-9.
9. Ligthart-Melis GC, Luiking YC, Kakourou A, Cederholm T, Maier AB, De Van Der Schueren MAE. Frailty, Sarcopenia, and Malnutrition Frequently (Co-)occur in Hospitalized Older Adults: A Systematic Review and Meta-analysis. J Am Med Direct Assoc. 2020;21(9):1216-28.
10. Moisey LL, Mourtzakis M, Cotton BA, Premji T, Heyland DK, Wade CE, et al. Skeletal muscle predicts ventilator-free days, ICU-free days, and mortality in elderly ICU patients. Crit Care. 2013;17(5):R206.
11. Baggerman MR, Van Dijk DPJ, Winkens B, Van Gassel RJJ, Bol ME, Schnabel RM, et al. Muscle wasting associated co-morbidities, rather than sarcopenia are risk factors for hospital mortality in critical illness. J Crit Care. 2020;56:31-6.
12. Lambell KJ, Tierney AC, Wang JC, Nanjayya V, Forsyth A, Goh GS, et al. Comparison of Ultrasound-Derived Muscle Thickness With Computed Tomography Muscle Cross-Sectional Area on Admission to the Intensive Care Unit: A Pilot Cross-Sectional Study. JPEN J Parenter Enteral Nutr. 2021;45(1):136-45.
13. Puthucheary ZA, Rawal J, McPhail M, Connolly B, Ratnayake G, Chan P, et al. Acute Skeletal Muscle Wasting in Critical Illness. JAMA. 2013;310(15):1591.
14. Kemp PR, Paul R, Hinken AC, Neil D, Russell A, Griffiths MJ. Metabolic profiling shows pre-existing mitochondrial dysfunction contributes to muscle loss in a model of ICU-acquired weakness. J Cachexia, Sarcopenia Muscle. 2020;11(5):1321-35.
15. Dimopoulos S, Raidou V, Elaiopoulos D, Chatzivasiloglou F, Markantonaki D, Lyberopoulou E, et al. Sonographic muscle mass assessment in patients after cardiac surgery. WJC. 2020;12(7):351-61.
16. Toledo DO, Freitas BJD, Dib R, Pfeilsticker FJDA, Santos DMD, Gomes BC, et al. Peripheral muscular ultrasound as outcome assessment tool in critically ill patients on mechanical ventilation: An observational cohort study. Clin Nutr ESPEN. 2021;43: 408-14.
17. Lee ZY, Ong SP, Ng CC, Yap CSL, Engkasan JP, Barakatun-Nisak MY, et al. Association between ultrasound quadriceps muscle status with premorbid functional status and 60-day mortality in mechanically ventilated critically ill patient: A single-center prospective observational study. Clin Nutr. 2021;40(3):1338-47.
18. Zhou DC, Yang XH, Zhan XL, Gu YH, Guo LL, Jin HM. Association of lean body mass with nutritional parameters and mortality in hemodialysis patients: A long-term follow-up clinical study. Int J Artif Organs. 2018;41(6):297-305.
19. Shibahashi K, Sugiyama K, Kashiura M, Hamabe Y. Decreasing skeletal muscle as a risk factor for mortality in elderly patients with sepsis: a retrospective cohort study. J Intensive Care. 2017;5(1):8.
20. Fuchs G, Thevathasan T, Chretien YR, Mario J, Piriyapatsom A, Schmidt U, et al. Lumbar skeletal muscle index derived from routine computed tomography exams predict adverse post-extubation outcomes in critically ill patients. Journal of Critical Care. 2018;44:117-23.
21. Looijaard WGPM, Dekker IM, Stapel SN, Girbes ARJ, Twisk JWR, Oudemans-van Straaten HM, et al. Skeletal muscle quality as assessed by CT-derived skeletal muscle density is associated with 6-month mortality in mechanically ventilated critically ill patients. Crit Care. 2016;20(1):386.
22. Lin J, Zhang W, Chen W, Huang Y, Wu R, Chen X, et al. Muscle Mass, Density, and Strength are Necessary to Diagnose Sarcopenia in Patients with Gastric Cancer. J Surg Res. 2019;241:141-8.
23. Formenti P, Umbrello M, Coppola S, Froio S, Chiumello D. Clinical review: peripheral muscular ultrasound in the ICU. Ann Intensive Care. 2019;9(1):57.
24. Van Aerde N, Meersseman P, Debaveye Y, Wilmer A, Gunst J, Casaer MP, et al. Five-year impact of ICU-acquired neuromuscular complications: a prospective, observational

25. Peñuelas O, Muriel A, Frutos-Vivar F, Fan E, Raymondos K, Rios F, et al. Prediction and Outcome of Intensive Care Unit-Acquired Paresis. J Intensive Care Med. 2018;33(1):16-28.
26. Millan I, Hill J, Wischmeyer P. Measurement of skeletal muscle glycogen status in critically ill patients: a new approach in critical care monitoring. Crit Care. 2015;19(Suppl 1):P400.
27. Thibault R, Makhlouf AM, Mulliez A, Cristina Gonzalez M, Kekstas G, Kozjek NR, et al. Fat-free mass at admission predicts 28-day mortality in intensive care unit patients: the international prospective observational study Phase Angle Project. Intensive Care Med. 2016;42(9):1445-53.
28. Stapel SN, Looijaard WGPM, Dekker IM, Girbes ARJ, Weijs PJM, Oudemans-van Straaten HM. Bioelectrical impedance analysis-derived phase angle at admission as a predictor of 90-day mortality in intensive care patients. Eur J Clin Nutr. 2018;72(7):1019-25.
29. Guglielmi G, Ponti F, Agostini M, Amadori M, Battista G, Bazzocchi A. The role of DXA in sarcopenia. Aging Clin Exp Res. 2016;28(6):1047-60.
30. Abdalla PP, Silva AM, Venturini ACR, Santos APD, Carvalho ADS, Siqueira VAAA, et al. Cut-off points of appendicular lean soft tissue for identifying sarcopenia in older adults in Brazil: a cross-sectional study. Nutr Hosp [Internet]. 202016;37(2):306-12.
31. Kalinkovich A, Livshits G. Sarcopenia - The search for emerging biomarkers. Ageing Res Rev. 2015;22:58-71.
32. Vatic M, Von Haehling S, Ebner N. Inflammatory biomarkers of frailty. Exper Gerontol. 2020;133:110858.
33. Cruz-Jentoft AJ, Sayer AA. Sarcopenia. The Lancet. 2019;393(10191):2636-46.
34. Kashani K, Rosner MH, Ostermann M. Creatinine: From physiology to clinical application. Eur J Internal Med. 2020;72:9-14.
35. Kashani KB, Frazee EN, Kukrálová L, Sarvottam K, Herasevich V, Young PM, et al. Evaluating Muscle Mass by Using Markers of Kidney Function: Development of the Sarcopenia Index. Crit Care Med. 2017;45(1):e23-9.
36. Barreto EF, Poyant JO, Coville HH, Dierkhising RA, Kennedy CC, Gajic O, et al. Validation of the sarcopenia index to assess muscle mass in the critically ill: A novel application of kidney function markers. Clin Nutr. 2019;38(3):1362-7.
37. Rahman A, Hasan RM, Agarwala R, Martin C, Day AG, Heyland DK. Identifying critically-ill patients who will benefit most from nutritional therapy: Further validation of the "modified NUTRIC" nutritional risk assessment tool. Clin Nutr. 2016;35(1):158-62.
38. Barreto EF, Kanderi T, DiCecco SR, Lopez-Ruiz A, Poyant JO, Mara KC, et al. Sarcopenia Index is a Simple Objective Screening Tool for Malnutrition in the Critically Ill. JPEN J Parenter Enteral Nutr. 2019;43(6):780-8.
39. Suzuki K, Furuse H, Tsuda T, Masaki Y, Okazawa S, Kambara K, et al. Utility of creatinine/cystatin C ratio as a predictive marker for adverse effects of chemotherapy in lung cancer: A retrospective study. J Int Med Res. 2015;43(4):573-82.
40. Borges RC, Barbeiro HV, Barbeiro DF, Soriano FG. Muscle degradation, vitamin D and systemic inflammation in hospitalized septic patients. J Crit Care. 2020;56:125-31.
41. Zhang XM, Chen D, Xie XH, Zhang JE, Zeng Y, Cheng AS. Sarcopenia as a predictor of mortality among the critically ill in an intensive care unit: a systematic review and meta-analysis. BMC Geriatr. 2021;21(1):339.
42. Hwang F, McGreevy CM, Pentakota SR, Verde D, Park JH, Berlin A, et al. Sarcopenia is Predictive of Functional Outcomes in Older Trauma Patients. Cureus [Internet]. 201911(11):e6154.
43. Joyce PR, O'Dempsey R, Kisby G, Anstey C. A retrospective observational study of sarcopenia and outcomes in critically ill patients. Anaesth Intensive Care. 2020;48(3):229-35.
44. Akahoshi T, Yasuda M, Momii K, Kubota K, Shono Y, Kaku N, et al. Sarcopenia is a predictive factor for prolonged intensive care unit stays in high-energy blunt trauma patients. Acute Med Surg. 2016;3(4):326-31.

CHAPTER 43

Feeding Options in Patients with Intra-abdominal Hypertension

Sunil Karanth, Mahesha P

INTRODUCTION

Intra-abdominal hypertension and abdominal compartmental syndrome is a common complication due to a plethora of ICU-requiring illnesses. Intra-abdominal hypertension (IAH) is defined as an abdominal pressure ≥12 mm Hg. When IAH is associated with organ failure, the syndrome is called as abdominal compartmental syndrome (ACS). IAH or ACS based on the cause is classified as "Primary ACS" or "Secondary ACS". Primary ACS includes abdominal trauma (blunt or penetrating), hemorrhage, abdominal aortic aneurysm, intestinal obstruction, retroperitoneal hematoma, etc. On the other hand, secondary causes include ileus, burns, ascites, pregnancy, intraabdominal sepsis, large-volume fluid replacement (>3 L), etc.[1-3]

It is a well-known fact that the mortality and morbidity more than doubles when ACS complicates the underlying illness. Furthermore, ACS itself in turn causes alteration of gut functioning causing intolerance to enteral feeding. In this situation, avoiding enteral nutrition and proceeding with parenteral nutrition further disadvantages the patient from the benefits of enteral nutrition such as gut motility, integrity of the intestinal epithelium, and microcirculation of the intestinal lining. This increases the risk of bacterial translocation and other associated complications.

In summary, ACS sets up a vicious cycle enhancing the risk of bacterial translocation while feeding can increase abdominal distention and worsen the ACS.[4-6]

In this context, it is also important to consider the nutritional needs of the acutely ill patient where the energy expenditure is increased by a mean of 1.49. Literature is sparse in regard to the timing and mode of feeding in this subset of patients developing ACS.[4,7]

It is proven without doubt that enteral nutrition decreases mortality, especially by reducing the incidence of infectious complications, decreasing organ failure, and necessity for surgical intervention. In comparison to parenteral nutrition, feeding through the enteral route is shown to decrease length of hospital stay and is shown to be safer.[8] However, on the contrary enteral nutrition may increase the risk of intraluminal pressure and worsen intraabdominal pressure resulting in severe complications.[9,10]

In view of these contradicting evidences, certain questions that need to be addressed include:
1. When is it safe to feed in patients with IAH?
2. When should enteral nutrition be stopped and alternative routes of feeding considered?

In an observational study of 274 patients with acute pancreatitis of whom

103 developed ACS Marcos-Neira et al. observed that intolerance to enteral nutrition was more in patients who had Grade 3 or 4 IAH with about 59% showing signs of intolerance requiring parenteral nutrition. In general, it is recommended that enteral nutrition can be administered until an IAP of around 15 mm Hg. Once the IAP goes over 15 mm Hg, continuation of enteral nutrition has to be done with caution.[11] In a small RCT of about 60 patients, Sun et al. noted that patients with IAH due to severe acute pancreatitis when started on early enteral nutrition seemed to have a better clinical course of the disease though they had a higher incidence of feed intolerance.[12]

The basic principles regarding the mode of feeding would largely follow the same sequence of escalation as in any other critically ill patient. Most patients with IAH will have gastrointestinal symptoms and signs such as large gastric residual volume, abdominal distention, ileus, etc. If the gastric residues are of large volume, consider nasojejunal feeding. In addition to the mode of feeding, other measures also need to be considered for improving feed tolerance. One of the important methods is to consider starting at a low rate of administration such as 20 mL/h. Two aspects to be carefully considered during enteral nutrition include gastric residual volume and IAP during the feeding. If the IAP increases to a value between 15 and 20 mm increasing the feeds above 20 mL/h can be detrimental. In fact, we may have to actually reduce the highest rates of feeding in such a situation to 20 mL/h or lower.[13] If the goals of nutrition are not met, it may be appropriate to consider parenteral nutrition.

Many of these patients may require decompressive laparotomy (called laparostomy) may often be necessary in patients with ACS as a life-saving procedure. In addition, these are hypercatabolic states with high nitrogen losses and a negative nitrogen balance. Several observational cohort studies have reported the feasibility and safety of initiating enteral feeds in patients with laparostomy. In fact, studies have shown a higher fascial closure rate (odds ratio of 5.3; $p < 0.01$), lower fistula rates, reduced nosocomial infections and lower hospital costs when enteral nutrition is commenced in patients with laparostomy. About 39% of patients with laparostomy were established on full enteral nutrition and tolerated the same well.[14-19]

CONCLUSION

Abdominal compartmental syndrome provides a unique challenge to enteral feeding in critically ill patients. Inability or absence of enteral feeding sets up the vicious cycle of bacterial translocation and further worsening mortality and multiorgan failure consequent to the lack of protective effects of enteral feeding on the intestinal epithelium. However, initiation of enteral feeding should be carefully balanced against the risk of feed intolerance and worsening of IAP. If feed intolerance is significant, a nasojejunal route of feeding may be considered.

REFERENCES

1. Vatankhah S, Sheikhi RA, Heidari M, Moradimajd P. The relationship between fluid resuscitation and intra-abdominal hypertension in patients with blunt abdominal trauma. Int J Crit Illn Inj Sci. 2018;8(3):149-53.
2. Gray S, Christensen M, Craft J. The gastro-renal effects of intra-abdominal hypertension: implications for critical care nurses. Intensive Crit Care Nurs. 2018;48:69-74.
3. Miranda E, Manzur M, Han S, Ham SW, Weaver FA, Rowe VL. Postoperative Development of Abdominal Compartment

Syndrome among Patients Undergoing Endovascular Aortic Repair for Ruptured Abdominal Aortic Aneurysms. Ann Vasc Surg. 2018;49:289-94.
4. Meier RF, Beglinger C. Nutrition in pancreatic diseases. Best Pract Res Clin Gastroenterol. 2006;20:507-29.
5. Dickerson RN, Vehe KL, Mullen JL, Feurer ID. Resting energy expenditure in patients with pancreatitis. Crit Care Med. 1991;19: 484-90.
6. van Brunschot S, Schut AJ, Bouwense SA, Besselink MG, Bakker OJ, van Goor H, et al. Abdominal compartment syndrome in acute pancreatitis: a systematic review. Pancreas. 2014;43(5):665-74.
7. Dickerson RN, Vehe KL, Mullen JL, Feurer ID. Resting energy expenditure in patients with pancreatitis. Crit Care Med. 1991;19: 484-90.
8. McClave SA, Taylor BE, Martindale RG, Warren MM, Johnson DR, Braunschweig C, et al. Guidelines for the provision and assessment of nutrition support therapy in the adult critically ill patient: Society of Critical Care Medicine (SCCM) and American Society for Parenteral and Enteral Nutrition (ASPEN). JPEN J Parenter Enter Nutr. 2016;40:159-211.
9. Marvin RG, McKinley BA, McQuiggan M, Cocanour CS, Moore FA. Nonocclusive bowel necrosis occurring in critically ill trauma patients receiving enteral nutrition manifests no reliable clinical signs for early detection. Am J Surg. 2000;179:7-12.
10. Reintam Blaser A, Starkopf J, Alhazzani W, Berger MM, Casaer MP, Deane AM, et al. Early enteral nutrition in critically ill patients: ESICM clinical practice guidelines. Intensive Care Med. 2017;43:380-98.
11. Marcos-Neira P, Zubia-Olaskoaga F, Lopez-Cuenca S, Bordeje-Laguna L. Epidemiology of Acute Pancreatitis in Intensive Care Medicine Study G. Relationship between intra-abdominal hypertension, outcome and the revised Atlanta and determinant-based classifications in acute pancreatitis. BJS Open. 2017;1:175-81.
12. Sun JK, Li WQ, Ke L, Tong ZH, Ni HB, Li G, et al. Early enteral nutrition prevents intra-abdominal hypertension and reduces the severity of severe acute pancreatitis compared with delayed enteral nutrition: a prospective pilot study. World J Surg. 2013;37:2053-60.
13. Reintam Blaser A, Malbrain M, Regli A. Abdominal pressure and gastrointestinal function: an inseparable couple? Anaesthesiol Intensive Ther. 2017;49:146-58.
14. Tsuei BJ, Magnuson B, Swintosky M, Flynn J, Boulanger BR, Ochoa JB, et al. Enteral nutrition in patients with an open peritoneal cavity. Nutr Clin Pract. 2003;18:253-8.
15. Cothren CC, Moore EE, Ciesla DJ, Johnson JL, Moore JB, Haenel JB, et al. Postinjury abdominal compartment syndrome does not preclude early enteral feeding after definitive closure. Am J Surg. 2004;188: 653-8.
16. Byrnes MC, Reicks P, Irwin E. Early enteral nutrition can be successfully implemented in trauma patients with an "open abdomen". Am J Surg. 2010;199:359-62. discussion 63.
17. Burlew CC, Moore EE, Cuschieri J, Jurkovich GJ, Codner P, Nirula R, et al. Who should we feed? Western Trauma Association multi-institutional study of enteral nutrition in the open abdomen after injury. J Trauma Acute Care Surg. 2012;73:1380-7. discussion 7e8.
18. Collier B, Guillamondegui O, Cotton B, Donahue R, Conrad A, Groh K, et al. Feeding the open abdomen. J Parenter Enter Nutr. 2007;31:410-5.
19. Dissanaike S, Pham T, Shalhub S, Warner K, Hennessy L, Moore EE, et al. Effect of immediate enteral feeding on trauma patients with an open abdomen: protection from nosocomial infections. J Am Coll Surg. 2008;207:690-7.

CHAPTER 44

Nutrition and Wound Healing

Sónia Maria Cabral

■ INTRODUCTION

The formation of wounds results from a disarrangement of the integrity of the skin, the upper layers of the mucous membrane, or organ tissue. Wounds occur as a part of a disease process or have accidental or intentional causes. The wound healing process is a natural physiological response to tissue damage, and upon injury, numerous cellular and extracellular pathways are activated to restore tissue integrity.[1]

Wound healing is a process that implicates a complex coordination of biological and molecular events that involve cell migration, cell proliferation, and extracellular matrix deposition (ECM).[2] Cellular responses to inflammatory mediators, to growth factors and cytokines, and to mechanical forces must be appropriate and precise.[3]

The normal wound healing includes four phases, hemostasis, inflammation, proliferation, and remodeling. Each phase is distinct and continuous with each phase overlapping the next.[3] Successful wound healing requires adequate blood and nutrients to be supplied to the site of damage, so the overall health and nutritional status of the patient has an enormous influence on the outcome of the damaged tissue.[4] Precisely because of so many factors that influence wound healing, the wound patients should have a holistic approach that considers coexisting physical and psychological factors, including nutritional status and disease states such as diabetes, cancer, and arthritis.

Best practice requires exploring all possible contributing factors to a physiologic environment conducive to tissue repair and regeneration.

■ ACUTE AND CHRONIC WOUNDS

The repair processes are similar besides the etiology of the wound. A wound results in tissue damage which stimulates a coordinated physiological response to provide hemostasis and initiate the processes of inflammation, proliferation, and remodeling.[5]

The type, size, and depth of wounds have significant repercussions on cellular and molecular events that occur after cutaneous injury, Falanga[3] mentioned the importance of the division of the wound-healing process into four overlapping steps of coagulation, inflammation, migration-proliferation, and remodeling because while acute wounds show a linear progression of these overlapping events, the progression in chronic wounds does not occur in synchrony, with some areas being in different phases at the same time. The growing prevalence of diabetes, obesity, changing lifestyle, and the aging population contributes to an increase in the incidence of chronic wounds.[6] They are described by an extended inflammatory response with low levels of growth factors and an increased wound bioburden,[7] so wounds usually heal in 4-6 weeks but chronic wounds are those that fail to heal within this period of time.[8]

FOUR PHASES OF WOUND HEALING

Wound healing involves a complex interaction between numerous cell types, cytokines, mediators, and the vascular system as a natural physiological response to a tissue injury. The initial phase is the achievement of *hemostasis* which is characterized by an efflux of lymphatic fluid and blood.[8] The primary goal is to stop the bleeding, so initially it takes part the cascade of vasoconstriction of blood vessels and platelet aggregation, which creates a transient ischemic state at the wound site through thrombosis.[8,9] This vasoconstriction is a sudden mechanism that is soon followed by vasodilation, which favors the influx of white cells and more thrombocytes.[8]

The inflammatory phase generally lasts up to 6 days and uses neutrophils, monocytes, and other inflammatory cells to promote phagocytosis and eliminate bacteria to finally clean the wound.[8,10] Simultaneously, fibroblast cells initiate surfacing a collagen network to stabilize the wound and organize the wound for epithelialization.[10] At the very same time, angiogenesis progresses. So, the proliferative phase is identified and it establishes in 5-7 days. The proliferative or granulation phase does not appear at a discrete time but is continuing all the time in the background.

About 2-3 weeks after the initial injury, the wound commences to mature, remodeling the collagen made during the proliferative phase and contracting to minimize defects. Wound contraction appears to a much higher extent in secondary healing than in primary healing. This mechanism takes longer than 12 months and is recognized as the maturation or remodeling phase.[8,10]

Describing all these wound healing phases it seems that wound healing is a continuous process, but this is not regularly what happens. Wounds usually fluctuate between different stages of healing beneath the influence of various internal and external factors.[2,10]

FACTORS THAT INFLUENCE WOUND HEALING

Many clinically significant factors are known to lead to impair wound healing. The main causes are hypoxia, bacterial colonization, ischemia, reperfusion injury, altered cellular response, and collagen synthesis defects. These can arise from a systemic illness, such as diabetes, or chronic conditions, such as smoking or malnutrition. Local causes that can decrease wound healing are pressure, tissue edema, hypoxia, infection, maceration, and dehydration.[8]

Age is also a risk factor for an impair in wound healing because the elderly people have a mole fragile epidermal layer and have slower inflammatory, migratory, and proliferation responses. They are more likely to have chronic disease that combined with having a slower wound healing makes them at higher risk of wound complications.[1]

In addition, a healing wound has high metabolic demands, made by the inflammation and cellular activity, which may require increased protein or amino acids, vitamins, and minerals.[7]

NUTRITION

It has long been admitted that nutritional status can influence wound healing. In the 15th century, the Portuguese explorer, Vasco da Gama, noted that sailors with scurvy had multiple and nonhealing skin lesions.

It was only in 1747 that James Lind, a Scottish surgeon, described that citrus fruits could successfully treat scurvy and enhance wound repair.[1]

Because the wound healing process has long-term potential, nutrition must be considered in wound prevention (e.g., pressure sores in inpatients) in wound preparation (e.g., preoperative evaluation) and in wound management, acute and chronic.[7] Malnutrition is a prevalent donor to wound chronicity.

Certain nutritional risk factors can lead to impaired wound healing by maintaining inflammation, inhibiting fibroblast function, and lessening angiogenesis and collagen deposition.

Malnutrition consists of limited intake, excessive intake, and specific nutritional deficiencies. Risk factors for malnutrition consist of loss of appetite, impotence of eating or needing help with eating, impaired taste and smell, and too little or too much energy, protein, body fluids, or micronutrients. Older adults are at higher risk of malnutrition due to medical, psychological, physiological, and social and economic problems associated with old age.[7]

There are some nutrients which role is the most relevant for wound healing, the macronutrients: proteins, carbohydrates and lipids, amino acids (arginine and glutamine), and the micronutrients: vitamins A, C, D, zinc, and copper.

ROLE OF MACRONUTRIENTS: PROTEINS, CARBOHYDRATES, AND LIPIDS

Proteins

Proteins are a crucial building block for tissue growth, cell renewal, and repair. They play a fundamental role in all four moments of the wound healing process because of their physiological functions in reinforcing the immune system, participating in epidermal growth and keratinization, creating collagen and elastic tissue, and synthesizing deoxyribonucleic acid (DNA) and ribonucleic acid (RNA).[9]

Some patient populations such as older adults (>65 years), patients with difficult-to-heal wounds, with venous insufficiency wounds and ambulatory outpatients with leg ulcers have a higher risk of protein deficiency. To calculate protein requirements, one must consider the patient's actual weight, wound proportions, and the type of wound. The general recommendations for protein intake and for patients with wounds are 1–2 g/kg and 1 mL/(kcal/day) of fluid intake but may differ according to wound severity.[9] Patients with pressure ulcers, the average protein requirement is 0.95 g/(kg/day) but it may vary between 0.75 and 1.30 g/(kg/day) according to wound severity.[9] In older patients, these protein requirements may be underestimated because of three main reasons: polypharmacy, social factors, such as reduced income or a difficulty in getting food provisions, leading to a lower intake and development of achlorhydria related to gastric mucosal atrophy, resulting in pernicious anemia (B_{12} deficiency) and bacterial overgrowth in the small intestine, leading to nutrients malabsorption.

Chronic protein malnutrition is related with deficiencies that are responsible for a slow-healing time and an increased risk of new wounds.

To optimize the metabolism, it is important to add supplementation with zinc and copper, because they are cofactors that play an important role in promoting proper folding for proteins and maintaining the wound environment to induce tissue regeneration.

Carbohydrates

Particularly during the proliferative phase, carbohydrates stimulate insulin production, which is very important for the anabolic processes of wound healing. Carbohydrates also play a critical role in this particular phase by arranging energy in the form of adenosine 5'-triphosphate (ATP) for metabolic processes, such as fibroblast proliferation and regeneration.[7,9]

Glucose deficiency is a worry in malnourished patients with wounds; however, hyperglycemia in diabetic populations with wounds is also a worrying issue because of its association with an increased risk of infection.[9]

Older age, pancreatic tumors, low body mass index (BMI <18.5 kg/m^2), disorders of the adrenal and pituitary glands, and hepatitis are the contributing factors to hypoglycemia or glucose deficiency. There are also factors that indicate a higher risk for hyperglycemia which includes corticosteroids and antibiotic use, intravenous (IV) fluids with dextrose, physiological stress, counter-regulatory hormones, diabetes, and insulin resistance.[7,9]

Low-glucose levels have an influence in the ability of fibroblasts proliferation and have been recorded in the wound fluid of patients with difficult-to-heal wounds. Instead, patients with a wound, hyperglycemia has been demonstrated to higher their risk of infectious complications and reduce the ability of granulocytes to function. Maintaining homeostatic levels is of paramount importance when studying the effects of carbohydrate and blood sugar levels on the wound-healing process.[9]

Carbohydrate intake in wound patients is consistent with traditional dietary recommendations and represents 45–60% of total daily calories. Daily calorie intake should be determined on an individual basis, as recommendations vary based on gender, weight, and overall nutritional status. For patients who are underweight or at risk of weight loss, the caloric intake should be increased to 35–40 kcal/kg bodyweight.[9] This caloric intake must have a very low progression especially if the patient has risk of refeeding syndrome.

Lipids and Essential Fatty Acids

Lipids and essential fatty acids participate in the three phases of wound healing, the hemostatic, the inflammatory and the proliferative phase. They provide an extra source of energy, increase absorption of fat-soluble nutrients so important to the wound-healing process, and assist in structural functions during tissue growth.[9]

Lipid deficiency is associated with many risk factors and comorbidities, which consists the inflammatory bowel disease, massive bowel resection, particularly of the distal jejunum and ileum, enterocutaneous fistulas involving the small bowel, cystic fibrosis, pancreatic enzyme insufficiency, bariatric surgery, long-term parenteral nutrition with limited or no intravenous fat emulsion provision, intravenous fat emulsion shortage, carnitine deficiency, extreme oral diet, or enteral fat restriction.

Adequate fat intake in patients with acute or chronic wounds can provide additional energy for the wound-healing process as well as structural functions including axonal myelination and lipid bilayers of cell and organellar membranes during tissue growth. Dietary fat plays an important role in ATP production via beta oxidation, which leads to other energy consuming processes that store proteins for wound healing.

Fat intake also plays an important role in the absorption of fat-soluble micronutrients, including vitamin A and omega-3 and omega-6 fatty acids. Omega-6 fatty acids are important precursors for the production of prostaglandins, thromboxane, and leukotrienes in the inflammatory response, deriving in platelet aggregation and inflammatory vasoconstriction.[7]

While omega-6 fatty acids have a pro-inflammatory response, the omega-3 fatty acids result in the liberation of cytokines resulting in an anti-inflammatory response. This decreases tensile strength of the wound and finally obstructs the healing process.[9]

Supplements during the inflammatory phase in a 1:1 ratio of omega-6 to omega-3 have been recommended as useful, however, it stills unclear the entire effect of essential fatty acids on wound healing.[7]

The recommended lipid supplement to be delivered through enteral or parenteral methods is a formula enriched with vitamins C, E, and A, copper, manganese, zinc, eicosapentaenoic acid (EPA), and γ-linolenic acid.[9]

It continuous uncertain the exact way in which lipid deficiency would abnormally restrain the normal wound healing process, evidence suggests that lipid supplements may assist in expediting later stages of healing by minimizing tissue injury during the inflammatory response.[9]

Moreover, comparing with isonitrogenous/isocaloric formulas, lipid-enriched formulas appeared to decrease serum CRP levels and inhibit the development of pressure ulcers. This suggests that lipid supplementation will primarily promote and improve the normal wound-healing process, in contrast to the negative effects associated with lipid deficiency.[9]

More knowledge is required on when to supplement fatty acids, what types and in what ratio are needed, as many studies in such a way have been confounded due to a multisupplement approach.[7]

MICRONUTRIENTS: VITAMINS A, C, D, ZINC, AND COPPER

The micronutrient category includes organic (vitamin) and inorganic (mineral) compounds required in small amounts.

Studies on supplemental amounts of each micronutrient have yet to be determined.

Micronutrient supplementation in healthy individuals can be determined based on recommendations, while adequate micronutrient supplementation in a patient population requires individual consideration as micronutrient levels may be compromised.[9]

Vitamin A

Vitamin A, a fat-soluble vitamin found in plant foods, in its active form, retinol, plays an important role in the inflammatory and proliferative phases of wound healing. In the initial stages of wound healing, deficiency of vitamin A can lead to B- and T-cell dysfunction and consequent antibody production.[7,9] Retinol also helps to initiate epidermal proliferation and re-epithelialization in the proliferative phase by binding to retinoic acid receptors on cell surface membranes. Vitamin A has been shown to promote dermal growth by inhibiting collagenase and surely affect collagen stability required during the proliferation and maturation phases, respectively. Finally, vitamin A also helps to alleviate the detrimental consequences of corticosteroids on wound healing.[7]

Dietary reference intake (DRI)[11] for daily intake of vitamin A is 700 mg/day for women and 900 mg/day for men (2,310 and 3,333 IU, respectively).[12] Documented recommendations to promote wound healing in injured patients include a range of 10,000–50,000 IU/day for 10 days or 10,000 IU intramuscularly.[12]

People more vulnerable to vitamin A deficiency include people with diabetes or those being treated with glucocorticoids, radiation, or chemotherapy. In patients with renal or hepatic insufficiency or protein deficiency, high vitamin A supplementation may be detrimental due to retinol-binding protein deficiency.[9]

It is important to know that vitamin A deficiency can also be caused by a lack of zinc, a cofactor needed for the body's oxidative synthesis of retinol to retinal.[9]

Vitamin A deficiency is harmful to the wound healing process because it can interfere with the production of the B-cells and T-cells needed to protect against initially infectious bacteria during the inflammatory phase and can also delay wound healing, and in the re-epithelialization and stability of collagen in proliferative and maturation stages.

Vitamin C

Vitamin C, a water-soluble vitamin found in fruits and vegetables, has an important role in the inflammatory, proliferative, and remodeling phases in its active form, ascorbic acid.[9] Throughout the inflammatory phase, vitamin C aids in immune regulation and antioxidant function. Along with vitamin A, vitamin C helps to maintain a healthy ratio of antioxidants to pro-oxidants. During proliferative and maturation phases, vitamin C raises capillary strength, collagen tensile strength, fibroblast proliferation, and wound matrix deposition.[12,13]

Research on recommended daily vitamin C supplements is inconclusive. However, based on general knowledge of the energy required for wound healing, 100-200 mg daily is recommended for patients with vitamin C deficiency or wounds including stage I or II pressure ulcers, and up to 1-2 g daily with more complex wounds, including stage III or IV pressure sores or severe trauma until healed.[12]

Vitamin C deficiency has been linked to adults over the age of 65 years, chronic smokers, and patients with chronic conditions such as cancer, cardiovascular disease, and rheumatoid arthritis.[13]

During the inflammatory phase, vitamin C deficiency gets itself evident by increasing the risk of infection. A clearer consequence of deficiency is seen during the proliferative and remodeling stages, when the risk of wound dehiscence increases.[9]

Vitamin D

Vitamin D, a fat-soluble vitamin found in milky products, poultry, and fish, plays an important role in hemostasis, inflammation, and proliferative phases.

In addition to helping the body absorb and use calcium and phosphorus to maintain bone and tooth density, vitamin D plays an important role in immune system function.[9,14]

Research on recommended daily vitamin C supplements is inconclusive. However, based on general knowledge, although research on vitamin D and wound healing is a new field, it is believed to have immunomodulatory effects that directly affect B- and T-cells and also increase the production of beneficial anti-inflammatory cytokines. Interleukin-10 (IL-10).[14] During the initial immune response in the hemostatic and inflammatory phases, vitamin D prepares B- and T-cells to respond by stimulating and suppressing the respective phenotypes of both cells.[14] Vitamin D affects the proliferative phase by inducing the antibacterial peptide cathelicidin, which promotes wound healing.[15] This study hypothesizes that vitamin D helps to prevent infection and maintain membrane structure integrity. Recently discovered vitamin D receptors in various tissue types also suggest that low levels of the trace element reduce membrane integrity and permeability to essential cell signals.[9]

Due to gaps in the literature, there is no consensus on the daily amount of vitamin D during wound healing, but a general guideline has been found to be around 5,000–50,000 IU.[9]

Vitamin D toxicity can lead to hypercalcemia, which can lead to kidney stones and other side effects. Populations at risk of vitamin D toxicity include those taking vitamin D supplements during wound healing and those already taking vitamin D supplements to treat hypoparathyroidism, osteomalacia, or end-stage renal disease.[16]

Zinc

Zinc plays several biochemical roles in wound healing, including catalysis and regulation of gene activity.[9] In general, zinc has two major functions in wound healing: ECM remodeling and ROS reduction. Zinc is a cofactor for matrix metalloproteinases (MMPs), which are responsible for breaking down ECM proteins.[17] Insufficient availability of zinc ions causes a lack of MMPs in wounds. As a result, zinc deficiency reduces the ability to degrade the extracellular matrix and reduces scar tissue cell turnover (i.e., the rate at which new cells are formed and old cells are shed or broken down).[9]

Zinc deficiency affects all stages of wound healing. In the inflammatory phase, immunity decreases and susceptibility to infections increases. In the proliferative phase, collagen synthesis and tensile strength are impaired, and in the remodeling phase, fibroblast proliferation, collagen synthesis, and epithelialization disappear.[7] However, excess zinc can interfere with the absorption of other cations, especially iron and copper, so supplements should be avoided unless deficient. The most common causes of zinc deficiency include diarrhea, malabsorption, and hypermetabolic conditions including stress, sepsis, and burns.[7]

Daily zinc intake is necessary as there is no known physiological mechanism for its accumulation. The recommended daily dose is 11 mg for males of 19 years old, 8 mg for females of 19 years old, and 11–13 mg for pregnant women, depending on age/time of breastfeeding.[18]

Recommendations for zinc supplementation in the zinc-deficient patient range from 40 mg/day up to 220 mg two times per day for 10–14 days.[7]

Copper

Copper is an essential mineral that plays an important role in connective tissue synthesis and angiogenesis in wound healing. Because of this, there are dozens of proteins that contribute to copper homeostasis in the face of stimuli such as trauma and stress. Copper supplementation is a concern of healthcare professionals. Because of its widespread distribution in various tissue types, there are few reliable methods for measuring actual body copper reserves.[19]

Ceruloplasmin is a common indicator of copper status, and serum copper is another commonly used indicator, but is insensitive and falsely elevated during the acute phase reaction. Copper deficiency can be caused by high doses of zinc supplements as well as conditions such as gastrointestinal malabsorption, severe burns, and cholestasis.[19,20]

The upper limit for copper intake is approximately 10 mg/day for adults.[20]

Amino Acids

Amino acids, especially arginine and glutamine, have been implicated in the role of wound healing.[7] Arginine is a conditionally essential amino acid synthesized by the kidneys and liver, normally from citrulline. Arginine is a precursor to nitric oxide, which is essential for the inflammatory process of wound healing, but is also used for collagen production. Arginine is also a precursor to proline, which is essential for collagen synthesis. Arginine supplementation has been shown to increase collagen deposition in wounds.

Administration of arginine to improve wound healing demonstrated that oral supplementation with up to 20 g/day is safe and relatively well tolerated in adults,[21] but to date there is no recommendation for maximum dose.

Like arginine, glutamine is also conditionally essential and can be produced endogenously. However, situations like increased demand and metabolic stress may require supplementation.[7] Glutamine decreases infectious complications and protects against inflammatory injury by inducing the expression of heat shock proteins.[22]

In critical situations such as trauma, burns, and sepsis, glutamine supplementation has been shown to improve intestinal function, reduce septic complications, and improve insulin sensitivity.[22] However, for chronic wounds without chronic inflammatory conditions, the role of glutamine supplementation is unclear. In conditions of chronic malnutrition, atrophy of the intestinal mucosa and general decrease in muscle mass may increase the replenishment role, reducing glutamine stores and thus increasing the need for exogenous glutamine. As with arginine, most researches on glutamine supplementation are confounded by the use of a combination supplement.[22] However, researchers repeatedly say that glutamine and arginine should not be considered substitutes for correcting malnutrition, and supplementation is not worthwhile without overall adequate protein intake.[7]

Fluids

The function of fluid in wound healing is to maintain skin turgor and promote tissue perfusion and oxygenation. The goal for fluid intake in patients with wounds is approximately 1 mL/kcal/day, but should be adjusted for insensible losses or comorbid renal or cardiac disease.[7]

CONCLUSION

Screening for the risk of malnutrition and diminishing nutritional deficiencies in susceptible patient groups must be a priority for reducing morbidity and healthcare costs associated with difficult healing wounds. Some of the most widely known nutrients involved in wound healing are the three macronutrients, glutamine and arginine, vitamins A, C, and D, and the minerals such as zinc and copper. An individualized nutritional assessment must be an integral part of a patient's treatment plan, so in addition to determining which supplement provides the greatest benefit for each patient, accurate daily recommendations tailored to individual needs can be created to optimize benefits and reduce associated risks with toxicity.

Recommendations for nutritional assessment and supplemental nutrition for patients at risk of experiencing wound healing must be followed.

REFERENCES

1. Young A, McNaught CE. The physiology of wound healing. Surgery [Internet]. 2011;29(10):475-9.

2. Barchitta M, Maugeri A, Favara G, San Lio RM, Evola G, Agodi A, et al. Nutrition and wound healing: an overview focusing on the beneficial effects of curcumin. Int J Mol Sci. 2019;20(5):1119.
3. Falanga V. Wound healing and its impairment in the diabetic foot. Lancet. 2005; 366(9498):1736-43.
4. MacKay D, Miller AL. Nutritional Support for Wound Healing. Altern Med Rev. 2003;8(4): 359-77.
5. Broughton G, Janis JE, Attinger CE. The basic science of wound healing. Plast Reconstr Surg. 2006;117(7 suppl):12S-34S.
6. Serena TE, Yaakov RA, DeLegge M, Mayhugh TA, Moore S. Nutrition in patients with chronic non-healing ulcers: a paradigm shift in wound care. Chronic Wound Care Manag Res. 2018;5:5-9.
7. Quain AM, Khardori NM. Nutrition in wound care management: a comprehensive overview. Wounds. 2015;27(12):327-35.
8. Wallace HA, Basehore BM, Zito PM. Wound Healing Phases. Treasure Island (FL): StatPearls Publishing; 2023.
9. Penny H, Flores R, Pennington E, Pedersen A, Tran S. The role of macronutrients and micronutrients in wound healing: a narrative review. J Wound Care. 2022;31(Suppl 5): S14-S22.
10. Ghaly P, Iliopoulos J, Ahmad M. The role of nutrition in wound healing: An overview. Br J Nurs. 2021;30(5):S38-42.
11. National Academies. (2023). Dietary Reference Intakes Collection. dietary-reference-intakes @ nap.nationalacademies.org [Internet]. [online] Available from: https://nap.nationalacademies.org/collection/57/dietary-reference-intakes [Last accessed June, 2023].
12. Stechmiller JK. Understanding the role of nutrition and wound healing. Nutr Clin Pract. 2010;25(1):61-8.
13. Doseděl M, Jirkovský E, Macáková K, Krčmová LK, Javorská L, Pourová J, et al. Vitamin C—sources, physiological role, kinetics, deficiency, use, toxicity, and determination. Nutrients. 2021;13(2):1-36.
14. Azrielant S, Shoenfeld Y. Vitamin D and the immune system. Isr Med Assoc J. 2017; 19(8):510-1.
15. Zhang Y, Wu S, Sun J. Vitamin D, vitamin D receptor and tissue barriers. Tissue Barriers. 2013;1(1):e23118.
16. Marcinowska-Suchowierska E, Kupisz-Urbanska M, Lukaszkiewicz J, Pludowski P, Jones G. Vitamin D Toxicity: a clinical perspective. Front Endocrinol (Lausanne). 2018;9:1-7.
17. Caley MP, Martins VLC, O'Toole EA. Metalloproteinases and wound healing. Adv Wound Care. 2015;4(4):225-34.
18. National Institute of Health. (2022). Health information: Zinc. a37d7b61312d05bd8804 13494eb8c28ece7bb585@ods.od.nih.gov[Internet].[online] Available from: https://ods.od.nih.gov/factsheets/Zinc-Health Professional/ [Last accessed June, 2023].
19. Livingstone C. Review of Copper Provision in the Parenteral Nutrition of Adults. Nutr Clin Pract. 2017;32(2):153-65.
20. National Institute of Health. (2022). Health information: Copper. c6a174e6089f f8538c4f22f5c1b44b8fe140d6f1 @ods.od.nih.gov [Internet]. [online] Available from: https://ods.od.nih.gov/factsheets/Copper-Consumer/ [Last accessed June, 2023].
21. Alexander JW, Supp DM. Role of Arginine and Omega-3 Fatty Acids in Wound Healing and Infection. Adv Wound Care. 2014;3(11):682-90.
22. Arribas-lópez E, Omorogieva O, Zand N, Snowden MJ, Kochhar T. A meta-analysis of the effect on wound healing of amino acids arginine and glutamine. Nutrients. 2021;13(8):2498.

SECTION 7: Organization of Nutritional Support Teams

45. **Nutrition Support Team**
    Bamini Arthi G Murugesh

46. **Is it Cost-effective to Feed Critically Ill Patients?**
    Sadanand Kulkarni, Sunil Honkalas

CHAPTER 45

Nutrition Support Team

Bamini Arthi G Murugesh

INTRODUCTION

The nutrition support teams (NSTs) are responsible for medical nutritional therapy and artificial nutrition support in hospitalized patients. The multidirectional and multidisciplinary approach improves the quality of treatment that helps to reduce the length of hospital stay and speedy recovery. NSTs were instituted to address the need for the safe implementation and management of parenteral and enteral nutrition (EN).[1] Nutritional therapy is urgently needed in malnourished patients to counteract negative metabolic and clinical consequences, to speed up recovery processes, and to improve patient outcomes.[2] Multifaceted clinical knowledge is required to ensure optimal nutritional support, according to a patient's individual situation and to avoid potential complications. Nutrition therapy has been declared as a basic global human right.[3]

EMERGENCE OF THE NUTRITION SUPPORT TEAMS

Only a few teams existed before 1975. Most countries formed teams after 1980. An examination of the results of two surveys performed in 1983 revealed the following facts about early NSTs. By 1975, the growing interest in nutrition support led to the formation of the American Society for Parenteral and Enteral Nutrition (ASPEN), dietitians in critical care, a dietetics practice of the American Dietetic Association (ADA), was established in 1978. After which many other guidelines have been published including from the European Society of Clinical Nutrition and Metabolism (ESPEN).[4]

A study in 2005 found that NSTs were present in 2.8% of the hospital in Germany, 7.9% in Austria, and 2.4% in Switzerland. 10 years later, a survey indicated that 62% hospitals had NST. Current data for Nutrition Day worldwide shows that most hospitals in Europe and the USA have NSTs with at least a physician and one dietitian. The composition of the team may vary according to local needs and options in terms of human resources. This highlights the rising importance of NST in industrialized countries.[5]

NEED FOR THE NUTRITION SUPPORT TEAMS

Nutrition support teams play a vital role to identifying the early detection of malnutrition and providing appropriate nutrition intervention for positive outcomes. Decreased waste and more appropriate use of parenteral nutrition (PN). Improved reimbursement and cost savings improved quality of care and outcomes optimized care in disease states including trauma, critical illness, coronavirus disease 2019 (COVID-19), esophageal cancer, liver cirrhosis, gastrostomy tube use, and maintenance were also improved.[6-10]

GOALS OF THE NUTRITION SUPPORT TEAMS

The major goals of NST include: Inpatient consultation, Home Nutrition Support Program, and Educational Program and Research.

Inpatient Consultation

Inpatient consultation includes: Assessment, therapy, monitoring, and standardization of practice.

One of the many things that distinguishes successful NST was nearly close coordination among team members to deliver comprehensive and cost-effective patient care. NSTs treat malnutrition: Assessing the patient's nutritional status using different tools, providing appropriate nutritional intervention, monitoring the progress of the patient's recovery closely for better outcomes, prevent or avoid complications including metabolic or mechanical problems.

Home Nutrition Support Program

Recent trends and protocols have been the shift in the use of PN and EN from the hospital to the home. As cost containment continues to focus on decreasing length of hospital stay, opportunities for home nutrition therapy will continue to increase. NST must ensure that the patient meets eligibility criteria for either EN or PN at home. As soon as a patient is identified as a home nutrition support candidate, the team begins assessing that person's discharge needs and educating the patient and the family in formula administration and care of the access site. NST should be visiting the patient at home or should at least encourage patients to visit nutrition support outpatient clinic regularly for monitoring.

Educational Program and Research

Nutrition support team should develop clinical nutrition guidelines and standards of care, and be a center of knowledge on education, training, and researches. NSTs must conduct and participate in research that contributes to the nutrition support knowledge, performing clinical efficacy, and cost-effectiveness studies. This helps to getting better data for documenting patterns of use of PN and EN in a variety of patient care settings.

NUTRITION SUPPORT TEAM MEMBERS

High-performing teams have three essential psychological needs: (1) Autonomy, (2) competence, and (3) relatedness.[11] NST includes one physician, a clinical dietitian, a nurse, and a clinical pharmacist, collaboration between whom requires a great deal effort on the part of all team members. The roles and responsibility of each professional must be clearly defined.

Nutrition support team policies and procedures are clearly detailed and must be codified in policy and procedure manuals that are periodically updated as needed. The goals, mission, vision, and values of the NST should be clearly articulated. The various functions to be accomplished should be outlined, including which member, practicing at "top of license," should usually be responsible for performing each function. Individuals of another discipline might need to conduct the function in a transdisciplinary fashion, provided it is within the scope of their license and/or certification.[12-14]

Physician

The NST physician (medicine, surgery, gastroenterology, nephrology, critical care, and anesthesiology) becomes the head and director of NST. They must be responsible for the medical direction of the team, overseeing all patients care activities. The physician must review the nutrition assessment form and approve the therapeutic nutrition plan. The physician also monitors the patient throughout therapy by evaluating the impacts of changes in clinical status on the nutrition support regimen. They also communicate with other professionals when there is a conflict of opinion regarding the plan of care and take appropriate decisions.

Clinical Dietitian

The clinical dietitian plays a key role in NST. The responsibility of the clinical dietitian begins after a patient identified through nutrition screening is referred to the NST for a more detailed assessment and decisions regarding specialized nutrition care. The first objective of the clinical dietitian is to determine the route of nutrition support whether oral enteral or parenteral, using established guidelines such as those of ASPEN.[15] Nutritional status is assessed and classified as borderline, mild, or severe. More recently a simplified and standardized tool is the Global Leadership in Malnutrition (GLIM) criteria to identify malnutrition, after intervention must be appropriate to the clinical condition.[2] The clinical dietitian monitors the patient daily for tolerance and balances the need for transitional feeds from PN to EN and then on to oral. Ensuring the requirement of calorie, protein, and other nutrients are met during the transition feed. Communication with all other team members by progress notes is documented in medical records, and also by verbal reports is important.[16]

Nurse

The NST nurse plays a major contribution in actual implementation of nutrition support, particularly in administration of feeding formulations and management of access devices. They assess the changes of nutrition requirements and clinical status of the patients and also support physicians during procedures and monitor the transition of care planning. Additional nursing duties and responsibilities include facilitating discharge planning, and educating patients and family in techniques of home nutrition support.

Clinical Pharmacist

The NST pharmacist is an expert on compounding PN formulation, ensuring the availability and stability of the PN products in the pharmacy. The pharmacist evaluates infusion for possible incompatibility with admixtures additives. Pharmacists provide expertise on nutrient-nutrient, drugs nutrient and drug-disease interactions, and drug-induced feeding intolerance, and other side effects.[17] Pharmacists help to teach home nutrition support techniques to patients and their families, especially when it comes to home PN. Again, communication with other team members is important.

NUTRITION SUPPORT TEAMS: EFFICACY AND EFFECTIVENESS

Innovation of NSTs would be progression to a transdisciplinary action and incorporation of all functions into the organized nutrition team's numerous responsibilities.[1] Involvement of NST results in more appropriate indications for PN or EN as a result, many labor—intensive intervention.[18] In the study of Sriram et al., the number of indicated parenteral therapies increased from 71.3 to 83.4% between 2003 and 2006.[19] At the same time, nonindicated interventions decreased from 16.5 to 8.9%, indicting a sign of higher quality of treatment.[19] Biotano et al. investigated compliance with the ASPEN guidelines for PN, which were implemented between 2007 and 2010.[20] Through the intervention of NST, metabolic complications could be significantly reduced from 66 to 34%. The percentage of patients receiving PN decreased to 35% which leads to more appropriate enteral tube feeding. Significant cost-saving was achieved due to NST involvement.[21] A more recent study by Park et al. showed that the early intervention of NST in critically ill patients with gastrointestinal diseases positively influences survival. NST involvement enabled reaching energy and protein requirements within 3 days, shortened the length of stay, quality of life, functional status, clinical outcomes were therefore significantly improved.[22]

An interdisciplinary approach to nutrition therapy is an effective cost-containment tool by improving quality of treatment, avoiding unnecessary interventions, and simplifying management. This is pertinent to modern healthcare policies. The key task of NST is to implement a comprehensive nutritional care system, so that every patient who could potentially benefit from nutritional support receives it rapidly, adequately, and with the highest standards of quality.[23]

FUTURE OF THE NUTRITION SUPPORT TEAMS

Nutrition support teams need to continually be abreast of technological advances in the field while simultaneously justifying their existence by demonstrating value, defined as the best quality in evidence-based outcomes for the minimum cost.[24-26] Likewise, individual nutrition support clinicians and nutrition-oriented societies should establish and promote nutrition care as a human right.[3,27]

Telenutrition

Technological advances in futures will likely involve computers and will drastically change the work environment for many healthcare practitioners. Physical location will no longer impose constraints on the practice setting. Practitioners will have digital access to patient records in distant hospitals to provide consultation to primary care providers and supervision for students and younger clinicians as preceptors. Expanded computerized information systems will greatly enhance NSTs ability to provide services within multihospital corporations.[28]

Molecular Biology

Equally important is the fact that molecular biology may change the practice of clinical nutrition in more indirect ways than using nutrients to regulate gene expression, nutrient requirements may be altered. Because the technology of molecular biology will bring new products and analytical methods to the field of clinical nutrition.

NUTRITION SUPPORT TEAMS IN CRITICAL CARE MEDICINE

Nutrition support teams in intensive care units (ICUs) have a four-step nutrition care process that align with the needs of critically ill patients.[29] First, NST possesses skills to use accurate tools and to conduct a nutrition assessment. Second, based on the nutrition assessment a diagnosis of malnutrition or malnutrition risk was identified and documented. This data will help appropriate to incorporate nutrition therapy into the overall ICU care plan. Third, NST will facilitate EN or PN. Fourth, monitoring (e.g., drug-nutrient interaction, metabolic complications) and evaluating indicators and outcomes related to the nutrition diagnosis and intervention strategies to achieve the desired outcomes of nutrition care while maintaining patient safety (e.g., monitoring electrolytes for risk of refeeding syndrome and glycemic control impacted by carbohydrate provision/insulin resistance).[30] An important role is to facilitate transitional feeds PN to EN to oral. NST improves the developing ICU educational curriculum, training, research, and administrative activities (e.g., continuous quality improvement).[31]

STRATEGIES FOR SUCCESS FOR THE NUTRITION SUPPORT TEAMS

The most critical task for team survival is to demonstrate reduced healthcare costs, reduced patient complications, and improved patient outcomes owing to team intervention. NST offers placement of central venous catheters and surgically placed enteral feeding tubes, facilitate fluoroscopy and endoscopy for placement of enteral feeding tubes, standardize PN and EN order entries and offer home nutrition support.[20] NST should stay in the spotlight, be accessible, communicative, work with clinicians and other allied staff to build and maintain their support.[32]

CONCLUSION

Looking at the effectiveness of NST and most importantly the benefits in ICU settings, it would be imperative to include NST in every hospital setting. NSTs provide the right nutrition support for the right patient at the right time and in the right way. Re-engineering of NSTs structure and role is inevitable, be tailor-made according to the institution, with clear delineation of roles and responsibilities. NST has proved to be an ideal model for quality care standards, and quality clinical outcome with cost effectiveness. Based on this, hospital administrators and medical staff committees will agree that hospitals cannot afford to be without organized NST.

REFERENCES

1. Barrocas A, Schwartz DB, Bistrian BR, Guenter P, Mueller C, Chernoff R, et al. Nutrition support teams: Institution, evolution, and innovation. Nutr Clin Pract. 2023;38:10-26.
2. Reber E, Strahm R, Bally L, Schuetz P, Stanga Z. Efficacy and Efficiency of Nutritional Support Teams. J Clin Med. 2019;8:1281.
3. Cárdenas D, Davisson Correia MIT, Hardy G, Ochoa JB, Barrocas A, Hankard R, et al. Consensus statement. Nutritional care is a human right: translating principles to clinical practice. Nutr Clin Pract. 2022;57:743-51.
4. Mueller C. The ASPEN Adult Nutrition Support Core Curriculum, 3rd edition. Silver, Spring, MD: American Society for Parenteral and Enteral Nutrition (ASPEN); 2017.
5. Shang E, Hasenberg T, Schlegel B, Sterchi AB, Schindler K, Druml W, et al. A European survey of structure and organization of nutrition support teams in Germany, Austria and Switzerland. Clin Nutr. 2005;24:1005-13.
6. Lee JS, Kang JE, Park SH, Jin HK, Jang SM, Kim SA, et al. Nutrition and clinical outcomes of nutrition support in multidisciplinary team for critically ill patients. Nutr Clin Pract. 2018;33:633-9.
7. Oh E, Shim H, Yon HJ, Moon JS, Kang DR, Jang JY. Effectiveness of a multidisciplinary team for nutrition support in a trauma intensive care unit. Acute Crit Care. 2020;35:142-8.
8. Taylor BR, Grant S, McCoy M, Hart T. Effect of early nutrition support on length of stay, mortality, and extubation in patients with COVID-19. Nutr Clin Pract. 2022;37:852-60.
9. Cong MH, Li SL, Cheng GW, Liu JY, Song CX, Deng YB, et al. An interdisciplinary nutrition support team improves clinical and hospitalized outcomes of esophageal cancer patients with concurrent chemoradiotherapy. Chin Med J. 2015;128:3003-7.
10. Iwasa M, Iwata K, Hara N, Hattori A, Ishidome M, Sekoguchi-Fujikawa N, et al. Nutrition therapy using a multidisciplinary team improves survival rates in patients with liver cirrhosis. Nutrition. 2013;29:1418-21.

11. Friedman R. (2021). 5 things high-performing teams do differently. Harvard Business Review. [online] Available from: https://hbr.org/2021/10/5-things-high-performing-teams-do-differently. [Last accessed June, 2023].
12. McClave SA. What does it mean to "own feeding tubes"? Nutr Clin Pract. 2009;24:430-2.
13. Hall BT, Englehart MS, Blaseg K, Wessel K, Stawicki SP, Evans DC. Implementation of a dietitian-led enteral nutrition support clinic results in quality improvement, reduced readmissions, and cost savings. Nutr Clin Pract. 2014;29:649-55.
14. Moawad H. (2017). Practicing at the top of your license. Medical Economics. [online] Available from: https:// www.medicaleconomics.com/view/practicing-at-the-top-ofyour-license. [Last accessed June, 2023].
15. Corrigan ML, Bobo E, Rollins C, Mogensen KM. Academy of nutrition and dietetics and American society for parenteral and enteral nutrition: Revised 2021 standards of professional performance for registered dietitian nutritionists (competent, proficient, and expert) in nutrition support. Nutr Clin Pract. 2021;36:1126-43.
16. Schneider PJ. Nutrition support teams: An evidence-based practice. Nutr Clin Pract. 2006;21:62-7.
17. Matarese LE, Gottschlich MM. Contemporary Nutrition Support Practice: A Clinical Guide. Eur J Clin Nutr. 1998;52:161.
18. A.S.P.E.N. Practice Management Task Force; Delegge M, Wooley JA, Guenter P, Wright S, Brill J, et al. The state of nutrition support teams and update on current models for providing nutrition support therapy to patients. Nutr Clin Pract. 2010;25:76-84.
19. Sriram K, Cyriac T, Fogg LF. Effect of nutritional support team restructuring on the use of parenteral nutrition. Nutrition. 2010;26:735-9.
20. Boitano M, Bojak S, McCloskey S, McCaul DS, McDonough M. Improving the safety and effectiveness of parenteral nutrition: Results of a quality improvement collaboration. Nutr Clin Pract. 2010;25:663-71.
21. Piquet MA, Bertrand PC, Roulet M. Role of a nutrition support team in reducing the inappropriate use of parenteral nutrition. Clin Nutr. 2004;3:437.
22. Park YE, Park SJ, Park Y, Cheon JH, Kim TI, Kim WH. Impact and outcomes of nutritional support team intervention in patients with gastrointestinal disease in the intensive care unit. Medicine. 2017;96:e8776.
23. Schuetz P, Fehr R, Baechli V, Geiser M, Deiss M, Gomes F, et al. Individualized nutritional support in medical inpatients at nutritional risk: A randomized clinical trial. Lancet. 2019;393:2312-21.
24. Barrocas A. Demonstrating the value of the nutrition support team to the C-suite in a value-based environment: rise or demise of nutrition support teams. Nutr Clin Pract. 2019;34:806-21.
25. Palmer LB, Limketkai BN. Modern challenges to gastrointestinal nutrition physicians and the nutrition support team: cautionary tales and call to action. Nutr Clin Pract. 2020;35:855-9.
26. Tyler R, Barrocas A, Guenter P, Araujo Torres K, Bechtold ML, Chan LN, et al. Value of nutrition support therapy: impact on clinical and economic outcomes in the United States. JPEN J Parenter Enter Nutr. 2020;44:395-406.
27. Cárdenas D, Toulson Davisson Correia MI, Hardy G, Ochoa JB, Barrocas A, Hankard R, et al. Nutritional care is a human right: translating principles to clinical practice. Clin Nutr. 2022;41:1613-8.
28. Mauldin K, Gleng J, Saarony D, Hu C. Performing nutritional assessment remotely via telehealth. Nutr Clin Pract. 2021;36:751-68.
29. Dhaliwal R, Cahill N, Lemieux M, Heyland DK. The Canadian critical care nutrition guidelines in 2013: an update on current recommendations and implementation strategies. Nutr Clin Pract. 2014;29:29-43.
30. Patel JJ, Mundi MS, Taylor B, McClave SA, Mechanick JI. Casting Light on the Necessary, Expansive, and Evolving Role of the Critical Care Dietitian: An Essential Member of the Critical Care Team. Crit Care Med. 2022;50(9):1289-95.
31. Noto MJ, Wheeler AP. Mechanical ventilation, clinical trials, and glaciers. Am J Respir Crit Care Med. 2013;188:128-30.
32. Sriram K, Cresci GAM. Dietitians' Role in Critical Care Interdisciplinary Team Needs Better Recognition. Crit Care Med. 2022;50(7):e658-e659.

CHAPTER 46

Is it Cost-effective to Feed Critically Ill Patients?

Sadanand Kulkarni, Sunil Honkalas

DISEASE-RELATED MALNUTRITION AND ITS COST IMPLICATIONS

Deficiency of various nutrients due to decreased intake, ongoing losses, and/or increased requirements leads to malnutrition in the patients. Pathophysiology of the disease itself, many diagnostic and therapeutic procedures, unawareness, and less interest in patients' nutritional status by the healthcare staff, and the lack of strategies to avoid fasting periods are among the main reasons behind hospital malnutrition. Due to all these, the need to identify patients at risk of malnutrition, periodic reassessment of the risk of malnutrition on an individual basis and, when necessary, employment of preventive measures and treatment has become important.[1]

Disease-related malnutrition (DRM) is associated with significant adverse clinical consequences, including increased risk of infectious and noninfectious complications, increased length of hospitalization, more frequent readmissions, and increased mortality. Therefore, malnourished patients consume an increased proportion of healthcare resources compared with those who are well nourished. Thus, DRM is a very much prevalent condition which may lead to a substantial, significant economic burden on hospitals, payers, and society.[2-4]

The estimated annual economic burden of disease-related malnutrition in public hospitals in Latin America was found to be is $10.19 billion. Critically ill patients accounted for a disproportionate share of the costs with a 6.5-fold higher average cost per patient compared with those in the ward ($5488.35 vs. $839.76).[5]

Recently, to calculate country-specific estimates of the economic burden of hospital malnutrition in Asia, an analysis was done. The data used for this analysis was country-specific cost and prevalence data. Based on this data, the incremental healthcare costs attributable to hospital malnutrition in 11 countries in Asia were calculated.

The reasons and sources of increased cost were increased length of hospital stay and increased antibiotic use in malnourished patients who develop a healthcare-associated infection. It is noteworthy that the costs were calculated separately for the patients in the wards and patients in the intensive care units (ICU). In this analysis, the estimated annual economic burden attributable to hospital malnutrition in Asia has been shown to be $30.1 billion out of which increased LOS accounts for the largest portion of the incremental cost, totalling $23.2 billion (77.2%) in the ward and $3.5 billion (11.5%) in the ICU. It has been depicted in this analysis that medication costs, i.e., costs attributable to antibiotics related to the treatment of infectious complications account for an additional $3.4 billion (11.3%).[6]

All these studies and research have emphasized the need for rigorous screening and assessment as well as continuous monitoring of nutrition status in hospitalized patients to facilitate early identification and proactive management of hospital malnutrition and in turn the attempts to reduce the healthcare costs.

IMPORTANCE OF NUTRITION IN HOSPITALIZED PATIENTS

In addition to primary treatment of the disease, proactive management of hospital malnutrition, designed, individualized nutrition support remains the mainstay in the treatment of patients in hospitals. An important question is whether the nutrition therapy or feeding interventions with any route to the patients improve the outcomes and thereby reduce the healthcare costs.

An emerging and compelling body of research indicates that such interventions delivered in the healthcare system might be associated with improved outcomes and reduced load on healthcare usage and costs.[7,8] Some other authors have concluded that identifying and treating malnutrition are critical to improving patient health outcomes and to reducing healthcare costs.[9]

NUTRITION-FOCUSED QUALITY IMPROVEMENT PROGRAMS

Nutrition-focused quality improvement programs can be used to (a) guide nutrition screening, (b) assessment to identify patients at risk of malnutrition, and (c) manage hospitalized patients at risk for malnutrition.

It is imperative that once decided to intervene with nutrition care when needed, ongoing monitoring and adjustment of nutrition are needed.[10,11]

Implementation of such programs has shown to be associated with improved patient outcomes and decreased healthcare costs, mainly due to reduced rates of hospital-acquired infections, shorter lengths of hospital stay, and lower rates of readmission.[10-13]

METHODS TO PROVIDE NUTRITION IN HOSPITALIZED PATIENTS

Nutritional support can be provided by both enteral and parenteral routes depending on the requirements and given medical circumstances.

The dietary components of a standard nutrition regimen (enteral or parenteral) are the macronutrients (proteins or amino acids, carbohydrate, and lipids or fats), the electrolytes, the micronutrients (trace elements and vitamins), and water. Carbohydrate, in the form of glucose or dextrose, and lipids are the major energy providers; proteins form the building blocks and act as resource in the synthesis of structural and visceral proteins in the body.

Enteral nutrition (EN) can be given by oral route or different types of tubes, viz., nasogastric, nasojejunal, jejunostomy, or gastrostomy tubes. Commonly used formulae in EN are kitchen feeds, polymeric diets, and oligomeric diets.

Parenteral nutrition (PN) can be given by peripheral veins or central veins. There are two ways of providing PN: Single bottle system and two chamber bags or three-chamber bags (3 CBs) or all-in-one (AIO) bags. They are also called as multichamber bags (MCBs). These bags may be compounded in hospital pharmacies, or they are available in the premixed form and are mixed at the bedside before administration.

In general, it has been widely studied as to which route and which modality employed in nutrition helps for cost savings. Economic and ergonomic aspects of the same have been studied.

What the important guidelines have to say?
For patients in ICUs, both American Society for Parenteral and Enteral Nutrition (ASPEN)[14] and the Society of Critical Care Medicine (SCCM)[15] advise to provide an increased amount of protein. Further, they suggest that when volitional intake is not possible, EN formulas containing supplemental immunonutrients can be used in surgical and trauma patients. Suggestion from these societies to employ routine use of postoperative immunonutrition (IM) formulae in the surgical ICU is also noteworthy.

In addition, largely data from randomized controlled clinical trials in patients who had major elective surgery suggest the same. Major elective surgery patients face decreased infectious complications and length of stay (LOS) after receiving high-protein formula containing supplemental L-arginine, ω-3 fatty acids, and nucleotides.

Incidentally, despite the guidelines and existing evidence, large numbers of surgical ICU patients receive lower-cost, and standard high-protein enteral feedings that do not contain added immunonutrients.[16]

IMPACT OF ENTERAL NUTRITION ON HEALTHCARE COSTS

Choice of high-protein EN for patients in the ICU has been shown to have an impact on healthcare resource utilization and daily hospital costs. There is a great correlation between formula ingredients and per-unit costs. That means EN products with added immunonutrients are the most cost-saving option as it may lead to lower total cost of hospitalization, cost per day, cost of ICU stay, and nutrition product cost compared with standard protein formulae.[16]

Gastrointestinal (GI) intolerance is always a concern while providing EN to patients in ICU. Some researchers have studied and quantified the cost of GI intolerance. They have also identified the cost implications of initiating EN with a semi-elemental versus standard polymeric EN formula in ICUs.

It has been shown that prolonged ICU stays are associated with an increased risk for hospital readmission along with death within 30 days of hospital discharge and long-term physical disability among the survivors. GI intolerance has been seen to be associated with frequent feeding interruptions leading to reduction in delivery of daily protein and calories which itself becomes an independent risk factor for prolonged ICU stay and higher mortality rate. In this analysis, they have also demonstrated that the use of a semi-elemental EN formula would be cost saving as it was tolerated better leading to fewer feeding interruptions due to GI intolerance, as compared to a standard polymeric EN formula.[17] However, this does not reduce the importance of the polymeric formulae as they are more commonly available and easy to administer.

Enteral nutrition is helpful in maintaining gut immunity because it has got a direct effect in promoting mucosa-associated lymphoid tissue (MALT) which provides IgA antibodies. Use of EN has been shown to be an important factor in reducing the incidence of pneumonia and intra-abdominal infections. This results in reducing the costs by reducing length of stay and lesser chances of infection.[18,19]

In India and many other Asian countries, specialized enteral feeding can be provided with blenderized kitchen feeds or reconstituted powder-based supplemental nutrition polymeric diets, also called as scientific formula feeds. Polymeric diets have got some advantages over blenderized kitchen diets which include minimization of feed contamination,[20-24] consistency in amount and supply of nutrients, prevention of viscosity-related blockage of enteral feeding tubes, etc.[20,21]

In an observational study in an ICU wherein nutrition is provided with specialized formula feed to 100% of its patients when indicated, it was shown that lesser the number of days the patient stays in the ICU more is the cost of scientific formula feeding. However, the cost of feeding per day is much lesser than the cost of antibiotics in the ICU.[22]

When it comes to nutrition therapy, the timing of the initiation of nutrition therapy—EN or PN becomes an important attribute. All hemodynamically stable patients can be fed as early as possible within 24 hours after the nutritional assessment and clinical and biochemical decision on the route and formula employed for feeding.

The provision of early and appropriate nutrition support to patients during a critical illness has been widely accepted to improve health outcomes with the preponderance of the clinical evidence suggesting that most benefit can be obtained from the provision of early enteral (gut) feeding.[23,24]

IMPACT OF PARENTERAL NUTRITION ON HEALTHCARE COSTS

It is important to understand that enteral feeding is often difficult to initiated early during critical illness. So, the use of early PN in critically ill patients with short-term relative contraindications to early EN may significantly and meaningfully reduce total costs of acute hospital care. It has been shown in an analysis using European cost data that cost savings are attributable to the use of early PN.[25]

Further, the Swiss supplemental parenteral nutrition study popularly called as "SPN" study demonstrated that optimized energy provision combining EN and SPN reduces nosocomial infections in critically ill adults who fail to achieve targeted energy delivery with EN alone.[26] The data from the SPN study was analyzed to characterize the relationships between SPN, cumulative energy deficit, nosocomial infection, and medical resource consumption. A significant cost reduction was found with SPN, suggesting that optimization of energy provision using SPN is a cost-effective strategy in selected critically ill adults. This pharmacoeconomic evaluation of the data showed that the SPN led to the savings in resource consumption mainly due to a reduction in infectious morbidity.[27]

For PN, either industrially premixed MCBs or hospital-compounded individualized admixtures are used. Industrially, premixed MCBs contain macronutrients and electrolytes in various amounts and volumes and they are widely available. Some hospital pharmacies that have appropriate facilities can locally produce PN solutions that are tailored to the patients' specific requirements. Hospitals can decide which approach meets their requirements in terms of clinical effectiveness and economic efficiency.

Widely studied aspect of PN has been its cost efficacy when employed either with MCBs or compounded bags. The hospital compounded PN preparation process is complex as it involves several different steps (prescription, order review, compounding, dispensing before administration, and monitoring). The complexity of the hospital-compounded PN process may lead to an increased risk of errors, contamination, and other potentially harmful complications. So, it has been suggested that MCBs may have several advantages over hospital compounded bags, such as decreased costs and compounding time and reduced risk of errors and incidence of bloodstream infections (BSIs).[28]

It is noteworthy that costs associated with compounding PN in hospitals are usually high due to the high manpower requirement and also the special facilities and equipment needed.[29]

Almost all the studies evaluating and comparing the cost of different PN application systems have demonstrated that industrial premixed bags (MCBs) are favorable in terms of the cost savings as compared to hospital-compounded bags due to the factors mentioned above.[30]

There is a growing body of evidence regarding clinical, ergonomic, and economic outcomes in patients receiving PN via MCBs. The use of MCBs has been widely associated with a lower risk of infectious complications compared with compounded bags. MCBs have been shown to be associated with a modest although statistically significant reduction in the length of hospitalization compared with compounded bags, despite the absence of a significant difference in the risk of BSI. Moreover, MCBs provide comparable nutrition efficacy, especially in terms of protein efficiency to compounded bags. Thus, the use of MCBs is associated with a meaningful cost benefit.[31]

CONCLUSION

Rigorous screening and assessment will lead to early identification of the patients at risk of malnutrition and its associated complications which impose economic burden due to infectious and noninfectious complications.

In addition to primary treatment of the disease, proactive management of hospital malnutrition, designed nutrition protocols, continuous monitoring of nutrition status in hospitalized patients, and individualized nutrition support remains the mainstay in the treatment of patients in hospitals. This is an effective modality in attempts to reduce the healthcare costs.

More importantly, irrespective of the choice of route and formula, feeding of the hospitalized patients imparts clinical benefits in terms of less infectious and non-infectious complications, metabolic benefits, and, in turn, reduce the lengths of hospital or ICU stays. This leads to significant cost reduction in the healthcare management of the patients. Mainly, early nutrition intervention either with EN or PN, especially with commercially available multiple chamber bags leads to significant reduction in the overall costs and thus becomes more cost effective.

REFERENCES

1. Kondrup J, Johansen N, Plum LM, Bak L, Larsen IH, Martinsen A, et al. Incidence of nutritional risk and causes of inadequate nutritional care in hospitals. Clin Nutr. 2002;21:461-8.
2. Snider JT, Linthicum MT, Wu Y, LaVallee C, Lakdawalla DN, Hegazi R, et al. Economic burden of community-based disease-associated malnutrition in the United States. J Parenter Enteral Nutr. 2014;38 (2 Suppl):77-85S.
3. Goates S, Du K, Braunschweig CA, Arensberg MB. Economic burden of disease-associated malnutrition at the state level. PLoS One. 2016;11:0161833.
4. Freijer K, Tan SS, Koopmanschap MA, Meijers JM, Halfens RJ, Nuijten MJ. The economic costs of disease related malnutrition. Clin Nutr. 2013;32:136-41.
5. Correia MITD, Perman MI, Pradelli L, Omaralsaleh AJ, Waitzberg DL. Economic burden of hospital malnutrition and the cost-benefit of supplemental parenteral nutrition in critically ill patients in Latin America. J Med Econ. 2018;21(11):1047-56.

6. Inciong JFB, Chaudhary A, Hsu HS, Joshi R, Seo JM, Trung LV, et al. Economic burden of hospital malnutrition: a cost-of-illness model. Clin Nutr ESPEN. 2022;48:342-50.
7. Berkowitz SA, Terranova J, Randall L, Cranston K, Waters DB, Hsu J. Association between receipt of a medically tailored meal program and healthcare use. JAMA Intern Med. 2019;179:786-93.
8. Berkowitz SA, Terranova J, Hill C, Ajayi T, Linsky T, Tishler LW, et al. Meal delivery programs reduce the use of costly health care in dually eligible Medicare and Medicaid beneficiaries. Health Aff (Millwood). 2018;37(4):535-42.
9. Kaegi-Braun N, Baumgartner A, Gomes F, Stanga Z, Deutz NE, Schuetz P. Evidence-based medical nutrition: a difficult journey, but worth the effort!. Clin Nutr. 2020;39:3014-8.
10. Meehan A, Partridge J, Jonnalagadda SS. Clinical and economic value of nutrition in healthcare: a nurse's perspective. Nutr Clin Pract. 2019;34:832-8.
11. McCauley SM, Barrocas A, Malone A. Hospital nutrition care Betters patient clinical outcomes and reduces costs: the malnutrition quality improvement initiative story. J Acad Nutr Diet. 2019;119:S11-4.
12. Sulo S, Feldstein J, Partridge J, Schwander B, Sriram K, Summerfelt WT. Budget impact of a comprehensive Nutrition-Focused quality improvement program for malnourished hospitalized patients. Am Health Drug Benefits. 2017;10:262-70.
13. Sriram K, Sulo S, VanDerBosch G, Partridge J, Feldstein J, Hegazi RA, et al. A comprehensive nutrition-focused quality improvement program reduces 30-day readmissions and length of stay in hospitalized patients. J Parenter Enteral Nutr. 2017;41:384-91.
14. McClave SA, Taylor BE, Martindale RG, Warren MM, Johnson DR, Braunschweig C, et al. Guidelines for the Provision and Assessment of Nutrition Support Therapy in the Adult Critically Ill Patient: Society of Critical Care Medicine (SCCM) and American Society for Parenteral and Enteral Nutrition (ASPEN). J Parenter Enteral Nutr. 2016;40(2):159-211.
15. Taylor BE, McClave SA, Martindale RG, Warren MM, Johnson DR, Braunschweig C, et al. Guidelines for the Provision and Assessment of Nutrition Support Therapy in the Adult Critically Ill Patient: Society of Critical Care Medicine (SCCM) and American Society for Parenteral and Enteral Nutrition (ASPEN). Crit Care Med. 2016;44(2):390-438.
16. Bozeman MC, Schott LL, Desai AM, Miranowski MK, Baumer DL, Lowen CC, et al. Healthcare resource utilization and cost comparisons of high-protein enteral nutrition formulas used in critically ill patients. JHEOR. 2022;9(1):1-10.
17. Curry AS, Chadda S, Danel A, Nguyen D. Early introduction of a semi-elemental formula may be cost saving compared to a polymeric formula among critically ill patients requiring enteral nutrition: a cohort cost-consequence model. Clinicoecon Outcomes Res. 2018;10:293-300.
18. Kudsk KA, Croce MA, Fabian TC, Minard G, Tolley EA, Poret HA, et al. Enteral *vs* parenteral feeding: Effects on septic morbidity following blunt and penetrating trauma. Ann Surg. 1992;215:511-3.
19. Kudsk KA. Beneficial effect of enteral feeding. Gastrointest Endosc Clin N Am. 2007;17:647-62.
20. Mokhalalati JK, Druyan ME, Shott SB, Comer GM. Microbial, nutritional and physical quality of commercial and hospital prepared tube feedings in Saudi Arabia. Saudi Med J. 2004;25:331-41.
21. Sullivan MM, Sorreda-Esguerra P, Santos EE, Platon BG, Castro CG, Idrisalman ER, et al. Bacterial contamination of blenderized whole food and commercial enteral tube feedings in the Philippines. J Hosp Infect. 2001;49:268-73.
22. Sanjith S, Apoorv T, Shah N. Cost of enteral formulae feed in critically ill patients in a tertiary care centre: an observational study from India. Indian J Nutr. 2019;6(3):207.

23. Doig GS, Heighes PT, Simpson F, Sweetman EA. Early enteral nutrition reduces mortality in trauma patients requiring intensive care: a meta-analysis of randomised controlled trials. Injury. 2011;42(1):50-6.
24. Doig GS, Heighes PT, Simpson F, Sweetman EA, Davies AR. Early enteral nutrition, provided within 24 h of injury or intensive care unit admission, significantly reduces mortality in critically ill patients: a meta-analysis of randomised controlled trials. Intensive Care Med. 2009;35(12):2018-27.
25. Doig GS, Simpson F. Early parenteral nutrition in critically ill patients with short-term relative contraindications to early enteral nutrition: a full economic analysis of a multicenter randomized controlled trial based on US costs. Clinicoecon Outcomes Res. 2013;5:369-79.
26. Heidegger CP, Berger MM, Graf S, Zingg W, Darmon P, Costanza MC, et al. Optimisation of energy provision with supplemental parenteral nutrition in critically ill patients: a randomised controlled clinical trial. Lancet. 2013;381:385-93.
27. Pradelli L, Graf S, Pichard C, Berger MM. Supplemental parenteral nutrition in intensive care patients: a cost saving strategy. Clin Nutr. 2018;37:573-9.
28. Hall JW. Safety, cost, and clinical considerations for the use of premixed parenteral nutrition. Nutr Clin Pract. 2015;30: 325-30.
29. Pontes-Arruda A, Zaloga G, Wischmeyer P, Turpin R, Liu FX, Mercaldi C. Is there a difference in bloodstream infections in critically ill patients associated with ready-to-use versus compounded parenteral nutrition. Clin Nutr. 2012;31(5): 728-34.
30. Berlana D, Almendral MA, Abad MR, Fernández A, Torralba A, Cervera-Peris M, et al. Cost, time, and error assessment during preparation of parenteral nutrition: multichamber bags versus hospital-compounded bags. J Parenter Enteral Nutr. 2019;43(4):557-65.
31. Alfonso JE, Berlana D, Ukleja A, Boullata J. Clinical, ergonomic, and economic outcomes with multichamber bags compared with (Hospital) pharmacy compounded bags and multibottle systems: a systematic literature review. J Parenter Enteral Nutr. 2017;41(7):1162-77.

Index

Page numbers followed by *b* refer to box, *f* refer to figure, *fc* refer to flowchart, and *t* refer to table

A

Abdominal compartment syndrome 151, 301, 306, 308, 456, 457
Abdominal hypertension 151
  management of 151
Absorption 222
Abundant cytoplasmic granules 24
Abundant dietary antioxidants 272
Acalculous cholecystitis 130
Accurate gas analyzer 93
Acetic acid 120
Acetyl coenzyme A 28
Acid–base imbalances 433
Acidosis 230
  metabolic 354, 367
Acitretin 214
Acquired immunodeficiency syndrome 426
Actinobacteria 440, 441
Actinomyces 441
Acute pancreatitis 121, 301-303
  incidence of 301
  prevalence of 301
Acute respiratory distress syndrome 3, 112, 249, 329, 366, 406
Adenosine triphosphate 15, 21, 129*fc*, 462
Adipose tissue 34
  subcutaneous 36
  total 36
  visceral 36
Adjuvant medical-nutritional therapy 293
Admixtures additives 473
Adrenal insufficiency 415
Adrenaline 17, 436
Adrenocorticotropic hormone 17, 18
Akkermansia 120
Alanine 405
Albumin 125, 162, 230, 231
  contraindications 231
  indications 231
  serum 253, 323, 362, 392, 433

Alcohol use disorder 426
Alendronate 214, 224
Aliskiren 214, 221
Alkaline phosphatase 316
Alkalosis 431
  metabolic 228
Allometry 216
Aluminum 214, 215
  contamination 131
Alveolar macrophages 25
Amiloride 220
Amino acids 17, 27, 28, 101, 119, 139, 219, 252, 257, 356, 391, 394, 403, 407, 442, 461, 465, 478
  branched-chain 29, 383
  essential 394
  higher levels of 102
  nonessential 322
  pathways 21, 23, 28
  precursors 22
  specific 322
  synthesis 15
Aminoglycosides, use of 11
Amiodarone 214
Amlodipine 221
Ammonia, increased brain levels of 383
Amoxicillin 125
Amphotericin B 224, 234
Amylase levels 301
Amyotrophic lateral sclerosis 371
Anabolic agents, role of 251
Anastomotic leaks 122
Anemia 65, 313, 330, 417
  pernicious 461
  severe 231
Angiotensin-converting enzyme 215
  inhibitors 220, 224
Angiotensin receptor blockers 220
Anorexia 5, 63, 285, 239, 272, 282, 285, 285*t*, 376, 378, 382
  bulimia 128
  nervosa 128, 426
Antacids 239

Anthropometric 43
  evaluation 286
  measurements 162, 391, 392
Anthropometry 253, 323, 362
Antiarrhythmics 214
Anti-asthmatic agent 214
Antibiotic 214
  therapy 148
Antibody 441
  production 401
Anticatabolic agents, role of 251
Anticoagulants, oral 195
Anticonvulsants 214
Antifungal agents 234
Antigens, dietary 60
Antihistamines 214
Antihypertensive agent 214
Anti-inflammatory cytokines 444
Antimalarial agent 214
Antimicrobial peptides 442, 443
Antineoplastic treatment 293
Antioxidant 114, 366
  cascade 407
  cocktail 408
  consumption of 269
  enzymes 120
  micronutrients 401, 402*t*, 407
  properties 112
  systems 272
    depletion of 322
  vitamin, level of 366
Aortic aneurysm, abdominal 456
Appendicular skeletal
  mass 284
  muscle 34
Appetite 285
Archaea 440
Arginine 29, 305, 352, 365, 401, 402*t*, 405, 461, 465, 466
  deficiency 366
  supplementation, role of 366
Arrhythmias 127, 239, 240, 322, 428
Artemether 214
Arterial blood gas 235
Arthritis 459
Ascites 92, 342
Ascorbic acid 407

Index

Aseptic technique,
    implementation of 172
Aspartate amino transaminase 15
Aspiration 172, 437
    pneumonia 177
    risk factors for 178*t*
Ataxia 180
Atenolol 214
Atherosclerosis, inflammatory
    process of 269
Atracurium 221
Attenuate skeletal muscle
    wasting 102
Autoimmune diseases 21
Autoimmune protocol diet 70
Autonomic nervous system 149
Autophagy 99, 104
Azilsartan medoxomil 220
Azoles 234
Azotemia 354, 394

B

Bacillus 443
Backbone nutritional components 262
Bacteria 440
    gram-positive 441
    luminal 442
    pathogenic 444
Bacterial translocation 302
    risk of 456
Bacteroides 441
Barbiturates 368
Bariatric surgery 462
Basal energy expenditure 61, 92, 323
Basal metabolic
    rate 92, 246
    pathways 21
B-cell 464
    dysfunction 463
Benazepril 220
Bepridil 221
Beriberi
    dry 180
    wet 428
Beta-blocker 214
Beta-carotene 408
Beta-hydroxy beta-
    methylglutaryl-CoA 214
Beta-methylglutaryl-CoA 215
Bifidobacterium 119-121, 441, 443
    percentage of 120

Bile
    acids 73*f*
    reinfusion 315
    salts 16
Biochemical data
    evaluation of 287
    interpretation of 287
Bioelectrical impedance analysis 49, 62, 94, 107, 253, 448, 450
    technique 34
Bioimpedance
    analysis 284
    technologies of 35
Biological therapy 294
Biopharmaceutical drug
    disposition
    classification
    system 213*f*
Biotherapy 294
Biotransformation, stages of 6, 6*fc*
Birth defects 338
Bisphosphonates 214, 215
Bleeding 172, 174, 322
    gastroesophageal 150, 382
Blind placement 157
Blood
    glucose 413, 416
        elevated 179
        measurements, frequency of 417
    polymorph numbers 402
    pressure, low 234
Bloodstream infection 126
    catheter-related 126, 194
    central line-associated 126
B-lymphocytes 25
    activation of 27
B-mode ultrasonography
    technique 50
Body
    cell mass, loss of 18
    composition 34, 49
        assessment 32, 322
        working group 48
    constitution, type of 336
    hydration 50
    mass 322
        index 32, 42, 43, 46, 47, 62, 63, 81*fc*, 128, 163, 246, 253, 272, 276, 283, 323, 334, 335, 343, 362, 377*f*, 391, 393, 462
    weight 282, 337

Bone
    density, loss of 61
    disease, metabolic 131
    marrow transplant 42
    morphogenetic proteins 451, 453
    pain 240
    resorption, inhibition of 241
Bowel
    atrophy 395
    ischemia 250, 436
    rest 75, 187
Bradycardia 240, 428
Brain injury 228
    traumatic 92, 229, 263, 276, 348, 355, 370, 403
Brain-derived neurotrophic
    factors 451
Breastfeeding 397
Breasts 440
Breath-by-breath basis 94, 162
British Society of
    Gastroenterology 80
Bundle branch block 240
Buried bumper syndrome 159
Burns 263, 351*f*, 366*t*, 393, 397, 465, 466
    major 348, 392
    management of 356
    nutritional support for 354
    percentage of 397
    physiological responses in 350
    severe 403, 465

C

Cachetin 385
Cachexia 272, 273, 281, 376
    stages of 283*f*
    syndrome, development of 281
Cajal interstitial cells 149
Calcineurin inhibitors 386
Calcitonin 241
    levels 162
Calcium 65, 131, 215, 248, 338, 371, 380, 381, 383, 385, 395, 427
    channel blockers 221
    deficiency 65
        prevalence of 65
    diet, low 241
    gluconate 240
    ionized 240
    phosphate 218
        precipitation 219

serum 240
supplement 224, 273
  oral 240
  utilization of 61
Caloric requirement, assessment of 363
Calorie 19
  non-nutritive 106
Campylobacter 148
Canadian Critical Care Nutrition Group Reveals 168
Canadian Nutrition Screening Tool 46
Cancer 21, 188, 281, 338, 426, 459
  cachexia 282t, 377, 377f
    pathophysiology of 281
    score 283
    stages of 377
  colon 292
  colorectal 292
  digestive system 290
  esophageal 290, 471
  gastric 290
  head 289
  hematologic 293
  hepatic 291
  malnutrition 376, 376f, 377, 378f
  neck 289
  pancreatic 291
  rectal 292
  treatment, type of 292
  types of 289, 290
Candesartan 220
Candida 126, 441
Capillary endothelium 17
Captopril 220
Carbamazepine 214, 224
Carbohydrates 14, 69, 165, 189, 254, 262, 323, 356, 365, 381, 382, 391, 393, 461, 462, 478
  consumption of 269
  diet 69b
    specific 68
  metabolism 14
  nature of 339
Carbon dioxide 93
  production 93, 382
Carcinoma, hepatocellular 347, 382
Cardiac arrest 444
Cardiac arrhythmia 234, 428
Cardiac failure 372, 433
  congestive 129fc

Cardiac hypercontraction 432
Cardiac surgery 273, 274b, 415
Cardiomyopathy 239, 269
Cardiopulmonary bypass, use of 274
Cardiothoracic intensive care 268
Cardiovascular diseases 268, 338, 347
Cardiovascular system 428
Catabolic metabolism 140
Catabolism 99
  inhibition of 274
Catecholamines 350
  use of 413
Catheter
  dislodgement 195
  management 194
  removal 196
Cavity, abdominal 196
Cefepime 125
Ceftriaxone 220
Celiac disease 121
Cell
  damage, prevention of 404
  wall fragments 119
Cellular components, biosynthesis of 24
Cellulose 118
Central nervous system 19, 25, 129fc, 376f, 378f
  symptoms 237
Central venous catheters 125, 126, 211
  placement of 475
Centrifugation step 218
Cerebrovascular diseases 268
Ceruloplasmin 392, 465
Cheilosis 428
Chemotherapeutic agents 294
Chemotherapy 188, 294, 426
Child-Turcotte-Pugh C category 344
Chloride 248
Cholecystitis 395
Cholecystokinin 442
Cholelithiasis 130
Cholestasis 314, 465
Cholestatic liver disease 130
Cholesterol 22
Cholestyramine 61, 76
Chromium 248
  amount of 354
Chronic obstructive pulmonary disease 4, 42, 329

acute exacerbation of 437
  severe 385
Chylomicrons 16
Chylothorax 395
Chyme 315
  reinfusion
    front facing 318f
    technology, limitations of 316
  therapy 315-319
Ciprofloxacin 224
Cirrhosis 342, 344, 346, 426
  advanced decompensated 342
  primary
    biliary 382
    scleroising 382
Cirrhotic failure 92
Cisatracurium 221
Citric acid cycle 22
Clavulanic acid 125
Clevidipine 221
Closed circuit systems 93
Clostridium 440
  difficile 121, 148, 175, 445
  infection 148, 314
  perfringens 120
Coenzyme Q10 22, 273
Cognitive dysfunction 237, 360
Colitis, severe acute 81
Collagen
  deposition 461
  stability of 464
  synthesis 465, 466
  defects 460
Colloids 230, 231
  characteristic of 230t
Colo-cutaneous fistula 160
Colonic pseudo-obstruction 436, 437
Colostomies 82
Coma 127
Commensal microbes, sets of 118
Compartment syndrome 151
Compensatory anti-inflammatory response syndrome 5
Complex venous access 199
Comprehensive nutritional assessment guide 342
Computed tomography 36, 284
  imaging 51
Confinement systems 93
Confusion 127, 180, 237, 240, 372
Conglomeration 447
Connective tissues 25

Consciousness, level of 368
Constipation 127, 149, 150, 240, 393
Continuous glucose monitoring 417
  advantages of 417
  components of 417
  limitations of 417
Continuous renal replacement therapy 380
Convulsions 127
Copper 112, 248, 328, 338, 357, 366, 380, 408, 463, 465
  amount of 354
  deficiency 408, 465
Coronavirus disease 2019 (COVID-19) 113, 331, 334, 417, 471
  pandemic 417
Corticosteroids 350, 418
  high-dose 11, 128
  use of 131
Cortisol 17
  levels 254
Corynebacterium 441
Coulter counter 218
Cranial nerve palsies 428
C-reactive protein 162, 253, 269, 314, 408
Creatinine 451
  serum 451, 452
Crohn's disease 58, 66, 75, 121
Cryptosporidium 148
Crystalloids 227, 230t
  balanced 229
  nonbalanced 229
  types of 228
Cushing syndrome 234
Cyclooxygenase-2 270
Cyclospora 148
Cyclosporine 214
Cystatin C 451, 452
Cystic fibrosis 385, 462
Cytochrome
  C 22
  P450 212-214
Cytokine 9, 350, 391
  induction of 29
  storm 302, 334
Cytotoxic functions 29

D

Dairy foods 270
Decarboxylation, oxidative 15

Decompensation, hepatic 347
Defensins 443
Dehydration 148, 224, 237, 314, 354, 382, 460
Delirium 372
Dendritic cells 442
Density, low-muscle 449
Deoxyribonucleic acid 441, 461
Detrimental diet 444
Dextran 230, 232
Dextrose 105, 229, 369, 462
  normal saline 228, 228fc
Diabetes 459, 462
  gestational 393
  history of 268
  insipidus 238fc
  mellitus 416, 418, 426
  prevalence of 459
Diarrhea 83, 122, 148, 175, 250, 436
  feed-associated 176b
  incidence of 148
  risk factors for 148
  severe 76
Dietary antioxidants, deficiency of 271
Dietary carbohydrates, subtypes of 118
Diets 58, 59, 68, 270
  anti-inflammatory 69, 69
  components of 139, 393
  therapy 295
Digestion 15
Digoxin 215, 224
Diltiazem 221
Dioxide production 162
Diphosphoglycerate 129fc
Disability-adjusted life years 268
Disaccharides 67
Dobutamine 436
Docosahexaenoic acid 189, 190, 355, 366, 402, 406
Dopamine 436
Double enterostomy, temporary 313
Double-labeled water method 94
Droplet size measurement techniques 218
Drug error reduction systems 204
Drug-nutrient interaction 212, 212t, 218, 222, 223t, 224b
  classification of 211t
  management of 223, 225fc

  mechanism of 211
  metabolic complications 474
  scope of 210
  working model of 211f
Dual placement tubes 155, 156
Dual-energy X-ray absorptiometry 32, 51, 62, 94, 107, 284, 450
Dumping syndrome 291, 294
Duodenum 141, 164, 224
Dynamic surface tension, measurement of 218
Dyselectrolytemia 384
Dysglycemia 142, 179, 413, 416, 418, 421, 429, 433
  consequences of 416
  management of 413, 418, 419f
  prevention of 421
  types of 414f
Dyslipidemia 269
Dysmotility, esophageal 426
Dysnatremia 430
  management of 430
Dysphagia 339, 426

E

Echinocandins 234
Echocardiography, transesophageal 194
Echogenicity 450
Edema 50
  peripheral 180, 200
  pulmonary 200
Egg allergy 394
Eicosapentaenoic acid 189, 190, 297, 355, 366, 402, 403, 406, 463
Elastic fibers 34
Elective gastrointestinal surgery 403
Electrocardiogram 428
  tests 205
Electrolyte 188, 189, 199, 205, 227, 248, 357, 381, 395, 431
  abnormalities 433
  balance, deviation of 230
  corrections 141
  imbalance 148, 180, 428
  interactions 220t
  monitoring of 475
  replacement 430t
  requirements 325
  salts 202

serum levels of 429
status 246
Electromagnetic image-guided placement 157
Electronic glucose management systems 419
Elemental preparation 249, 369
Emesis 148, 429
Emphysema 385
Emulsification 16
Enalapril 220
Enalaprilat 220
Endocrine
  disruptors 336
  messengers 149
  normalization of 137
  systems 142
Endogenous glucose production 426
Endoscopic technique 157
Endothelial dysfunction 405
Endotoxemia, portal 130
Energy 104, 336
  adequate calories of 255
  dense formulae 249
  expenditure 91, 99, 255, 323, 352b
    expenditure measurement 95, 96
  fixed weight-based calculations of 363
  needs, determination of 162
  prescription of 96
  production 16
  provision, quantity of 104
  requirements 327, 391
    estimation 246
  substrate 404
Entamoeba histolytica 148
Enteral access devices 155
Enteral feeding 141, 163, 163fc, 172t, 176t, 456
  complications of 172
  composition 164
  initiation of 161, 165, 167fc
  maintenance of 161, 168
  modes of 163
  progression of 161
Enteral formulas
  scientific 140
  standard 368
Enteral nutrition 73, 74, 77, 106f, 135, 137, 139, 168, 188, 188t, 218, 264f, 273, 303,
304, 308, 314, 328, 331fc, 349f, 355t, 357, 358, 363, 366, 367b, 368, 382, 395, 396, 402, 403, 427, 433, 471, 478, 479
  complications of 171
  early 436
  excessive 65, 67b
  impact of 479
  management of 171
  partial 70, 71t
  process of 163
  superiority of 171
  support 295
  use of 258
Enteral tube 368
Enteroendocrine cells 442
Enterostomy, double-barreled 313
Enzyme 119, 212
  pancreatic 385
  serum glutamate oxaloacetic aminotransferase 15
Epigenetics 336
Epinephrine 413
Epithelial barrier, loss of 302
Epithelial cells 59
Eplerenone 220
Eprosartan 220
Erector spinae 36
Erythrocytosis 417
Erythromycin 248
Erythropoiesis, crucial for 112
Escherichia coli 120, 175, 440
Esomeprazole 125
Euglycemia 274
European Crohn's and colitis organization 63b
European Society for Clinical Nutrition and Metabolism 81fc
Excretion, organs of 212
Expanded computerized information systems 474
Extracellular amino acid pools 322
Extracellular fluid 227
  accumulation 343
Extracellular matrix deposition 459
Extracellular water 50
  estimate of 35
  surplus of 107
Extracorporeal membrane oxygenation 106f, 330
Extracorporeal therapies 95
Extravascular lung water index 234
Eye 428, 440

F

Faecalibacterium prausnitzii 67, 119, 445
Fatigue 272
Fats 14, 101, 262, 356, 390, 391, 393, 394, 478
  absorption 15
    role of 16
  emulsion, parenteral 432
  free mass 33
  malabsorption 76
  mass 33
  metabolism 15
  storage of 17
  transport 16
Fatty acid 16, 366
  essential 247, 394, 395, 462
  monounsaturated 269
  long-chain 16
  medium-chain 16
  polyunsaturated 269, 371, 406
  synthesis 15, 21, 23
  short-chain 16, 59, 119, 139, 442
  oxidation 21, 23
Fatty liver 354
Fatty tissue, loss of 384
Feeding
  aggressive 105
  disease-specific 249
  interruption of 261
  interventions 478
  mode 59
  optimum 353
  options 456
  postpyloric 248
  prepyloric 164
  route of 324
  timing of 324
  trickle 436
  trophic 263
  tube 211, 224, 225b
    large-bore 156
    small-bore 155
Felodipine 221
Femoral venous catheterization 125, 126

Fexofenadine 214
Fiber 139
　consumption of 269
Fibrin sheath 195
Fibroblast 34
　cells 460
　proliferation 465
Fibronectin 393
Fibrosis 78, 450
Fick's method 94
Finerenone 220
Firmicutes 440
Fistula
　chronic 187
　enteroatmospheric 313
　enterocutaneous 313
　formation of 160
　gastrocutaneous 174
Fistuloclysis 315
Flavin adenine dinucleotide 22
Flavobacterium 441
Fluid 227, 466
　accumulation of 92, 450
　balance 140
　　maintenance of 140
　compartments 228
　intravenous 227
　overload 180
　　effect of 343
　requirement 203
　retention 385
　therapy 233
　　phases of 233
　type of 230
Fluoroquinolones 214, 215
Fluoroscopy 157
Folate 112, 395
　deficiency 380
Folic acid 65, 112, 215, 395
　antagonist 61
Follistatin 451
Food 211
　and immunosuppressive drug
　　interactions 386
　component 211
　frequency questionnaire 270
　intake, reduced 78
　texture, modification of 69
Formula feeding
　continuous 276
　scientific 248
Fosinopril 220
Frailty index 346
Frank muscle paralysis 235

Free-fatty acids 101
French gastronome 210
French scale 155
Fructose oligosaccharides 139
Full sterile barrier technique 193
Fungi 440
Furosemide 205

G

G tube
　low-profile 158
　standard 158
　nonballoon 158
Galveston's equation 397
Gamma-aminobutyric acid 443
Gamma-glutamyl transferase 316
Gamma-linolenic acid 406
Gastric
　acid secretion 159
　feeding intolerance 248
　juice 149
　outlet obstruction 160
　placement 155, 157
　residual volume 177, 276, 367
　　monitoring 248
　　measurement of 168
Gastrin 137
Gastrointestinal beriberi 428
Gastrointestinal diseases 301
Gastrointestinal dysfunction 101,
　　106f, 147f, 147t, 382
Gastrointestinal dysmotility 149
Gastrointestinal failure 149
Gastrointestinal nutrient loss 61
Gastrointestinal peptides 442
　neurocrine functions of 137
Gastrointestinal system 428
Gastrointestinal tract 124, 198,
　　315, 440, 442
　function 171
Gastrojejunostomy tubes 158
Gastroparesis 149
Gastropexy 159
Gastrostomy
　percutaneous endoscopic
　　163, 174
　tube 471
Gelatin polymer 231
Genital tract 440
Ghost biotics 119
Giardia 148
Gland, autodigestion of 301
Glasgow coma scale 367
Glomerular filtration rate 451

Glomerulonephritis 378
Glossitis 428
Glucagon 17, 119, 413
Glucocorticoids 413
Glucogenesis 282
Gluconeogenesis 15, 282, 413
　viscera for 394
Glucose 101, 219, 224, 391
　absorption 315
　administration of 205
　against, absorption of 14
　amount of 256
　clearance 282
　deficiency 462
　intake, parenteral 256
　intolerance, degrees of 161
　levels 384, 429
　　correction of 429
　　maintenance of 142
　monitoring 416
　overfeeding 130
　rich fluids 106
　transporters 14
　　expression of 29
Glutamine 28, 29, 249, 297, 305,
　　352, 358, 365, 401, 402t,
　　403, 408, 461, 465
　exogenous 466
　supplementation 263, 365, 466
Glutathione 22
　peroxide 120
Glycemic
　balance 421
　control 199
　management 417
　targets 418, 418t
　variability 413, 415, 416
Glycocalyx 443
Glycogen
　hepatic 101
　maternal 390
Glycogenic substrate, utilization
　　of 415
Glycogenolysis 282
Glycolytic pathway 21, 27
Goblet cells 442, 443
Graft acceptance 350
Grafted organ function 376
Growth
　hormone 17, 414f
　placental 390
Guillain-Barré syndrome 9, 428
Gut
　barrier function 308

brain axis 119, 443, 445
dysbiosis 444, 445
dysfunction 314
integrity, maintenance of 274
ischemia 181
microbiome 440, 441, 443-445
   common phyla of 441f
microbiota 138
motility 367
mucosa 137

H

Haemaccel 231
Handgrip dynamometer 48, 48f
Harris-Benedict equation 246, 363, 393
Head injury 42
   severe 403
Health stroke scale 367
Healthcare costs 478, 480
Heart
   disease 4
      coronary 269
      ischemic 268
      valvular 269
   failure 199, 269, 419, 451
      chronic 384
      congestive 272, 428
   transplantation 384
Heat
   killed probiotics 119
   shock protein 404
Helicobacter pylori 121
Hematologic malignancy 42
Hematoma 142
   mediastinal 395
Hemicellulose 118
Hemodialysis 380
Hemodynamic failure, severe 436, 437
Hemoglobin 272
   levels 246
Hemorrhage 395, 456
   gastroesophageal 149
   subarachnoid 360
Hemostasis 413, 460
Heparin 395
   use of 131
Hepatic dysfunction 415
Hepatic failure 249, 415
Hepatic glucose production 385
Hepatic protein synthesis 282
Hepatobiliary dysfunction 314
Hepatocarcinoma 291

Herbal dietary supplements 213
High-calorie-density tissue 390
High-protein
   diet 339
   nutritional regimen 339
High-sodium diets 60
Hip fracture 42
Histidine 352
Histiocytes 25
Hohn catheters 192
Home nutrition support 296
   program 472
Hormone 413
   antidiuretic 238fc
   counter-regulatory 462
   lipolytic 17
   secretion, maternal 391
   sensitive lipase 17
Host's tissues 401
Hounsfield unit 36
Human cells 440
Human microbiome project 118
Human milk
   oligosaccharides 441
Hydration 241, 274
   status 343
Hydrochloric acid 195
Hydrogen peroxide 407
Hydrothorax 395
Hydroxyethyl starch 220fc, 232
Hydroxyproline 405
Hypercalcemia 228, 240
   causes 240
   symptoms 240
Hypercapnia 372
Hypercatabolic state 161
Hyperchloremia 230
Hyperdynamic state 350
Hyperemesis 427
   gravidarum 426
Hyperglucagonemia 415
Hyperglycemia 9, 11, 142, 148, 254, 322, 354, 372, 382, 385, 393, 413, 417, 419
   pathophysiology of 414f
   risk for 462
Hyperinflammation, state of 334
Hyperkalemia 215, 220, 221, 235, 386
   causes 235
   management 235
   signs 235
   symptoms 235
Hyperlipidemia 372, 386

Hypermagnesemia 241
   causes 241
   management 241
   symptoms 241
Hypermetabolic state 92, 350, 352
Hypermetabolism 6, 188, 253
Hypernatremia 224, 236, 238, 238fc
   causes 237
   symptoms 237
Hyperoxaluria 76
Hyperphosphatemia 238, 239
   causes 238
   clinical features 238
   management 238
Hypertension 269, 385
   abdominal 151
   history of 268
   intra-abdominal 147, 151, 301, 308, 456
Hypertriglyceridemia 128, 254, 394
Hypoactive bowel sounds 367
Hypoalbuminemia 148, 165, 272, 313
Hypocalcemia 239, 433
   causes 239
   management 240
   symptoms of 240, 433
Hypocaloric feeding 168, 263
Hypocoagulability 142
Hypoglycemia 127, 294, 395, 413, 415, 420
   causes of 415
   complications of 335
   incidence of 415
   levels of 415t
   postnatal 396
Hypoglycemic episodes, higher incidence of 370
Hypokalemia 224, 234, 330
   causes 234
   management 235
   periodic paralysis 234
   symptoms 234
Hypomagnesemia 239, 241, 330, 386, 427, 431
   causes 241
   management 241
   symptoms 241
Hypomotility 149
   management of 150
Hyponatremia 224, 236, 237fc, 430

causes 236
symptoms 236
Hypoparathyroidism 465
Hypophosphatemia 239, 330, 353, 427, 428, 432
 causes 239
 clinical features 239
 management 239
 manifests 127
 mild-to-moderate 239
 severe 239, 372
Hypoproteinemia, correction of 231
Hypotension 180
Hypothalamus-pituitary-adrenal axis 443
Hypotonia 127
Hypovitaminosis D 114
Hypoxia 378, 460
 inducible factor-1, production of 28
 stress 377

I

Ideal body weight 216, 329t, 393
Ileostomy 76, 82
Immobility 254
Immobilization 5
Immune
 cells 24, 27, 28, 403, 404, 442, 444
 dysfunction 338, 392, 401
 dysregulation 445
 function 171, 401, 406
  gut-associated 353
 homeostasis 443
 inflammatory pathways 445
 modulating nutrients 402t
  supplementation 370
 nutrition, role of 395
 responses 21, 25, 377, 444
 system 27, 29, 401, 402, 408
Immunity 401
 cell-mediated 394, 401
 cellular 408
 humoral 408
 impaired innate 70
 innate 26
Immunoglobulin A 441
Immunometabolism 21, 29
Immunomodulation 121
Immunonutrition 81, 305, 328, 355, 365, 401

Immunosuppression 29, 283, 405
Immunosuppressive 214
 medications 385
Immunotherapy 294
Impaired cellular function 50
Implanted venous access devices 126
Indian Council of Medical Research 348
Indian Society for Parenteral and Enteral Nutrition 348
Indian Society of Clinical Nutrition 348
Indirect calorimetry 91, 93, 94, 100, 162, 255, 262, 323, 364, 364t
 principles of 92
Infections 4, 21, 148, 159, 314, 376, 460
 catheter-related 194
 risk of 395
Infectious disease 5
Inflammation 21, 78, 79, 171, 282, 283, 314
 mild-to-moderate 79
 worsening of 377
Inflammatory bowel disease 58, 59f, 63, 64t, 65, 66fc, 77fc, 79, 121
 pathophysiology of 59
Inflammatory cytokines 253, 350
Inflammatory diseases 81fc
Inflammatory eicosanoids 406
Injury 5
 acute gastroesophageal 146, 147
 reperfusion 460
 traumatic 264
Innate lymphoid cells 444
Inotropes 358, 436
Insoluble fibers 139, 177
Insulin 205, 413
 action of 14
 automated delivery of 417
 dosage 420
 infusion 420
  protocol 419
 nutrition mismatch 415
 overdose 415
 requirement, amount of 420
 resistance 19, 239, 372
  phenomenon of 19
 secretion 415
 solution 420

 subcutaneous 420
 therapy 419, 420fc
Intensive care unit 32, 45, 106f, 112, 124, 126, 148, 155, 161, 189, 224b, 229, 258, 276, 322, 323, 331fc, 334, 344, 349f, 413, 414f, 418, 426, 477
 associated weakness 447
 survivors 245
Intercellular functions 24
Interferon-gamma 282
Interleukin 45, 46, 162, 269, 282, 302, 349f, 361, 378f, 414f
Intermuscular adipose tissue 36
Internal jugular vein 191, 193f
Internal retention devices 158
International Clinical Nutrition Section 205
International Federation for Surgery of Obesity and Metabolic Disorders 334
International Fluid Academy, executive summary of 233f
International Organization for Study of Inflammatory Bowel Diseases 71
International Scientific Association for Probiotics and Prebiotics 118
Intestinal barrier, type of 443
Intestinal epithelial hemostasis leads, disturbance of 307
Intestinal epithelium 442, 443
Intestinal failure 187, 198, 313
Intestinal microbiota 137
 malfunction of 338
Intestinal motor inhibition 149
Intestinal obstruction 80, 456
Intestinal pseudo-obstruction 150
Intestine 25
Intra-abdominal pressure 147, 306
 raised 150
Intra-abdominal sepsis 456
 risk of 80
Intracellular amino acid pools 322

Intracellular electrolytes,
    depletion of 371
Intracellular fluid 227
Intracellular hormone sensitive
    lipase 17
Intracellular microbes,
    destruction of 26
Intracranial pressure 427
    risk of 456
Intravenous access
    choice of 192
    management of 193
Intravenous fluids 227
    therapy 233f
Intravenous insulin infusion 421
Intravenous lipid emulsion 256, 261
    toxicity 199
Inulin 139
Irbesartan 220
Ireton-Jones equation 363
Irisin 451
Iron 61, 112, 215, 338, 357, 380, 395
    deficiency 64
    dysmetabolism 112
    parenteral 433
    supplements 214
Irritable bowel syndrome 121
Ischemia 460
    reperfusion injury 112
Ischemic reperfusion injury 405
Isocaloric enteral nutrition 247
Isotonic saline 230
Isotretinoin 214
Isradipine 221
Itraconazole 224

J

Jejunostomy 301
    feeding 83
    high-output 76
    tube 158
Jejunum 164
Jugular vein catheterization 125, 126

K

Ketoacidosis 420
    diabetic 228
Ketogenic therapy 370
Ketone
    bodies 19
    serum 362

Kidney 378
    disease
        acute 322
        chronic 237, 323, 324, 427
    dysfunction 419
    failure 325
    function 415
    injury, acute 113, 115, 228, 237, 322, 323, 323t, 396, 427, 451
    replacement therapies 325
    transplant 378
Klebsiella pneumoniae 126
Krebs cycle 15, 22
Kupffer cells 25

L

Lactalbumin 441
Lactate production 282
Lactation 397
Lactic acid 15, 120
Lactic acidosis 180
Lacticaseibacillus
    casie 121
    paracasei 121
    rhamnosus 121
Lactiplantibacillus plantarum 121
Lactobacillus 71, 119, 120, 121, 441
    plantarum 120
Lactoferrin 441
Lactose 69
Lactulose 120
Lamina propria macrophages 25
Langerhans cells 25
Laparotomy, decompressive 457
Large gastric residual volumes 167
L-arginine 405
Laser diffraction 218
Lean body mass 32, 91
    loss of 252
Lean muscle tissue, catabolic breakdown of 102
Lean tissue mass extrapolation 216
Learning difficulties 338
Legionella 441
Leptin 17
Lethargy 234, 240
Leukocyte
    dysfunction 428
    migration, inhibition of 272
Leukotrienes 406

Levamlodipine 221
Levodopa 214
Levosimendan 436
Levothyroxine 215
Lignins 118
Limb injury 92
Limosilactobacillus reuteri 121
Linoleic acid 165
Lipid 189, 219, 262, 323, 365, 369, 382, 406, 461, 462, 478
    deficiency 462
    degrees of 161
    emulsion 219
        composition of 190t
        phospholipid part of 130
    intake 256
    metabolism 254, 282t
    supplements 383
Lipogenesis 382, 393
Lipolysis 282
    reduction of 322
Lipopolysaccharides 119
Lipoprotein
    high-density 16
    lipase 17, 282
    low-density 16, 270
    very low-density 16, 386
Lipoteichoic acid 120
Liquid magnesium 83
Lisinopril 220
Liver 25
    cancer 291
    cirrhosis 471
    disease 392
        chronic 342, 382
        end-stage 130
        undernutrition screening tool 344
    dysfunction 419
    failure 342, 382, 396
    frailty index 346, 346t
    function 395, 415
        tests 314
    transplant 382
Losartan 220
Low glycemic index 269, 421
Lower motor neuron paralysis 428
Low-molecular-weight heparin 195
Low-volume nutrition therapy 432
Luminal gut microbiota 59
Lung 25
    cancer 290

function 327
injury, acute 105
transplantation 385
Lymph nodes 401
Lymphocyte 402
  count, total 379
  function, normal 405
Lymphoid
  cells 442
  system 401
  tissue 137, 443
    gut-associated 26, 138, 171, 404
    mucosa-associated 26
Lysozymes 443

M

Maceration 460
Macronutrient 98, 140, 198, 246, 355, 364, 393
  deficiency 161
  load 262
  metabolism 217, 254, 282
  role of 461
Macrophages 25
  peritoneal 25
Macrosomia 396
Magnesium 141, 215, 240, 248, 338, 371, 380, 385, 387t, 425
  replacement 430
  salts 221, 222
  supplementation 315, 386
Magnetic resonance imaging 36
Major histocompatibility complex 26
Malabsorption 61, 148, 165, 239
Malnutrition 32, 63, 72, 161, 199, 245, 252, 330, 335, 342, 361b, 376, 461
  assessment of 61, 65
  causes of 342
  context of 33
  criteria 47t
  diagnosis of 41, 47, 474
  disease-related 98, 198, 376, 402, 477
  etiology of 62fc
  iatrogenic 273
  moderate 47, 78
  multifactorial mechanisms of 73f
  pretransplant 388

prevalence of 41, 342
risk of 477
screening 322, 335, 342, 361
  assessment 335
  tool 42, 42t, 46
severe 47, 78, 165, 188
universal screening 46
  tool 62, 162, 172, 322, 335
Malposition 172
Manganese 463
Mass spectrometry 94
Matrix metalloproteinases 465
Maturation, phases of 27
Mechanical ventilation 330, 403, 438, 448
Medical nutrition therapy 324, 339
Mediterranean diet 70
Medium-chain triglycerides 190, 165, 249
  higher concentration of 128
Mental instability 240
Metabolic acidosis 354, 367
Metabolic alkalosis 228
Metabolic complications 127, 179, 181, 314, 392
  acute 127
  chronic 127
  long-term 129
Metabolic disorders 21
Metabolic disturbances 6, 283
Metabolic function 392, 413
Metabolic parameters 395
Metabolic pathways 27
  multiple 405
Metabolism 348
  failure of 5
  maintenance of 274
Metformin 419, 444
Methicillin-resistant
  Staphylococcus aureus 444
Methylcellulose 139
Methyldopa 215
Metoclopramide 248
  use of 179
Microbial killing 24
Microbiome 67, 118
  dysbiosis 314
  management 264
Microbiota
  composition 60
  reservoir of 440

Microfold cells 25, 442
Micronutrient 112, 113, 141, 188, 189, 198, 199, 247, 328, 338, 365, 383, 393, 394, 463
  chronic 247
  deficiency 64, 64t, 116, 161
    prevalence of 112
  essential 356
  fat-soluble 462
  monitoring 205
  physiology 112
  protective effect of 271
  provision 205
  requirement 325, 328
  supplementation 408, 463
Mid-arm circumference 362
Milrinone 436
Mineral 112, 213, 338, 355, 357, 366, 380, 381, 390, 393, 463
  consumption of 269
  deficiency 382
  supplement 214, 395
Mini nutritional assessment 62, 172
Minimum daily enteral protein 257
Mininutrition assessment 43, 43t, 46
Mitochondrial electron transport chain 10
Mitochondrial function 112
Mivacurium 221
Mobility 43
Modern intensive care unit 98
Moexipril 220
Molecular patterns
  damage-associated 26
  nature of 26
Molecules, anti-inflammatory 29
Monocyte chemoattractant protein 269
Monohydrate dextrose 393
Mononeuritis multiplex 9
Monosaccharides 67
Motilin 137
Mouth 440
Mucins 118
Mucosal cytokine modulation 67
Mucosal membranes 26
Multichamber bags 201, 478
Multifactorial syndrome 281
Multi-ingredient medicinal product 198

Multiorgan dysfunction 407,
    415, 448
  score 147
  sepsis-induced 112
  syndrome 3
Multiorgan system 426
  failure 11, 457
Multiple sclerosis 6, 371
  prevention of 371
Multiple trace element
    admixtures 141
Multivitamin 395
  preparations 141
Muscle 19, 254
  breakdown 382
  consumption 352
  density 449
  dysfunction 447
  echo intensity 51
  fiber membrane disruption 8
  function 346
  growth, markers for 453
  loss 376
    quantification of 343
  mass 47, 284, 322
    assessment methods of
      47, 49
    functional 52
    loss of 259
    low 336, 447
    normal 448
    reduced 47, 78
    wasting 253
  membranes, excitability of 9
  metabolism 453
  pain 433
  protein
    kinesis 103
    loss 253
  proteolysis 282
  strength 47, 284
    evaluation of 447
  tissue changes 162
  wasting 331, 447
    excessive 350
  weakness 240
Muscular tissues 19
Muscular weakness 127
Musculoskeletal stress markers
    284
Mycobacteria 441
Myelin membrane 371
Myeloid
  cells 406
  derived suppressor cells 29

Myonecrosis 450
Myopathy 4, 7, 7*fc*, 8*fc*
Myosin, lack of 8
Myostatin 451

N

Nails 440
Naïve T cells 444
Nasal tubes 76
Nasoenteral tube feeding 296
Nasogastric tube 437
  output 367
  presence of 179
  syndrome 172, 174
National Health Service 199
National Institute of Nutrition 348
Natremia, hypovolemic 228
Natural killer cells 24, 25, 119,
    408, 444
Nausea 429
Negative protein balance 453
Neonatal intensive care unit 316
Nephrocalcinosis 240
Nephrolithiasis 240
Neural testing 394
Neuroaxonal degeneration 447
Neurocritical care 370
Neurodegenerative disorders 338
Neuroendocrine 252
Neurological diseases 360
Neuromuscular junction
    blockers 11
Neuropathy, peripheral 180
Neuropeptides 442
Neutrophil 24
  extracellular traps 25, 444
  recruitment of 444
Next-generation sequencing 118,
    440
Niacin 215, 380
Nicardipine 221
Nicotinamide adenine
    dinucleotide pathways
    28, 120, 428
Nifedipine 221
Nimodipine 221
Nisoldipine 221
Nitric oxide 366, 405
  generation of 29
Nitrogen
  balance 18, 362, 393, 394, 396
  urinary excretion of 18
Nondepolarizing neuromuscular
    blocker 221

Noninvasive ventilation 330, 395,
    436, 437
Nonketotic hyperosmolar
    coma 420
Nonocclusive bowel ischemia 181
Nonprotein energy, source of 406
Nonsteroidal anti-inflammatory
    drugs 125, 444
Noradrenaline 17, 436
Nosocomial infections 457
  rate of 96
N-terminal pro-brain natriuretic
    peptide, levels of 270
Nucleated cells 451
Nucleotides 401
  synthesis of 27
NUTRIC score scoring system 46*t*
Nutrient 297, 355, 378
  absorption 442
  deficiencies 127
    prevention of 295
  delivery 256
  drug
    classification 211
    clinical significance 210
    interactions 214*t*
    risk factors 210
  metabolism 14, 217
  multiple 210
  specific 217
Nutrition 243, 250, 259, 268, 301,
    348, 358, 379*t*, 381*t*, 388,
    401, 436, 459, 460, 478
  adequate 383, 390
  administration, route of 353
  advancement of 366
  assessment 44, 161, 259, 361
  backbones 98
  care 478
    changes, trajectory of 101
  components of 364
  considerations 269
  delivery 164*f*, 438
  diagnosis 474
  disease-specific 396
  initiation of 366
  intervention 255
  monitoring of 366
  parenteral 74, 106*f*, 124, 127,
      163, 167, 171, 185, 187,
      188*t*, 198, 200*f*, 201*f*,
      217, 247, 249, 258, 261*f*,
      303, 304, 328, 349*f*, 363,
      368, 368*t*, 369, 369*t*, 382,
      395, 403, 426, 433, 456,
      478

pathophysiology of 3
peripheral parenteral 74
planning 376
polymeric diets 479
quantity of 438
risk screening 46, 162, 188, 331*fc*
route of 247
screening 41
status, monitoring of 396, 481
supplements, oral 72, 73, 77, 168, 377*f*
support 274*b*, 275, 384, 427, 431
  actual implementation of 473
  goals of 161
  therapy 205, 383*t*
support teams 471-474
  emergence of 471
  future of 474
  goals of 472
  role of 431
  strategies for 475
survey 168
therapy 137, 140, 363*t*, 370, 388, 401, 408, 429, 431, 433, 434, 478, 480
  complications of 250
  significance of 98
Nutritional deficiency 61, 63
  assessment of 65
Nutritional factors influencing weaning process 330*b*
Nutritional intervention 72, 81*fc*, 89
Nutritional management 246, 302, 313, 342
  concepts of 301
Nutritional requirement 203, 327, 344
Nutritional risk 32
  scores 162
  screening 41, 42*t*, 62, 81*fc*, 172, 322, 361
Nutritional screening 344, 344*t*
Nutritional status 211, 215, 378, 384, 401, 477
  assessment of 245, 252, 285, 362*t*
  deterioration 253
Nutritional strategies 328
Nutritional supplementation 72, 360
  types of 368

Nutritional support 79, 82, 155, 265, 295, 330, 331, 390, 397, 421, 478
  adequacy of 396
  assessment of 353
  early 432
Nutritional therapy 76, 77, 258, 327, 331, 335, 337*t*, 349*f*, 357, 471
  education and training in 332
  implementation of 331, 331*fc*
  long-term of 330
  monitoring of 328
  role of 330
  standard 354
  timing of 353

O

Obesity 50, 199, 200, 328, 334, 338, 339, 346, 386, 396
  complications of 335
  prevalence of 459
  severe 334
Obligatory protein loss 18
Ogilvie syndrome 250
Oligomeric diets 165
Oligosaccharides, fermentable 67
Oliguria 237
Olmesartan 220
Omega-3 fatty acids 305, 358, 366, 371, 401, 406, 463
  amount of 352
  use of 329
Oncology 298
Open circuit indirect systems 93
Opioids 368
Organ
  dysfunction 6, 425
  systems 139, 427
Organic acids 120
Organic anion transporting polypeptides 214
Ornithine, synthesis of 406
Oropharyngeal dysphagia, higher incidence of 360
Osmotic pressure 228
Osteoclasts 25
Osteodystrophy 240
Osteoporosis 61, 338, 386
Overfeeding 127, 250, 353, 372
Overhydration, risk of 200
Oxaloacetate 15

Oxygen
  consumption 93, 162, 391
  dissociation curve 129*fc*
  production of 407

P

Pain
  abdominal 67, 240
  control 301
  muscle 433
  scales 285
Paleolithic diet 70
Pancreas
  inflammatory process of 301
  transplantation 385
Pancreatic dysfunction 165
Pancreatic enzymes 385
  activation of 301
  insufficiency 462
Pancreatitis 121, 301-303, 342, 396, 403
Pancuronium 221
Pantoprazole 125
Paracrine 137
  hormones 442
Paralysis 150
Paralytic ileus 181
Parapsychobiotics 119
Parathyroid hormone, synthetic form of 240
Parenteral nutrition 74, 106*f*, 124, 127, 163, 167, 171, 185, 187, 188*t*, 198, 200*f*, 201*f*, 217, 247, 249, 258, 261*f*, 303, 304, 328, 349*f*, 363, 368, 368*t*, 369, 369*t*, 382, 395, 403, 426, 433, 456, 478
  administration 204
  central 77
  components 189*t*
  dispensing 202
  impact of 480
  initiation of 188
  intravenous access for 191
  metabolic complications of 124
  mitigates 314
  monitoring 204
  osmolality of 369
  partial 124
  peripheral 72, 77
  safety recommendations 206
  solutions 219, 219*t*
  supplemental 100*f*, 258

support 296
therapy 198
total 75, 124, 218, 383, 395
use of 471
Paresthesia 127
Parkinson's disease 371
Parturient, assessment of 392
Pectin 139
fiber 118
Pediatric critical illness 252
Pediatric intensive care settings 252
Pentose phosphate pathway 21, 22, 28
Peptides, gastrointestinal 442
Peptidoglycan 120
Perindopril 220
Peripheral nerves, axons of 9
Peripheral venous line 430
Peripherally inserted central catheter 125, 187, 192
Peroxide levels, measurement of 218
Peroxynitrites 10
Persistent inflammatory catabolic syndrome 245
Peyer's patches 442
Phagocytes, functions of 401, 408
Phagocytosis 24, 29
Pharmacodynamic interactions 212
Pharmacokinetic interactions 212
Phenotypic criteria 47
Phenytoin 214, 224
Phosphate 131, 248, 371
serum 396
Phosphodiesterase 214
Phospholipid 16
membrane 406
Phosphorous level 430
Phosphorus 61, 141, 380, 381, 383, 387t, 425
levels 240
metabolism 428
replacement 430t
tests 235
Phosphorylation, oxidative 21, 22
Physiorehabilitation 348
Placental steroid 391
Plasma
cells 27
complement, levels of 408
glucose 415
volume expansion 231

Plasmalyte 230
composition of 230
Platelet aggregation 460
Pneumonia 80, 445
severe 42
ventilatory-associated 121
Pneumothorax 173
Polyamines, production of 405
Polycystic kidney disease 378
Polymeric diet 305
Polymeric formula 165, 369
Polyneuromyopathy 4, 7, 10, 10f
Polyneuropathy 4, 7, 7fc, 8fc, 9
acute inflammatory demyelinating 9
diabetic 9
Polyphenols, consumption of 269
Polysaccharide 139
Polytrauma 339, 358, 392
Polyunsaturated fatty acids 269, 371, 406
long chain of 15
Polyurethane 156
catheters 125
nasojejunal feeding 427
Porphyromonas 441
Positive end-expiratory pressure 95
Postbiotics 118, 119
Postoperative ileus, incidence of 315
Postpyloric tube 158
Post-transplant nutrition 384
Potassium 83, 215, 224, 235, 248, 371, 380, 425
metabolism of 378
phosphate 430
replacement 430
serum levels of 141
sparing diuretics 220
Prealbumin 253
levels 362
Prebiotics 71, 118
Precachexia 376
Pregnancy, twin 391
Prepyloric tube 158
Pressure sores 461
Prevotella 441
Proatherogenic genes, expression of 270
Probiotics 71, 118, 305, 306
beneficial roles of 119
organisms, metabolic pathways of 120
role of 301

Proinflammatory cytokines, effects of 282
Prokinetic agents 178, 248
Promote nutrition care 474
Propionic acids 139
Propofol 105, 106
infusion 372
Protein 14, 17, 19, 26, 104, 165, 189, 257, 262, 323, 336, 356, 364, 369, 383, 387b, 390, 391, 393, 394, 461, 478
accretion 139
administration, route of 102
breakdown 403
catabolic rate 323
catabolism 254, 322, 393
cytokine effects on 282t
deficiency 464
risk of 461
energy
deficiency 168
malnutrition 64, 378, 401
formula, high 249
hemostasis 447
malnutrition, chronic 461
metabolism 17, 254
oxidation 282
receptor-related 270
requirements 325, 327, 331, 393, 394t, 397
retinol-binding 393
rich food 387
serum 287
synthesis 8, 254
acute phase 394
total serum 392
Proteobacteria 440
Proteolysis 282
Proximal jejunum 141
Pseudomembranous enteritis 175
Pseudomonas 441, 445
Psoas 36
muscle 449
Psychiatric scales 285
Psychotic behavior 240
Pull technique 159
Push technique 159
Pylorus 164
Pyridoxine 214
Pyruvate, importance of 14

Q

Quadrates lumborum 36
Quinapril 220
Quinolones 224

R

Radiotherapy 294
Ramipril 220
Randomized controlled trials 276
Rapid urbanization trends 60
Reactive oxygen species 7*fc*, 8*fc*, 120
Red blood cell production process 112
Refeeding syndrome 101, 107, 128, 141, 179, 180*b*, 239, 250, 353, 371, 384, 425, 431, 433
   management of 432
   pathophysiology of 129*fc*
   risk of 205
Reflux, gastroesophageal 146
Rehabilitation 450
Rehydration, intravenous 314
Renal cortex 19
Renal disease, end-stage 465
Renal dysfunction 415
Renal failure 92, 240, 415
Renal insufficiency 427, 464
Renal replacement therapy 323, 349*f*
Renal tubular
   acidosis 234
   disorders 234
Renin–angiotensin system inhibitors 221
Respiratory complications 233
Respiratory failure 322, 327, 372, 396
Respiratory illnesses, chronic 385
Respiratory insufficiency 354
Respiratory muscle
   endurance 396
   weakness 234
Respiratory status 354
Respiratory system 428
Respiratory tract 440
Resuscitation 233
   intravascular 228
Retinoids 214
Rhabdomyolysis 372, 451
Rheumatic heart disease 268
Rhinosinusitis 179
Riboflavin 395
Ribonucleic acid 461
Ringer's lactate 229, 230
Rocuronium 221
Russell method 159

S

Saccharomyces 441
   boulardii 121
Saline, normal 229
Saliva 440
Salmonella 120, 148, 441
Sarcopenia 139, 259, 283, 284*t*, 336, 343, 376, 388, 447, 448, 451, 453
   assessment of 449
   diagnostic criteria for 284*t*
   evaluation of 447
   index 451, 452
   obesity 376
   presence of 344
   primary 447
   secondary 447
Scar tissue cell, reduced 465
Sclerosis, multiple 6, 371
Scoring system 63
Seizures 237, 239, 372
Selenium 112, 115, 248, 275, 328, 357, 366, 383, 408
   amount of 354
   supplementation 115
Semielemental diet 165, 305
   role of 305
Seminal fluid 440
Semi-synthetic colloids 231, 232
Semivegetarian diet 69
Sepsis 3, 21, 29, 92, 322, 339, 392, 397, 415, 444, 451, 465, 466
   diagnosis of 397
   severe 11, 415
Septic shock 113, 366
Septicemia, incidence of 122
Sequential organ failure assessment 45, 361
   score 114
Serum bilirubin levels 316
Serum creatinine 451, 452
   phosphokinase 235
Serum electrolytes, plasma concentrations of 287
Severe acute respiratory syndrome coronavirus 2 334
Severe malnutrition 47, 78, 165, 188
   category 344
Shock 3, 6, 419, 432
   pathophysiology of 6*fc*
   types of 6

Short bowel syndrome 187, 313
Short physical performance battery 343
Sildenafil 214
Single-slice regional analysis 36
Skeletal muscle 33, 447
   quality 284
Skin 440
   fold thickness 362
   lesions, nonhealing 460
   rashes 428
Sleep, lack of 336
Small bowel
   diseases 187
   ileus 248
   stomal fluid 314
Small intestinal
   bacterial overgrowth 73*f*
   mucosal thickness 138
   placement 157
Smooth muscle layers 442
Sodium 224, 248, 380
   channel inactivation 9
   concentration 314
   glucose cotransporter-2 419
   hydroxide 195
   phosphate 239, 430
Solid organ transplantation 376
Somatic protein stores 392
Sparsentan 220
Spectroscopy analysis 35
Speech, abnormal 237
Sphincter, esophageal 291
Spinal cord injury 366, 370
Spironolactone triamterene 220
Spleen 401
Splenic macrophages 25
Staphylococcus aureus 126
Starvation 254
   ketosis 391
Statins 444
Steatohepatitis, nonalcoholic 347
Steatosis 354, 428
ST-elevation myocardial infarction 268, 418
Steroids
   cessation 415
   use of 413
Stigma 335
Stoma 313
   obstructive 83
Stomach 224
Stress 254, 465
   hormones 390

hyperglycemia 352, 413, 415
  pathophysiology of 414
  oxidative 112, 269, 407
  pathophysiological 4
  physiological 414, 462
  response 4, 102, 252, 253
Stroke 42, 268, 370
Stupor 240
Subclavian vein thrombosis 395
Subjective global assessment 81*fc*
  components of 44*f*
Sudden death, causes of 428
Sulfasalazine 61
Sulfonylureas 419
Superoxide dismutase 120
Superoxide molecule
      production 10
Surgery 294
  abdominal 42, 339
  oropharyngeal 294
Surgical site infections 122
Swallowing, endoscopic
      evaluation of 285
Swiss supplemental parenteral
      nutrition 480
Synbiotics 118, 119
Syndrome of inappropriate
      antidiuretic hormone
      secretion 237
Systemic inflammation 269, 301,
      331, 377*f*, 378*f*
Systemic inflammatory response
      syndrome 5

T

Tachycardia 180, 234, 237
Tailor-made stock formulations
      203
Taste, evaluation of 285
T-cell 401, 408, 464
  dysfunction 463
  function, regulation of 366
Telenutrition 474
Telmisartan 220
Tetracyclines 215, 224
Tetrapolar bioelectrical
      impedance analysis 343
Tetrastarch 232
T-helper 1 cytokines 405
Thermogenesis, diet-induced 92
Thiamine 113, 395, 425, 428, 431
  cosupplementation of 114
  deficiency 180, 380, 425, 426,
      427

signs of 141
  symptoms of 141
  role of 431
  supplementation of 113
Thromboembolic complications,
      incidence of 125
Thrombolytics 195
Thrombosis 195, 314
  management of 195
Thyroid-stimulating hormone
      253
Tissue 212
  breakdown 376
  edema 460
  maternal 391
  proteins, formation of 18
T-lymphocyte 25
  activation of 26
Tonicity 228
Tonsils 401
Total body
  electrical conductivity 62
  surface 352, 405
  water 216
      distribution of 227*f*
  weight 227
Total energy expenditure 104, 344
Total parenteral nutrition 75, 124,
      218, 383, 395
  use of 303
Trace element 116, 189, 247, 401,
      407, 433, 478
  deficiencies 354, 433
Trandolapril 220
Transferrin 392
  level 362
Transplant surgeries 376
Trauma 263, 348, 351*f*, 355, 355*t*,
      397, 413, 466
  abdominal 92, 456
  management of 356
  multiple 102, 395
  nutritional support for 354
  physiological responses in 348
  severe 402, 403
Treitz ligament 164
Tricarboxylic acid cycle 21, 22
Triglycerides 17
  levels 17
  long-chain 188
  resynthesis of 16
Trimethoprim 221
Tryptophan 29
Tubular necrosis, acute 428

Tumor
  growth 281
  indirect effects of 378
  microenvironment 377
  necrosis factor 269, 282, 349*f*,
      378*f*, 414*f*
    alpha 138, 214, 302
  pancreatic 462
  seeding 160
  solid 281
Tyrosine 322

U

Ulcerative colitis 58, 121
Ultrasonography, musculoskeletal
      449, 450
Ultrasound 37, 50, 157
Ultraviolet B radiation, influence
      of 114
Upper limb veins, anatomy of
      191*f*
Uric acid
  cycle 15
  serum 235
Urine myoglobin test 235
Utility tubes
  long-term 159
  short-term 159

V

Valsartan 220
Vascular endothelial growth
      factor 9
Vasopressin 436
Vasopressors 307, 358, 368
  high-dose 11, 261
Vasospasm, incidence of 360
Vecuronium 221
Ventilated open-circuit
      systems 93
Ventilator 428
Verapamil 221, 234
Viruses 440
Visual analog pain scale
      questionnaire 285
Visual testing, neonatal 394
Vitamin 73, 114, 116, 189, 213,
      214, 247, 328, 355, 357,
      365, 380, 390, 393, 401,
      407, 408, 433, 442, 463,
      478
  A 64, 112, 214, 247, 338, 352,
      357, 383, 384, 395, 463,
      466

deficiency 380, 463
supplementation 408, 464
B 112, 113, 120, 214
B1 deficiency 180
B12 61, 112, 338, 380, 383
  deficiency 65, 294, 461
B6 112, 380
C 112, 114, 271, 328, 352, 357, 366, 383, 395, 407, 408, 463, 464, 466
  amount of 354
  deficiency 380, 464
  supplementation 114
consumption of 269
D 114, 131, 239, 240, 273, 328, 338, 357, 381, 385, 395, 464, 466
  deficiency 65, 114, 294, 380
  group 115
  supplement 240, 383
  toxicity 131
deficiency 382, 395, 432
E 112, 215, 271, 357, 366, 380, 383, 407, 408, 463
essential 112
fat-soluble 61, 73f, 385, 390
folate 338
K 120, 215
  deficiency 380, 383
  regeneration, regulation of 407
  requirement 394
  supplementation of 328
Vomiting 148, 167, 436, 437

W

Warfarin 215, 224
Warm saline flushes 173
Water retention 426
Weight
  change 32, 44
  gain 386, 387b
  loss 43, 46, 47, 63, 78, 283, 290, 313, 362, 376, 387b
Weir's equation 350
Wernicke's encephalopathy 180, 428
White cell count, elevated 148
Whole-food restricted diets 67
Wound
  acute 459
  chronic 459
  contraction 460
  dehiscence 200
  formation of 459
  healing 274, 350, 376, 385, 459, 460, 464-466
    four phases of 460
    mechanisms 350
    normal 459
    poor 405
    stages of 463
  large 393
  severity 461

Y

Yale insulin infusion protocol 420

Z

Zinc 61, 64, 112, 115, 202, 247, 248, 328, 338, 357, 366, 380, 408, 463, 465
  amount of 354
  deficiencies 115, 271, 384, 465
  supplementation of 83, 116